Autoimmune Diseases: Current Research

Autoimmune Diseases: Current Research

Edited by Chloe Weber

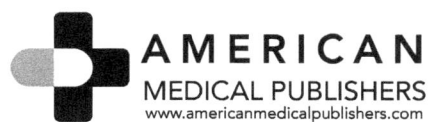

AMERICAN
MEDICAL PUBLISHERS
www.americanmedicalpublishers.com

American Medical Publishers,
41 Flatbush Avenue,
1st Floor, New York,
NY 11217, USA

Visit us on the World Wide Web at:
www.americanmedicalpublishers.com

ISBN: 978-1-63927-209-9

Cataloging-in-Publication Data

Autoimmune diseases : current research / edited by Chloe Weber.
    p. cm.
Includes bibliographical references and index.
ISBN 978-1-63927-209-9
1. Autoimmune diseases. 2. Autoimmunity. 3. Immunologic diseases. I. Weber, Chloe.
RC600 .A88 2022
616.978--dc23

Table of Contents

Permissions

List of Contributors

Index

Preface

This book has been a concerted effort by a group of academicians, researchers and scientists, who have contributed their research works for the realization of the book. This book has materialized in the wake of emerging advancements and innovations in this field. Therefore, the need of the hour was to compile all the required researches and disseminate the knowledge to a broad spectrum of people comprising of students, researchers and specialists of the field.

Autoimmune diseases are conditions arising from abnormal immune response of the body to a healthy body part. There can be many types of autoimmune diseases and nearly every body part can be involved. Some common examples are celiac disease, psoriasis, inflammatory bowel disease, rheumatoid arthritis, multiple sclerosis and systemic lupus erythematosus. Symptoms such as low grade fever and exhaustion are common. An autoimmune disease is quite difficult to diagnose and requires direct evidence from transfer of disease-causing T lymphocyte white blood cells or disease-causing antibodies, or circumstantial evidence from clinical clues. Its treatment depends upon the type and severity of the condition. Frequently, immunosuppressants and nonsteroidal anti-inflammatory drugs are prescribed. A major research direction in autoimmune diseases is the mitigation of inflammation by activating anti-inflammatory genes and suppressing inflammatory genes in immune cells for therapy. Another major intervention that is widely being investigated for its effect on autoimmune diseases is stem cell transplantation. This book explores the emerging aspects of autoimmunity and autoimmune diseases. It provides significant information of autoimmune diseases to help develop a good understanding of their diagnosis and management. It aims to equip students and experts with the advanced topics and upcoming concepts in these medical conditions.

At the end of the preface, I would like to thank the authors for their brilliant chapters and the publisher for guiding us all-through the making of the book till its final stage. Also, I would like to thank my family for providing the support and encouragement throughout my academic career and research projects.

Editor

Comparative Effects of n-3, n-6 and n-9 Unsaturated Fatty Acid-Rich Diet Consumption on Lupus Nephritis, Autoantibody Production and CD4+ T Cell-Related Gene Responses in the Autoimmune NZBWF1 Mouse

James J. Pestka[1,2,3]*, Laura L. Vines[1,2], Melissa A. Bates[1,2], Kaiyu He[2,3], Ingeborg Langohr[4]

1 Department of Food Science and Human Nutrition, Diagnostic Center for Population and Animal Health, Michigan State University, East Lansing, Michigan, United States of America, 2 Center for Integrative Toxicology, Diagnostic Center for Population and Animal Health, Michigan State University, East Lansing, Michigan, United States of America, 3 Department of Microbiology and Molecular Genetics, Diagnostic Center for Population and Animal Health, Michigan State University, East Lansing, Michigan, United States of America, 4 Division of Anatomic Pathology, Diagnostic Center for Population and Animal Health, Michigan State University, East Lansing, Michigan, United States of America

Abstract

Mortality from systemic lupus erythematosus (SLE), a prototypical autoimmune disease, correlates with the onset and severity of kidney glomerulonephritis. There are both preclinical and clinical evidence that SLE patients may benefit from consumption of n-3 polyunsaturated fatty acids (PUFA) found in fish oil, but the mechanisms remain unclear. Here we employed the NZBWF1 SLE mouse model to compare the effects of dietary lipids on the onset and severity of autoimmune glomerulonephritis after consuming: 1) n-3 PUFA-rich diet containing docosahexaenoic acid-enriched fish oil (DFO), 2) n-6 PUFA-rich Western-type diet containing corn oil (CRN) or 3) n-9 monounsaturated fatty acid (MUFA)-rich Mediterranean-type diet containing high oleic safflower oil (HOS). Elevated plasma autoantibodies, proteinuria and glomerulonephritis were evident in mice fed either the n-6 PUFA or n-9 MUFA diets, however, all three endpoints were markedly attenuated in mice that consumed the n-3 PUFA diet until 34 wk of age. A focused PCR array was used to relate these findings to the expression of 84 genes associated with CD4+ T cell function in the spleen and kidney both prior to and after the onset of the autoimmune nephritis. n-3 PUFA suppression of autoimmunity in NZBWF1 mice was found to co-occur with a generalized downregulation of CD4+ T cell-related genes in kidney and/or spleen at wk 34. These genes were associated with the inflammatory response, antigen presentation, T cell activation, B cell activation/differentiation and leukocyte recruitment. Quantitative RT-PCR of representative affected genes confirmed that n-3 PUFA consumption was associated with reduced expression of CD80, CTLA-4, IL-10, IL-18, CCL-5, CXCR3, IL-6, TNF-α and osteopontin mRNAs in kidney and/or spleens as compared to mice fed n-6 PUFA or n-9 MUFA diets. Remarkably, many of the genes identified in this study are currently under consideration as biomarkers and/or biotherapeutic targets for SLE and other autoimmune diseases.

Editor: Wolf-Hagen Schunck, Max Delbrueck Center for Molecular Medicine, Germany

Funding: This work was supported by National Institute of Environmental Health Sciences (ES021265) to JJP, and National Institute of Diabetes, Digestive, and Kidney Disorders (DK058833) to JJP. The funders had no role in study design, data collection and analysis, decision to publish, or preparation of the manuscript.

Competing Interests: The authors have declared that no competing interests exist.

* Email: pestka@msu.edu

Introduction

Systemic lupus erythematosus (SLE), a debilitating chronic autoimmune disease affecting approximately 1 in 1000 persons in the U.S., has a complex etiology that involves genetic, environmental and nutritional interactions [1]. Critical events in the initiation of SLE include the impaired clearance of apoptotic cells by macrophages and aberrant presentation of self-antigens to T and B cells. This results in formation of autoantibody-autoantigen complexes and their subsequent deposition in the kidney and other tissues [2]. Collectively, these changes elicit cytokine/chemokine production, complement activation and infiltration with monocyte/macrophages, CD4+ T cells, CD8+ T cells, B cells and

plasma cells that together evoke irreparable tissue damage [3]. CD4+ T cell activation is a hallmark of SLE and has been previously reported in autoimmune-prone mice [4]. CD4+ T cells compromise the majority of infiltrating cells in the kidneys of patients with active lupus nephritis and urinary concentrations of CD4+ T cells are correlated to severity of lupus nephritis [5]. Importantly, SLE mortality correlates with the development of autoimmune glomerulonephritis [6]. Because many SLE patients have untoward side effects from or are unresponsive to conventional drugs and biological therapeutics, they often seek complementary or alternative therapy options that include diet modification and use of nutritional supplements [7,8]. Consumption of fish oil is one such approach that has potential to prevent and/or ameliorate SLE and other types of autoimmune glomerulonephritis [9].

Since humans and other mammals require but do not synthesize polyunsaturated fatty acids (PUFAs), it is essential that they consume these in their diet [10]. Linoleic acid (C18:2n-6), is the major PUFA found in food oils derived from plants (e.g. corn and soybean) that are extensively used in Western diets. Following consumption and metabolism, linoleic acid elongates and desaturates to yield arachidonic acid (C20:4n-6; AA). The $\Delta 15$-desaturase found in plants converts linoleic acid to α-linolenic acid which can be elongated to eicosapentaenoic acid (c20:5n-3) (EPA) and docosahexaenoic acid (22:6n-3) (DHA). While these latter two conversions occur slowly in mammals, they are readily carried out by marine algae. Fish consuming these algae readily incorporate EPA and DHA into their tissue, making fish and fish oils a source of preformed long chain n-3 PUFAs for human foods and dietary supplements. A CDC-NHIS survey found that nearly 30 million individuals of U.S. adults consume fish oil supplements because of perceived health benefits [11].

n-3 PUFAs suppress proinflammatory cytokine production, lymphocyte proliferation, cytotoxic T cell activity, natural killer cell activity, macrophage-mediated cytotoxicity, neutrophil/monocyte chemotaxis, MHCII expression and antigen presentation [10]. The potential of n-3 PUFAs to specifically delay, prevent and ameliorate SLE has been investigated extensively in mouse models. The female New Zealand Black White (F1) mouse (NZBWF1), a widely used model that closely resembles human SLE, spontaneously develops the characteristics of lupus nephritis between approximately 30 to 40 wk of age resulting in a drastically shortened lifespan [12]. Early studies with NZBWF1 mice demonstrated that initiating feeding of menhaden oil, DHA ethyl ester or EPA ethyl ester early in life markedly reduced severity and incidence of renal disease as well as extended lifespan compared to mice fed beef tallow [13,14,15]. These findings coincided with reductions of anti-ds-DNA and circulating immune complexes, biomarkers positively correlated with SLE disease activity. Elegant studies from the Fernandes laboratory have related the delayed onset and decreased severity of renal disease exhibited in fish oil-fed NZBWF1 mice to reduced IL-1β, TNF-α, TGFβ1, ICAM-1 and fibronectin expression and increased expression of antioxidant enzymes [16,17,18,19,20]. The ameliorative effects of n-3 PUFAs have been similarly replicated in two other murine SLE models, BXSB/MpJ and MRL-1pr/1pr, as evidenced by decreased proteinuria and glomerular injury as well as increased lifespan [14,21,22]. Effects of fish oil in MRL-1pr/1pr mice were linked to altered eicosanoid metabolism as well as decreased plasma IL-6, IL-10, IL-12 and TNF-α [23,24,25].

There is clinical evidence that consumption of fish oil benefits SLE patients. In a prospective double blind crossover study, 27 SLE patients were given either 20 g of fish oil daily or 20 g of olive oil for 12 wk as part of a standardized isoenergetic low fat diet [26]. When outcome measures were assessed, 14 out of 17 compliant patients who received fish oil showed benefits when evaluated for generalized lupus disease criteria. Wright and coworkers [27] conducted a 24 wk double-blind placebo-controlled parallel trial in which the effects of daily consumption of 3 g of n-3 PUFA (1.2 g DHA plus 1.8 g EPA) by SLE patients for 24 wk were compared to SLE patients consuming an olive oil placebo. There were significant improvements in systemic lupus scores and disease activity for SLE in those consuming n-3 PUFAs. It must be noted that, in contrast to the aforementioned studies, two other clinical trials reported that n-3 PUFAs were not effective in treating lupus nephritis [28,29].

Many questions remain regarding the use of n-3 PUFA-containing oils to prevent or counter autoimmune responses in SLE and other autoimmune diseases concerning their efficacy relative to comparative effects of other unsaturated fatty acids, molecular mechanisms, cellular targets, potential biomarkers of effect and requisite dosages. In this investigation, we used the NZBWF1 SLE model to compare the effects on of autoimmunity onset as reflected by autoantibody production and glomerulonephritis in animals consuming: 1) an n-3 PUFA-rich diet containing docosahexaenoic acid enriched fish oil (DFO), 2) an n-6 PUFA-rich Western-style diet containing corn oil (CRN) or 3) an n-9 monounsaturated fatty acid (MUFA)-rich Mediterranean-style diet containing high oleic safflower oil (HOS). In addition, a focused PCR array was used to relate these findings to the expression of genes associated with CD4$^+$ T cell function in spleen and kidney both prior to and after the onset of the autoimmune nephritis. Finally, the downregulation of selected genes from the array was confirmed by quantitative RT-PCR. Marked autoantibody and nephritic responses were observed to the same extent in mice fed either n-6 PUFA or n-9 MUFA diets, however, these effects were remarkably suppressed in mice consuming the n-3 PUFA diet. Notably, this suppression was concurrent with generalized downregulation of CD4$^+$ T cell-related gene expression of in kidney and/or spleen. Many of the genes identified in this study are under consideration as potential biomarkers and/or therapeutic targets for human SLE.

Materials and Methods

Animals

All animal protocols were reviewed and approved by Michigan State University's Institutional Animal Care and Use Committee. Three-week-old female NZBWF1/J mice were purchased from Jackson Laboratory (Bar Harbor, ME) and provided food and water *ad lib*. Mice were housed 4 per cage under specific pathogen-free conditions using a HEPA filtered Innorack IVC cages (Innovive Inc., San Diego, CA).

Diets

Standard purified isocaloric AIN-93G diets [30] (Dyets, Inc., Bethlehem, PA) containing 70 g total oil per kg were prepared (Table 1). Experimental diets were modified to contain 60 g/kg diet of oils from three different sources. DHA ethyl ester-enriched fish oil (DFO) from Ocean Nutrition Canada (Dartmouth, Nova Scotia) containing 540 g/kg DHA and 50 g/kg EPA was used for the n-3 PUFA- rich diet. Corn oil (CRN) from Dyets containing 612 g/kg linoleic acid (n-6) and 26 g/kg of oleic acid (n-9) was employed as a source of n-6 PUFA. High-oleic safflower oil (HOS) from Hain Celestial Group (Boulder, CO) containing 750 g/kg oleic acid and 140 g/kg linoleic acid was utilized as the n-9 MUFA source. To provide basal essential fatty acids, all diets were supplemented with corn oil (10 g/kg diet).

Experimental Design

Beginning at 4 wk of age, mice (n = 16 per group) were randomly assigned to DFO, CRN or HOS treatments and maintained on diet until sacrifice. Diets were prepared weekly and stored at -20°C to avoid oxidation. After assignment, all mice were further subdivided (n = 8 per group) into a pre-nephritis cohort that was terminated at 16 wk of age or a post-nephritis cohort that was terminated at 34 wk of age. Body weights were measured biweekly. Urine for proteinuria determination was obtained at regular intervals using the animal spot-urine collection method [31]. Blood was collected for plasma autoantibody and

Table 1. Composition of experimental diets.

| Ingredients[a] | Experimental Diet | | |
| | CRN | HOS | DFO |
	g/kg	g/kg	g/kg
Casein	200.00	200.00	200.00
Dyetrose	132.00	132.00	132.00
Cornstarch	397.49	397.49	397.49
Sucrose	100.00	100.00	100.00
Cellulose	50.00	50.00	50.00
t-Butylhydroquinone (TBHQ)	0.01	0.01	0.01
AIN 93-G Salt Mix	35.00	35.00	35.00
AIN-93G Vitamin Mix (with vitamin E)	10.00	10.00	10.00
LCystiene	3.00	3.00	3.00
Choline Bitartrate	2.50	2.50	2.50
Corn Oil[a,b]	70.00	10.00	10.00
High-Oleic Safflower Oil[a,c]	-	60.00	-
DHA-Enriched Fish Oil[a,d]	-	-	60.00
Unsaturated fatty acid composition			
n-3 (DHA plus EPA)	0	0	35.4
n-6 (linoleic acid)	42.8	14.5	6.1
n-9 (oleic acid)	18.2	47.6	2.6

[a]As reported by the manufacturer.
[b]Corn oil contained 612 g/kg linoleic acid and 26 g/kg of oleic acid.
[c]High oleic acid safflower oil contained 140 g/kg linoleic acid and 750 g/kg oleic acid.
[d]DHA-enriched fish oil contained 540 g/kg DHA and 50 g/kg EPA.

immunoglobulin analysis at selected intervals from the saphenous vein using lithium-heparin-treated microvettes (Sarstedt, Numbrecht, Germany) [32]. At termination, animals were euthanized via an injection of sodium pentobarbital (60 mg/kg body weight) and cervical dislocation. Terminal blood collection was made by cardiac puncture using heparinized (100 IU/ml) syringes. The left kidney was excised and immersed in 10% (v/v) neutral buffered formalin for histopathology. The right kidney and spleen were immersed in RNAlater (Ambion, Inc., Austin, TX) for mRNA analysis by PCR array and quantitative RT-PCR.

Glomerulonephritis Assessment

Protein in urine was assessed utilizing Multistix's 10 SG Urine Strips (Siemens Healthcare Diagnostics, Deerfield, IL). Readings greater than 300 mg/dL were considered indicative of proteinuria. For histopathological analysis, formalin-fixed paraffin-embedded kidneys were sectioned at 5 μm and stained with either Hematoxylin and Eosin [H&E] or Periodic acid Schiff [PAS]. Identifications were masked and glomerular injury was scored blindly by a board certified veterinary pathologist using the International Society of Nephrology-Renal Pathology Society Lupus Nephritis Classification [33].

Measurement of Anti-dsDNA Autoantibodies and Immunoglobulins in Plasma

Whole heparinized blood was centrifuged at 2000×g for 5 min and the resultant plasma was collected and stored at −80C until analysis. Plasma anti-dsDNA IgG autoantibodies were determined using dsDNA ELISA kits (Alpha Diagnostic International, San Antonio, TX). Total IgM, IgG1, IgG2a, IgG2b, IgG3, IgA was assessed utilizing a Milliplex bead assay (Millipore Corp., Billerica, MA).

Analysis of CD4+T Cell-related mRNA Expression in Kidney and Spleen by Focused PCR Array

Kidney and spleen samples were held in RNAlater at 4°C overnight and then stored at −80°C until analysis. Extraction of total renal and splenic RNA was performed with TriReagent (Sigma Aldrich Co., St. Louis, MO) according to manufacturer instructions. Genomic DNA was removed employing an RNeasy Mini Kit with DNase treatment (Qiagen Valencia, CA). Total RNA was dissolved in Ambion nuclease-free water and quantified using a NanoDrop-1000 (Thermo Fisher Scientific, Wilmington, DE). The SA Biosciences Mouse Profiler Th1-Th2-Th3 PCR Array (Frederick, MD) was used to assess impact of dietary treatments on CD4+ T cell-related mRNA expression. Prior to array analysis, samples were pooled (n = 8) using equal concentrations of RNA. cDNAs were prepared and arrays loaded according to manufacturer instructions. PCR was conducted using ABI 7900 HT Fast Real-Time PCR System (Foster City, CA) under universal RNA cycling conditions (10 min at 95°C, 15 s at 95°C, 1 min 60°C for 40 cycles). Data analysis was performed using SA Bioscience's proprietary online program (http://pcrdataanalysis.sabiosciences.com/pcr/arrayanalysis.php, (last accessed 2/19/2014) which utilizes the ΔΔCt method for reporting expression changes.

Quantitative PCR of Selected CD4[+] T Cell-related mRNAs in Kidney and Spleen

Quantitative RT-PCRs using specific primer-probes obtained from Applied Biosystems (Foster City, CA) were performed on selected genes that were identified in the array study (CD80, CTLA-4, IL-10, IL-18, CCL-5, CXCR3, IL-6, TNF-α and OPN). Data were analyzed with ABI 7900 HT Fast Real-Time PCR System Applied Biosystems SDS 2.3 software and the absolute quantification method [34]. HPRT1 was used as the housekeeping gene. Data were normalized to expression of the target gene at wk 16 in the HOS-fed group.

Statistics

Data are presented as mean +/− standard error of the mean (SEM). Statistical differences (p-value<0.05) were assessed using one-way ANOVA (Systat Software, Inc., San Jose, CA) and Tukey post hoc test for multiple comparisons. When normality or equality of variance failed, the Kruskal-Wallis ANOVA and/or Dunn's post hoc test was applied.

Results

DFO Consumption Suppresses Glomerulonephritis and Body Weight Increase

The effects of consuming DFO, CRN and HOS diets enriched in n-3, n-6 and n-9 unsaturated fats, respectively, on proteinuria, an indicator of glomerulonephritis, were compared in female NZBWF1 mice. Proteinuria was initially observed in 13% of the CRN-fed animals at wk 26 and this increased to 63% by wk 34 (Fig. 1A). The HOS treatment group exhibited proteinuria in 13% of the mice beginning at wk 30 which increased to 75% by wk 34.

In contrast to these two groups, proteinuria was not observed in mice that consumed the DFO diet up to and including wk 34. Interestingly, HOS- and CRN-fed mice began to exhibit greater body weights than the DFO-fed group beginning at 20 wk of age (Fig. 1B). Upon termination at the age of 34 wk, DFO-fed mice weighed 8 and 12% less than HOS- and CRN-fed animals, respectively.

To confirm effects of the three dietary regimens on glomerulonephritis, kidney sections from the 34 wk cohort were assessed histopathologically following H&E and PAS staining. Both CRN and HOS fed mice exhibited: 1) moderate to severe diffuse glomerular hypercellularity, 2) mesangial expansion, and 3) tubular proteinosis characteristic of glomerulonephritis. Additionally, the mice had moderate to severe lymphocytic inflammation at the renal pelvis (Fig. 2A–D). In contrast, these endpoints were modest or absent in DFO-fed mice (Fig. 2E, F). Mice were individually graded for severity of lupus nephritis lesions using the ISN-RPS classification system. 5 out of 8 mice in the CRN group and 4 out of 8 in the HOS group had lesions categorized as class IV, which is indicative of severe glomerulonephritis (Fig. 3). In comparison, all DFO-fed mice had lesions classified as II or lower. Thus, consistent with proteinuria data, consumption of n-3 PUFA attenuated both the onset and severity of glomerulonephritis as compared to the n-6 PUFA or n-9 MUFA diet groups.

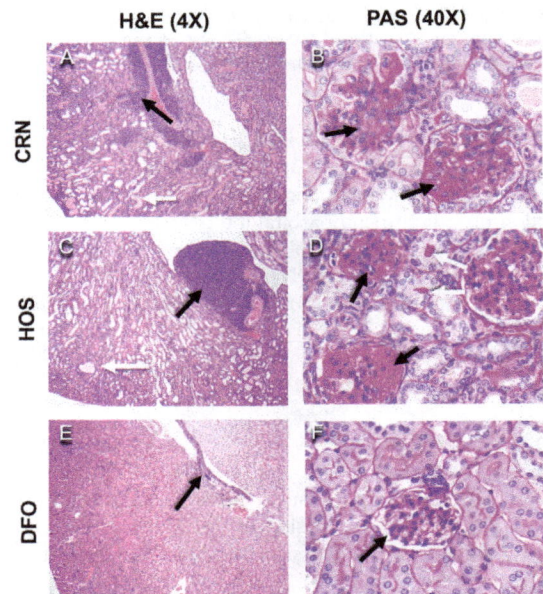

Figure 2. n-3 PUFA consumption attenuates glomerulonephritis. Female NZBWF1/J mice were fed CRN, HOS, or DFO diets for 30 wk beginning at 4 wk. At wk 34, renal histopathology was assessed. Panels A, C and F show representative hematoxylin and eosin (H&E)-stained sections (4X). Note the variable degree of tubular dilation and proteinosis (white arrow) and lymphocyte infiltration at the pelvis (black arrows). Panels B, D and F depict Periodic Acid-Schiff (PAS)-stained sections (40X). Note the tubular proteinosis (white arrows) and the thickened tubular basement membrane and mesangial cell hyperplasia-related glomerular hypercellularity with extensive adhesions to the Bowman's capsule (black arrows). Lesions were moderate to severe in mice fed CRN and HOS diets and were mild in the mice fed DFO diet.

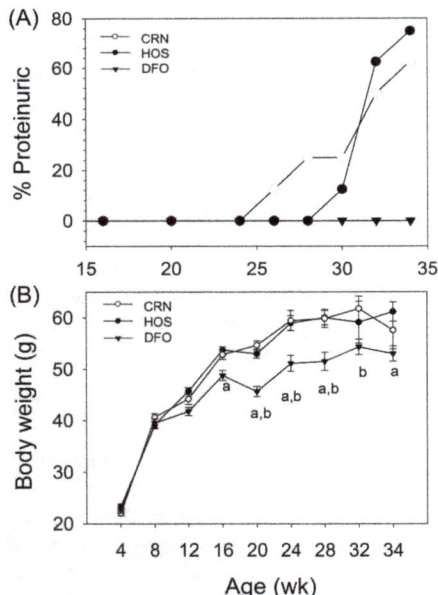

Figure 1. n-3 PUFA consumption prevents proteinuria onset and reduces weight gain. Female NZBWF1/J mice were fed DFO, CRN or HOS diets beginning at 4 wk of age. (A)Urinary protein was assessed using urinalysis reagent strips. Mice exhibiting ≥300 mg/dL were considered positive for proteinuria. (B) Effect of experimental diets on body weight. Values are mean ± SEM (n = 16) until 16 wk of age and n = 8, thereafter Letters a and b indicate body weights of DFO-fed mice differ significantly from those of CRN- and HOS-fed mice, respectively (p<0.05).

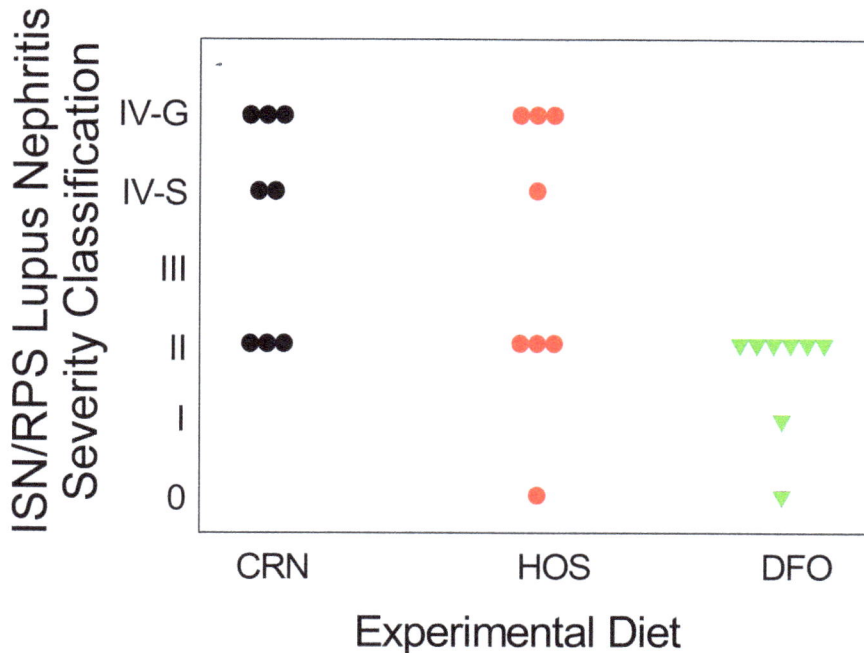

Figure 3. Summary of histopathological findings. Figure depicts summary of histopathological findings using ISN/RPS lupus nephritis classification system.

DFO Dietary Regimen Inhibits Autoantibody Production

Elevation of circulating autoantibodies is known to precede and/or co-occur with nephritis in NZBWF1 mice and is a key contributing factor in human SLE [3]. Consistent with this notion, mice fed CRN and HOS diets exhibited elevated anti-dsDNA IgGs in plasma beginning at wk 20 to 24, with concentrations increased 6- and 7-fold from wk 16 to wk 34, respectively (Fig. 4). By comparison, plasma anti-dsDNA IgG concentrations in the DFO treatment group were significantly lower (P<0.05) than those in the CRN and HOS treatment groups at all weeks tested.

Since polyclonal B cell activation and differentiation to IgG-secreting plasma cells occurs during SLE [35,36], the effects of the different dietary regimens on plasma Ig isotype levels were also assessed. Compared to wk 16, concentrations of plasma IgG1, IgG2a, IgG2b, IgG3, IgM and IgA were increased by 2- to 12-fold

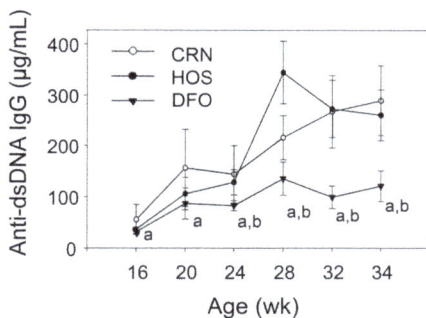

Figure 4. n-3 PUFA consumption delays autoantibody production. Female NZBWF1/J mice were fed CRN, HOS, or DFO diets beginning at 4 wk of age. Plasma anti-dsDNA autoantibody formation was monitored by ELISA. Data are expressed as mean ± SEM (n = 8). Letters a and b denote significant differences (p<0.05) from CRN- and HOS-fed mice, respectively.

at wk 34 in the CRN and HOS treatment groups (Fig. 5A–F). In contrast, concentrations of all isotypes in the DFO treatment group were significantly lower (p<0.05) than the CRN and HOS groups at wk 34.

DFO Consumption Downregulates Expression of CD4+ T Cell-related Genes in Kidney and Spleen

Relative expression of 84 CD4+-T cell-related genes in kidneys and spleens from the three treatment groups were compared at wk 16 and wk 34 using a proprietary mouse profiling PCR array. While differences among groups at wk 16 were modest (see Fig. S1 and Table S1), they were markedly robust at wk 34 (Fig. 6, Table 2). A total of 33 genes on the array were found to be downregulated ≥1.5-fold while 3 were upregulated ≥1.5 fold in kidneys of DFO-fed mice as compared to HOS-fed mice (Fig. 6A). A similar comparison of DFO-fed mice with CRN-fed mice identified 37 downregulated and 2 upregulated genes (Fig. 6B). In spleens of 34 wk old mice, 26 genes were downregulated and 1 upregulated at 34 wk in DFO-fed mice as compared to HOS-fed mice. Similarly, 25 genes were downregulated and 7 were upregulated as compared to CRN-fed mice (Fig. 6D, E). In contrast to the aforementioned effects, comparison of CD4+ T cell-related gene expression between the HOS and CRN group revealed more modest differences with 7 and 8 genes being downregulated and upregulated, respectively, in kidney, (Fig. 6C) and 1 and 10 genes being downregulated and upregulated, respectively, in spleen (Fig. 6F).

Overall, expression of many CD4+ T cell-related genes was suppressed by DFO consumption at wk 34 (Table 2). These included 1) cytokines (IFN-γ, IL-2, IL-10, IL-18, IL-27, TNF-α, osteopontin [OPN]), 2) chemokines (CCL5, CCL7), 3) chemokine receptors (CCR2, CCR3, CCR4, CCR5, CXCR3), 4) T cell membrane proteins (CD4, CD28, CD40L, CTLA 4) and 5) accessory and B cell membrane proteins (CD27 and CD80). As described in the following sections, representatives from each of

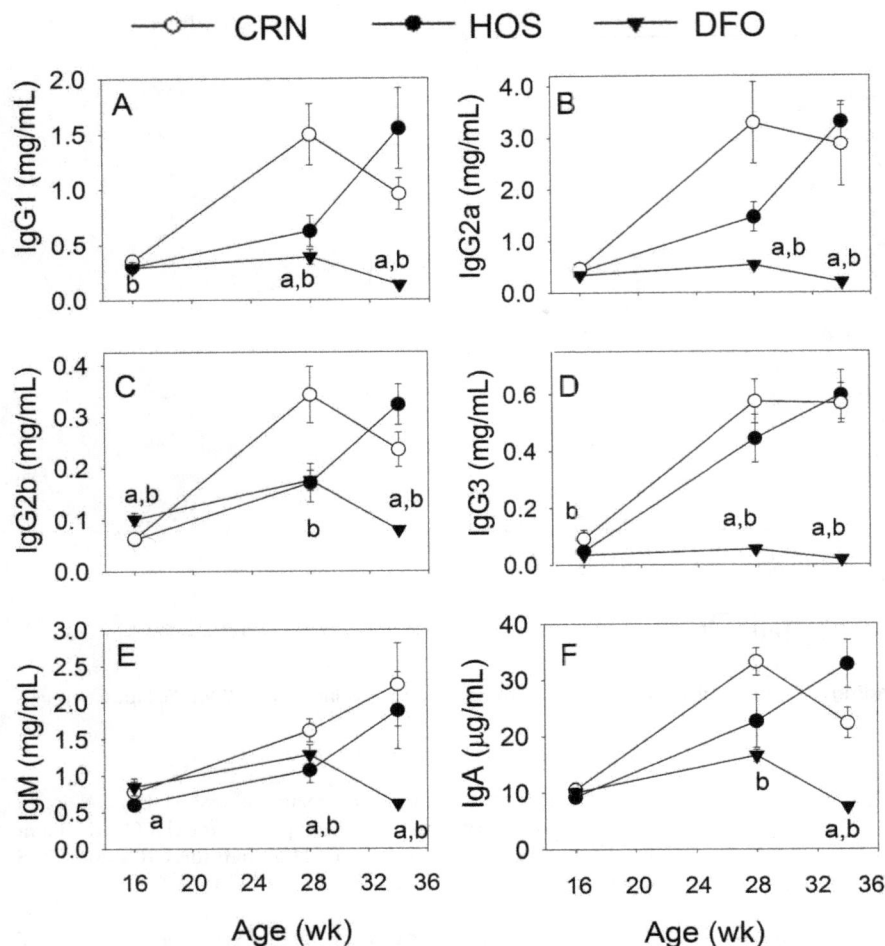

Figure 5. n-3 PUFA consumption inhibits plasma IgG1, IgG2a, IgG2b, IgG3, IgM and IgA elevation. Female NZBWF1/J mice were fed CRN, HOS, or DFO diets beginning at 4 wk of age. Concentrations of immunoglobulin isotypes were measured at wks 16 (n = 16), 28 (n = 8) and 34 (n = 8) using Milliplex Bead assay. Data are expressed as mean ± SEM. Letters *a* and *b* denote significant differences (p<0.05) from CRN- and HOS-fed mice, respectively.

these gene families were selected and their mRNAs measured by quantitative real-time PCR in kidney and spleens at 16 and 34 wks.

DFO Treatment Downregulates CD80 and CTL4A mRNA Expression in Kidney and Spleen

CD80 and CTL4A are integral membrane proteins on antigen-presenting cells and $CD4^+$ T cells, respectively, that were downregulated in the array of DFO fed mice compared to either CRN- or HOS-fed mice. Quantitative RT-PCR indicated that, in the kidney, expression of CD80 mRNA in the CRN and HOS treatment groups increased by 52- and 153-fold, respectively from wk 16 to wk 34 (Fig. 7A). However, CD80 mRNA expression in the DFO treatment group was attenuated at both wk 16 (2- to 3-fold) and wk 34 (5- to 15-fold) as compared to CRN and HOS groups. CD80 expression was also modestly suppressed in the spleens of DFO-fed mice at wk 16 but not wk 34 (Fig. 7B). CTLA-4 mRNA expression in kidney increased from wk 16 to wk 34 by 14- and 15-fold in CRN- and HOS-treated mice, respectively (Fig. 7C), while DFO treatment attenuated these responses by 2- to 3-fold. Although increases in splenic CTLA4 mRNA expression

from wk 16 to wk 34 were more modest than kidney, relative mRNA levels for this gene at wk 34 were again 2- to 3-fold lower in the DFO group than the CRN and HOS groups (Fig. 7D).

Expression of IL-10 and IL-18 mRNA in Kidney and Spleen is Attenuated following N-3 PUFA Consumption

IL-10 and IL-18 are examples of regulatory cytokines that impact T cell function, both of which were downregulated in the PCR array. Quantitative RT-PCR revealed that IL-10 mRNA expression in kidney robustly increased from wk 16 to wk 34 in CRN and HOS treatment groups by 17- and 22-fold, respectively (Fig. 8A), whereas IL-18 mRNAs for these groups increased more modestly (Fig. 8C). Elevated expression at wk 34 of both genes in the kidney was significantly attenuated in the DFO treatment group. Consumption of CRN and HOS elevated IL-10 mRNA expression from 16 to 34 wk by 2- to 3-fold (Fig. 8B) in spleen. Consistent with the kidney, increases in IL-10 mRNA were largely ablated in mice that consumed DFO. However, dietary unsaturated fat regimens largely did not affect IL-18 mRNA expression in spleen (Fig. 8D).

KIDNEY　　　　　**SPLEEN**

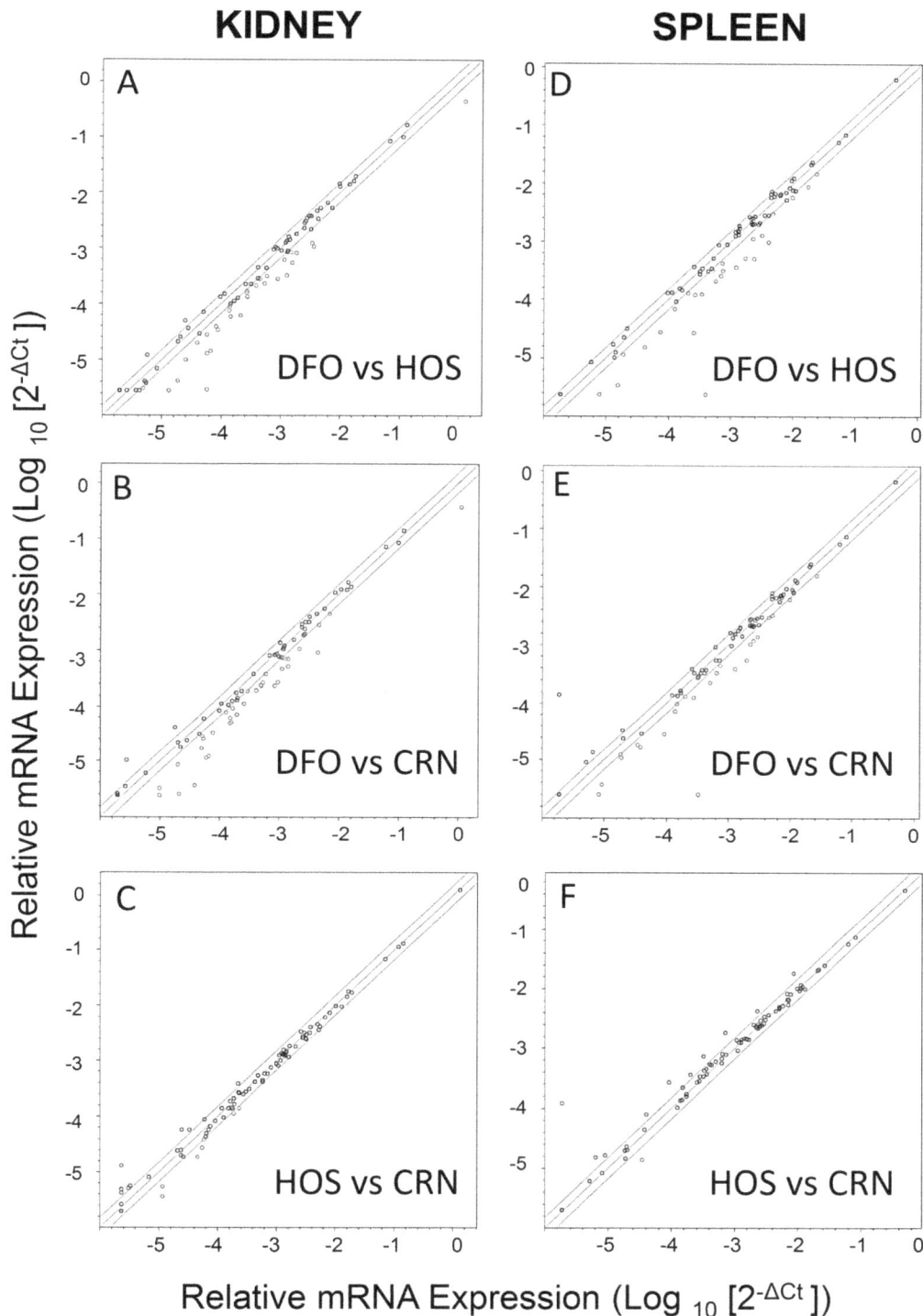

Figure 6. Comparative effects of n-3 PUFA consumption on CD4[+] T cell-related gene expression in kidneys and spleens of 34 wk old NZBWF1/J mice. Cohorts of female mice were fed CRN, HOS, or DFO diets for 30 wk beginning at 4 wk. At wk 34, mice were euthanized and mRNA isolated from kidneys. Extracted mRNA were pooled and analyzed using a SABioscience Mouse Th1-Th2-Th3 PCR Array. Points outside of solid line are >1.5–fold difference.

DFO Diet Suppresses CCL5 and CXCR3 mRNA Expression in Kidney and Spleen

Downregulated expression of CCL5 and CXCR3 mRNAs, prototypical examples of a chemokine and chemokine receptor, respectively, in DFO-treated mice was verified by quantitative PCR. CCL5 mRNA was found to increase from wk 16 to 34 by 11- and 15-fold in the kidneys of CRN and HOS fed mice, respectively and these responses were suppressed in DFO fed mice

Table 2. Differential effects of consuming n-3, n-6 and n-9 PUFAs on expression of CD4[+] T cell-related genes in kidneys and spleens of 34 wk old female NZBWF1 mice[a,b].

Gene ID	Gene Description	KIDNEY		SPLEEN	
		DFO vs CRN	DFO vs HOS	DFO vs CRN	DFO vs HOS
Integral Membrane Protein					
Ccr2	Chemokine (C-C motif) receptor 2	−2.0	−2.2	1.3	1.4
Ccr3	Chemokine (C-C motif) receptor 3	−2.4	−2.8	1.5	1.6
Ccr4	Chemokine (C-C motif) receptor 4	−10.6	−4.4	−1.0	1.0
Ccr5	Chemokine (C-C motif) receptor 5	−2.1	−2.7	−2.2	−4.2
Ccr10	Chemokine (C-C motif) receptor 10	−1.3	1.3	−2.2	−2.2
Cd4	CD4 antigen	−2.3	−2.1	1.2	1.3
Cd27	CD27 antigen	−3.0	−2.0	1.2	−1.0
Cd28	CD28 antigen	−1.5	−1.7	−1.2	−1.1
Cd40	CD40 antigen	−1.6	−1.3	−1.2	−1.4
Cd40lg	CD40 ligand	−1.8	−2.6	−1.2	−1.0
Cd80	CD80 antigen	−5.4	−4.7	−1.2	1.0
Cd86	CD86 antigen	−1.6	−1.5	−1.2	−1.0
Ctla4	Cytotoxic T-lymphocyte-associated protein 4	−5.3	−4.5	−3.3	−3.3
Cxcr3	Chemokine (C-X-C motif) receptor 3	−2.1	−2.3	−2.2	−2.5
Icos	Inducible T cell co-stimulator	−2.1	−1.6	−1.6	−1.6
Igsf6	Immunoglobulin superfamily, member 6	−1.8	−1.8	−1.0	−1.1
Il1r1	Interleukin 1 receptor, type I	−1.6	−1.5	1.2	1.2
Il2ra	Interleukin 2 receptor, alpha chain	3.7	2.1	−1.4	−2.7
Il4ra	Interleukin 4 receptor, alpha	−2.9	−2.4	−130.0	−168.8
Il12rb2	Interleukin 12 receptor, beta 2	ND	−1.5	74.9	1.2
Il13ra1	Interleukin 13 receptor, alpha 1	−1.0	1.1	1.2	1.1
Il18r1	Interleukin 18 receptor 1	−1.8	−1.5	1.5	1.4
Il27ra	Interleukin 27 receptor, alpha	−1.6	−1.4	−1.1	−1.0
Ptprc	Protein tyrosine phosphatase, receptor type C	−3.5	−3.9	1.1	−2.0
Tlr4	Toll-like receptor 4	−1.4	−1.5	−1.0	−1.1
Tlr6	Toll-like receptor 6	−1.1	−1.8	1.1	1.1
Tmed1	Transmembrane emp24 domain containing 1	1.2	1.3	−1.0	−1.0
Tnfrsf4	Tumor necrosis factor receptor superfamily, member 4	−1.4	−1.6	−2.1	−2.1
Tnfrsf8	Tumor necrosis factor receptor superfamily, member 8	−4.1	−1.3	−1.9	−1.9
Kinases					
Jak1	Janus kinase 1	−1.2	−1.1	1.2	1.2
Jak2	Janus kinase 2	1.1	1.2	1.4	1.5
Jak3	Janus kinase 3	−1.1	1.0	−1.5	−1.5
Junb	Jun-B oncogene	−2.1	−1.5	−1.2	−2.7
Mapk8	Mitogen-activated protein kinase 8	1.3	1.2	1.5	1.2
Mapk9	Mitogen-activated protein kinase 9	1.2	1.3	1.2	1.2
Tyk2	Tyrosine kinase 2	−1.0	1.0	−1.0	1.1
Cytokine/Chemokine					
Ccl5	Chemokine (C-C motif) ligand 5	−4.9	−3.4	−1.4	−1.5
Ccl7	Chemokine (C-C motif) ligand 7	−2.7	−1.9	−3.3	−9.6
Ccl11	Chemokine (C-C motif) ligand 11	2.4	2.0	−1.9	1.3
Csf2	Colony stimulating factor 2 (granulocyte-macrophage)	ND	ND	ND	ND
Ifng	Interferon gamma	−8.3	−19.5	−1.5	−2.7
Il2	Interleukin 2	ND	−4.7	−1.5	−1.7
Il4	Interleukin 4	1.0	−1.2	−1.8	−1.4

Table 2. Cont.

Gene ID	Gene Description	KIDNEY		SPLEEN	
		DFO vs CRN	DFO vs HOS	DFO vs CRN	DFO vs HOS
Il5	Interleukin 5	−1.2	−1.4	1.2	1.2
Il6	Interleukin 6	−1.5	1.3	−2.3	−2.7
Il7	Interleukin 7	1.1	1.4	−1.1	−1.2
Il9	Interleukin 9	1.1	1.4	ND	ND
Il10	Interleukin 10	−3.1	−3.4	−3.7	−4.8
Il12b	Interleukin 12B	−2.1	−1.5	−1.1	−1.4
Il13	Interleukin 13	1.3	−1.6	1.8	1.5
Il15	Interleukin 15	1.0	1.2	1.2	1.2
IL17a	Interleukin 17A	ND	ND	ND	ND
Il18	Interleukin 18	−2.0	−1.9	1.0	1.1
Il23a	Interleukin 23, alpha subunit p19	1.1	1.3	−2.5	−4.6
Il27	Interleukin 27	−1.2	−2.1	−1.5	−1.4
Opn	Osteopontin	−3.1	−2.9	−2.0	−2.4
Tgfb3	Transforming growth factor, beta 3	−1.3	−1.5	−1.1	−1.6
Tnf	Tumor necrosis factor	−2.3	−2.1	−1.2	−1.4
Tnfsf4	Tumor necrosis factor superfamily, member 4	−3.1	−1.4	1.1	1.3
Transcription Factors and Regulators					
Bcl6	B cell leukemia/lymphoma 6	−1.1	1.1	−1.4	−1.4
Cebpb	CCAAT/enhancer binding protein (C/EBP), beta	−1.1	−1.0	−1.6	−1.7
Crebbp	CREB binding protein	1.1	1.1	1.2	1.3
Gata3	GATA binding protein 3	−1.3	−1.1	−1.1	−1.2
Gfi1	Growth factor independent 1	−2.4	−2.6	−1.2	−1.7
Irf1	Interferon regulatory factor 1	−1.6	−1.2	−1.4	−1.3
Irf4	Interferon regulatory factor 4	−2.7	−1.7	−1.1	1.0
Maf	V-maf AS42 oncogene homolog	1.1	1.5	−1.2	−1.2
Nfatc1	NF of activated T cells, cyto., calcineurin-dep. 1	−1.2	−1.0	−1.1	1.2
Nfatc2	NF of activated T cells, cyto., calcineurin-dep. 2	−1.0	1.1	−1.2	−1.0
Nfatc2ip	Natc2 interacting protein	1.0	1.1	1.3	1.3
Nfatc3	NF of activated T cells, cyto., calcineurin-dep. 3	1.2	1.3	1.1	1.2
Nfkb1	NF of K light PP gene enhancer in B cells 1, p105	−1.4	−1.1	1.0	1.3
Pcgf2	Polycomb group ring finger 2	1.3	−1.3	ND	ND
Stat1	Signal transducer and activator of transcription 1	−1.6	−1.4	−1.7	−1.6
Stat4	Signal transducer and activator of transcription 4	ND	1.1	2.1	−1.1
Tbx21	T-box 21	−1.2	1.1	−2.3	−2.8
Tcfcp2	Transcription factor CP2	−1.0	1.3	1.5	1.4
Yy1	YY1 transcription factor	1.3	1.3	1.1	1.2
Miscellaneous					
Inha	Inhibin alpha	−1.2	−1.1	1.7	1.5
Il18bp	Interleukin 18 binding protein	−1.1	1.1	−1.1	−1.2
Socs1	Suppressor of cytokine signaling 1	−1.6	−1.5	−1.7	−1.8
Socs3	Suppressor of cytokine signaling 3	−3.6	−3.2	−1.3	−3.4
Socs5	Suppressor of cytokine signaling 5	1.2	1.2	−1.0	1.1
Sftpd	Surfactant associated protein D	−2.4	−1.9	−3.3	−3.4

[a]For qRT-PCR array comparisons, RNA expression values obtained from the kidneys of female NZBWF1/J mice fed docosahexaenoic acid-enriched diets were made relative to specified feeding group values and expressed as fold change. Expression ≥1.5 fold change was considered noteworthy.
[b]Abbreviations are: CRN, corn oil-enriched diet; HOS, high-oleic safflower oil-enriched diet; DFO, docosahexaenoic acid ethyl ester-enriched diet; ND, not detected.

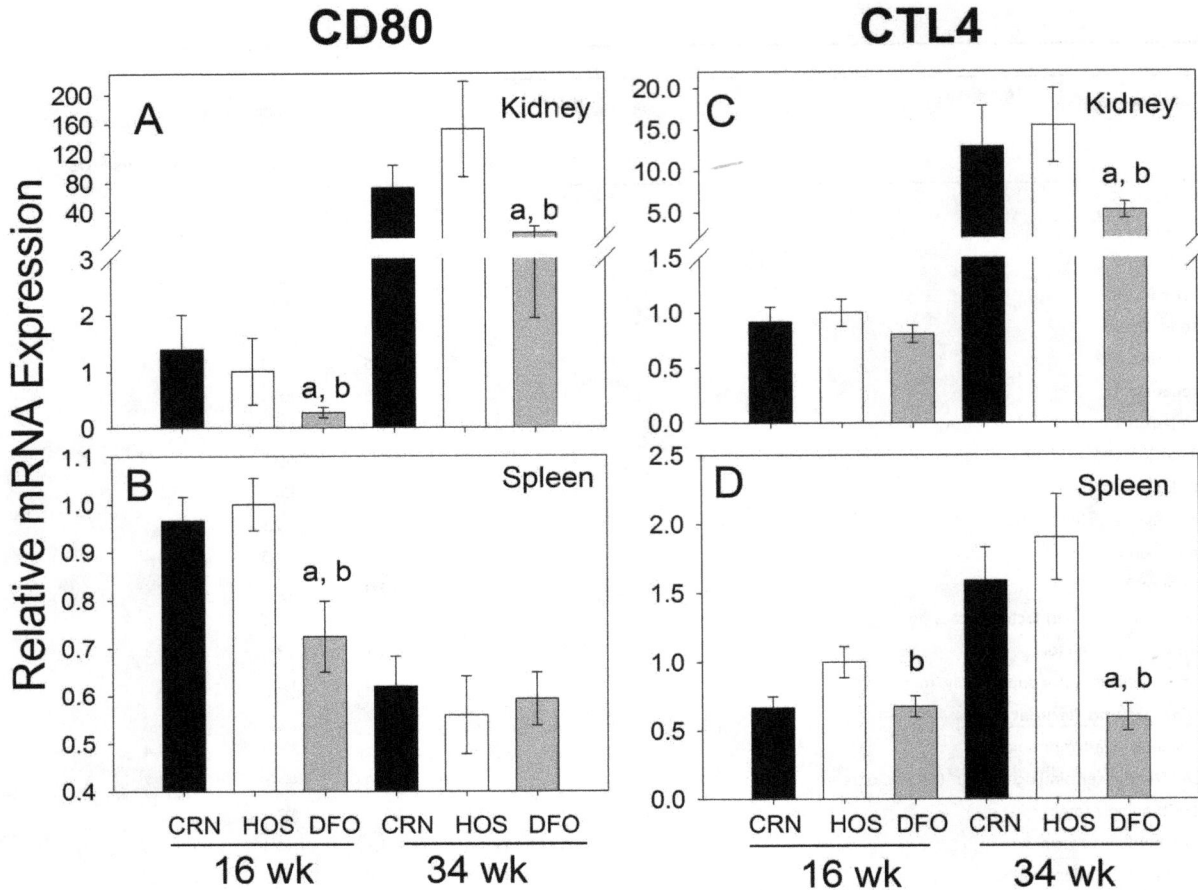

Figure 7. Differential effects of n-3, n-6 and n-9 PUFA consumption on CD80 and CTLA4 mRNA expression. Cohorts of 4 wk old female NZBWF1/J mice were fed diets enriched in n-3 (DFO), n-6 (CRN) or n-9 (HOS) for 30 wk. At wk 16 (pre-nephritis) and wk 34 (post-nephritis), mRNA was isolated from (A, C) kidneys and (B, D) spleens and analyzed for gene expression of CD80 (A, B) and CTLA4 (C, D) by real-time PCR. Data are expressed as mean ±SEM (n = 8). Letters *a* and *b* denote significant differences (p<0.05) from CRN- and HOS-fed mice, respectively.

by 4- to 7-fold (Fig. 9A). Splenic expression of this chemokine at 16 wk was also lower in DFO treatment animals than in CRN or HOS treatment groups, whereas no effects were observed at 34 wk (Fig. 9B). CXCR3 mRNA expression in the kidney also increased from 16 to 34 wk in mice fed CRN (4-fold) and HOS (6-fold) diets, but this elevation was suppressed by 3-fold in those mice fed DFO (Fig. 9C). Similar but more modest effects were observed in the spleen (Fig. 9D).

DFO Consumption Impairs IL-6 and TNF-α mRNA Expression in Kidney and Spleen

The proinflammatory cytokines IL-6 and TNF-α were markedly upregulated from wk 16 to 34 in the kidneys of mice consuming the CRN (6- and 15-fold, respectively) and HOS (6- and 14-fold, respectively) diets (Fig. 10A, C). In contrast, consumption of the DFO diet attenuated expression of IL-6 and TNF-α mRNAs in the kidneys by 3- to 5-fold. In spleen, while dietary treatment effects on IL-6 mRNA expression were not evident (Fig. 10B), DFO consumption modestly suppressed TNF-α mRNA expression at 16 wk but not at 34 wk (Fig. 10D).

Osteopontin mRNA Expression is Inhibited in Kidneys

and Spleens of DFO-fed Mice

The dietary effects of n-3 PUFAs on expression of the pleotropic cytokine OPN were measured by quantitative PCR. In the kidney, mRNA levels of this gene increased from wk 16 to wk 34 by 7- to 8-fold in CRN- and HOS-fed mice, whereas these elevations were attenuated by DFO-feeding (Fig. 11A). In analogous fashion, DFO treatment reduced expression of osteopontin mRNA in the spleen at both wk 16 and wk 34 when compared to CRN or HOS treatment groups (Fig. 11B).

Discussion

Preclinical models such as the female NZBWF1 mouse have been invaluable to unraveling the complex mechanisms involved in human SLE as well as identifying biomarkers and cellular targets for directing potential therapies. This chronic disease involves defects in the negative selection of autoreactive B and T cells as well as immune hyperactivity. Together these defects evoke aberrant activation of self-reactive lymphocytes, production of autoreactive antibodies and immune complex deposition in the kidney that result in glomerulonephritis. The CRN diet employed in this study was chosen to mimic the fatty acid profile of a typical Western diet in which individuals eat a high concentration of the

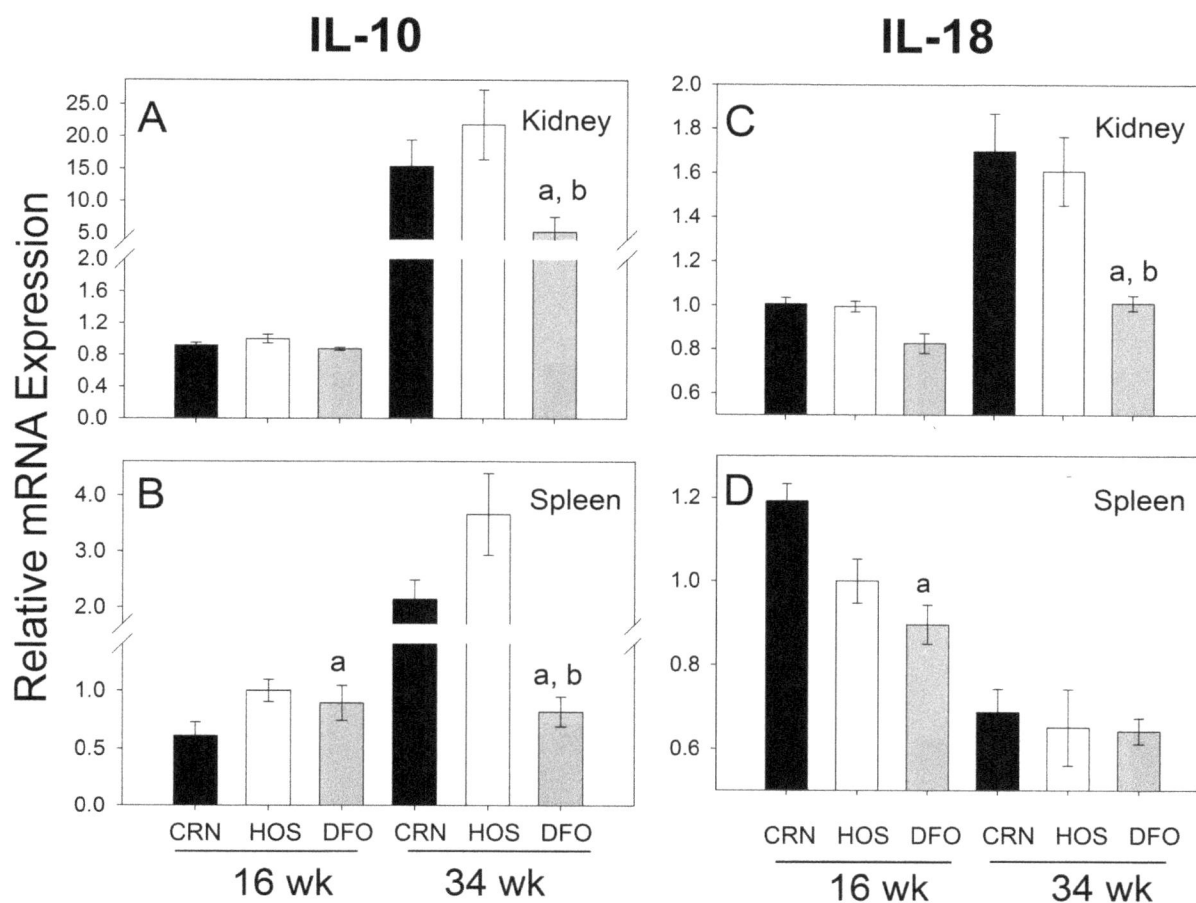

Figure 8. Differential effects of n-3, n-6 and n-9 PUFA consumption on IL-10 and IL-18 mRNA expression. Experiment conducted as described in Fig. 7 legend except that IL-10 (A, B) and IL-18 (C, D) mRNAs were measured by quantitative RT-PCR.

n-6 PUFA linoleic acid, favoring formation of arachidonic acid and its inflammatory eicosanoids. The HOS diet was used to recapitulate consumption of high levels of oleic acid, primarily from olive oil, that are present in a Mediterranean diet. Consumption of this n-9 MUFA per se has been suggested to reduce inflammatory responses [37]. This diet also provided insight to whether simply reducing n-6 PUFA-derived arachidonic acid pools could be responsible for any observed protective effects of the n-3 PUFA diet. The results presented herein demonstrate that autoantibody production, polyclonal B cell activation and lupus nephritis were similarly evident in mice fed diets rich in n-6 or n-9 unsaturated fats. However, the onset and/or severity of these responses were markedly suppressed in mice consuming the n-3 PUFA diet. Thus, the effects of n-3 PUFAs could not be replicated by substitution with the n-9 MUFA oleic acid.

The focused PCR array study revealed that n-3 PUFA suppression of the autoimmune responses co-occurred with generalized downregulation of gene expression in kidney and/or spleen of CD4+ T cell-related genes associated with inflammation including leukocyte recruitment, antigen presentation, T cell activation, and B cell activation/differentiation. Furthermore, effects of replacing n-6 PUFAs with the n-9 MUFAs on gene expression responses were negligible. Downregulation of these genes by n-3 PUFAs in kidney and spleen could be explained by inherently lower expression by cells that populate these tissues and/or by decreased infiltration by T cells, B cells, antigen-

presenting cells and other leukocytes. Importantly, genes down-regulated by the n-3 PUFA regimen included CD80, CTLA-4, IL-10, IL-18, CCL-5, CXCR3, OPN, IL-6 and TNF-α. Many of these are under consideration as biomarkers and/or potential targets for specific monoclonal antibody or receptor antagonist treatments of SLE and other autoimmune diseases.

n-3 PUFAs likely exert the pleiotropic effects observed here via both eicosanoid-dependent and eicosanoid-independent pathways [10]. Eicosanoids are a diverse group of chemical mediators produced by immune cells that depend upon the cell membrane PUFA composition [38]. For example, the eicosanoid prostaglandin E2 (PGE2), a cyclooxygenase (COX) metabolite of AA, can be proinflammatory and modulate cytokine production. Likewise, the 4-series leukotrienes (LTs) are lipooxygenase (LOX) metabolites of AA that have chemotactic properties, and upregulate proinflammatory cytokine production promoting inflammation. DHA and EPA competitively displace AA as a substrate for oxygenation by both COX-2 and 5-LOX. This reduces inflammation through eicosanoid-dependent pathways by: 1) decreasing membrane AA levels, 2) suppressing generation of proinflammatory eicosanoids (2 series PGs and 4-series LTs), 3) inhibiting COX-2 and 5-LOX expression and 4) promoting production of novel metabolites. Regarding the latter, studies over the last decade from the Serhan lab have shown that n-3 PUFAs convert to a novel series of lipid mediators termed specialized proresolving lipid mediators. These include resolvins, protectins, and maresins that can elicit,

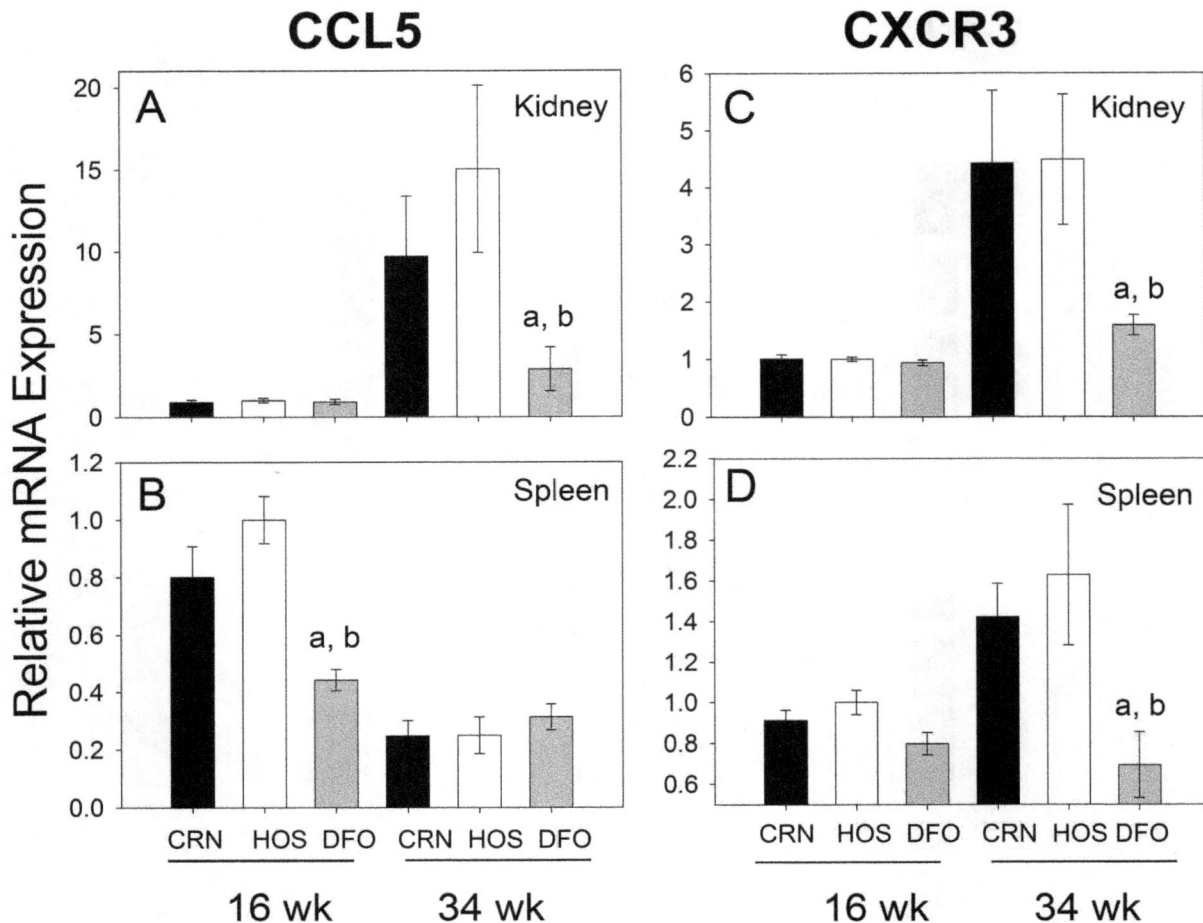

Figure 9. Differential effects of n-3, n-6 and n-9 PUFA consumption on CCL5 and CXCR3 mRNA expression. Experiment conducted as described in Fig. 7 legend except that CCL5 (A, B) and CXCR3 (C, D) mRNAs were measured by quantitative RT-PCR.

sometimes at very low concentrations, protective and beneficial effects in the resolution of inflammation [39]. Eicosanoid-independent mechanisms also play critical roles in n-3 PUFA suppression of gene expression. These include: 1) changes in membrane lipid/lipid raft composition that alter G-protein receptor or tyrosine-kinase linked receptor signaling [40,41], 2) interference with membrane receptors such as the TLR family [42], 3) alteration of transcription factor activity or abundance as has been described for PPAR, LXR, NNF-4, NF-κβ, AP-1 and CREB [43,44,45]and 4) interference with activity of critical second messenger-regulated kinases such as PKA, PKC, CaMKII, AKT and mitogen-activated protein kinases [45,46,47].

Another important consideration is the potential for n-3 PUFA consumption to inhibit inflammagenic mediator production associated with the increased fat mass and metabolic changes in NZBWF1 mice. White adipose tissue is composed of not only adipocytes, but also cells of the innate and adaptive immune systems that collectively secrete numerous cytokines and chemokines [48] that could contribute to development of SLE. Indeed numerous characteristics of obesity and metabolic syndrome have been observed in 36 wk old NZBWF1 mice that included increased body weight, hypertension, elevated plasma leptin, insulin resistance, and central adiposity with macrophage infiltration [49]. A study in B6.Sle.1Sle2.Sle3 SLE-prone mice reported significantly worsened glucose tolerance, increased adipose tissue

insulin resistance, increased β-cell insulin secretion, and increased adipocyte size compared with their respective B6 controls [50]. B cells isolated from the white adipose tissue of B6.SLE mice were skewed toward IgG production, and the level of IgG1 was elevated in the serum of SLE-prone mice. In the study presented herein, DFO-fed NZBWF1 mice weighed 8 and 12% less than HOS- and CRN-fed animals, respectively. Thus, reduced body weight and fat mass could be factors in reduced SLE severity observed in mice that consumed DFO. Although we did not specifically measure food intake or adiposity in this study, Bargut et. al [51] recently reported that B6 mice fed high fat fish oil diet exhibit reductions in body weight, adiposity index and plasma IL-6 as compared to mice fed high fat soybean oil diets. Importantly, no differences in food intake were observed between the two groups, and, furthermore, fish oil-fed mice exhibited higher energy expenditure. Thus, it might be speculated that reduced body weights in DFO-fed NZBWF1 mice in the present study resulted from lower feed efficiency than that for CRN- and HOS-fed animals and that this reduction contributed to reduced adipose tissue inflammation. It will therefore be critical in future studies to relate n-3 PUFA attenuation of autoimmunity to the potential effects on food intake, feed efficiency, metabolism, obesity and leukocyte infiltration/gene expression to adipose tissue.

CD80, also known as B7-1, is constitutively expressed on dendritic cells and is inducible in other antigen-presenting cells

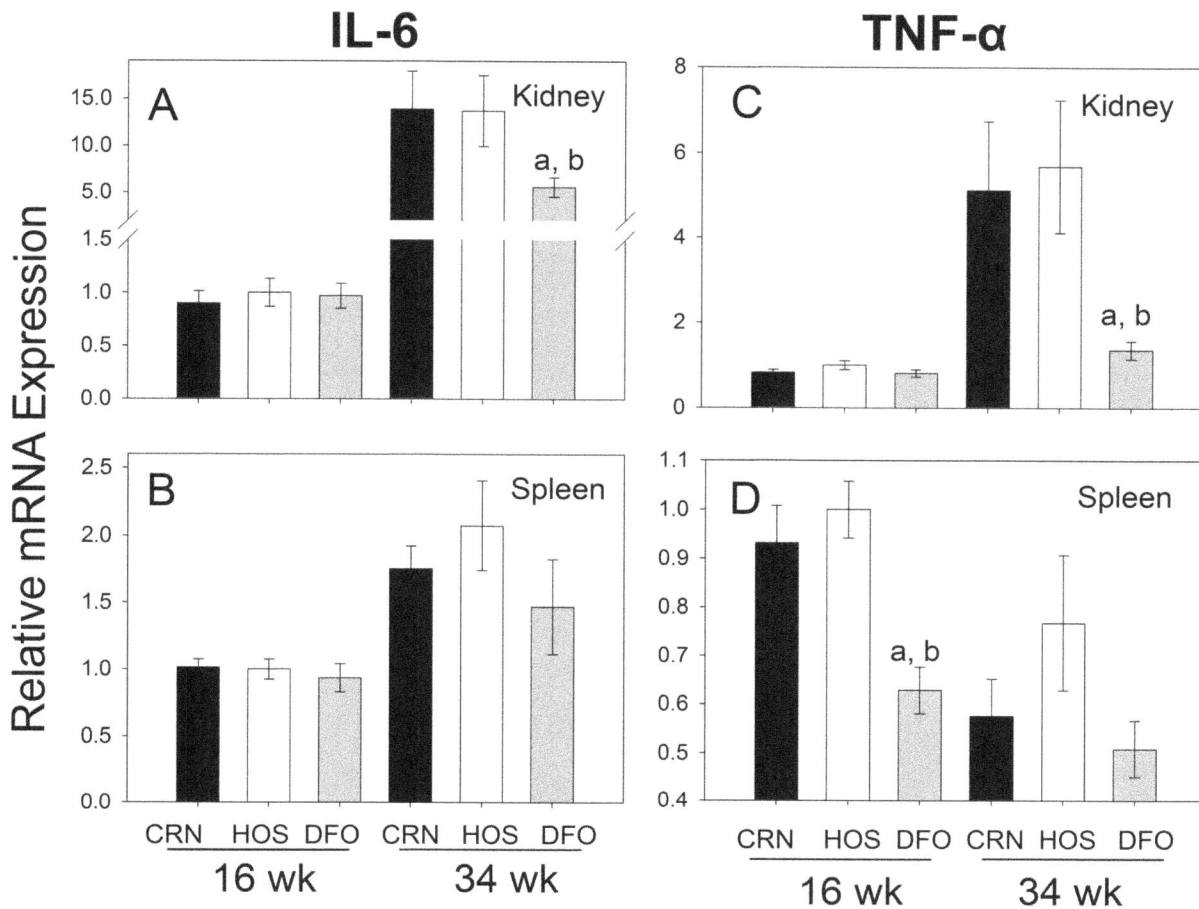

Figure 10. Differential effects of n-3, n-6 and n-9 PUFA consumption on IL-6 and TNF-α mRNA expression. Experiment conducted as described in Fig. 7 legend except that IL-6 (A, B) and TNF-α (C, D) mRNAs were measured by quantitative RT-PCR.

such as B cells and monocytes [52]. This integral membrane protein provides the requisite costimulatory signal for T cell activation and survival. CD80 works in tandem with CD86 to prime T cells by serving as ligand for CD28 and CTLA-4 on the T cell surface [53]. CD28 is upregulated early during T cell activation and its stimulation can: 1) augment and prolong IL-2 secretion by T cells as well as delay the onset of peripheral immune tolerance, 2) enable T cells to signal B cells to proliferate and differentiate into antibody-producing plasma cells, and 3) enhance other cognate costimulatory interactions between antigen-presenting cells and T cells thereby intensifying proinflammatory gene expression. While structurally similar to CD28, CTLA-4 differs because it is expressed after prolonged T cell activation and transduces an inhibitory signal to T cells rather than a stimulatory signal [54].

Several lines of evidence indicate that impairment of the CD80 costimulatory pathway attenuates autoimmune effects associated with SLE. Blockade of CD80 by monoclonal antibody has been shown in the pristane-induced lupus mouse model to attenuate both the inflammatory response and the severity of SLE hallmarks [55]. It has been further shown in a murine SLE model that following treatment with CTLA4-Ig (Abatacept), a recombinant fusion protein that contains the Fc fragment of human IgG1 and binds either to CD80 or CD86 with a much higher avidity than CD28, that there is a reduction in both numbers of autoreactive B cells and autoantibodies [56]. CTLA4-Ig has been shown in

clinical studies to dampen the interaction between T and B lymphocytes, resulting in the attenuation of autoimmune-driven inflammation [57]. Accordingly, CD80 mRNA downregulation observed here in spleens at wk 16 and kidneys at wk 16 and wk 34 of DFO-fed mice compared to CRN- and HOS-fed mice is of profound significance, because it implies that DHA inhibits the capacity of antigen-presenting cells to stimulate T cells and evoke both humoral and cell-mediated autoimmune sequelae. These findings are consistent with decreased CD80 and CD86 expression in peripheral blood mononuclear cells found previously in fish oil-fed NZBWF1 mice [58]. While the observation that DFO treatment also suppressed upregulation of CTLA-4 mRNA expression in spleen and kidney appears to be counterintuitive to this notion, these findings might rather reflect generalized downregulation of T cell activation, with tolerance-inducing late-stage CTLA-4 upregulation being particularly vulnerable to the immunosuppressive effects of DHA.

IL-10 is produced by many types of leukocytes including regulatory T cells, macrophages, dendritic cells and B cells [59]. This protein suppresses the capacity of macrophages and dendritic cells to present antigen and stimulate T cells, thereby limiting and controlling subsequent T cell responses [60]. In B cells, IL-10 acts as a potent growth factor that induces class switching and differentiation into Ig-secreting plasma cells [61]. SCID mice injected with PBMCs from human lupus patients produced less IgG when treated with anti-IL-10 antibodies [62] and similarly-

OPN

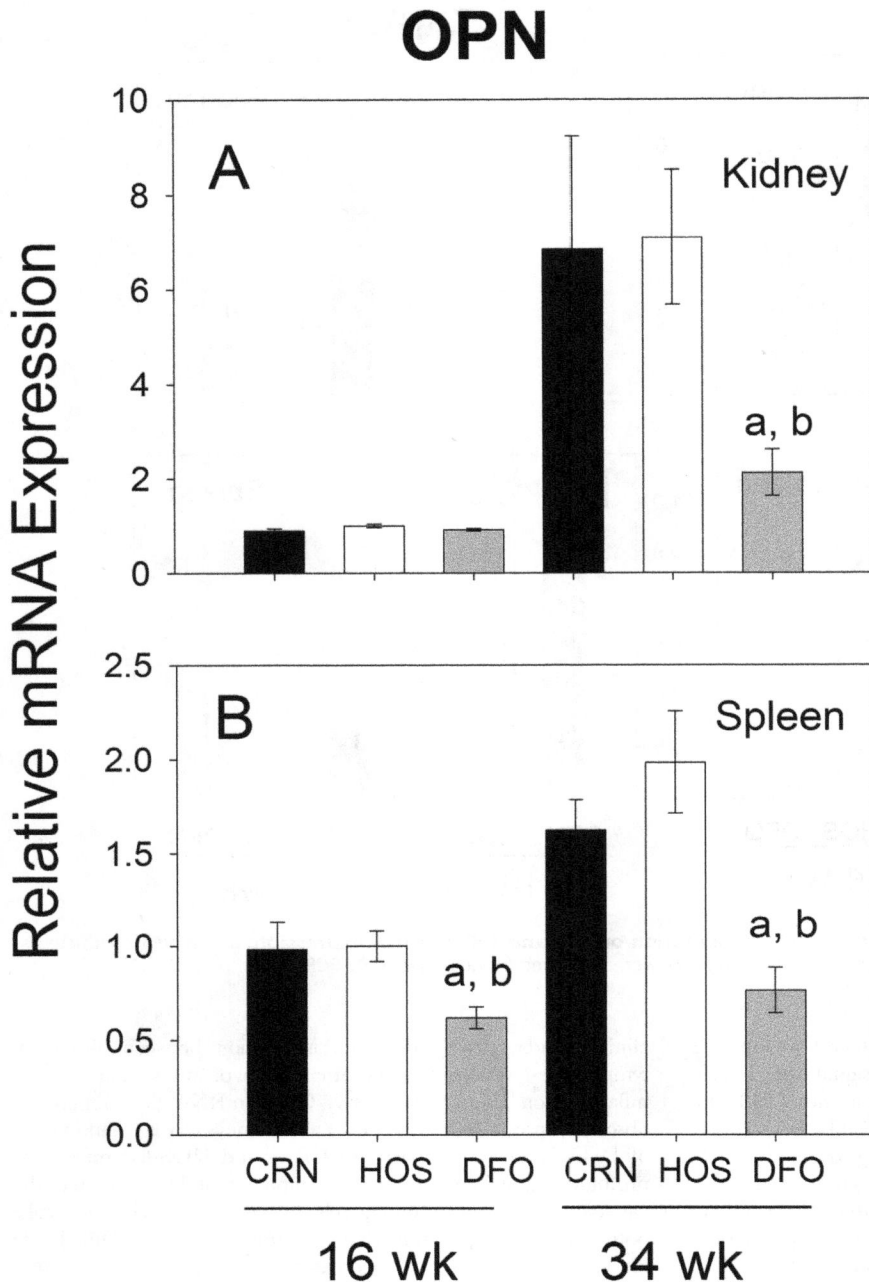

Figure 11. Differential effects of n-3, n-6 and n-9 PUFA consumption on OPN mRNA expression. Experiment conducted as described in Fig. 7 legend except that OPN mRNAs were measured by quantitative RT-PCR.

treated mice showed less renal impairment after IL-10 blockade [63]. The finding that IL-10 is present in higher concentrations in lupus patients than controls, and is elevated in SLE patients with active disease compared to inactive, further supports the notion that IL-10 contributes to lupus pathogenesis [64]. One clinical trial of IL-10 blocking antibodies as a therapy for lupus has been reported that suggests there were benefits from this approach [65]. Accordingly, reduced IL-10 expression in kidneys and spleens of mice fed DFO could be another contributing factor to the reduced autoantibody production and nephritis observed in that treatment group.

IL-18, a proinflammatory cytokine produced by dendritic cells and macrophages, exerts pleiotropic effects on T cells, dendritic cells and natural killer cells [66] [67]. IL-18 contributes to the onset and severity of lupus indicating a critical pathogenic role of this cytokine [68,69]. Decreased IL-18 gene expression observed here at wk 34 in kidneys of DFO-fed mice as compared to HOS- or CRN-fed mice therefore might be a factor in reduced lupus manifestations. Relatedly, the Fernandes group found that NZBWF1 mice fed DHA-enriched fish oil exhibited reduced serum and kidney IL-18 responses following LPS-challenge as compared to corn oil-fed mice [70]. It is important to note that IL-18 is a potent inducer of IFN-γ which can both skew the Th response towards a Th1 pattern and promote inflammation in lupus [71]. Interestingly, we observed in the PCR array 8- to 19-fold and 2- to 3-fold decreases in IFN-γ mRNA expression in kidneys and spleens of the DFO treatment group, respectively (Table 2). In future studies, it will therefore be important to link the suppressive effects of n-3 PUFA on IL-18 to Th1 polarization and IFN-γ expression.

Chemokines produced in inflamed tissues, and corresponding chemokine receptors expressed on the surface of the leukocytes, are essential for leukocyte infiltration at sites of inflammation. A number of chemokine genes (CCL5, CCL7, CCL11) were downregulated in DFO-fed mice. CCL5, also known as RANTES (regulated on activation, normal T cell expressed and secreted), is a C–C chemokine that plays a role in regulating Th-cell cytokine production and leukocyte trafficking. CCL5 is expressed by renal epithelial and mesangial cells, activated T cells, airway epithelial cells, fibroblasts, platelets and lymphocytes [72]. Importantly, CCL5 induces both leukocyte migration and activation and mediates the recruitment of lymphoid cells such as CD4+ and CD8+ T cells and monocytes to sites of inflammation [73]. *In vitro* studies have confirmed CCL5 produced by cytokine-activated proximal tubular epithelial cells in kidney promote selective recruitment of activated T cells via receptors on these cells specific for CCL5 [74]. Plasma CCL5 concentrations are significantly elevated in SLE patients when compared with normal controls and correlate with autoantibody levels, indicating that this chemokine might be involved in SLE pathogenesis [75]. Thus, decreased expression of CCL5 is likely to contribute to attenuated autoimmune and nephritic responses observed in n-3 PUFA-fed mice.

Expression of several chemokine receptors (CXCR3, CCR2, CCR3, CCR4, CCR5, CCR10) was depressed in the kidneys and/or spleens of the DFO treatment group. CXCR3 is a G protein–coupled receptor superfamily member that is expressed on activated T cells [76]. Natural ligands to CXCR3 are CXCL9, CXCL10, and CXCL11. Both the receptor and its ligands are considered potential therapeutic targets for treatment of lupus nephritis. CXCR3 deficiency ameliorates T cell infiltration and nephritic damage in the MRL/lpr model of SLE [77]. Similarly, lack of CXCR3 also reduces renal T cell infiltrates and nephritis after induction of nephrotoxic serum nephritis in non-autoimmune C57BL/6 mice [78,79]. It is further notable that plasma cells expressing CXCR3 also localize into inflamed kidneys of lupus mice [80].

In human patients with lupus nephritis, CXCR3 is similarly expressed on subpopulations of activated T cells and plasma cells [81,82] as well as in a large proportion of CD4+ T cells that infiltrate the kidney [83]. Both systemic and kidney levels of CXCR3's cognate ligands are elevated in SLE patients, all of which correlate with disease activity [84,85]. CXCR3+CD4+ T cells are significantly elevated in the urine of lupus patients with active nephritis flares and are a useful biomarker for renal disease activity [83]. CXCR3 is also expressed on subpopulations of memory B cells and plasma cells from lupus patients and it has been demonstrated that plasma cell precursors migrate toward gradients of CXCR3 ligands [86]. Taken together, reduced expression of CXCR3 in kidneys and spleens of DFO-fed NZBWF1 mice observed here might reflect decreased populations of activated T and/or B cells that mediate autoimmune sequelae and nephritis observed in this model.

IL-6, one of the initial cytokines investigated in SLE pathogenesis, is produced by the monocytes, fibroblasts and endothelial cells as well as by T and B cells [67]. n-3 PUFA consumption has recently been shown in NZBWF1 mice to decrease both kidney

IL-6 mRNA expression and ex vivo IL-6 secretion by LPS-induced splenocytes [87]. IL-6 induces 1) CD4 + T cell differentiation, 2) B cell maturation into plasma cells, 3) antibody secretion, 4) production of acute phase proteins and 5) promotion of macrophage and osteoclast differentiation [88]. Studies in lupus-prone mice support an important role for IL-6 in evoking autoimmune sequelae [89]. IL-6 is found at increased levels in SLE patients [90], and furthermore, IL-6 and its receptors can serve as biomarkers to monitor disease activity and treatment response [91,92]. IL-6 blockade significantly abrogates spontaneous immunoglobulin secretion by B cells isolated from SLE patients, which is restorable with exogenous IL-6 [90]. An anti-IL-6 receptor antibody, Tocilizumab, approved for use in rheumatoid arthritis, shows promise in treating lupus, with effects that seemed directed at autoantibody production [93]. Therefore, decreased IL-6 expression in kidneys of DFO-fed mice might further contribute to the decreased autoimmune and nephritic responses observed here.

TNF-α is expressed after the activation of macrophages and dendritic cells and can promote expression of many genes related to inflammation. TNF-α concentrations are elevated in both sera and renal tissue of lupus-prone mice and SLE patients alike and its levels correlate with disease activity and glomerulonephritis [94,95]. Accordingly, decreased TNF-α expression in kidney and spleens of mice fed DFO might also be important in the downregulation of autoimmune sequelae.

This is the first report of decreased OPN expression in a model of SLE following n-3 PUFA supplementation. OPN, also known as secreted phosphoprotein 1 (SPP1), is a pluripotent cytokine that is secreted by dendritic cells, macrophages, T cells, and B cells [96,97]. OPN can be induced by several inflammatory cytokines including IL-1β, TNF-α and IFN-γ [98]. Because OPN enhances macrophage migration, survival and cytokine production, it plays an important role in chronic inflammation [99,100] and pathogenesis of autoimmunity [101]. OPN contributes to activation of dendritic cells, enhancement of Th1 and inhibition of Th2 cytokine expression [102]. Importantly, OPN is also a polyclonal B cell activator [103,104]. In murine lupus nephritis, a specialized subset of macrophages known as alternatively activated macrophages, which participate in tissue repair, express OPN and mediate aggressive proliferative lesions with enhanced crescent formations [105]. OPN deficiency in autoimmune models causes delayed onset of polyclonal B cell activation [100,106]. Anti-dsDNA antibodies arise spontaneously in mice that overexpress OPN and have no other genetic abnormalities contributing to autoimmune disease phenotype [103]. In further support of the role of OPN in lupus nephritis, humans with SLE and autoimmune-prone mice have increased OPN systemically and in tissue lesions that correlate with disease activity [107,108]. Elevation of OPN in human SLE precedes increased cumulative disease activity and organ damage [101]. Accordingly, OPN is an important factor in lupus, making its downregulation in DFO-fed mice a highly relevant finding.

The n-3 PUFA (DHA+EPA) concentration used here, 35.4 g/kg, was selected because this approximate level has been previously demonstrated to be efficacious by our laboratory for ameliorating both deoxynivalenol-induced IgA nephropathy and ex vivo IL-6 expression [43,109,110]. We have shown that consumption of this dietary n-3 PUFA level by mice for 2 wk was sufficient to increase splenic n-3 PUFA content by 6-fold (from 2.7 to 16.3%) and reduce n-6 PUFA content by 2-fold (from 21.9 to 11.5%) compared to HOS-fed mice [111]. Further changes in the n-3 PUFA content of splenocytes were not observed after 4 or 6 wk of feeding. Relatedly, Halade and coworkers [112] used the same commercial source of DHA-enriched fish oil as here to prepare a diet containing an approximate n-3 PUFA concentration of 58.5 g/kg that effectively inhibited autoimmune nephritis in the NZBWF1 mouse.

Typical n-3 PUFA intake recommendations for healthy people range from 0.5 to 2 g/d, but higher levels of consumption ranging from 3 to 20 g/d have been used in clinical trials for SLE therapy [26,27,113]. The combined DHA and EPA concentration in the DFO diet employed in the present study would account for 8.2% of total energy intake. Upon extrapolation, a human consuming 2000 kcal/d (8.368 MJ/d) would require 18 g/d to correlate with the amount consumed in this experiment. Thus, while these concentrations exceed normal human diet recommendations in terms of energy percentage in the diet, they are consistent with high-end therapeutic use of (n-3) PUFAs. It will be nevertheless be desirable in future studies to determine the dose response effects of DFO on autoimmune nephritis and expression of the genes identified here.

Conclusion

We have demonstrated in the NZBWF1 preclinical SLE mouse model that consumption of n-3 PUFA-enriched diet effectively blunted the marked autoantibody and nephritic responses that were observed in mice consuming either an n-6 PUFA-enriched Western-style or an n-9 MUFA-enriched Mediterranean-style diets. Remarkably, these attenuating effects co-occurred with generalized downregulation of CD4$^+$ T cell-associated genes in the kidney and, to a lesser extent, in spleen that are associated with antigen presentation, T cell activation, leukocyte recruitment, B cell activation/differentiation and inflammatory responses. Many of these genes are under consideration as potential targets for development of expensive biological therapeutics for human SLE

including monoclonal antibodies and receptor antagonists. Supplementation with n-3 PUFAs might be a lower cost alternative that could impact many of these therapeutic targets simultaneously. A major concern with this strategy would be whether doses needed to suppress autoimmunity and inflammation will adversely impact health by interfering with innate and adaptive immune responses to pathogens or neoplastic events [114]. Accordingly, further clarification is needed on the underlying mechanisms and dose-response effects of n-3 PUFAs on expression of genes associated with prevention and intervention of SLE in the NZBWF1 mouse and other autoimmune models.

Supporting Information

Figure S1 Comparative effects of n-3 PUFA consumption on CD4$^+$ T cell-related gene expression in kidneys and spleens of 16 wk old NZBWF1/J mice. Cohorts of mice were fed CRN, HOS, or DFO diets for 30 wk beginning at 4 wk. At wk 34, mice were euthanized and mRNA isolated from kidneys. Extracted mRNA were pooled and analyzed using a SABioscience Mouse Th1-Th2-Th3 PCR Array. Points outside of solid line are >1.5-fold difference.

Table S1 Differential effects of consuming n-3, n-6 and n-9 PUFAs on expression of CD4+ T cell-related genes in kidneys and spleens of 16 wk old female NZBWF1 mice.

Author Contributions

Conceived and designed the experiments: JJP LLV IL. Performed the experiments: LLV KH IL. Analyzed the data: JJP LLV KH IL. Contributed to the writing of the manuscript: JJP LLV KH IL MB.

References

1. Furst DE, Clarke AE, Fernandes AW, Bancroft T, Greth W, et al. (2013) Incidence and prevalence of adult systemic lupus erythematosus in a large US managed-care population. Lupus 22: 99–105.

2. Muñoz LE, Janko C, Schulze C, Schorn C, Sarter K, et al. (2010) Autoimmunity and chronic inflammation - Two clearance-related steps in the etiopathogenesis of SLE. Autoimmun Rev 10: 38–42.

3. D'Agati VDAGB, Wallace DJHBH (2007) Lupus nephritis: Pathology and pathogenesis. Dubois' Lupus Erythematosus. Philadelphia: Lippincott Williams & Wilkins. pp. 1094–1110.

4. Okamoto A, Fujio K, Tsuno NH, Takahashi K, Yamamoto K (2012) Kidney-infiltrating CD4+ T-cell clones promote nephritis in lupus-prone mice. Kidney Int 82: 969–979.

5. Enghard P, Rieder C, Kopetschke K, Klocke JR, Undeutsch R, et al. (2014) Urinary CD4 T cells identify SLE patients with proliferative lupus nephritis and can be used to monitor treatment response. Ann Rheum Dis 73: 277–283.

6. Borchers AT, Leibushor N, Naguwa SM, Cheema GS, Shoenfeld Y, et al. (2012) Lupus nephritis: a critical review. Autoimmun Rev 12: 174–194.

7. Haija AJ, Schulz SW (2011) The role and effect of complementary and alternative medicine in systemic lupus erythematosus. Rheum Dis Clin N Amer 37: 47–62.

8. Greco CM, Nakajima C, Manzi S (2013) Updated review of complementary and alternative medicine treatments for systemic lupus erythematosus. Current Rheumatol Rep 15: 378.

9. Pestka JJ (2010) n-3 Polyunsaturated fatty acids and autoimmune-mediated glomerulonephritis. Prost Leukotriene Essent Fatty Acids 82: 251–258.

10. Calder PC (2010) The 2008 ESPEN Sir David Cuthbertson Lecture: Fatty acids and inflammation–from the membrane to the nucleus and from the laboratory bench to the clinic. Clin Nutr 29: 5–12.

11. Barnes PM, Bloom B, Nahin RL (2008) Complementary and alternative medicine use among adults and children: United States, 2007. Nat Health Stat Rep: 1–23.

12. Sang A, Yin Y, Zheng YY, Morel L (2012) Animal models of molecular pathology systemic lupus erythematosus. Prog Mol Biol Transl Sci 105: 321–370.

13. Prickett JD, Robinson DR, Steinberg AD (1983) Effects of dietary enrichment with eicosapentaenoic acid upon autoimmune nephritis in female NZB X NZW/F1 mice. Arthritis Rheum 26: 133–139.

14. Robinson DR, Prickett JD, Makoul GT, Steinberg AD, Colvin RB (1986) Dietary fish oil reduces progression of established renal disease in (NZB x NZW)F1 mice and delays renal disease in BXSB and MRL/1 strains. Arthritis Rheum 29: 539–546.

15. Robinson DR, Prickett JD, Polisson R, Steinberg AD, Levine L (1985) The protective effect of dietary fish oil on murine lupus. Prostaglandins 30: 51–75.

16. Bhattacharya A, Lawrence RA, Krishnan A, Zaman K, Sun D, et al. (2003) Effect of dietary n-3 and n-6 oils with and without food restriction on activity of antioxidant enzymes and lipid peroxidation in livers of cyclophosphamide treated autoimmune-prone NZB/W female mice. J Am Coll Nutr 22: 388–399.

17. Chandrasekar B, Fernandes G (1994) Decreased pro-inflammatory cytokines and increased antioxidant enzyme gene expression by omega-3 lipids in murine lupus nephritis. Biochem Biophys Res Commun 200: 893–898.

18. Chandrasekar B, Troyer DA, Venkatraman JT, Fernandes G (1995) Dietary omega-3 lipids delay the onset and progression of autoimmune lupus nephritis by inhibiting transforming growth factor beta mRNA and protein expression. J, Autoimmun 8: 381–393.

19. Chandrasekar B, Troyer DA, Venkatraman JT, Fernandes G (1996) Tissue specific regulation of transforming growth factor beta by omega-3 lipid-rich krill oil in autoimmune murine lupus. Nutr Res 16: 489–503.

20. Kim YJ, Kim FJ, No JK, Chung HY, Fernandes G (2006) Anti-inflammatory action of dietary fish oil and calorie restriction. Life Sci 78: 2523–2532.

21. Westberg G, Tarkowski A, Svalander C (1989) Effect of eicosapentaenoic acid rich menhaden oil and MAXEPA on the autoimmune-disease of MRL/L mice Int Arch Allergy Appl Immunol 88: 454–461.

22. Theofilopoulos AN, Dixon FJ (1985) Murine models of systemic lupus erythematosus. Adv Immunol 37: 269–390.

23. Venkatraman JT, Chu WC (1999) Effects of dietary omega-3 and omega-6 lipids and vitamin E on serum cytokines, lipid mediators and anti-DNA antibodies in a mouse model for rheumatoid arthritis. J Am Coll Nutr 18: 602–613.

24. Kelley VE, Ferretti A, Izui S, Strom TB (1985) A fish oil diet rich in eicosapentaenoic acid reduces cyclooxygenase metabolites, and suppresses lupus in MRL-lpr mice. J Immunol 134: 1914–1919.

25. Spurney RF, Ruiz P, Albrightson CR, Pisetsky DS, Coffman TM (1994) Fish oil feeding modulates leukotriene production in murine lupus nephritis. Prostaglandins 48: 331–348.

26. Walton AJE, Snaith ML, Locniskar M, Cumberland AG, Morrow WJW, et al. (1991) Dietary fish oil and the severity of symptoms in patients with systemic lupus-erythematosus.

27. Wright SA, O'Prey FM, McHenry MT, Leahey WJ, Devine AB, et al. (2008) A randomised interventional trial of omega-3-polyunsaturated fatty acids on endothelial function and disease activity in systemic lupus erythematosus. Ann Rheum Dis 67: 841–848.

28. Westberg G, Tarkowski A (1990) Effect of MAXEPA in patients with SLE - a double-blind, crossover study. Scand J Rheumatol 19: 137–143.

29. Clark WF, Parbtani A, Philbrick DJ, Spanner E, Huff MW, et al. (1993) Dietary protein restriction versus fish oil supplementation in the chronic remnant nephron model. Clin Nephrol 39: 295–304.

30. Reeves PG, Nielsen FH, Fahey GC Jr (1993) AIN-93 purified diets for laboratory rodents: final report of the American Institute of Nutrition ad hoc writing committee on the reformulation of the AIN-76A rodent diet. J Nutr 123: 1939–1951.

31. Kurien BT, Scofield RH (1999) Mouse urine collection using clear plastic wrap. Lab Anim 33: 83–86.

32. Hem A, Smith AJ, Solberg P (1998) Saphenous vein puncture for blood sampling of the mouse, rat, hamster, gerbil, guinea pig, ferret and mink. Lab Anim 32: 364–368.

33. Weening JJ, D'Agati VD, Schwartz MM, Seshan SV, Alpers CE, et al. (2004) The classification of glomerulonephritis in systemic lupus erythematosus revisited. Kidney Int 65: 521–530.

34. Schmittgen TD, Livak KJ (2008) Analyzing real-time PCR data by the comparative C-T method. Nature Protocols 3: 1101–1108.

35. Starke C, Frey S, Wellmann U, Urbonaviciute V, Herrmann M, et al. (2011) High frequency of autoantibody-secreting cells and long-lived plasma cells within inflamed kidneys of NZB/W F1 lupus mice. Eur J Immunol 41: 2107–2112.

36. Hiepe F, Doerner T, Hauser AE, Hoyer BF, Mei H, et al. (2011) Long-lived autoreactive plasma cells drive persistent autoimmune inflammation. Nat Rev Rheumatol 7: 170–178.

37. Sales-Campos H, Souza PR, Peghini BC, da Silva JS, Cardoso CR (2013) An overview of the modulatory effects of oleic acid in health and disease. Mini Rev Med Chem 13: 201–210.

38. Yang R, Chiang N, Oh SF, Serhan CN (2011) Metabolomics-lipidomics of eicosanoids and docosanoids generated by phagocytes. Current protocols in immunology/edited by John E Coligan [et al] Chapter 14: Unit 14 26.

39. Villalta D, Bizzaro N, Bassi N, Zen M, Gatto M, et al. (2013) Anti-dsDNA antibody isotypes in systemic lupus erythematosus: IgA in addition to IgG anti-dsDNA help to identify glomerulonephritis and active disease. PLoS ONE 8.

40. Turk HF, Chapkin RS (2013) Membrane lipid raft organization is uniquely modified by n-3 polyunsaturated fatty acids. Prost Leuk Essent Fat Acids 88: 43–47.

41. Shaikh SR, Jolly CA, Chapkin RS (2012) n-3 Polyunsaturated fatty acids exert immunomodulatory effects on lymphocytes by targeting plasma membrane molecular organization. Mol Aspects Med 33: 46–54.

42. Lee JY, Plakidas A, Lee WH, Heikkinen A, Chanmugam P, et al. (2003) Differential modulation of Toll-like receptors by fatty acids: preferential inhibition by n-3 polyunsaturated fatty acids. J Lipid Res 44: 479–486.

43. Jia Q, Zhou HR, Shi Y, Pestka JJ (2006) Docosahexaenoic acid consumption inhibits deoxynivalenol-induced CREB/ATF1 activation and IL-6 gene transcription in mouse macrophages. J Nutr 136: 366–372.

44. Jump DB (2004) Fatty acid regulation of gene transcription. Crit Rev Clin Lab Sci 41: 41–78.

45. Shi Y, Pestka JJ (2009) Mechanisms for suppression of interleukin-6 expression in peritoneal macrophages from docosahexaenoic acid-fed mice. J Nutr Biochem 20: 358–368.

46. Kim HFS, Weeber EJ, Sweatt JD, Stoll AL, Marangell LB (2001) Inhibitory effects of omega-3 fatty acids on protein kinase C activity in vitro. Mol Psych 6: 246–248.

47. Mirnikjoo B, Brown SE, Kim HF, Marangell LB, Sweatt JD, et al. (2001) Protein kinase inhibition by omega-3 fatty acids. J Biol Chem 276: 10888–10896.

48. Kalupahana NS, Claycombe KJ, Moustaid-Moussa N (2011) (n-3) Fatty acids alleviate adipose tissue inflammation and insulin resistance: Mechanistic insights. Advances in Nutrition: An International Review Journal 2: 304–316.

49. Ryan MJ, McLemore GR Jr, Hendrix ST (2006) Insulin resistance and obesity in a mouse model of systemic lupus erythematosus. Hypertension 48: 988–993.

50. Gabriel CL, Smith PB, Mendez-Fernandez YV, Wilhelm AJ, Ye AM, et al. (2012) Autoimmune-mediated glucose intolerance in a mouse model of systemic lupus erythematosus. Lipids. pp. E1313–E1324.

51. Bargut TC, Frantz ED, Mandarim-de-Lacerda CA, Aguila MB (2014) Effects of a Diet Rich in n-3 Polyunsaturated Fatty Acids on Hepatic Lipogenesis and Beta-Oxidation in Mice. Lipids 49: 431–444.

52. Pollard KM, Arnush M, Hultman P, Kono DH (2004) Costimulation requirements of induced murine systemic autoimmune disease. J Immunol 173: 5880–5887.

53. Rudd CE, Taylor A, Schneider H (2009) CD28 and CTLA-4 coreceptor expression and signal transduction. Immunol Rev 229: 12–26.

54. Fu SM, Deshmukh US, Gaskin F (2011) Pathogenesis of systemic lupus erythematosus revisited 2011: End organ resistance to damage, autoantibody initiation and diversification, and HLA-DR. J Autoimmun 37: 104–112.

55. Shi Q, Gao ZY, Xie F, Wang LF, Gu YP, et al. (2011) A novel monoclonal antibody against human CD80 and its immune protection in a mouse lupus-like disease. Int J Immunopathol Pharmacol 24: 583–593.

56. Mihara M, Tan I, Chuzhin Y, Reddy B, Budhai L, et al. (2000) CTLA4Ig inhibits T cell-dependent B-cell maturation in murine systemic lupus erythematosus. J Clin Invest 106: 91–101.

57. Davidson A, Diamond B, Wofsy D, Daikh D (2005) Block and tackle: CTLA4Ig takes on lupus. Lupus 14: 197–203.

58. Muthukumar A, Sun D, Zaman K, Barnes JL, Haile D, et al. (2004) Age associated alterations in costimulatory and adhesion molecule expression in lupus-prone mice are attenuated by food restriction with n-6 and n-3 fatty acids. J Clin Immunol 24: 471–480.

59. Saraiva M, O'Garra A (2010) The regulation of IL-10 production by immune cells. Nat Rev Immunol 10: 170–181.

60. Moore KW, Ogarra A, Malefyt RD, Vieira P, Mosmann TR (1993) Interleukin-10. Ann Rev Immunol 11: 165–190.

61. Rousset F, Peyrol S, Garcia E, Vezzio N, Andujar M, et al. (1995) Long-term cultured CD40-activated B-lymphocytes differentiate into plasma-cells in response to IL-10 but not IL-4. Int Immunol 7: 1243–1253.

62. Blenman KRM, Duan B, Xu ZW, Wan SG, Atkinson MA, et al. (2006) IL-10 regulation of lupus in the NZM2410 murine model. Lab Invest 86: 1136–1148.

63. Ravirajan CT, Wang Y, Matis LA, Papadaki L, Griffiths MH, et al. (2004) Effect of neutralizing antibodies to IL-10 and C5 on the renal damage caused by a pathogenic human anti-dsDNA antibody. Rheumatol 43: 442–447.

64. Koenig KF, Groeschl I, Pesickova SS, Tesar V, Eisenberger U, et al. (2012) Serum cytokine profile in patients with active lupus nephritis. Cytokine 60: 410–416.

65. Llorente L, Richaud-Patin Y, Garcia-Padilla C, Claret E, Jakez-Ocampo J, et al. (2000) Clinical and biologic effects of anti-interleukin-10 monoclonal antibody administration in systemic lupus erythematosus. Arthritis Rheum 43: 1790–1800.

66. Clark DN, Markham JL, Sloan CS, Poole BD (2013) Cytokine inhibition as a strategy for treating systemic lupus erythematosus. Clin Immunol 148: 335–343.

67. Yap DY, Lai KN (2013) The role of cytokines in the pathogenesis of systemic lupus erythematosus - from bench to bedside. Nephrol 18: 243–255.

68. Favilli F, Anzilotti C, Martinelli L, Quattroni P, De Martino S, et al. (2009) IL-18 activity in systemic lupus erythematosus. In: Shoenfeld Y, Gershwin ME, editors. Contemporary Challenges in Autoimmunity. pp. 301–309.

69. Shimizu C, Fujita T, Fuke Y, Ito K, Satomura A, et al. (2012) High circulating levels of interleukin-18 binding protein indicate the severity of glomerular involvement in systemic lupus erythematosus. Mod Rheumatol 22: 73–79.

70. Halade GV, Rahman MM, Bhattacharya A, Barnes JL, Chandrasekar B, et al. (2010) Docosahexaenoic acid-enriched fish oil attenuates kidney disease and prolongs median and maximal life span of autoimmune lupus-prone mice. J Immunol 184: 5280–5286.

71. Calvani N, Richards HB, Tucci M, Pannarale G, Silvestris F (2004) Up-regulation of IL-18 and predominance of a Th1 immune response is a hallmark of lupus nephritis. Clin Exp Immunol 138: 171–178.

72. Ye DQ, Yang SG, Li XP, Hu YS, Yin J, et al. (2006) Polymorphisms in the promoter region of RANTES in Han Chinese and their relationship with systemic lupus erythematosus. Arch Dermatol Res 297: 108–113.

73. Lima G, Soto-Vega E, Atisha-Fregoso Y, Sanchez-Guerrero J, Vallejo M, et al. (2007) MCP-1, RANTES, and SDF-1 polymorphisms in Mexican patients with systemic lupus erythematosus. Hum Immunol 68: 980–985.

74. Cockwell P, Calderwood JW, Brooks CJ, Chakravorty SJ, Savage COS (2002) Chemoattraction of T cells expressing CCR5, CXCR3 and CX3CR1 by proximal tubular epithelial cell chemokines. Nephrol Dialysis Transplant 17: 734–744.

75. Lu MM, Wang J, Pan HF, Chen GM, Li J, et al. (2012) Increased serum RANTES in patients with systemic lupus erythematosus. Rheumatol Int 32: 1231–1233.

76. Loetscher M, Gerber B, Loetscher P, Jones SA, Piali L, et al. (1996) Chemokine receptor specific for IP10 and Mig: Structure, function, and expression in activated T-lymphocytes. J Exp Med 184: 963–969.

77. Steinmetz OM, Turner JE, Paust HJ, Lindner M, Peters A, et al. (2009) CXCR3 mediates renal Th1 and Th17 immune response in murine lupus nephritis. J Immunol 183: 4693–4704.

78. Menke J, Zeller GC, Kikawada E, Means TK, Huang XR, et al. (2008) CXCL9, but not CXCL10, promotes CXCR3-dependent immune-mediated kidney disease. J Am Soc Nephrol 19: 1177–1189.

79. Panzer U, Steinmetz OM, Paust H-J, Meyer-Schwesinger C, Peters A, et al. (2007) Chemokine receptor CXCR3 mediates T cell recruitment and tissue injury in nephrotoxic nephritis in mice. J Amer Soc Nephrol 18: 2071–2084.

80. Lacotte S, Decossas M, Le Coz C, Brun S, Muller S, et al. (2013) Early differentiated CD138(high) MHCII(+) IgG(+) pasma cells express CXCR3 and localize into inflamed kidneys of lupus mice. PLoS ONE 8.

81. Amoura Z, Combadiere C, Faure S, Parizot C, Miyara M, et al. (2003) Roles of CCR2 and CXCR3 in the T cell-mediated response occurring during lupus flares. Arthritis Rheum 48: 3487–3496.

82. Nicholas MW, Dooley MA, Hogan SL, Anolik J, Looney J, et al. (2008) A novel subset of memory B cells is enriched in autoreactivity and correlates with adverse outcomes in SLE. Clin Immunol 126: 189–201.

83. Enghard P, Humrich JY, Rudolph B, Rosenberger S, Biesen R, et al. (2009) CXCR3+CD4+ T cells are enriched in inflamed kidneys and urine and provide a new biomarker for acute nephritis flares in systemic lupus erythematosus patients. Arthritis Rheum 60: 199–206.

84. Segerer S, Banas B, Wornle M, Schmid H, Cohen CD, et al. (2004) CXCR3 is involved in tubulointerstitial injury in human glomerulonephritis. AmJ Pathol 164: 635–649.

85. Lit LC, Wong CK, Tam LS, Li EK, Lam CW (2006) Raised plasma concentration and ex vivo production of inflammatory chemokines in patients with systemic lupus erythematosus. Ann Rheum Dis 65: 209–215.

86. Hauser AE, Debes GF, Arce S, Cassese G, Hamann A, et al. (2002) Chemotactic responsiveness toward ligands for CXCR3 and CXCR4 is regulated on plasma blasts during the time course of a memory immune response. J Immunol 169: 1277–1282.

87. Halade GV, Williams PJ, Veigas JM, Barnes JL, Fernandes G (2013) Concentrated fish oil (Lovaza (R)) extends lifespan and attenuates kidney disease in lupus-prone short-lived (NZBxNZW)F1 mice. Exp Biol Med 238: 610–622.

88. Tackey E, Lipsky PE, Illei GG (2004) Rationale for interleukin-6 blockade in systemic lupus erythematosus. Lupus 13: 339–343.

89. Cash H, Relle M, Menke J, Brochhausen C, Jones SA, et al. (2010) Interleukin 6 (IL-6) deficiency delays lupus nephritis in MRL-Fas(lpr) mice: the IL-6 pathway as a new therapeutic target in treatment of autoimmune kidney disease in systemic lupus erythematosus. J Rheumatol 37: 60–70.

90. Linker-Israeli M, Deans RJ, Wallace DJ, Prehn J, Ozeri-Chen T, et al. (1991) Elevated levels of endogenous IL-6 in systemic lupus erythematosus. A putative role in pathogenesis. J Immunol 147: 117–123.

91. Brugos B, Vincze Z, Sipka S, Szegedi G, Zeher M (2012) Serum and urinary cytokine levels of SLE patients. Pharmazie 67: 411–413.

92. De La Torre M, Urra JM, Blanco J (2009) Raised expression of cytokine receptor gp130 subunit on peripheral lymphocytes of patients with active lupus. A useful tool for monitoring the disease activity? Lupus 18: 216–222.

93. Illei GG, Shirota Y, Yarboro CH, Daruwalla J, Tackey E, et al. (2010) Tocilizumab in systemic lupus erythematosus data on safety, preliminary efficacy, and impact on circulating plasma cells from an open-label phase I dosage-escalation study. Arthritis Rheum 62: 542–552.

94. Kontoyiannis D, Kollias G (2000) Accelerated autoimmunity and lupus nephritis in NZB mice with an engineered heterozygous deficiency in tumor necrosis factor. Eur J Immunol 30: 2038–2047.

95. Brennan DC, Yui MA, Wuthrich RP, Kelley VE (1989) Tumor necrosis factor and IL-1 in New-Zealand Black-White mice - enhanced gene-expression and acceleration of renal injury. J Immunol 143: 3470–3475.

96. Patarca R, Freeman GJ, Singh RP, Wei FY, Durfee T, et al. (1989) Structural and functional-studies of the early lymphocyte-t activation-1 (ETA-1) gene - definition of a novel t-cell-dependent response associated with genetic-resistance to bacterial-infection. JExpMed 170: 145–161.

97. Rothstein TL, Guo B (2009) Receptor crosstalk: reprogramming B cell receptor signalling to an alternate pathway results in expression and secretion of the autoimmunity-associated cytokine, osteopontin. J Intern Med 265: 632–643.

98. Ogawa D, Stone JF, Takata Y, Blaschke F, Chu VH, et al. (2005) Liver X receptor agonists inhibit cytokine-induced osteopontin expression in macro-

phages through interference with activator protein-1 signaling pathways. Circulation Res 96: 59–67.

99. Nystrom T, Duner P, Hultgardh-Nilsson A (2007) A constitutive endogenous osteopontin production is important for macrophage function and differentiation. Exp Cell Res 313: 1149–1160.

100. Weber GF, Cantor H (2001) Differential roles of osteopontin/Eta-1 in early and late lpr disease. CliniExp Immunol 126: 578–583.

101. Rullo OJ, Woo JM, Parsa MF, Hoftman AD, Maranian P, et al. (2013) Plasma levels of osteopontin identify patients at risk for organ damage in systemic lupus erythematosus. Arthritis Res Ther 15: R18.

102. Shinohara ML, Jansson M, Hwang ES, Werneck MBF, Glimcher LH, et al. (2005) T-bet-dependent expression of osteopontin contributes to T cell polarization. ProcNatAcadSci 102: 17101–17106.

103. Iizuka J, Katagiri Y, Tada N, Murakami M, Ikeda T, et al. (1998) Introduction of an osteopontin gene confers the increase in B1 cell population and the production of anti-DNA autoantibodies. LabInvest 78: 1523–1533.

104. Lampe MA, Patarca R, Iregui MV, Cantor H (1991) Polyclonal b-cell activation by the ETA-1 cytokine and the development of systemic autoimmune-disease. J Immunol 147: 2902–2906.

105. Triantafyllopoulou A, Franzke C-W, Seshan SV, Perino G, Kalliolias GD, et al. (2010) Proliferative lesions and metalloproteinase activity in murine lupus nephritis mediated by type I interferons and macrophages. ProcNatAcadSci 107: 3012–3017.

106. Yumoto K, Ishijima M, Rittling SR, Tsuji K, Tsuchiya Y, et al. (2002) Osteopontin deficiency protects joints against destruction in anti-type II collagen antibody-induced arthritis in mice. Proc Nat Acad Sci 99: 4556–4561.

107. Patarca R, Wei FY, Singh P, Morasso MI, Cantor H (1990) Dysregulated expression of theT-cell cytokine ETA-1 in CD4-8-lymphocytes during the development of murine autoimmune-disease. J Exp Med 172: 1177–1183.

108. Wong CK, Lit LCW, Tam LS, Li EK, Lam CWK (2005) Elevation of plasma osteopontin concentration is correlated with disease activity in patients with systemic lupus erythematosus. Rheumatol 44: 602–606.

109. Jia Q, Shi Y, Bennink MB, Pestka JJ (2004) Docosahexaenoic acid and eicosapentaenoic acid, but not alpha-linolenic acid, suppress deoxynivalenol-induced experimental IgA nephropathy in mice. J Nutr 134: 1353–1361.

110. Jia Q, Pestka JJ (2005) Role of cyclooxygenase-2 in deoxynivalenol-induced immunoglobulin a nephropathy. Food Chem Toxicol 43: 721–728.

111. Beli E, Li M, Cuff C, Pestka JJ (2008) Docosahexaenoic acid-enriched fish oil consumption modulates immunoglobulin responses to and clearance of enteric reovirus infection in mice. J Nutr 138: 813–819.

112. Halade GV, Rahman MM, Williams PJ, Fernandes G (2010) High fat diet-induced animal model of age-associated obesity and osteoporosis. J Nutr Biochem 21: 1162–1169.

113. Duffy EM, Meenagh GK, McMillan SA, Strain JJ, Hannigan BM, et al. (2004) The clinical effect of dietary supplementation with omega-3 fish oils and/or copper in systemic lupus erythematosus. J Rheumatol 31: 1551–1556.

114. Fenton JI, Hord NG, Ghosh S, Gurzell EA (2013) Immunomodulation by dietary long chain omega-3 fatty acids and the potential for adverse health outcomes. Prostag Leukotr Ess Fatty Acid 89: 379–390.

2

Altered Development of NKT Cells, γδ T Cells, CD8 T Cells and NK Cells in a PLZF Deficient Patient

Maggie Eidson[1,♙,¤a], **Justin Wahlstrom**[1,♙,¤b], **Aimee M. Beaulieu**[2], **Bushra Zaidi**[3], **Steven E. Carsons**[4], **Peggy K. Crow**[5,6], **Jianda Yuan**[3], **Jedd D. Wolchok**[7], **Bernhard Horsthemke**[8], **Dagmar Wieczorek**[8], **Derek B. Sant'Angelo**[2,6,9]*

1 Department of Pediatrics, Memorial Sloan-Kettering Cancer Center, New York, New York, United States of America, 2 Immunology Program, Sloan-Kettering Institute, Memorial Sloan-Kettering Cancer Center, New York, New York, United States of America, 3 Ludwig Center for Cancer Immunotherapy, Immunology Program, Memorial Sloan-Kettering Cancer Center, New York, New York, United States of America, 4 Division of Rheumatology, Allergy and Immunology, Department of Medicine, Winthrop-University Hospital, Mineola, New York, United States of America, 5 Rheumatology Division, Mary Kirkland Center for Lupus Research, Hospital for Special Surgery, New York, New York, United States of America, 6 Weill Graduate School of Medical Sciences of Cornell University, New York, New York, United States of America, 7 Department of Medicine, Memorial Sloan-Kettering Cancer Center, New York, New York, United States of America, 8 Institut fuer Humangenetik, Universitaetsklinikum Essen, Essen, Germany, 9 Gerstner Graduate School of Biomedical Sciences, Memorial Sloan-Kettering Cancer Center, New York, New York, United States of America

Abstract

In mice, the transcription factor, PLZF, controls the development of effector functions in invariant NKT cells and a subset of NKT cell-like, γδ T cells. Here, we show that in human lymphocytes, in addition to invariant NKT cells, PLZF was also expressed in a large percentage of CD8+ and CD4+ T cells. Furthermore, PLZF was also found to be expressed in all γδ T cells and in all NK cells. Importantly, we show that in a donor lacking functional PLZF, all of these various lymphocyte populations were altered. Therefore, in contrast to mice, PLZF appears to control the development and/or function of a wide variety of human lymphocytes that represent more than 10% of the total PBMCs. Interestingly, the PLZF-expressing CD8+ T cell population was found to be expanded in the peripheral blood of patients with metastatic melanoma but was greatly diminished in patients with autoimmune disease.

Editor: Lishomwa C. Ndhlovu, University of Hawaii, United States of America

Funding: This work was supported by National Institutes of Health/National Institute of Allergy and Infectious Diseases (NIH/NIAID) R01s AI059739 and AI083988 (D.B.S.) and T32 CA009149 (A.M.B.). The funders had no role in study design, data collection and analysis, decision to publish, or preparation of the manuscript.

Competing Interests: The authors have declared that no competing interests exist.

* E-mail: santangd@mskcc.org

♙ These authors contributed equally to this work.

¤a Current address: Department of Pediatric Hematology-Oncology, Miami Children's Hospital, Miami, Florida, United States of America
¤b Current address: Department of Pediatrics, University of California San Francisco, San Francisco, California, United States of America

Introduction

The promyelocytic leukemia zinc finger (PLZF, $ZBTB16$) transcriptional regulator is a member of the BTB/POZ-ZF (Broad complex, tramtrack, bric-à-brac or poxvirus and zinc finger-zinc finger; BTB-ZF) family of proteins that have a wide variety of biological activities [1]. Over the last few years, it has become apparent that BTB-ZF proteins are critical regulators of immune system development and function. For example, Bcl6 has been shown to be necessary for both the B cell germinal center reaction [2,3] as well as for the development of follicular helper T cells [4,5]. ThPok has been shown to be necessary and sufficient for CD4 T cell development [6] and the B cell versus T cell commitment step is controlled by LRF (leukemia/lymphoma related factor) [7]. Mazr influences CD8 T cell development, in part by regulating the expression of ThPok [8].

PLZF was first identified due to a t(11;17)(q23;q21) translocation that fused PLZF with RARα(retinoic acid receptor alpha) in some patients with acute promyelocytic leukemia (APL) [9]. The fusion protein that results from this translocation was subsequently shown to be an important determining factor in the development

APL and its response to therapy with retinoic acid [10]. The transcription factor has since been implicated in a wide variety of developmental processes, including axial skeletal patterning [11], CNS development [12], male spermatogenesis [13,14], and immune function [15].

Recently it was shown that PLZF is highly expressed in mouse and human invariant natural killer T (iNKT) cells [16,17]. NKT cells represent a subset of CD3+ lymphocytes that serve as a bridge between the innate and adaptive immune systems. Invariant NKT cells represent a subset that expresses a CD1d-restricted Vα24Jα18 TCR in humans [18,19]. Both variant and invariant subsets are capable of rapid and copious secretion of a wide variety of Th1 and Th2 cytokines upon initial stimulation, although evidence suggests that the specific roles of each subset may differ [20]. The invariant TCR expressed by iNKT cells recognizes lipid antigens presented in the context of the MHC class I-like molecule CD1d. Invariant NKT cells, which have been extensively studied in mice, are, comparatively, quite rare in humans. For example, in mice 30–40% of T cells in the liver are iNKT cells; in humans only ~1% of hepatic T cells are iNKT cells [21,22,23]. Only 0.008–1.1% of human peripheral blood T cells and only 0.001–0.01% of human thymocytes have been reported to be iNKT cells [24,25,26].

Our lab, and others, have shown that in mice, PLZF controls the development of essentially all of the innate-like features of NKT cells [16,17]. For example, PLZF-deficient NKT cells do not acquire the typical "activated" phenotype characterized by high expression of CD44 and CD69 [16,17]. PLZF deficient NKT cells also do not constitutively express granzyme B or the mRNA transcript for IL-4 [16] and fail to acquire the capacity to secrete multiple cytokines upon primary stimulation [16,17]. Furthermore, the frequency of NKT cells is substantially reduced in PLZF-deficient mice and the cells accumulate in the lymph nodes and spleen rather than in the thymus and liver. Overall, the phenotype of PLZF-deficient NKT cells is highly reminiscent of naïve, conventional CD4 T cells [16]. In contrast, ectopic expression of PLZF in conventional T cells results in the acquisition of innate T cell-like characteristics such as an activated phenotype, the rapid secretion of Th1 and Th2 cytokines in response to an initial stimulus and homing to non-lymphoid tissues [17,27,28].

Recent studies have shown that PLZF expression is not strictly limited to invariant NKT cells in mice, but can also be found in a specific subset of γδ T cells that express a Vγ1.1Vδ6.3 TCR [29,30,31]. This subset of "NKT" γδ T cells functionally resemble invariant NKT cells in that they co-secrete both IFN-γ and IL-4 upon primary activation. Importantly, PLZF has been shown to be required for the innate T cell-like characteristics of NKT γδ T cells [29]. These studies, together with the findings in NKT cells, highlight an essential and non-redundant role for PLZF in the development of innate T cell effector functions.

In addition to directly controlling the function of the cells it is expressed within, PLZF impacts immune function in trans. Of great interest, studies show that the IL-4 produced by these PLZF-expressing cells profoundly alters the CD8 T cell compartment [32,33]. In mice with an expanded PLZF-expressing T cell compartment, CD8 T cells were found to take on an innate-like phenotype, represented by increased expression of CD44, Eomes and an enhanced capacity to secrete IFN-γ. Such mice also harbor increased numbers of germinal center B cells and high serum levels of IgE, in concordance with their heightened Th2 responses [31]. These data show that innate-like T cells, such as NKT cells, have a broad impact on the immune response.

The role of NKT cells in disease is complex and appears to be dependent on both the NKT cell subtype and the microenvironmental context. In mice, NKT cells have been shown to be important in the suppression of solid tumors as a consequence of interactions with dendritic cells and other lymphocytes [34,35,36,37,38,39,40]. In contrast, the immunomodulatory activity of NKT cells can also influence the immune response against autoantigens. For example, autoimmunity in the Type 1 diabetes-susceptible NOD mouse appears to be exacerbated by a deficiency of invariant NKT cells since it is alleviated by NKT activation [41]. In humans with autoimmune diseases, including systemic lupus erythematosus (SLE) [42], diabetes mellitus, and rheumatoid arthritis, decreases in circulating NKTs have, in some studies, been shown to correlate with the frequency of disease [43].

Spurred by recent reports of a broader expression pattern of, and functional relevance for, PLZF in mouse lymphocytes, we examined the full breadth of PLZF expression in human T cells. Furthermore, analysis of the only known person to harbor a biallelic loss of PLZF enabled us, for the first time, to examine the role of this transcription factor in the development of human T cells. We found that in addition to iNKT cells, nearly all γδ T cells and natural killer (NK cells) expressed PLZF. Furthermore, more than 5% of CD8$^+$ T cells and ~2% of CD4$^+$ T cells were found to express the transcription factor. Therefore, in total, more than 10% of human PBLs express PLZF. Finally, to study the importance of PLZF for the development of these various cell types, we obtained peripheral blood samples from the only person known to harbor a biallelic loss of functional PLZF [44]. Overall, our data suggest that differences in PLZF expression represent a significant divergence between the mouse and human immune system.

Materials and Methods

Blood Draw

Blood draw protocols and ethics were reviewed and approved by the Internal Review Board's (IRB) at Memorial Sloan-Kettering Cancer Center (New York, NY), the Hospital for Special Surgery (New York, NY), the Winthrop-University Hospital (Mineola, NY) and Universitaetsklinikum Essen (Essen, Germany). Written informed consent forms were obtained from all donors.

Flow Cytometry

Anti-CD3-Pacific Blue-CD4-PerCPCy5.5, -CD8-AlexaFluor700, CD56-PECy7, -CD161-APC, -γδTCR-PE, -Vα24-Jα18-PE, and −CD4-AlexaFluor488, were obtained from BD, eBioscience or BioLegend. Mags.21F7 (anti-PLZF) was described [16]. Dead cells were excluded by DAPI when possible and doublets were excluded. Cell sorts were done by MSKCC's Flow Cytometry Core Facility. Post-sort analysis confirmed cell purity >95%.

Cytokine Expression

T cells were plated in X-vivo media with PMA (100 ng/ml) and ionomycin (500 ng/ml) or beads coated with anti-CD3/CD28 (Miltenyi Biotec). Brefeldin A was added for the last five hours of a 6 hour culture. Cells were stained for surface markers, fixed, made permeable and stained with anti-IFNγ AlexaFluor 488 (BD). NK cells were activated with beads coated with anti-NKp46 and anti-CD2 (Miltenyi Biotec). Cytokines were analyzed with cytokine bead arrays (BD).

Patient Samples

Patients with an established diagnosis of systemic lupus erythematosus (SLE, n = 6), primary Sjögren's syndrome (n = 3), or metastatic melanoma (n = 10) and healthy controls (n = 8) were consented in accordance with local institutional review board guidelines. Lymphocytes were isolated from patients with stage III-IV melanoma by leukapheresis. Lymphocytes from fresh peripheral blood for other samples were isolated by Ficoll extraction.

Real Time PCR

Sorted cells were suspended in 1 ml Trizol and frozen at -80 degrees. RNA was isolated using Qiagen's RNeasy mini kit. Following reverse transcription, the abundance of PLZF cDNA was quantified by real-time PCR using the MasterMix (2X) HotStart-IT Syber kit (USB). Expression levels were normalized against the housekeeping gene GAPDH, according to the formula: relative PLZF induction $= 2^{CT(GAPDH) - CT(PLZF)}$.

Statistical Methods

Statistical analysis was done either with a two-tailed, unpaired Student's t-test or the Mann-Whitney U-test, which is a more robust for small sample sizes.

Results

PLZF expression in human T cells

PLZF is expressed both in mouse and human invariant NKT cells [16]. Recent studies in mice, however, show that PLZF expression is not limited to this cell type [29,30,31]. Therefore, we more carefully examined the expression of PLZF in PBLs from healthy volunteers by FACS. Similar to mice, PLZF was not detected in "conventional" T cells (**Fig. 1A**). The γδ TCR and iNKT cell-negative, CD3$^+$ T-cell compartment can be demarcated by the expression of CD161 and CD56. These cells are found at fairly high frequencies, with CD56$^+$ T cells on average at 1.7% (+/−2.5%) and CD161$^+$ T cells often found at more than 10% of the total T cells (**Fig. 1B**). CD56$^+$ T cells, which are often are considered to be non-invariant NKT cells, did not express PLZF (**Fig. 1C**). Similarly, CD161^{lo} cells (white box, **Fig. 1B**) also did not express PLZF. Of particular interest, however, was a distinct population of T cells (3.4% +/−2.5%) marked by high levels of CD161 (**Fig. 1B**) that clearly expressed PLZF (**Fig. 1C**).

The majority of the PLZF-expressing CD161^{hi} T cells were found to be CD8$^+$ (**Fig. 1D**). Furthermore, the CD161^{hi}CD8$^+$ T cells (**Fig. 1E**), expressed higher levels of PLZF as compared to the CD161^{hi}CD4$^+$ T cells (**Fig. 1F**). PLZF expression was lower than in iNKT cells (**Fig. 1F**). PLZF expression levels were consistent among cells from eight healthy donors (**Fig. 1G**). Expression levels were also confirmed by rtPCR of sorted cell populations (**Fig. 1H**). The CD161^{hi}CD8$^+$ population represented, on average, ~6% of the total CD8$^+$ T cells (**Figs. 1B, 1E**). PLZF is not expressed in any identified CD8$^+$ T cell population in mice [16]and unpublished data). Therefore, PLZF expression defines an abundant T cell subgroup in humans that does not exist in mouse peripheral blood.

To determine if the CD161^{hi} subset arose from the CD161$^-$ population as a result of activation, CD8$^+$ and CD4$^+$ T cells that were CD161$^-$ (**Fig. 1I**, black lines) or CD161^{hi} (**Fig. 1I**, red lines) were sorted and cultured with beads coated with antibodies against CD3 and CD28. After three days, low levels of CD161 were induced on the CD161$^-$ T cells (**Fig. 1J**, black lines). CD161^{hi} CD8$^+$ T cells were found to retain high levels of CD161 expression post-activation (**Fig. 1J**, red lines). The CD161^{hi} CD4$^+$ T cells, however, downregulated CD161 post-activation (**Fig. 1J**, red lines). Therefore, the CD161hi phenotype is specific to the PLZF-expressing CD8$^+$ T cells and expression of high levels of CD161 cannot be induced by activation. Furthermore, PLZF was not induced in non-PLZF expressing T cells by activation (data not shown).

Next we activated PBMCs with either PMA/ionomycin or anti-CD3 and anti-CD28, followed by FACS analysis for IFN-γ production. Surprisingly, unlike PLZF-expressing cells in mice [16,29], few PLZF-expressing CD161^{hi}CD8$^+$ T cells produced IFN-γ (**Fig. 1K**). As expected, many PLZF-negative CD161$^-$CD8$^+$ T cells produced IFN-γ upon stimulation (**Fig. 1K**).

The frequency of PLZF-expressing CD161^{hi}CD8$^+$ T cells is altered in patients with autoimmunity or advanced melanoma

To begin to study the role of PLZF-expressing CD161^{hi}CD8$^+$ T cells in the human immune response, we obtained peripheral blood samples from patients with systemic autoimmune diseases or malignancy. Patient samples were collected based only on availability; no selection criteria were utilized and treatment status was unknown. Monocyte-depleted PBMCs were stained with antibodies against CD3, CD4, CD8, CD161, CD56 and γδ TCR, then analyzed by flow cytometry. Two representative samples

acquired from patients diagnosed with systemic lupus erythematosus (SLE) is shown in **Fig. 2A**. CD161^{hi} T cells appeared to be reduced, but not to a level that reached statistical significance, when the SLE samples were compared to healthy donors (**Fig. 2A**). The apparent reduced frequency of CD56$^+$ T cells also did not reach statistical significance (data not shown). There was, however, a clear reduction in the percentage of CD8$^+$ cells within the CD161^{hi} population in patients with SLE (**Fig. 2B**). Similarly, the frequency of CD161^{hi} cells within the CD3$^+$CD8$^+$ T cell population was significantly reduced in the SLE samples, as compared to healthy controls (**Fig. 2C**). Again, the apparent reduction of CD3$^+$CD8$^+$CD56$^+$ was not statistically significant (data not shown). A similar trend was seen in a limited survey of patients with primary Sjogren's syndrome (data not shown). Finally, the residual CD161^{hi}CD8$^+$ T cells in the SLE patients expressed little or no PLZF (**Fig. 2D**).

Next, we evaluated the frequency of CD161$^+$ T-cells in blood samples from ten patients with advanced melanoma. In contrast to our findings in SLE and Sjogren's patients, we observed a substantial increase in the frequency of CD161^{hi} T cells in the melanoma cohort as compared to healthy controls (**Fig. 3A**). Different than the patients with autoimmunity, there was no change in the frequency of the CD8 to CD4 ratio within the CD161^{hi} T cells (**Fig. 3B**). Among the CD8$^+$ T cells, however, there was a substantial increase in the percentage of CD161^{hi} T cells (**Fig. 3C**). Also different than the SLE samples, the CD161^{hi}CD8$^+$ T cells in the patient samples were found to express PLZF at levels similar to healthy donors (**Fig. 3D**). These data, along with published studies [45], show that the PLZF-expressing PBL T cell population changes in patients with disease.

T cell subset deficiencies as a consequence of a biallelic loss of functional PLZF

Recently, the first and, to our knowledge, only person with a biallelic loss of functional PLZF was identified [44]. The maternal allele of PLZF was found to have a missense mutation that resulted in a methionine to valine substitution within a zinc finger domain. This mutation is paired with the paternal chromosome harboring a *de novo* deletion of ~8 Mbp, resulting in the loss of the gene encoding PLZF. Peripheral blood from this person was obtained and analyzed by FACS. In the absence of PLZF, the total percentage of CD3$^+$ T cells among PBLs and the percentage of CD4$^+$ and CD8$^+$ T cells were similar to healthy controls (**Fig. 4A**). The frequency of the CD56$^+$ and the CD161^{hi} T cell populations, however, were reduced as compared to the mean frequency found in healthy controls (**Fig. 4B,C**) and the few CD56$^+$ and CD161^{hi} cells found did not express PLZF (**Fig. 4D**). The few CD161^{hi} cells observed in this donor were strongly skewed towards CD4 rather than CD8 expression, which contrasted with the pattern observed in healthy controls (**Fig. 4E,F**). Additionally, there was a decrease in frequency of CD161^{hi} DN T cells, as compared to controls (**Fig. 4E,F**).

Human iNKT cells require PLZF for normal development

In mice, iNKT cells develop in the absence of PLZF, but they do not acquire innate T cell characteristics [16,17]. For example, in mice, PLZF-deficient iNKT cells accumulate in the lymph nodes rather than in the liver, do not express high levels of CD44 and CD69 and, also, fail to make cytokines upon primary activation. PLZF-deficient mouse iNKT cells are highly skewed towards CD4 and express low levels of NK1.1 [16]. iNKT cells are also present in the peripheral blood of PLZF-deficient mice, but at a reduced frequency as compared to wild type mice (data not shown). The frequency of human iNKT cells in the PLZF-deficient donor was

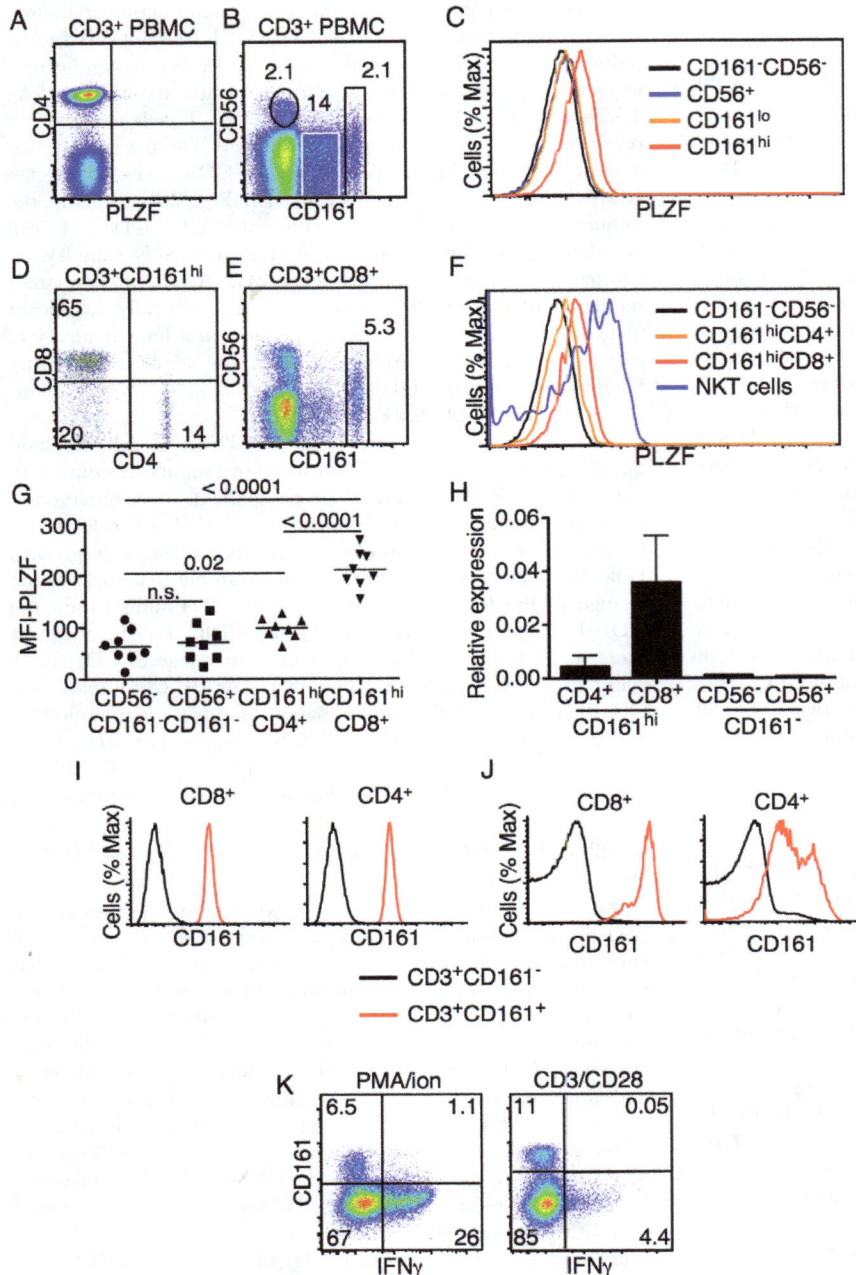

Figure 1. Expression of PLZF in peripheral T cell subsets. (**A**) Intranuclear FACS analysis of PLZF expression in total CD3$^+$ T cells; (**B**) CD161 and CD56 expression on CD3$^+$, NKT cell$^-$, $\gamma\delta$ TCR$^-$ lymphocytes; (**C**) PLZF expression in the indicated cell populations. Expression is compared to that of PLZF negative CD3$^+$CD161$^-$CD56$^-$ conventional T cells (black line). (**D**) CD4 and CD8 expression on electronically gated CD3$^+$CD161^{hi} T cells. (**E**) CD161 expression on electronically gated CD3$^+$CD8$^+$ T cells. (**F**) PLZF expression in the indicated cell populations. (**G**) Mean fluorescence intensity (MFI) of PLZF expression in indicated cells (N = 8). P values are indicated (n.s. = not significant); (**H**) cDNA made from RNA collected from the indicated populations was analyzed by real-time quantitative rtPCR. Units are relative to the expression of GAPDH. Data are the average of two independent experiments with an N = 4. (**I**) Healthy donor lymphocytes were sorted into four T cell subsets: CD161$^-$CD4$^+$, CD161$^-$CD8$^+$, CD161^{hi}CD4$^+$ and CD161^{hi}CD8$^+$. Representative data for CD161 expression on the four populations analyzed immediately post-sort is shown (black line = CD161$^-$ cells; red line = CD161^{hi} cells). (**J**) CD161 levels of the indicated sorted cells, analyzed three days after activation with anti-CD3/CD28 coated beads, is shown (black line = CD161$^-$ cells; red line = CD161^{hi} cells). (**K**) IFN-γ expression by peripheral blood T cells 6 hours after activation with PMA/Ionomycin or anti-CD3/C28 coated beads. Numbers indicate percentage of cells within the indicated gate. Data in A–G are representative of eight donors, each analyzed at least two times. Data in I and J are representative of two individuals done in two independent experiments. Data shown in K are from two different individuals and were two independent experiments.

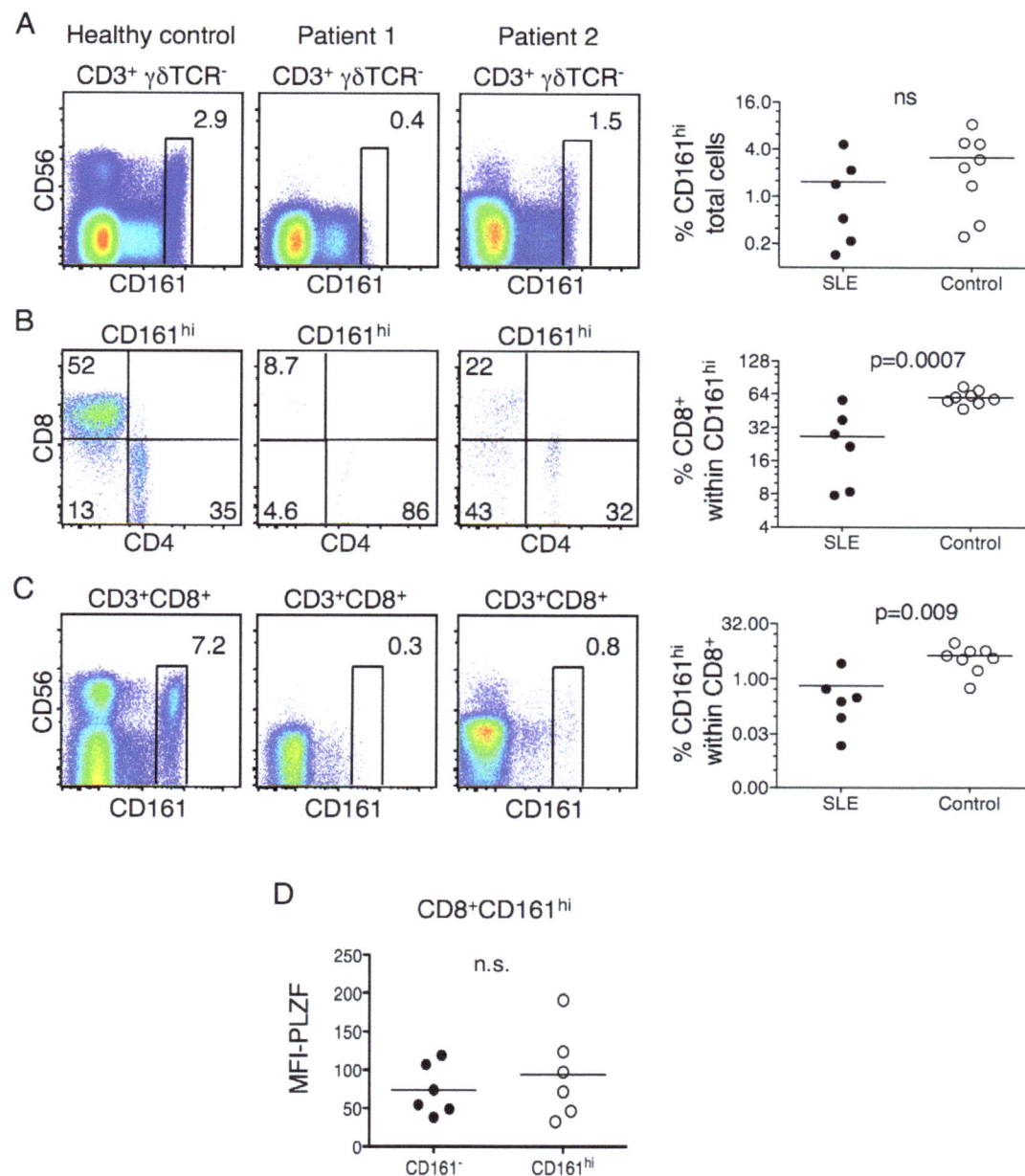

Figure 2. Patients with systemic lupus erythematosus show decreased circulating have altered frequencies of PLZF-expressing T cells. (**A**) The frequency of CD161^{hi} lymphocytes within the CD3$^+$ γδ TCR$^-$ population. (**B**) The CD4/CD8 profile of the CD161^{hi} T cells as identified in (A). (**C**) The frequency of CD161^{hi} T cells within the CD3$^+$CD8$^+$ γδ TCR$^-$ lymphocyte gate. (**D**) The remaining CD161^{hi}CD8$^+$ T cells in SLE patients express low levels of PLZF. PBMC's were collected from six patients with SLE and stained as previously described. A representative control and two patient samples are shown for each analysis. Data from the control and patient groups are summarized in scatter plots. P values are shown in figures (n.s. = not significant).

only slightly reduced as compared to the mean frequency found in healthy controls (**Fig. 5A**). However, the phenotype of the PLZF-deficient iNKT cells clearly resembled that of iNKT cells from PLZF-deficient mice. In particular, PLZF-deficient human iNKT cells were strongly skewed towards expressing CD4 at the expense of the DN population (**Fig. 5B**). Furthermore, the PLZF deficient iNKT cells were largely CD161 (NK1.1) low (**Fig. 5C**). These data suggest that, similar to the findings in mice, PLZF impacts the development of iNKT cells in humans.

Human γδ T cells express PLZF

The reduction in the frequency of CD161^{hi} DN T cells in the absence of PLZF (**Fig. 4E,F**) prompted us to more carefully examine this population of T cells. A large percentage of the CD161^{hi} DN T cells proved to be γδ T cells (data not shown). We, and others, recently reported the existence of a minor subset of NKT cell-like γδ T cells in mice that express high levels of PLZF [30,31]. Unlike the subset-restricted pattern of PLZF expression in mouse γδ T cells, all human peripheral blood γδ T cells were

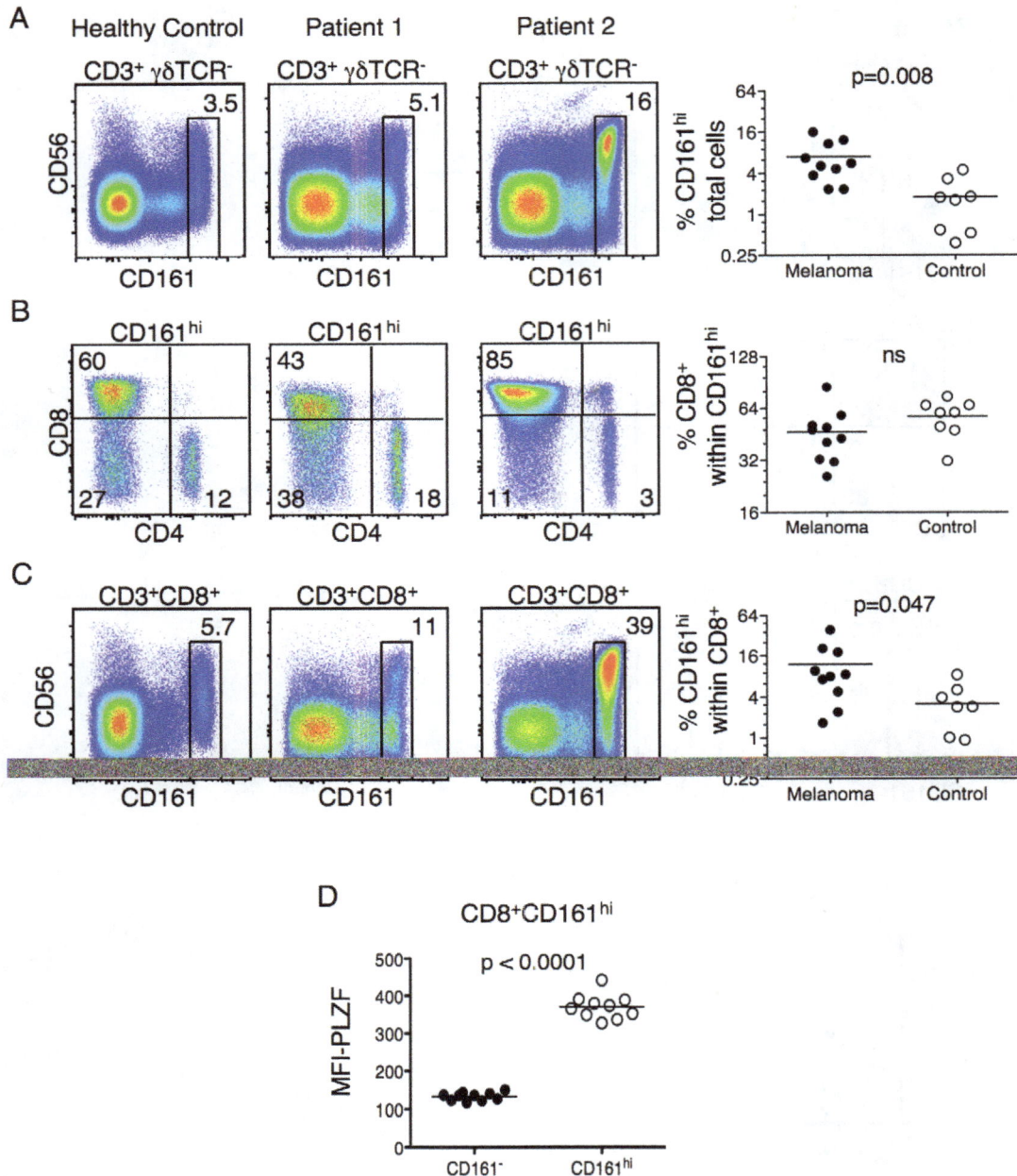

Figure 3. Patients with advanced melanoma have expanded circulating CD8$^+$ CD161^{hi} T cell populations. (A) The frequency of CD161^{hi} lymphocytes within the CD3$^+$ $\gamma\delta$ TCR$^-$ population. (B) The CD4/CD8 profile of the CD161^{hi} T cells as identified in (A). (C) The frequency of CD161^{hi} T cells within the CD3$^+$CD8$^+$ $\gamma\delta$ TCR$^-$ lymphocyte gate. (D) CD161^{hi}CD8$^+$ T cells from patients with advanced melanoma retain PLZF expression, as compared to conventional CD8 T cells. PBMC's from ten patients with metastatic melanoma were isolated via leukapheresis. The cells were stained and analyzed by FACS as described above. A representative control and two patient samples are shown for each analysis. Data from the control and patient groups are summarized in scatter plots. P values are shown in figures (n.s. = not significant).

found to express PLZF (**Fig. 6A**). The expression of PLZF was confirmed by comparing $\gamma\delta$ T cells from healthy donors to $\gamma\delta$ T cells from the PLZF-deficient donor (**Fig. 6A**). $\gamma\delta$ T cells were found to develop in the absence of PLZF and were present at a frequency similar to that published by others ($\sim$4%) [46] and to a larger panel of samples we analyzed (**Fig. 6B and data not shown**). The data suggests that the frequency of CD161^{hi} $\gamma\delta$ T cells was reduced in the absence of PLZF, while the frequency of CD8$^+$ $\gamma\delta$ T cells was increased (**Fig. 6B**), however, $\gamma\delta$ T cell

phenotypes were found to be highly variable among healthy donors.

Human NK cells express PLZF

Less than 5% of mouse NK cells constitutively express PLZF [16] and PLZF is not induced in mouse NK cells by activation (data not shown). Furthermore, mouse NK cells develop and appear to function normally in PLZF-deficient mice ([16] and data not shown). Therefore it was very surprising to find that nearly all

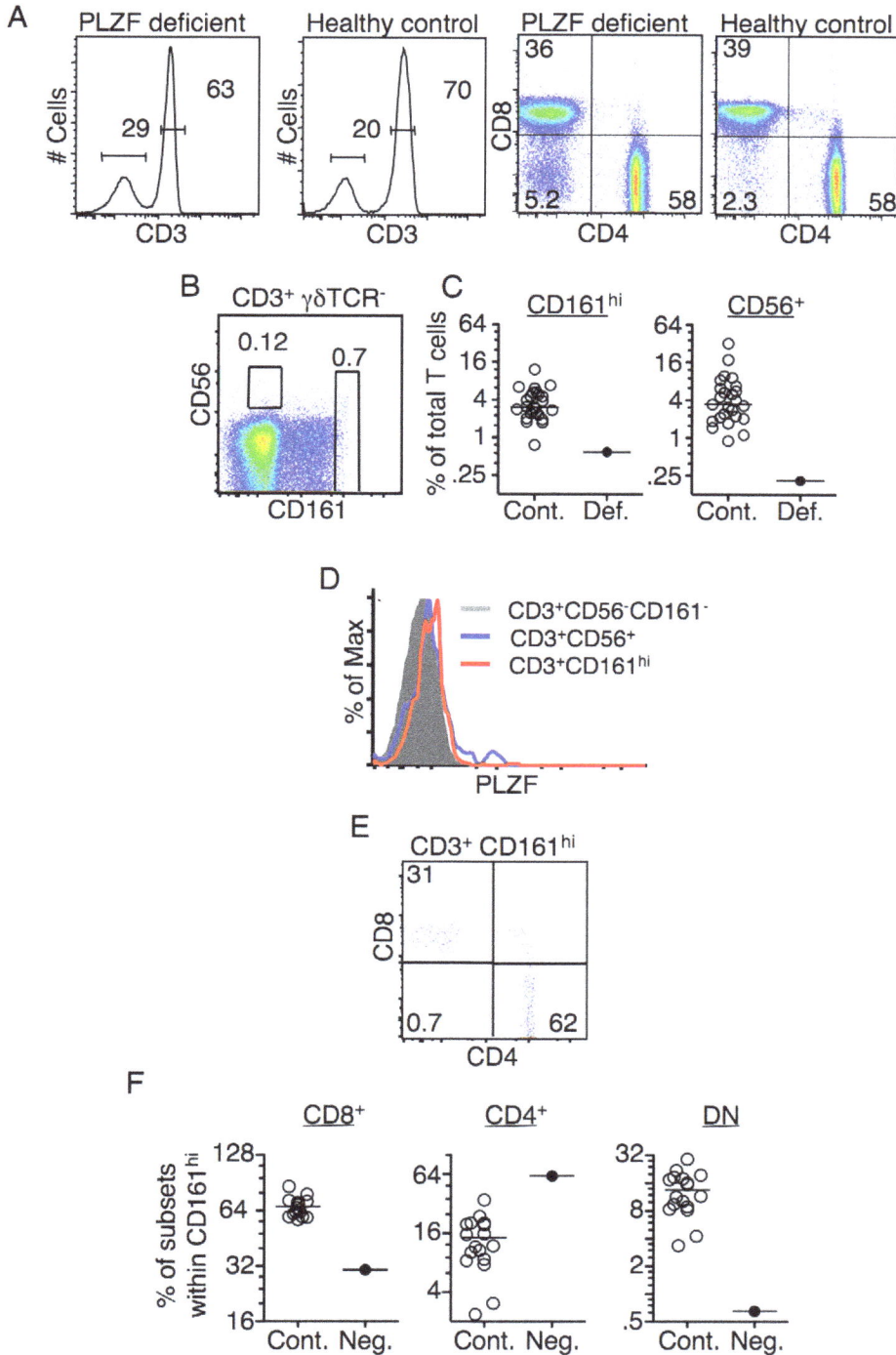

Figure 4. PBMCs from a person with a biallelic loss of functional PLZF were analyzed by FACS. (**A**) The frequency of CD3$^+$ T cells and the CD4/CD8 of the CD3$^+$ T cells was not altered as compared to healthy donor samples. Results shown are representative of three experiments. (**B**) Dot plot shows the frequency of CD161^{hi} and CD56$^+$ expression on CD3$^+$ T cell from the PLZF-deficient donor. γδ T cells were excluded from the analysis. (**C**) Scatter plot shows the frequency of the CD161^{hi} and CD56$^+$ T cell subsets from the PLZF-deficient donor in comparison to healthy controls (Cont. = healthy control; Def. = PLZF-deficient). (**D**) Histogram shows PLZF expression in CD3$^+$ CD161^{hi} and CD56$^+$ T cells from the PLZF deficient donor in comparison to the donor's conventional T cells (CD56$^-$CD161$^-$). (**E**) CD8 versus CD4 expression on NKT cell$^-$, γδ T cell$^-$, CD161^{hi} T cells from the PLZF-deficient donor. (**F**) Scatter plot shows CD8, CD4 and DN distribution of CD161^{hi} T cells from the PLZF-deficient donor as compared to healthy controls. Numbers within FACS plot represent the percentage of events in the indicated gate. Results were consistent in three samples that were obtained from the PLZF deficient donor.

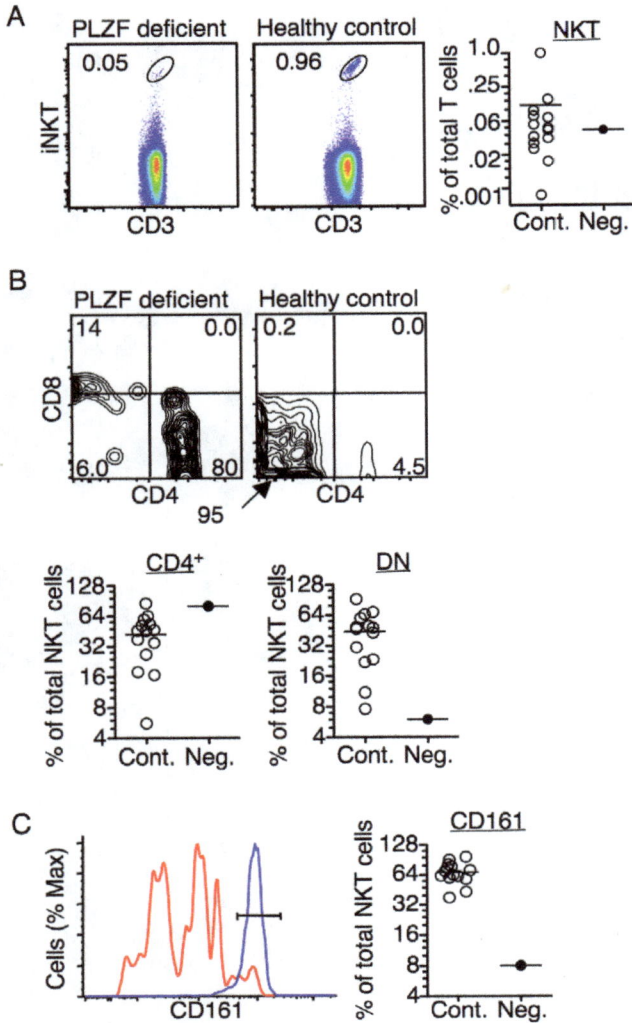

Figure 5. Invariant NKT cell development is altered in the absence of PLZF. (A) Invariant NKT cells from the PLZF-deficient and a healthy control donor identified with antibodies against the Vα24Jα18 iTCR antibody (6B11) and CD3. The scatter plot shows the frequency of iNKT cells in the PLZF-deficient as compared to healthy donors. The healthy control sample shown in the dot plot was acquired in the same experiment as the PLZF deficient sample. Therefore, this sample is shown although the frequency of iNKT cells is higher than the median for all samples. (B) Dot plots show the expression of CD4 and CD8 on iNKT cells identified in (A). The scatter plots show the frequency of CD4+ and CD4−CD8− double negative (DN) iNKT cells from the PLZF-deficient donor as compared to healthy controls. (C) Histogram shows a comparison of CD161 expression on iNKT cells from the PLZF-deficient donor to healthy controls. iNKT cells were identified as shown in (A). The scatter plot compares the frequency of CD161hi iNKT cells from the PLZF-deficient donor as compared to healthy controls. High expression of CD161 was defined by the black bar shown in the histogram. Cont.= health control; Neg. = PLZF deficient.

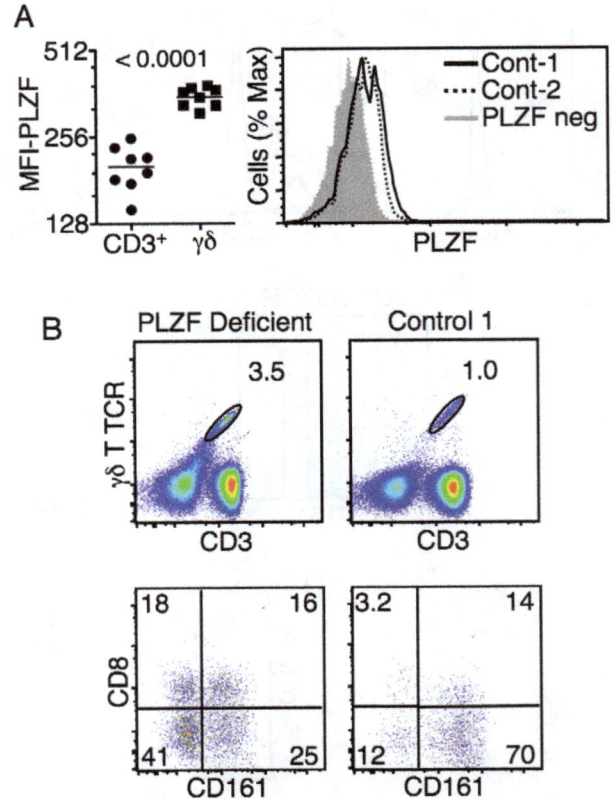

Figure 6. Human γδ T cells express PLZF. (A) The MFI of PLZF expression in γδ T cells as compared to CD3+CD56−CD161− T cells (P value is shown). Histogram shows PLZF expression in γδ T cells collected from two healthy donors in comparison to γδ T cells from the PLZF-deficient donor. (B) The frequency of γδ T cells from a healthy control and the PLZF deficient donor is shown in the panels at the top. Although the frequency of γδ T cell in PLZF deficient sample appears higher than the controls, the percentage is actually consistent with a broader analysis (data not shown) and with published reports. The bottom panels show CD161 and CD8 expression on γδ T cells from the healthy control and the PLZF deficient donor. γδ T cells were identified as shown in the top panels. Data from PLZF deficient donor were consistent from three independent blood samples. Numbers indicate the frequency of cells within each panel.

human NK cells expressed the transcription factor. The expression of PLZF was made clear by comparing samples from healthy donors to the PLZF-deficient donor (Fig. 7A)

PLZF-deficient NK cells were found to express lower levels of CD56, CD16 and CD161 (Fig. 7B). To assess the functional relevance of PLZF in human NK cells, NK cells from healthy controls and the PLZF-deficient donor were activated with beads coated with antibodies against CD335 (NKp46) and CD2. Supernatants were collected after three days for cytokine analysis. There was a clear increase in the amount of secreted IFN-γ, TNF and Granzyme B in the PLZF-deficient sample as compared to the control samples (Fig. 7C). GM-CSF was also found to be increased, but to a lesser degree. Therefore, PLZF expression appears to subdue cytokine secretion by human NK cells.

Discussion

We show that in people, CD8+ and CD4+ CD161hi T cells, all γδ T cells, NKT cells and all NK cells express PLZF. Collectively, these populations represent more than 10% of the total human peripheral blood lymphocytes. In contrast, PLZF expression in mice is limited to NKT cells and a minor subset of γδ T cells, which combined, account for ~1% of the total lymphocytes. Furthermore, few, if any, mouse NK cells express PLZF. Therefore, PLZF arguably plays a far more significant role in the human immune system than in that of the mouse.

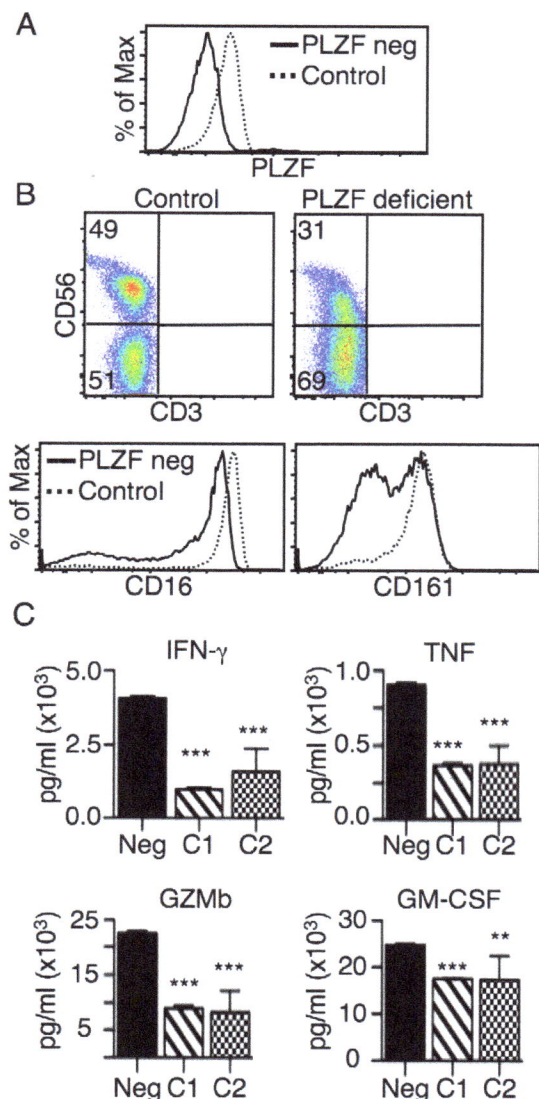

Figure 7. PBMCs from a healthy control and the PLZF-deficient donor were analyzed by FACS. (A) Histogram shows PLZF levels in permeabilized CD3⁻CD56⁺ NK cells. (B) CD56 levels on CD3⁻ PBMCs from a healthy control or the PLZF-deficient donor. CD16 and CD161 levels on CD3⁻CD56⁺ NK cells (solid line = PLZF-deficient donor; dotted line = healthy control). (C) CD3⁻CD56⁺ NK cells were sorted and then activated with beads coated with anti-NKp46 and anti-CD2. Supernatants were collected after 72 hours and analyzed by cytokine bead array. Control-1 was obtained from a healthy donor the day of the sort; control-2 was obtained from a healthy donor and the sample was shipped with the PLZF-deficient sample. FACS analysis was consistent for eight healthy controls. Samples from the PLZF-deficient donor were collected three times and were analyzed in three independent FACS experiments. Cells for the cytokine release experiment were collected from one sample. Sorted cells were split into multiple wells (between 3 and 8 wells) and treated as independent samples for statistical purposes. (** P value = 0.0080; *** P value < 0.0001).

The frequency, phenotype and/or function of all of the PLZF-expressing cell types were altered in some way in samples obtained from a person with a biallelic loss of functional PLZF. For example, the phenotype of CD1d-restricted NKT cells was altered and the frequency of CD161ʰⁱCD8⁺ T cells was reduced, suggesting that these T cells are dependent upon PLZF for

development. γδ T cells were present in the PLZF-deficient donor, but appeared to have altered CD161 and CD8 expression. In the absence of PLZF, NK cells expressed lower levels of CD56 and the activating receptors CD16 and CD161. Surprisingly, we found that PLZF-deficient NK cells produced substantially greater amounts of several different cytokines. No obvious alterations in the PLZF-expressing cell types were detected in a limited analysis of the donor's mother, who carries a point mutation in one copy ZBTB16 (data not shown). As mentioned above, the donor's father carries two non-mutated copies of the PLZF gene and, therefore, blood samples were not obtained. Finally, the donor has not shown overt signs of autoimmunity nor increased susceptibility to infectious disease. Indeed, although the donor is EBV positive, he does not display signs of active disease.

Rather surprisingly, we found that PLZF was not expressed in CD3⁺CD56⁺ T cells. Nevertheless, the frequency of CD3⁺CD56⁺ T cells was reduced in the PLZF-deficient donor, implicating PLZF in the development of these cells. It is possible that expression of PLZF in CD3⁺CD56⁺ T cells may occur during T cell development, when it directs the acquisition of an innate T-cell phenotype in this population, but is then downregulated prior to the migration of these cells into the periphery, similar to what was found for embryonic CD4 T cells [47]. Alternatively, the reduced frequency of CD56⁺ T cells may be due to cell extrinsic factors, such as altered cytokine expression by other PLZF-expressing cells.

Recently published data suggests that a large percentage of CD161ʰⁱ CD8⁺ and CD161ʰⁱ double negative T cells express an invariant Vα7.2 TCRα chain [48]. T cells expressing this invariant TCR belong to a subset known as mucosal-associated invariant T cells (MAIT cells). The finding that human, but not mouse, MAIT cells express PLZF suggests a functional divergence in this T cell subset.

To begin to understand the role of PLZF-expressing CD161ʰⁱCD8⁺ T cell lineage in the human immune system, we analyzed the frequency of this population in blood obtained from patients with either autoimmunity or cancer. Patients with SLE were found to have a highly significant decrease in the percentage of CD8⁺ T cells within the CD161ʰⁱ subpopulation. Similar results were obtained from a small cohort of patients with primary Sjögren's syndrome. Interestingly, patients with advanced melanoma were found to have a significant increase in the frequency of CD161ʰⁱ T cells. In one extreme example, ~16% of the total T cells were CD161ʰⁱ and, in particular, nearly 40% of the patient's CD8 T cells were CD161ʰⁱ. While these data have not been correlated with clinical outcomes, it is clear that the PLZF-expressing population is dynamic and that it changes with different types of immunological stress.

The patient data are consistent with a previous report showing that CD161ʰⁱ CD8⁺ T cells are reduced in patients with a variety of rheumatic diseases including SLE, MCTD (mixed connective-tissue disease), SSc (systemic sclerosis) and PM/DM (polymyositis/dermatomyositis) [45]. Our data are also consistent with a report showing that CD161ʰⁱCD8⁺ T cells do not produce IFN-γ, TNF-α or IL-2 following TCR activation [49]. A more recent paper suggests that CD161ʰⁱCD8⁺ T cells contain an IL-17 producing subset as well as IL-22 producing cells [50]. Interestingly, it was found that the IL-17 producing cells were enriched in the livers of patients during chronic hepatitis. The PLZF-expressing CD161ʰⁱCD8⁺ T cells also express high levels of the IL-18 receptor α chain (data not shown). Therefore it is possible that the cells we study here are the same or similar to those described as having the capacity to efflux and, therefore, survive treatments involving chemotherapy drugs [51]. It was suggested that the

CD161^{hi} T cells are actually precursors of CD161^{lo} cells and, thus, might represent self-renewing stem cell-like memory CD8 T cells [51]. It will be interesting to determine if these proposed functions are dependent on PLZF.

Overall, we have found that PLZF is expressed in a greater variety of lymphocytes and in a higher percentage of lymphocytes in humans as compared to mice. The function of PLZF-expressing cells appears to be diverse. For example, CD161^{hi}CD8$^+$ T cells clearly do not make abundant levels of cytokines following activation. Furthermore, PLZF expression in human NK cells appears to limit cytokine production. Therefore, in sharp contrast to other PLZF-expressing lymphocytes, PLZF expression in human CD8$^+$ T cells and NK cells appears to inhibit cytokine expression.

References

1. Kelly KF, Daniel JM (2006) POZ for effect--POZ-ZF transcription factors in cancer and development. Trends Cell Biol 16: 578–587.
2. Dent AL, Shaffer AL, Yu X, Allman D, Staudt LM (1997) Control of inflammation, cytokine expression, and germinal center formation by BCL-6. Science 276: 589–592.
3. Fukuda T, Yoshida T, Okada S, Hatano M, Miki T, et al. (1997) Disruption of the Bcl6 gene results in an impaired germinal center formation. J Exp Med 186: 439–448.
4. Nurieva RI, Chung Y, Martinez GJ, Yang XO, Tanaka S, et al. (2009) Bcl6 mediates the development of T follicular helper cells. Science 325: 1001–1005.
5. Yu D, Rao S, Tsai LM, Lee SK, He Y, et al. (2009) The transcriptional repressor Bcl-6 directs T follicular helper cell lineage commitment. Immunity 31: 457–468.
6. He X, Park K, Kappes DJ (2010) The role of ThPOK in control of CD4/CD8 lineage commitment. Annu Rev Immunol 28: 295–320.
7. Maeda T, Merghoub T, Hobbs RM, Dong L, Maeda M, et al. (2007) Regulation of B versus T lymphoid lineage fate decision by the proto-oncogene LRF. Science 316: 860–866.
8. Sakaguchi S, Hombauer M, Bilic I, Naoe Y, Schebesta A, et al. (2010) The zinc-finger protein MAZR is part of the transcription factor network that controls the CD4 versus CD8 lineage fate of double-positive thymocytes. Nat Immunol 11: 442–448.
9. Scaglioni PP, Pandolfi PP (2007) The theory of APL revisited. Curr Top Microbiol Immunol 313: 85–100.
10. He LZ, Guidez F, Triboli C, Peruzzi D, Ruthardt M, et al. (1998) Distinct interactions of PML-RARalpha and PLZF-RARalpha with co-repressors determine differential responses to RA in APL. Nat Genet 18: 126–135.
11. Barna M, Hawe N, Niswander L, Pandolfi PP (2000) Plzf regulates limb and axial skeletal patterning. Nat Genet 25: 166–172.
12. Avantaggiato V, Pandolfi PP, Ruthardt M, Hawe N, Acampora D, et al. (1995) Developmental analysis of murine Promyelocyte Leukemia Zinc Finger (PLZF) gene expression: implications for the neuromeric model of the forebrain organization. J Neurosci 15: 4927–4942.
13. Buaas FW, Kirsh AL, Sharma M, McLean DJ, Morris JL, et al. (2004) Plzf is required in adult male germ cells for stem cell self-renewal. Nat Genet 36: 647–652.
14. Costoya JA, Hobbs RM, Barna M, Cattoretti G, Manova K, et al. (2004) Essential role of Plzf in maintenance of spermatogonial stem cells. Nat Genet 36: 653–659.
15. Doulatov S, Notta F, Rice KL, Howell L, Zelent A, et al. (2009) PLZF is a regulator of homeostatic and cytokine-induced myeloid development. Genes Dev 23: 2076–2087.
16. Kovalovsky D, Uche OU, Eladad S, Hobbs RM, Yi W, et al. (2008) The BTB-zinc finger transcriptional regulator PLZF controls the development of invariant natural killer T cell effector functions. Nat Immunol 9: 1055–1064.
17. Savage AK, Constantinides MG, Han J, Picard D, Martin E, et al. (2008) The transcription factor PLZF directs the effector program of the NKT cell lineage. Immunity 29: 391–403.
18. Bendelac A, Savage PB, Teyton L (2007) The biology of NKT cells. Annu Rev Immunol 25: 297–336.
19. Kronenberg M, Gapin L (2002) The unconventional lifestyle of NKT cells. Nat Rev Immunol 2: 557–568.
20. Berzofsky JA, Terabe M (2009) The contrasting roles of NKT cells in tumor immunity. Curr Mol Med 9: 667–672.
21. Benlagha K, Weiss A, Beavis A, Teyton L, Bendelac A (2000) In vivo identification of glycolipid antigen-specific T cells using fluorescent CD1d tetramers. J Exp Med 191: 1895–1903.
22. Matsuda JL, Naidenko OV, Gapin L, Nakayama T, Taniguchi M, et al. (2000) Tracking the response of natural killer T cells to a glycolipid antigen using CD1d tetramers. J Exp Med 192: 741–754.
23. Hammond KJ, Pellicci DG, Poulton LD, Naidenko OV, Scalzo AA, et al. (2001) CD1d-restricted NKT cells: an interstrain comparison. J Immunol 167: 1164–1173.
24. Marsh RA, Villanueva J, Kim MO, Zhang K, Marmer D, et al. (2009) Patients with X-linked lymphoproliferative disease due to BIRC4 mutation have normal invariant natural killer T-cell populations. Clin Immunol 132: 116–123.
25. Baev DV, Peng XH, Song L, Barnhart JR, Crooks GM, et al. (2004) Distinct homeostatic requirements of CD4+ and CD4- subsets of Valpha24-invariant natural killer T cells in humans. Blood 104: 4150–4156.
26. Berzins SP, Cochrane AD, Pellicci DG, Smyth MJ, Godfrey DI (2005) Limited correlation between human thymus and blood NKT cell content revealed by an ontogeny study of paired tissue samples. Eur J Immunol 35: 1399–1407.
27. Kovalovsky D, Alonzo ES, Uche OU, Eidson M, Nichols KE, et al. (2010) PLZF induces the spontaneous acquisition of memory/effector functions in T cells independently of NKT cell-related signals. J Immunol 184: 6746–6755.
28. Raberger J, Schebesta A, Sakaguchi S, Boucheron N, Blomberg KE, et al. (2008) The transcriptional regulator PLZF induces the development of CD44 high memory phenotype T cells. Proc Natl Acad Sci U S A 105: 17919–17924.
29. Alonzo ES, Gottschalk RA, Das J, Egawa T, Hobbs RM, et al. (2010) Development of promyelocytic zinc finger and ThPOK-expressing innate gamma delta T cells is controlled by strength of TCR signaling and Id3. J Immunol 184: 1268–1279.
30. Kreslavsky T, Savage AK, Hobbs R, Gounari F, Bronson R, et al. (2009) TCR-inducible PLZF transcription factor required for innate phenotype of a subset of gammadelta T cells with restricted TCR diversity. Proc Natl Acad Sci U S A 106: 12453–12458.
31. Felices M, Yin CC, Kosaka Y, Kang J, Berg LJ (2009) Tec kinase Itk in gammadeltaT cells is pivotal for controlling IgE production in vivo. Proc Natl Acad Sci U S A 106: 8308–8313.
32. Verykokakis M, Boos MD, Bendelac A, Adams EJ, Pereira P, et al. (2010) Inhibitor of DNA binding 3 limits development of murine slam-associated adaptor protein-dependent "innate" gammadelta T cells. PLoS One 5: e9303.
33. Weinreich MA, Odumade OA, Jameson SC, Hogquist KA (2010) T cells expressing the transcription factor PLZF regulate the development of memory-like CD8+ T cells. Nat Immunol 11: 709–716.
34. Renukaradhya GJ, Khan MA, Vieira M, Du W, Gervay-Hague J, et al. (2008) Type I NKT cells protect (and type II NKT cells suppress) the host's innate antitumor immune response to a B-cell lymphoma. Blood 111: 5637–5645.
35. Swann JB, Uldrich AP, van Dommelen S, Sharkey J, Murray WK, et al. (2009) Type I natural killer T cells suppress tumors caused by p53 loss in mice. Blood 113: 6382–6385.
36. Teng MW, Sharkey J, McLaughlin NM, Exley MA, Smyth MJ (2009) CD1d-based combination therapy eradicates established tumors in mice. J Immunol 183: 1911–1920.
37. Teng MW, Yue S, Sharkey J, Exley MA, Smyth MJ (2009) CD1d activation and blockade: a new antitumor strategy. J Immunol 182: 3366–3371.
38. Tahir SM, Cheng O, Shaulov A, Koezuka Y, Bubley GJ, et al. (2001) Loss of IFN-gamma production by invariant NK T cells in advanced cancer. J Immunol 167: 4046–4050.
39. van der Vliet HJ, Pinedo HM, von Blomberg BM, van den Eertwegh AJ, Scheper RJ, et al. (2002) Natural Killer T cells. Lancet Oncol 3: 574.
40. Motohashi S, Nakayama T (2009) Invariant natural killer T cell-based immunotherapy for cancer. Immunotherapy 1: 73–82.
41. Novak J, Griseri T, Beaudoin L, Lehuen A (2007) Regulation of type 1 diabetes by NKT cells. Int Rev Immunol 26: 49–72.
42. Wither J, Cai YC, Lim S, McKenzie T, Roslin N, et al. (2008) Reduced proportions of natural killer T cells are present in the relatives of lupus patients and are associated with autoimmunity. Arthritis Res Ther 10: R108.
43. Van Kaer L (2006) Role of invariant natural killer T cells in immune regulation and as potential therapeutic targets in autoimmune disease. Expert Rev Clin Immunol 2: 745–757.
44. Fischer S, Kohlhase J, Bohm D, Schweiger B, Hoffmann D, et al. (2008) Biallelic loss of function of the promyelocytic leukaemia zinc finger (PLZF) gene causes severe skeletal defects and genital hypoplasia. J Med Genet 45: 731–737.

Acknowledgments

We thank Dr. Lisa Denzin for critical reading of the manuscript and Dr. Thorsten Rosenbaum for taking blood samples from the PLZF-deficient donor.

Author Contributions

Conceived and designed the experiments: ME JW DBS. Performed the experiments: ME JW AMB BZ. Analyzed the data: ME JW AMB JY JDW DBS. Contributed reagents/materials/analysis tools: BZ SEC PKC JY JDW BH DW DBS. Wrote the paper: ME JW AMB DBS.

45. Mitsuo A, Morimoto S, Nakiri Y, Suzuki J, Kaneko H, et al. (2006) Decreased CD161+CD8+ T cells in the peripheral blood of patients suffering from rheumatic diseases. Rheumatology (Oxford) 45: 1477–1484.
46. Kosub DA, Lehrman G, Milush JM, Zhou D, Chacko E, et al. (2008) Gamma/ Delta T-cell functional responses differ after pathogenic human immunodeficiency virus and nonpathogenic simian immunodeficiency virus infections. J Virol 82: 1155–1165.
47. Lee YJ, Jeon YK, Kang BH, Chung DH, Park CG, et al. (2010) Generation of PLZF+ CD4+ T cells via MHC class II-dependent thymocyte-thymocyte interaction is a physiological process in humans. J Exp Med 207: 237–246.
48. Martin E, Treiner E, Duban L, Guerri L, Laude H, et al. (2009) Stepwise development of MAIT cells in mouse and human. PLoS Biol 7: e54.
49. Takahashi T, Dejbakhsh-Jones S, Strober S (2006) Expression of CD161 (NKR-P1A) defines subsets of human CD4 and CD8 T cells with different functional activities. J Immunol 176: 211–216.
50. Billerbeck E, Kang YH, Walker L, Lockstone H, Grafmueller S, et al. (2010) Analysis of CD161 expression on human CD8+ T cells defines a distinct functional subset with tissue-homing properties. Proc Natl Acad Sci U S A 107: 3006–3011.
51. Turtle CJ, Swanson HM, Fujii N, Estey EH, Riddell SR (2009) A distinct subset of self-renewing human memory CD8+ T cells survives cytotoxic chemotherapy. Immunity 31: 834–844.

3

Mutually Positive Regulatory Feedback Loop between Interferons and Estrogen Receptor-α in Mice: Implications for Sex Bias in Autoimmunity

Ravichandran Panchanathan[1,2], Hui Shen[1,2], Xiang Zhang[1], Shuk-mei Ho[1], Divaker Choubey[1,2]*

1 Department of Environmental Health, University of Cincinnati, Cincinnati, Ohio, United States of America, **2** Cincinnati Veterans Affairs Medical Center, Cincinnati, Ohio, United States of America

Abstract

Background: Systemic lupus erythematosus (SLE), an autoimmune disease, predominantly affects women of childbearing age. Moreover, increased serum levels of interferon-α (IFN-α) are associated with the disease. Although, the female sex hormone estrogen (E2) is implicated in sex bias in SLE through up-regulation of IFN-γ expression, the molecular mechanisms remain unknown. Here we report that activation of IFN (α or γ)-signaling in immune cells up-regulates expression of estrogen receptor-α (ERα; encoded by the *Esr1* gene) and stimulates expression of target genes.

Methodology/Principal Findings: We found that treatment of mouse splenic cells and mouse cell lines with IFN (α or γ) increased steady-state levels of ERα mRNA and protein. The increase in the ERα mRNA levels was primarily due to the transcriptional mechanisms and it was dependent upon the activation of signal transducer and activator of transcription-1 (STAT1) factor by IFN. Moreover, the IFN-treatment of cells also stimulated transcription of a reporter gene, expression of which was driven by the promoter region of the murine *Esr1* gene. Notably, splenic cells from pre-autoimmune lupus-prone (NZB × NZW)F₁ female mice had relatively higher steady-state levels of mRNAs encoded by the IFN and ERα-responsive genes as compared to the age-matched males.

Conclusions/Significance: Our observations identify a novel mutually positive regulatory feedback loop between IFNs and ERα in immune cells in mice and support the idea that activation of this regulatory loop contributes to sex bias in SLE.

Editor: Derya Unutmaz, New York University, United States of America

Funding: Work was supported by a grant (AI066261) from the National Institutes of Health to D.C. The funders had no role in study design, data collection and analysis, decision to publish, or preparation of the manuscript.

Competing Interests: The authors have declared that no competing interests exist.

* E-mail: Divaker.choubey@uc.edu

Introduction

Systemic lupus erythematosus (SLE) is a prototype autoimmune disease in which patients develop pathogenic autoantibodies against nuclear antigens and the disease involves multiple organs, including the kidneys [1,2]. The disease has a strong sex bias and develops at a female-to-male ratio of 10:1 [3–6]. The sex bias in SLE is thought to be influenced by sex hormones, such as estrogen and androgen [4–6]. Additionally, it has been noted [7] that ERα mRNA levels are significantly higher in peripheral blood mononuclear cells (PBMCs) from SLE patients as compared to normal controls. Moreover, the female sex hormone estrogen (E2) is known to have immunomodulatory effects [5]. For example, in vitro treatment of PBMCs from SLE patients with estrogen results in polyclonal activation, secretion of antibodies to double-stranded DNA, and defects in apoptosis of immune cells [5,6].

Sex hormones also influence the pathogenesis of murine lupus [8–11]. For example, in (NZB × NZW) F₁ mouse model of SLE disease, female mice develop the disease earlier and have shorter life spans than males [8]. In contrast, castrated male (NZB × NZW) F₁ mice have earlier onset of lupus and shorter life span than their intact littermates [9]. In addition treatment with estrogen exacerbates disease activity and causes early mortality [10,11].

Estrogen functions by activating one of its two nuclear receptors, ERα and ERβ [12,13]. Both receptors are expressed in most immune cells [14]. Several recent studies involving mouse models of SLE disease have provided evidence for a prominent role of ERα in the development of lupus disease [10,11,15,16]. Interestingly, the ERα deficiency in (NZB × NZW) F1 female mice attenuated glomerulonephritis and increased survival of mice [15]. Of note, the increased survival of ERα deficient female mice was associated with reduced development of anti-chromatin and anti-dsDNA antibodies as well as reduced serum levels of IFN-γ [15]. Moreover, E2 is known to promote IFN-γ production by invariant natural killer T cells [17], dendritic cells [18], and splenocytes [19]. Interestingly, the participation of IFN-γ in lupus pathogenesis has been demonstrated in mice [20] and in SLE patients [21]. Consistent with a role for IFN-γ in the development of lupus disease, deletion of the IFN-γ receptor [22] or depletion of IFN-γ in lupus-prone (NZB × NZW)F₁ mice [23] prevents autoantibody production and glomerulonephritis. These observations have demonstrated a role for both estrogen and IFN-γ signaling in the development of lupus disease in mouse models.

Studies have indicated that SLE patients with active disease have elevated serum levels of type I IFNs (IFN-α/β) [20,24]. It has been proposed that tissue damage, either as a result of infections or sterile injuries could be source of apoptotic debris and, thus, autoantigen, which in turn can induce the type I IFN production [25]. Moreover, consistent with increased serum levels of IFN-α in SLE patients, PBMCs from SLE patients also exhibit a gene expression profile indicative of an active IFN-α signaling [24,25]. The role of type I IFN-signaling has also been investigated in mouse models of SLE [20]. It is known that mice that are deficient in the type I receptor do not develop the disease [20]. Interestingly, a comparison of gene expression analysis between pre-autoimmune (NZB × NZW) F$_1$ and MRL/lpr mice has suggested that mononuclear cells from (NZB × NZW) F$_1$ female mice express higher levels of IFN-α and IFN-γ-inducible genes than the MRL/lpr mice [26]. Moreover, our work revealed that the type I interferon receptor deficiency reduces lupus-like disease in the lupus-prone NZB mice [27]. Although, the above studies using mouse models of SLE and human SLE patients have also provided evidence for a role for IFN-signaling in lupus disease, it remains unclear whether the increased levels of IFNs contribute to sex bias in SLE.

Type I IFNs are multifunctional cytokines with potent immuno-modulatory activities [20]. In IFN-responsive cells, binding of Type I IFNs to cell surface receptor results in activation of the receptor-associated Janus tyrosine kinases, Jak1 and Tyk2, which in turn leads to tyrosine phosphorylation and activation of latent transcription factors termed STATs [28]. The activated STATs then form homodimers or heterodimers and translocate into the nucleus, bind to conserved promoter sequences termed <u>i</u>nterferon <u>s</u>timulated <u>r</u>esponse <u>e</u>lement (ISRE), and induce the transcription of IFN-responsive genes. The IFN-stimulated gene factor 3 (ISGF3), which includes IRF9, and Stat1:Stat2 heterodimers binds to the ISRE sequence and activates transcription of the target genes. Notably, the type IFNs can also activate transcription of certain IFN-responsive genes independent of the Jak/STAT pathway [29].

Numerous studies have suggested role for IFN [20,24,25] and estrogen [4–6] signaling in the development of SLE. Moreover, the female hormone estrogen is known to up-regulate the expression of IFN-γ in immune cells [15,17–19]. Therefore, we explored whether IFNs could regulate expression of ERα. Here, we report that the IFNs (α or γ) up-regulate the expression of ERα and stimulate the ERα-mediated transcriptional activation of genes.

Materials and Methods

Mice and Cells

All mice were handled in accordance with good animal practice as defined by the requirement of the National Institutes of Health and the University of Cincinnati's animal committee, and all experimental protocols that are used in this manuscript were approved (approval #07-05-24-01) by the University of Cincinnati's Animal Care and Use Committee. Age-matched (~6–8 weeks old) male and female C57BL/6J and (NZB × NZW) F1 mice were purchased from The Jackson Laboratory. Age-matched wild type and homozygous Stat1-null 129S6/SvEv-Stat1tm1Rds mice (age ~6–8 weeks) [30] were purchased from Taconic Farm (Hudson, NY). All mice were housed in a germ-free Laboratory Animal and Medical Services facility of the University of Cincinnati.

Splenocyte Isolation, Cell culture, and Hormone Treatment

Total single cell splenocytes were prepared from male or female mice as described previously [31]. Unless, otherwise indicated, splenic cells from two or more age-matched male or female mice were pooled to prepare total RNA or protein extracts. Splenic B or T cells were purified from total splenic cells using magnetic beads from Miltenyi Biotech (Auburn, CA) as described previously [31]. Estrogen-responsive mouse breast cancer cell line WT276 [31] was generously provided by Dr. JoEllen Welsh, University of Notre Dame, Notre Dame, IN. Mouse RAW264.7 macrophage cell line was purchased from ATCC. Cells were maintained in DMEM medium supplemented with 10% fetal bovine serum and 1× antibiotic-antimycotic solution (Invitrogen, Carlsbad, CA). When indicated, mouse splenic cells or mouse cell lines were treated with either IFN-α (1,000 u/ml; Universal IFN-α, from R & D Systems, Minneapolis, MN) or murine IFN-γ (10 ng/ml) for the indicated duration. For treatment of mouse splenocytes or cell lines with 17-β-estradiol (E2; 1–10 nM), cells were cultured in phenol red-free RPMI 1640 medium (Invitrogen) and the medium was supplemented with 10% charcoal-stripped fetal bovine serum (Invitrogen). Splenocytes (5-8×10^6 cells) were used to isolate total RNA using TRIzol (Invitrogen).

Plasmids

The ERE-luc-reporter plasmid has been described previously [32]. The ISRE-luc-reporter plasmid was purchased from B D Biosciences (San Jose, CA). A plasmid reporter construct in which the murine $Esr1$ gene promoter-region (~5-kb) is linked to the β-galactosidase reporter gene was generously provided by Dr. Alessandro Weisz (Seconda Università degli Studi di Napoli, Italy) and the plasmid construct has been described [33].

Reporter Assays

For reporter assays, sub-confluent cultures of WT276 cells (in 6-well plates) were transfected with the indicated reporter plasmids (either ERE-luc or ISRE-luc; 1.8 µg plasmid DNA) and a second reporter plasmid pRL-TK (0.2 µg;), as an internal control to normalize the transfections efficiency, using the FuGENE 6 transfection reagent (Roche, Indianapolis, IN), as suggested by the supplier. When indicated, cells were either treated with ethanol (vehicle), the indicated concentration of E2, or IFN-α (1,000 u/ml) for 18 h. Unless, otherwise indicated, cells were harvested between 40 and 45 h after transfections. Cells were lysed, and the firefly and $Renilla$ dual luciferase activities were determined using a dual luciferase assay kit (Promega, Madison, WI) as described previously [31]. For β-galactosidase assay, a Galacto-Light Plus Systems kit (Applied Biosystems, Bedford, MA) was used following the manufacturer's instructions. For this assay, the units were normalized for total protein content measured with the Bio-Rad protein assay reagent.

RT-PCR and Quantitative Real-Time PCR Analysis

Splenocytes (5-8×10^6 cells) or purified (93–95% pure) splenic B or T cells (2-3×10^6 cells) were used to isolate total RNA using TRIzol (Invitrogen). Total RNA (2.0 µg) was used for or RT-PCR reaction. We used the Superscript one-step RT-PCR system from Invitrogen. Primers for the murine $Esr1$ gene that were used (forward: 5′-aattctgacaatcgacgccag- 3′; backward: 5′-gtgcttcaa-cattctccctcctc-3′) gave a single band of 345 base pair. Quantitative real-time TaqMan PCR technology (Applied Bio-systems, Foster City, CA, USA) was used to quantitate the steady-state levels of mRNAs. The PCR cycling program consisted of denaturation at 95°C for 10 min, 40 cycles at 95°C for 15 seconds, followed by annealing and elongation at 60°C for 1 min. The TaqMan assays for $Serpinb2$ (Assay Id# Mm00440905_m1), $Rab10$ (#Mm00489481_m1), $Ifi202$ (#Mm03048198 _m1), $Mx1$ (#Mm00487796_m1), $Syn25A$ (#Mm00836412_m1), $Esr1$ (Assay

Id#Mm00433 149_m1), and the endogenous control β2-micro-globulin (Assay Id#Mm00437762_ m1) were purchased from Applied Bio-systems (Foster City, CA) and used as suggested by the supplier.

Immunoblot Analysis

Total splenocytes, purified splenic B or T cells, WT276, or RAW264.7 cells were collected in PBS and re-suspended in a modified radio-immune precipitation assay (RIPA) lysis buffer (50 mM Tris-HCl, pH 8.0, 250 mM NaCl, 1% Nonidet P-40, 0.5% sodium deoxycholate, 0.1% SDS), supplemented with protease inhibitors (Roche Diagnostics, Mannheim, Germany) and phosphatase inhibitors (Sigma) and incubated at 4°C for 30 min. Cell lysates were sonicated briefly before centrifugation at 14,000 rpm in a microcentrifuge for 10 min at 4°C. The supernatants were collected, and the protein concentration was measured by Bio-Rad protein assay kit. Equal amounts of protein were processed for immunoblotting. Antibodies to detect mouse ERα (sc-542; MC-20), c-Jun (sc-1694; H-79), p-c-Jun (sc-822; KM-1), and β2-mcroglobulin (sc-13565) were purchased from Santa Cruz Biotechnology (Santa Cruz, CA). Antibodies to detect STAT1 (#9172), p-STAT1 (#9177), and β-actin (#4967) were purchased from Cell Signaling Technology (Danvers, MA).

Statistical Analysis

Data are presented as the means ± S.E. For statistical comparisons between two groups, Student's two-tailed t test was used. $p < 0.05$ was considered significant.

Results

IFN-Treatment Increases Steady-state Levels of ERα mRNA and Protein

To explore whether IFNs could regulate the expression of ERα, we treated total splenic cells from non lupus-prone C57BL/6 female mice with either the murine IFN-α (1,000 u/ml) or IFN-γ (10 ng/ml) and compared steady-state levels of ERα mRNA by quantitative real-time PCR. As shown in Fig. 1A, treatment of cells with IFN-α or IFN-γ measurably increased the steady-state levels of ERα mRNA. Interestingly, the increase was more pronounced (~50% versus 30%) after the IFN-α than IFN-γ treatment. Next, we compared the IFN-mediated increase in ERα mRNA levels between C57BL/6 male and age-matched female mice. As shown in Fig. 1B, treatment of total splenic cells with IFN-α measurably increased the steady-state levels of ERα mRNA (Fig 1B) and protein (Fig. 1C) in both male and female mice. Notably, the extent of IFN-α-mediated increase in ERα mRNA (Fig. 1B) and protein (Fig. 1C) was more appreciable (~2-4-fold) in male splenic cells than the age-matched females. Moreover, basal levels of ERα protein were reproducibly ~2-fold higher in splenic cells from females than the age-matched males in several experiments. Because we recently reported that the murine splenic B cells express relatively higher levels of ERα than T cells [31], we also compared ERα mRNA levels between purified splenic T and B cells. As shown in Fig. 1D, as compared to T cells, the B cells had significantly (~4-fold) higher levels of ERα mRNA. Together, these observations revealed that IFN-α or γ treatment of C57BL/6 splenic cells increases steady-state levels of ERα mRNA and protein.

We also tested whether IFN-treatment of splenic cells from pre-autoimmune (age ~8-weeks) lupus-prone (NZB × NZW) F₁ mice also increases ERα expression. As shown in Fig. 2, the IFN-α treatment of splenic cells from both male and female mice increased the steady-state levels of ERα mRNA as determined by

both semi-quantitative (Fig. 2A) and quantitative real-time PCR (Fig. 2B). Consistent with these observations, IFN-α treatment of splenic cells also increased ERα protein levels ~2-4-fold (Fig. 2C). Interestingly, basal levels of ERα mRNA (Fig. 2A, compare lane 3 with 1) and protein (Fig. 2C, compare lane 3 with 1) were measurably higher in (NZB × NZW) F₁ female mice as compared to the age-matched male mice. Furthermore, consistent with our above and the previous [31] observations, the basal levels of ERα protein were about two-fold higher in purified splenic B cells from female mice than the age-matched male mice and IFN-α treatment of B cells further increased the levels of ERα protein ~2-4-fold (Fig. 2D).

Binding of type I IFNs to the cell surface receptor activates multiple signaling pathways, including the classical Jak/STAT pathway, which lead to the transcriptional activation of the IFN-inducible genes [28,29]. Therefore, we explored whether the IFN-treatment of splenic B cells activates the STAT1 transcription factor. As shown in Fig. 2E, treatment of splenic B cells from (NZB × NZW) F₁ mice with IFN-α increased the activating phosphorylation of STAT1 and basal levels of STAT1 protein in both male and female splenic cells. Again, the extent of IFN-α-mediated increase in the phosphorylation of STAT1 and increase in the levels of ERα protein were more appreciable in male B cells than the age-matched females. Moreover, the basal levels of phospho-STAT1 and ERα protein were reproducibly higher in splenic cells from females than the age-matched males. Together, these observations suggested that the basal levels of ERα mRNA and protein are relatively higher in splenic cells from lupus-prone (NZB × NZW) F₁ females than the age and strain-matched males and IFN-α (or IFN-γ) treatment of splenic cells increases the steady-state levels of ERα mRNA and protein in both males and females. Additionally, these observations suggested that the basal levels of phospho-STAT1 and ERα in female B cells were relatively higher than the age-matched males and the IFN-α treatment of B cells increased the steady-state levels of both phospho-STAT1 and ERα further.

To investigate the molecular mechanisms by which IFN-signaling increases the steady-state levels of ERα mRNA and protein in mouse splenic cells, we investigated the effect of IFN-treatment of WT276 mouse breast cancer cell line (an ERα-positive cell line; ref. 31) on steady-state levels of ERα mRNA and protein. As shown in Fig. 3A, treatment of cells with either IFN-α or IFN-γ increased the ERα protein levels and the extent of the increase was dependent on the dose of IFN-α or IFN-γ. Moreover, steady-state levels of ERα mRNA were also increased after IFN-α or IFN-γ treatment as determined by semi-quantitative RT-PCR (Fig. 3B) and quantitative real-time PCR (Fig. 3C). Similarly, treatment of mouse macrophage cell line RAW264.7 with IFN-α or IFN-γ also increased steady-state levels of ERα mRNA and protein in a dose-dependent manner (data not shown). Together, these observations revealed that IFN-α or IFN-γ treatment of mouse cell lines that express ERα also increased the steady-state levels of ERα mRNA and protein.

Interferon-signaling Increases ERα mRNA Levels Primarily by Transcriptional Mechanism

Regulation of steady-state levels of ERα mRNA and protein is complex and the regulation may depend on the cell type [10–13]. Moreover, the promoter of the murine Esr1 gene is reported to be relatively weak and does not contain a TATA box [32,33,34]. Therefore, to investigate the molecular mechanisms by which IFN-α treatment of cells increased the expression of ERα, we compared levels of ERα mRNA in WT276 cells that were treated with IFN-α alone or along with actinomycin-D, an inhibitor of

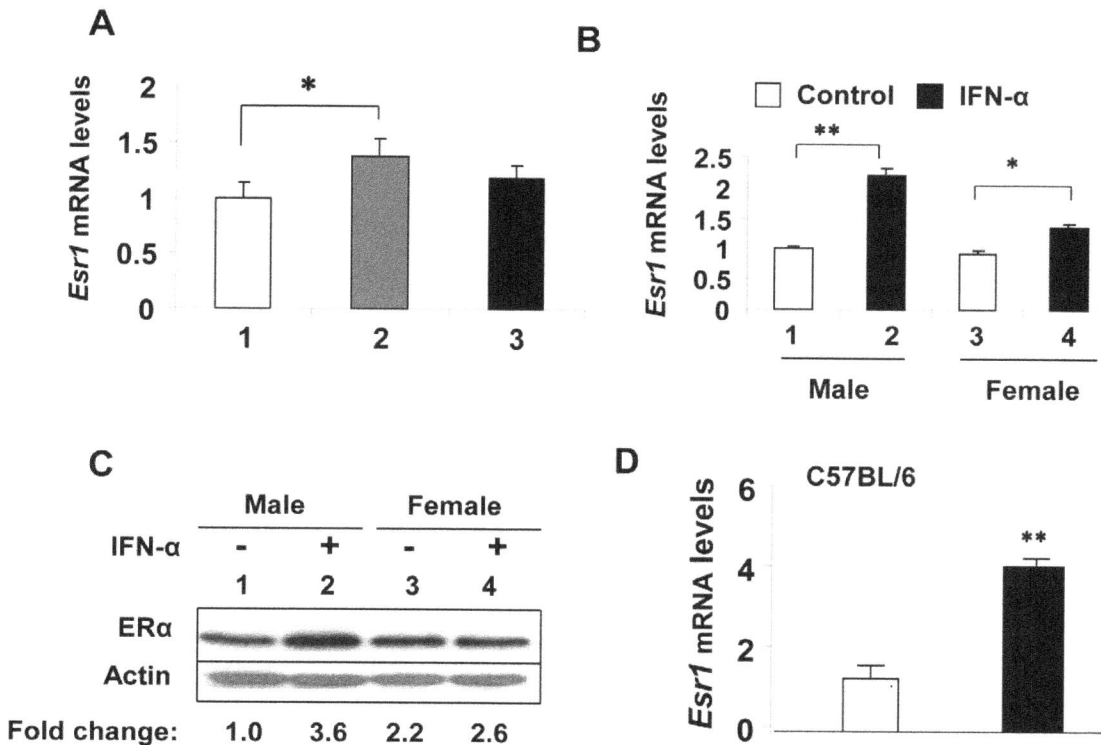

Figure 1. IFN-treatment increases steady-state levels of ERα mRNA and protein in C57BL/6 splenic cells. (A) Total RNA was isolated from control (column 1), IFN-α (column 2), or IFN-γ (column 3) treated total splenic cells that were prepared from female (age ~8 weeks) C57BL/6 mice. The RNA was analyzed for steady-sate levels of Esr1 mRNA by quantitative real-time PCR. The ratio of the Esr1 mRNA to β2-microglobulin mRNA was calculated in units (one unit being the ratio of Esr1 mRNA to β2-microglobulin mRNA). Results are mean values of triplicate experiments and error bars represent standard deviation ($^*p<0.05$). (B) Total RNA was isolated from control (column 1 and 3) or IFN-α (column 2 and 4) treated splenic cells that were prepared from either male (age ~8 weeks) or age-matched female C57BL/6 mice. The RNA was analyzed by quantitative real-time PCR for the steady-sate levels of Esr1 mRNA as described in (A). Results are mean values of triplicate experiments and error bars represent standard deviation ($^*p<0.05$; $^{**}p<0.005$). (C) Total protein extracts were prepared from control (lanes 1 and 3) or IFN-α (lanes 2 and 4) treated splenic cells that were isolated from either male (age ~8 weeks) or age-matched female C57BL/6 mice. The total cell extracts were analyzed by immunoblotting using antibodies specific to the indicated proteins. Fold change in ERα protein levels is indicated below the Figure. (D) Total RNA was isolated from purified splenic T cells (column 1) or B cells (column 2) isolated from female (age ~8 weeks) C57BL/6 mice. The RNA was analyzed by quantitative real-time PCR for steady-sate levels of Esr1 mRNA. Results are mean values of triplicate experiments and error bars represent the standard deviation ($^{**}p<0.005$).

gene transcription [35]. As shown in Fig. 4A, treatment of cells with the inhibitor alone decreased basal steady-state levels of ERα mRNA about 60% (compare column 3 with 1). Interestingly, co-treatment of cells with IFN-α plus the inhibitor abrogated the IFN-α-mediated increase in the ERα mRNA levels (compare column 4 with 2). Moreover, treatment of WT276 cells with IFN-α, cycloheximide (an inhibitor of protein synthesis) or both IFN-α plus cycloheximide increased steady-state levels of ERα mRNA (Fig. 4B) and protein (Fig. 4C). Together, these observations suggested that the IFN-α treatment of WT276 cells increases ERα mRNA levels primarily through a transcriptional mechanism and protein synthesis is required for a rapid turnover of the ERα mRNA in WT276 cells.

Expression of the Esr1 gene is STAT1-dependent

Transcription-dependent increase in ERα mRNA levels in IFN-treated cells (Fig. 4A) and an increased activating phosphorylation of STAT1 in IFN-α treated B cells, which associated with increased expression of ERα (Fig. 2E), prompted us to determine whether the IFN-treatment indeed activates the transcriptional of the Esr1 gene. As shown in Fig. 5A (Top panel), consistent with the presence of three potential interferon-sensitive response elements (ISREs) consensus

sequence (TTCCCGGAA) in the 5′-regulatory region of the Esr1 gene, treatment of WT276 cells with IFN-α stimulated the activity of a reporter gene, the transcription of which was driven by the 5′-reglatory region of the murine Esr1 gene [32]. Interestingly, consistent with our earlier observations (Fig. 1A) the stimulation of the reporter activity was relatively more in the IFN-α treated cells than IFN-γ. To further investigate how IFN-signaling activates the transcription of the Esr1 gene, we compared basal steady-sate levels of ERα mRNA and protein between wild type and STAT1-null male and female splenocytes. As shown in Fig. 5, steady-state levels of ERα mRNA (Fig. 5B) and protein (Fig. 5C) were significantly lower in STAT1-null male and females as compared to the wild-type age-matched mice. Consistent with a role for STAT1 in IFN-mediated signaling in transcriptional activation of the Esr1 gene, we noted that treatment of C57BL/6 splenocytes with fludarabine, an inhibitor of STAT1 phosphorylation [36], which resulted in inhibition of STAT1 phosphorylation (Fig. 5D), was associated with significantly reduced levels of ERα protein (Fig. 5D) and mRNA (Fig. 5E). Moreover, treatment of cells with JNK inhibitor II (SP600125, 60 nM in DMSO) did not result in any measurable decreases in the ERα protein levels (data not shown). Thus, ruling out IFN-mediate regulation of Esr1 expression through the JNK/AP-1 pathway.

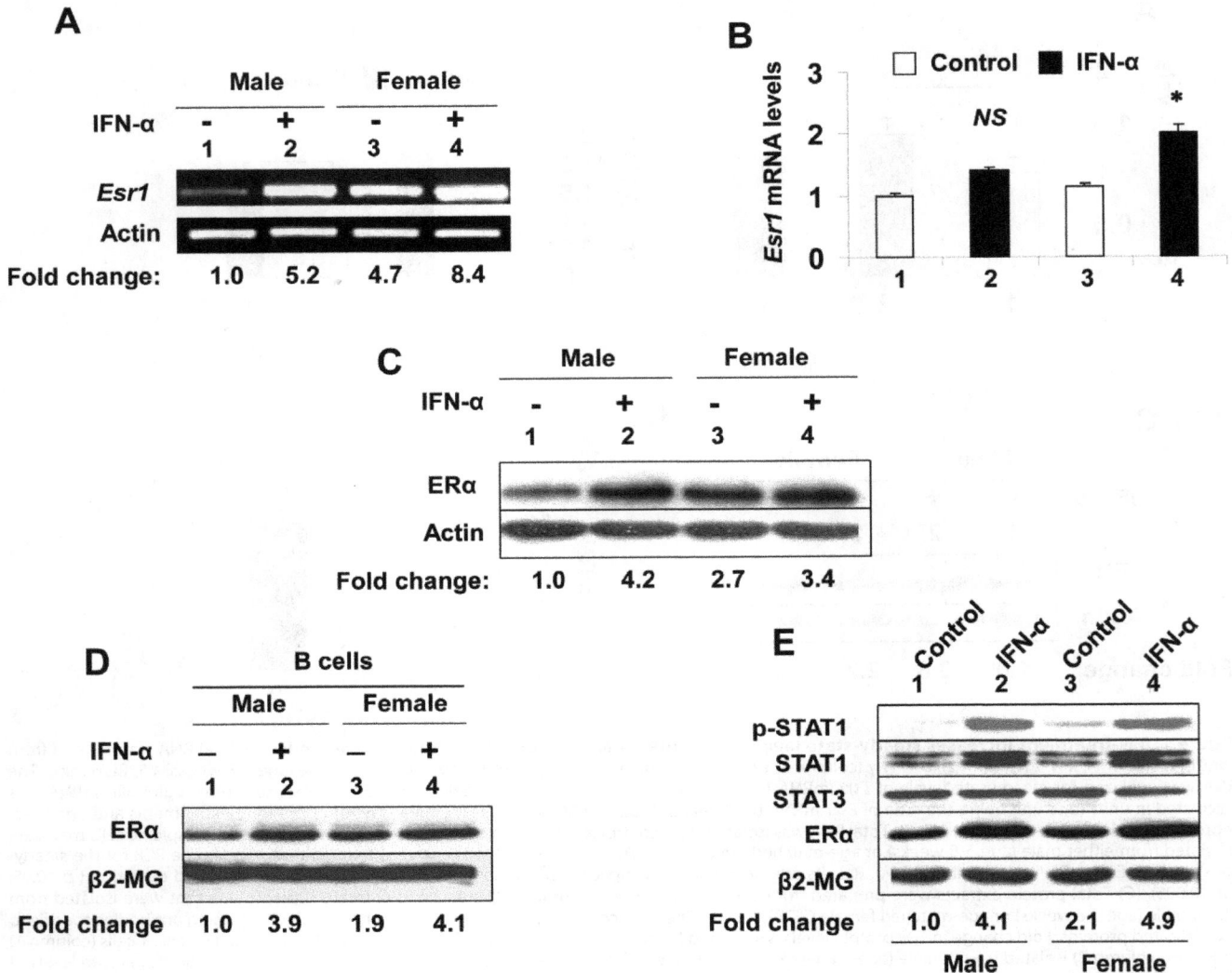

Figure 2. IFN-treatment increases steady-state levels of ERα mRNA and protein in splenic cells from lupus-prone (NZB × NZW) F₁ mice. (A) Total RNA isolated from control (lanes 1 and 3) or IFN-α (lanes 2 and 4) treated total splenic cells that were isolated from either male (age ~8 weeks) or age-matched female (NZB × NZW) F₁ mice. The total RNA was analyzed for steady-state levels of Esr1 mRNA by semi-quantitative RT-PCR. Fold change in Esr1 mRNA levels is indicated below the Figure. (B) Total RNA isolated from control (columns 1 and 3) or IFN-α (columns 2 and 4) treated total splenic cells that were isolated from either male (age ~8 weeks) or age-matched female (NZB × NZW) F₁ mice. The total RNA was analyzed for the steady-state levels of Esr1 mRNA by quantitative real-time PCR. Results are mean values of triplicate experiments and error bars represent standard deviation (*$p < 0.05$; NS, not significant). (C) Total protein extracts were prepared from control (lanes 1 and 3) or IFN-α (lanes 2 and 4) treated splenic cells that were isolated from either male (age ~8 weeks) or age-matched female (NZB × NZW)F₁ mice. The total cell extracts were analyzed by immunoblotting using antibodies specific to the indicated proteins. Fold change in ERα protein levels is indicated below the Figure. (D and E) Total protein extracts were prepared from control (lanes 1 and 3) or IFN-α (lanes 2 and 4) treated purified splenic B cells that were isolated from either male (age ~8 weeks) or age-matched female (NZB × NZW) F₁ mice. The total cell extracts were analyzed by immunoblotting using antibodies specific to the indicated proteins. Fold change in ERα protein levels is indicated below the Figures.

Our observations that basal levels of pSTAT1 are relatively higher in (NZB × NZW) F₁ females than the age-matched males (Fig. 2E) and STAT1-null mice express relatively low levels of ERα (Fig. 5C) prompted us to compare the specific DNA-binding activities of STAT1 between males and female B cells. This approach revealed that the specific DNA-binding activity of STAT1 in nuclear extracts from C57BL/6 female B cells was measurably higher than the age-matched males in gel-mobility shift assays (data not shown). Moreover, IFN-treatment of cells increased the DNA-binding relatively in extracts from both female and male mice; however, the increase in the DNA-binding was

higher in extracts from females than males. Together, these observations demonstrated that IFN-signaling up-regulates the expression of the murine Esr1 gene in gender-dependent manner through the activation of STAT1.

The IFN and E2-signaling Cooperate to Activate Transcription

Up-regulation of ERα expression by IFN-signaling in the murine cells in the above experiments prompted us to determine whether the IFN and E2-signaling cooperate with each other to

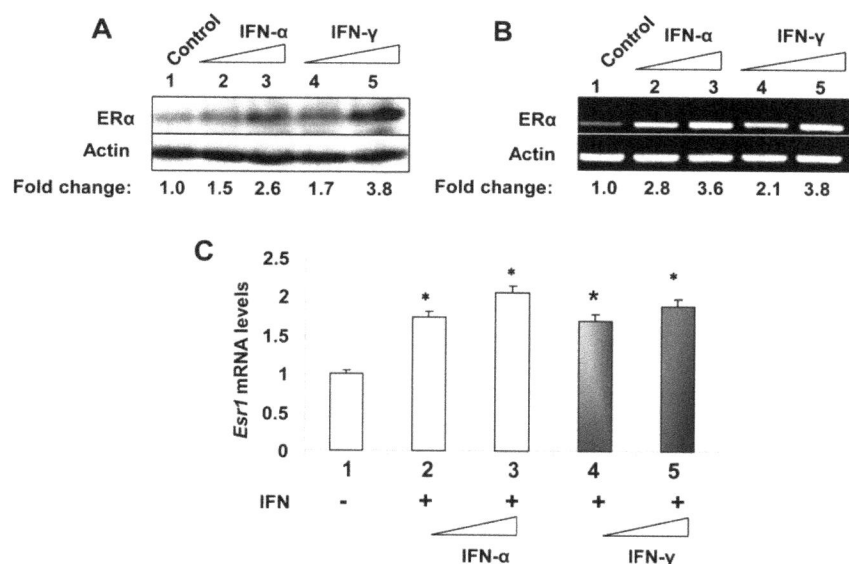

Figure 3. IFN-treatment increases steady-state levels of ERα mRNA and protein in mouse breast cancer cell line WT276. (A) Total protein extracts were prepared from control (lane 1), increasing concentrations (1,000 or 2000 u/ml) of IFN-α (lanes 2 and 3, respectively) or IFN-γ (5 or 10 ng/ml; lanes 4 and 5, respectively) treated WT276 cells. As a negative control, we also included extracts from AKR-2B cells. The extracts were analyzed by immunoblotting using the antibodies specific to the indicated proteins. Fold change in ERα protein levels is indicated below the Figure. (B) Total RNA was isolated from control (lane 1), increasing concentrations of IFN-α (lanes 2 and 3) or IFN-γ (lanes 4 and 5) treated WT276 cells. As a positive control, we also included RNA from splenic cells. The total RNA was analyzed for steady-state levels of *Esr1* mRNA by semi-quantitative RT-PCR. Fold change in ERα mRNA levels is indicated below the Figure. (C) Total RNA was isolated from control (column 1), increasing concentrations of IFN-α (columns 2 and 3) or IFN-γ (columns 4 and 5) treated WT276 cells. The total RNA was analyzed for steady-state levels of *Esr1* mRNA by quantitative real-time PCR. Results are mean values of triplicate experiments and error bars represent standard deviation ($^*p<0.05$).

activate transcriptional of target genes. As shown in Fig. 6A, treatment of WT276 cells with E2 stimulated the activity of an E2-responsive reporter about 3-fold (compare column 2 with 1).

However, treatment of cells with IFN-α (in the absence of E2) did not result in stimulation of the activity of the reporter (compare column 3 with 1). Interestingly, treatment of cells with both E2 and

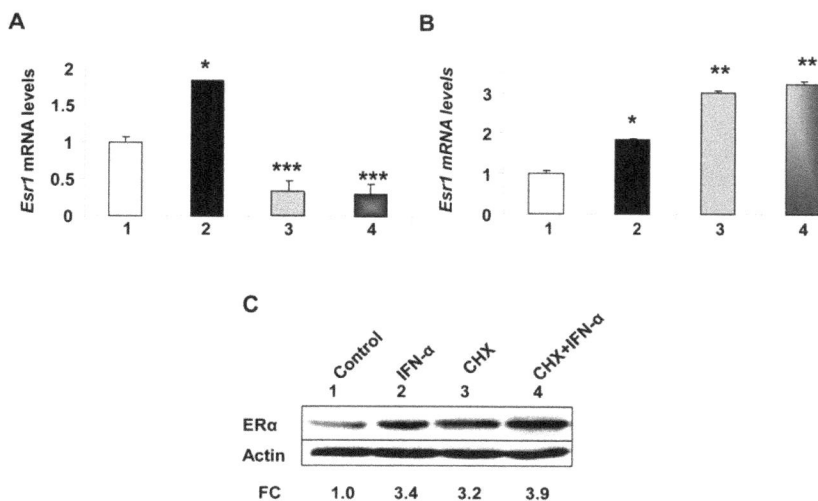

Figure 4. Interferon-signaling increases ERα mRNA levels primarily by Transcriptional mechanism. (A) Total RNA was isolated from control (column 1), IFN-α (column 2), actinomycin D (column 3), or both IFN-α and actinomycin D (column 4) treated WT276 cells. The RNA was analyzed by quantitative real-time PCR for steady-state levels of *Esr1* mRNA. Results are mean values of triplicate experiments and error bars represent standard deviation ($^*p<0.05$; $^{***}p<0.0005$). (B) Total RNA was isolated from control (column 1), IFN-α (column 2), cycloheximide (column 3), or both IFN-α and cycloheximide (column 4) treated WT276 cells. The RNA was analyzed by quantitative real-time PCR for steady-sate levels of Esr1 mRNA. Results are mean values of triplicate experiments and error bars represent standard deviation ($^*p<0.05$; $^{**}p<0.005$). (C) Total cell extracts were prepared from control (lane 1), IFN-α (lane 2), cycloheximide (lane 3), or both IFN-α and cycloheximide (lane 4) treated WT276 cells. The cell extracts were analyzed by immunoblotting using antibodies specific to the indicated proteins. Fold change in ERα protein levels is indicated below the Figure.

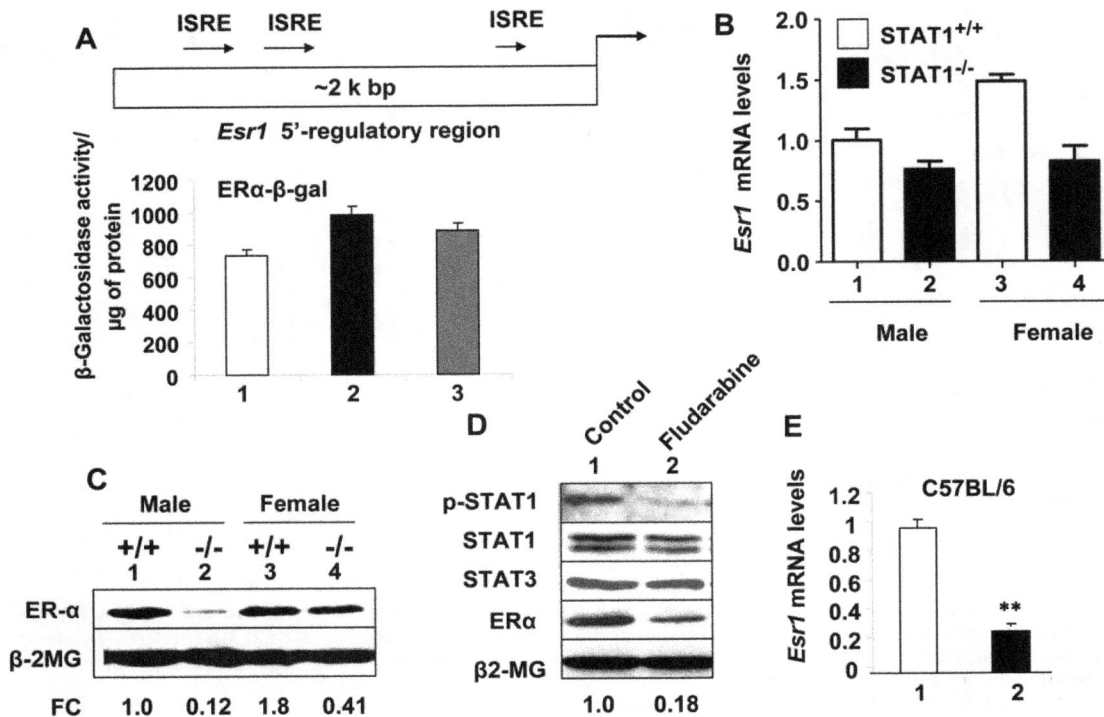

Figure 5. Expression of the *Esr1* gene is dependent on activation of STAT1. (A) Top panel: Schematic presentation of the 5′-regulatory region of the murine *Esr1* gene (the NCBI accession # for the sequence: NT_039490.7) and potential *cis*-elements that are predicted to render the gene responsive to the IFN treatment. The regulatory sequence for the gene is derived from the C57BL/6J strain of mice. The regulatory region includes three potential ISREs for binding of activated STAT1 (ISGF3) transcription factor. Bottom panel: Sub-confluent cultures of WT276 cells in a 6-well plate were transfected with ERα promoter-β-galactosidase plasmid (2 µg) along with pRL-TK (0.2 µg) plasmid using the FuGene 6 transfection agent. 24 h after transfections, cells were either left untreated treated (column1), treated with IFN-α (column 2), or IFN-γ (column 3). 40–45 h after transfections, cells were lysed and the lysates were processed for estimation of protein followed by β-galactosidase activity assays. (B) Total RNA was isolated from wilt-type (columns 1 and 3) or STAT1-null (columns 2 and 4) total splenic cells that were prepared from male or age-matched female (age ~8 weeks) mice. The RNA was analyzed by quantitative real-time PCR for steady-sate levels of *Esr1* mRNA. (C) Total cell extracts were prepared from wilt-type (lanes 1 and 3) or STAT1-null (lanes 2 and 4) total splenic cells that were prepared from male or age-matched female (age ~8 weeks) mice. The RNA was analyzed by quantitative real-time PCR for steady-sate levels of *Esr1* mRNA. Fold change in ERα protein levels is indicated below the Figure. (D) Total cell isolated from C57BL/6 were either left untreated (lane 1) or treated with fludarabine (lane 2) for 24 h. Total cell extracts were prepared and analyzed by immunoblotting using antibodies specific to the indicated proteins. Fold change in ERα protein levels is indicated below the Figure. (E) Total cell isolated from C57BL/6 were either left untreated (lane 1) or treated with fludarabine (lane 2) for 24 h. Total RNA was prepared and steady-state levels of Esr1 mRNA were analyzed by quantitative real-time PCR. Results are mean values of triplicate experiments and error bars represent standard deviation ($^{**}p<0.005$).

IFN-α resulted in significantly increased stimulation of the activity of reporter (compare column 4 with 2). Because treatment of WT276 cells with E2 did not result in measurable increases (or decreases) in the ERα mRNA levels (data not shown), the above observations indicated that the IFN-induced levels of ERα increase the E2-mediated transcription of the ERα target genes.

Because E2 treatment of ER-positive cells is known to result in production of IFN-γ in a variety of cells [17–19], which up-regulates expression of IRF9 (a component of the ISGF3 transcription factor; ref. 29), we also tested whether treatment of cells with E2 alone or both E2 and IFN-α has any effect on expression of an IFN-responsive reporter gene. As shown in Fig. 6B, treatment of WT276 cells with E2 alone resulted in ~3-fold stimulation of the activity of the ISRE-luc-reporter, an IFN-responsive reporter. Furthermore, treatment of cells with IFN-α alone stimulated the activity of the reporter ~5-fold. Interestingly, treatment of cells with both IFN-α and E2 stimulated the activity of reporter ~14-fold. Together, our observations indicated that both E2 and IFN-α signaling cooperate with each other to activate the transcription of certain ERα and IFN-responsive genes.

Sex Bias in the Expression of IFN and E2-responsive Genes

Increased steady-state levels of ERα mRNA (Fig. 2A) protein (Fig. 2B and C) in splenic cells from (NZB × NZW) F1 female mice as compared to age-matched male mice and cooperation between the IFN and E2-signaling in cells to activate transcription of reporter genes (Fig. 6) prompted us to investigate whether the expression of E2 or IFN-responsive genes is differentially regulated between male and female (NZB × NZW) F1 lupus-prone mice. As shown in Fig. 7A, we noted that steady-state levels of mRNAs encoded by two E2-responsive genes were relatively higher in female (NZB × NZW) F1 mice than the age-matched males (Fig. 7A). Similarly, steady-state levels of mRNA encoded by three IFN-responsive genes were relatively higher in female mice than the age-matched male mice (Fig. 7B). Together, these observations demonstrated a sex bias in the expression of both E2 and IFN-responsive genes.

Discussion

The development of SLE is known to have a strong sex bias [3–6]. Moreover, peak SLE disease incidence in women occurs

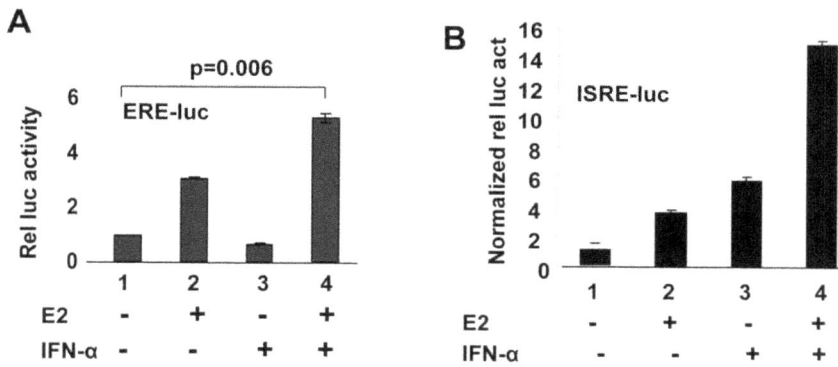

Figure 6. The IFN and E2-signaling cooperate to activate transcription of genes. (A) Sub-confluent cultures of WT276 cells in a 6-well plate were transfected with ERE-luc-reporter plasmid (2 μg) along with pRL-TK (0.2 μg) plasmid using FuGENE 6 transfection reagent. 24 h after transfections, cells were either left untreated (column 1), treated with E2 (column 2), IFN-α (column 3) or E2 and IFN-α (column 4). 40–45 h after transfections, cells were processed for dual luciferase activity. Result are mean values of triplicate experiments and error bars represent standard deviation (p value is 0.006). (B) Sub-confluent cultures of WT276 cells in a 6-well plate were transfected with ISRE-luc-reporter plasmid (2 μg) along with pRL-TK (0.2 μg) plasmid using FuGENE 6 transfection reagent. 24 h after transfections, cells were either left untreated (column 1), treated with E2 (column 2), IFN-α (column 3) or E2 and IFN-α (column 4). 40–45 h after transfections, cells were processed for dual luciferase activity.

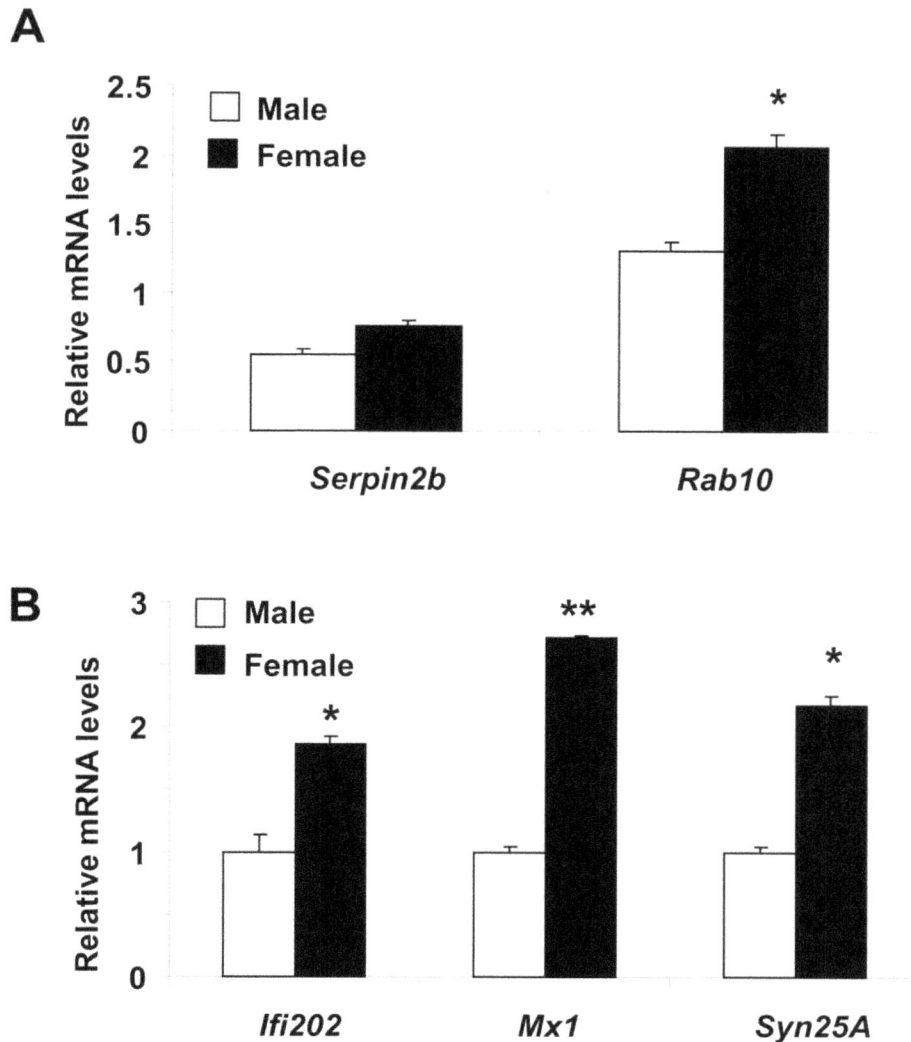

Figure 7. Sex bias in the expression of IFN and E2-responsive genes. (A and B) Total RNA isolated from pre-autoimmune (age ~8 weeks) male or age-matched female (NZB × NZW) F_1 mice was analyzed for steady-state levels of the indicated known estrogen-responsive (A) and IFN-responsive (B) genes by quantitative real-time PCR. Results are mean values of triplicate experiments and error bars represent standard deviation ($^*p < 0.05$; $^{**}p < 0.005$).

during the early reproductive years (ages 20–30 years) [37]. Additionally, risk of SLE development is associated with the use of combined oral contraceptives [38]. Studies have revealed that PBMCs from SLE patients overexpress IFN-α-inducible genes as compared with healthy individuals [7] and high serum IFN-α level is a heritable risk factor for SLE development [37]. Notably, activation of TLR7-induced signaling is associated with higher IFN-α production in females [39] and the peak time frame for lupus onset in women coincides with an increase in IFN-α activity [37]. In light of the above observations, our observations that: (i) activation of IFN-signaling up-regulates the expression of ERα (Figs. 1, 2 and 3); and (ii) E2 and IFN-signaling cooperate to activate transcription of certain target genes (Figs. 6 and 7) provide support for the idea that the female sex hormone estrogen and increased levels of IFN-α contribute to sex bias in SLE through the activation of a mutually positive feedback loop.

A recent study [40] has revealed that estrogen treatment of splenocytes enhances STAT1 DNA-binding activity without increasing the levels of phosphorylated and total STAT1. Furthermore, the study also noted that estrogen induces serine protease-mediated proteolysis of STAT1, which may alter and enhance the activity of the transcription factor. In contrast to this report, we noted that steady-state levels of phospho-STAT1 and total STAT1 were consistently higher in splenocytes from female mice than the age-matched males. Moreover, we did not detect any additional forms of the STAT1 in extracts from female mice as compared to males (data not shown). Therefore, further work will be needed to resolve this apparent discrepancy.

A study [10] revealed that treatment of BALB/c mice with ER-subtype-selective agonists that results in activation of ERα, but not ERβ, plays a major role in estrogen-induced thymic atrophy and thymic T cell and splenic B cell phenotype alterations. Moreover, the study also revealed that ERα, but not ERβ, mediates the estrogen-induced up-regulation of IFN-γ. Similarly, a recent study has demonstrated a role for ERα in E2-induced development of the lupus phenotype in mice [16]. Consistent with these studies, generation of ERα knockout (NZB × NZW)F$_1$ mice and their characterization revealed that E2 through ERα promotes lupus disease, in part, by inducing the IFN-γ production [15]. Moreover, estrogen is known to enhance IFN-γ production by CD11c$^+$ cells [18]. Together, these observations raise the possibility that estrogen signaling through ERα in certain strains of female mice up-regulates expression of IFN-inducible genes, in part, by increasing the production of IFN-γ (Fig. 8).

The murine Esr1 gene is transcribed from a complex transcription unit with multiple potential promoters and upstream regulatory sequences [32,34]. Consistent with this observation, multiple transcription start sites have been identified in the regulatory region of the gene. Moreover, the promoter of the Esr1 gene is reported to be relatively weak [33]. Therefore, our observations that treatment of cells with IFN-α or IFN-γ resulted in a modest stimulation of the activity of the reporter, the expression of which was driven by the 5'-regulatory region (~5-kb) of the Esr1 gene (Fig. 5A), are consistent with the above reports.

A study [26] has noted differences in estrogen receptors levels between BALB/c mice, which do not get autoimmune disease and two strains that do (MRL/MP-lpr/lpr and NZB/W mice). Therefore, our observations that basal as well as IFN-induced levels of ERα were relatively higher in non lupus-prone (C57BL/6) as well as lupus-prone (NZB × NZW) F$_1$ female mice as compared to the age and strain-matched males will require further work to determine whether other factors, such as promoter polymorphisms in the Esr1 gene, also contribute to differential expression of ERα in certain strains of mice.

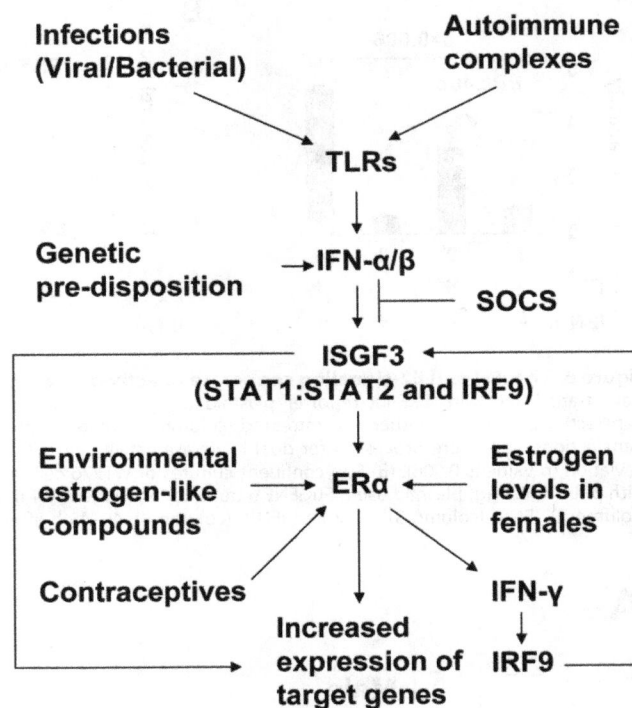

Figure 8. Cooperation between the IFN and E2-signaling in sex bias in SLE in mice. Increased levels of type I IFNs up-regulate expression of ERα. Activation of ERα by the female sex hormone estrogen leads to up-regulation of IFN-γ and IFN-γ-inducible IRF9. Increased levels of the IRF9 potentiate ISGF3-mediated transcription of IFN-inducible genes, which mediate the immunomodulatory functions of the IFNs.

Notably, a study has provided evidence that the XX sex chromosome complement, as compared with XY, confers greater susceptibility to certain autoimmune diseases, such as experimental autoimmune encephalomyelitis (EAE) and pristane-induced lupus [41]. However, it remains unclear whether the XX sex chromosome complement also contributes to sex bias in mouse models of lupus disease, such as (NZB × NZW) F$_1$, which spontaneously develop the disease. Therefore, further work will be needed to investigate the role of XX sex chromosomes in these mouse models of the disease.

In summary, our observations provide support for our model (Fig. 8). The model predicts that increased levels of IFNs (IFN-α or IFN-γ) in serum of SLE patients and certain lupus-prone strains of female mice, by up-regulating the expression of ERα, potentiate the expression of certain E2 and IFN-responsive genes. Notably, increased expression of the IFN-inducible genes is associated with the active disease in SLE patients [20,24] and certain lupus-prone strains of mice [26]. Importantly, increased expression of these IFN-inducible genes is associated with increased survival of autoreactive immune cells and autoimmunity [20,24,31]. Therefore, our observations concerning a mutually positive feedback loop between IFNs and ERα in mice provide a potential molecular basis for the sex bias in SLE. Further work will be needed to determine whether increased levels of type I IFN in SLE patients are associated with up-regulation of ERα expression and active SLE.

Author Contributions

Conceived and designed the experiments: RP DC. Performed the experiments: RP HS XZ. Analyzed the data: HS XZ SmH DC. Contributed reagents/materials/analysis tools: SmH. Wrote the paper: RP DC.

References

1. Kotzin BL (1996) Systemic lupus erythematosus. Cell 85: 303–306.
2. Crispín JC, Liossis SN, Kis-Toth K, Lieberman LA, Kyttaris VC, et al. (2010) Pathogenesis of human systemic lupus erythematosus: recent advances. Trends Mol Med 16: 47–57.
3. Whitacre CC (2001) Sex differences in autoimmune disease. Nat Immunol 2: 777–780.
4. Rider V, Abdou NI (2001) Gender differences in autoimmunity: molecular basis for estrogen effects in systemic lupus erythematosus. Int Immunopharmacol 1: 1009–1024.
5. Cohen-Solal JF, Jeganathan V, Grimaldi CM, Peeva E, Diamond B (2006) Sex hormones and SLE: influencing the fate of auto reactive B cells. Curr Top Microbiol Immunol 305: 67–88.
6. Zandman-Goddard G, Peeva E, Shoenfeld Y (2007) Gender and autoimmunity. Autoimmun Rev 6: 366–372.
7. Inui A, Ogasawara H, Naito T, Sekigawa I, Takasaki Y, et al. (2007) Estrogen receptor expression by peripheral blood mononuclear cells of patients with systemic lupus erythematosus. Clin Rheumatol 26: 1675–1678.
8. Roubinian JR, Papoian R, Talal N (1977) Androgenic hormones modulate autoantibody response and improve survival in murine lupus. J Clin Invest 59: 1066–1070.
9. Roubinian JR, Talal N, Greenspan JS, Siiteri PK (1978) Effect of castration and sex hormone treatment on survival, anti-nucleic acid antibodies, and glomerulonephritis in NZB/NZW F1 mice. J Exp Med 147: 1568–1583.
10. Li J, McMurray RW (2006) Effects of estrogen receptor subtype-selective agonists on immune functions in ovariectomized mice. Int Immunopharmacol 6: 1413–1423.
11. Li J, McMurray RW (2007) Effects of estrogen receptor subtype-selective agonists on autoimmune disease in lupus-prone NZB/NZW F1 mouse model. Clin Immunol 123: 219–226.
12. Carroll JS, Brown M (2006) Estrogen receptor target gene: an evolving concept. Mol Endocrinol 20: 1707–1714.
13. Deroo BJ, Korach KS (2006) Estrogen receptors and human disease. J Clin Invest 116: 561–570.
14. Erlandsson MC, Ohlsson C, Gustafsson JA, Carlsten H (2001) Role of oestrogen receptors-α and -β in immune organ development and in oestrogen-mediated effects on thymus. Immunology 103: 17–25.
15. Bynote KK, Hackenberg JM, Korach KS, Lubahn DB, Lane PH, et al. (2008) Estrogen receptor-α deficiency attenuates autoimmune disease in (NZB × NZW)F1 mice. Genes Immun 9: 137–152.
16. Feng F, Nyland J, Banyai M, Tatum A, Silverstone AE, et al. (2009) The induction of the lupus phenotype by estrogen is via an estrogen receptor-alpha-dependent pathway. Clin Immunol 134: 226–236.
17. Gourdy P, Araujo LM, Zhu R, Garmy-Susini B, Diem S, et al. (2005) Relevance of sexual dimorphism to regulatory T cells: estradiol promotes IFN-γ production by invariant natural killer T cells. Blood 105: 2415–2420.
18. Siracusa MC, Overstreet MG, Housseau F, Scott AL, Klein SL (2008) 17β-Estradiol alters the activity of conventional and IFN-producing killer dendritic cells. J Immunol 180: 1423–1431.
19. Nakaya M, Tachibana H, Yamada K (2006) Effect of estrogens on the interferon-gamma producing cell population of mouse splenocytes. Biosci Biotechnol Biochem 70: 47–53.
20. Theofilopoulos AN, Baccala R, Beutler B, Kono DH (2005) Type I interferon (α/β) in immunity and autoimmunity. Annu Rev Immunol 23: 307–336.
21. Harigai M, Kawamoto M, Hara M, Kubota T, Kamatani N, et al. (2008) Excessive production of IFN-γ in patients with systemic lupus erythematosus and its contribution to induction of B lymphocyte stimulator/B cell activating Factor/TNF ligand superfamily-13B. J Immunol 181: 2211–2219.
22. Theofilopoulos AN, Koundouris S, Kono DH, Lawson BR (2001) The role of IFN-γ in systemic lupus erythematosus: a challenge to the Th1/Th2 paradigm in autoimmunity. Arthritis Res 3: 136–41.
23. Haas C, Ryffel B, Hir ML (1998) IFN-receptor deletion prevents autoantibody production and glomerulonephritis in lupus-prone (NZB × NZW) F1 mice. J Immunol 160: 3713–3718.
24. Banchereau J, Pascual V (2006) Type I interferon in systemic lupus erythematosus and other autoimmune diseases. Immunity 25: 383–392.
25. Baccala R, Hoebe K, Kono DH, Beutler B, Theofilopoulos AN (2007) TLR-dependent and TLR-independent pathways of type I interferon induction in systemic autoimmunity. Nat Med 13: 543–551.
26. Lu Q, Shen N, Li ZM, Chen SL (2007) Genomic view of IFN-α response in pre-autoimmune NZB/NZW and MRL/lpr mice. Genes Immunity 8: 590–603.
27. Santiago-Raber ML, Baccala R, Haraldsson KM, Choubey D, Stewart TA, et al. (2003) Type-I interferon receptor deficiency reduces lupus-like disease in NZB mice. J Exp Med 197: 777–88.
28. Stark GR, Williams BRG, Silverman RH, Schreiber RD (1999) How cells respond to interferons? Ann Rev Biochem 67: 227–262.
29. Platanias LC (2005) Mechanisms of type-I- and type-II-interferon-mediated signaling. Nat Rev Immunol 5: 375–386.
30. Meraz MA, White JM, Sheehan KC, Bach EA, Rodig SJ, et al. (1996) Targeted disruption of the Stat1 gene in mice reveals unexpected physiologic specificity in the JAK-STAT signaling pathway. Cell 84: 431–442.
31. Panchanathan R, Shen H, Gubbels Bupp M, Gould KA, Choubey D (2009) Female and male sex hormones differentially regulate expression of Ifi202, an interferon-inducible lupus susceptibility gene within the Nba2 interval. J Immunol 183: 7031–7038.
32. Kipp JL, Kilen SM, Woodruff TK, Mayo KE (2007) Activin regulates estrogen receptor gene expression in the mouse ovary. J Biol Chem 282: 36755–36765.
33. Cicatiello L, Cobellis G, Addeo R, Papa M, Altucci L, et al. (1995) In vivo functional analysis of the mouse estrogen receptor gene promoter: a transgenic mouse model to study tissue-specific and developmental regulation of estrogen receptor gene transcription. Mol Endocrinol 9: 1077–1090.
34. Ishibashi O, Kawashima H (2001) Cloning and characterization of the functional promoter of mouse estrogen receptor beta gene. Biochim Biophys Acta 1519: 223–229.
35. Clayman CH, Collett MS, Faras AJ (1977) In vitro transcription of the avian oncornavirus genome by the RNA-directed DNA polymerase: effect of actinomycin D on the extent of transcription. J Virol 23: 209–212.
36. Johnston JB, Jiang Y, van Marle G, Mayne MB, Ni W, et al. (2000) Lentivirus infection in the brain induces matrix metalloproteinase expression: role of envelope diversity. J Virol 74: 7211–7220.
37. Niewold TB, Adler JE, Glenn SB, Lehman TJ, Harley JB, et al. (2008) Age- and sex-related patterns of serum interferon-alpha activity in lupus families. Arthritis Rheum 58: 2113–2119.
38. Bernier MO, Mikaeloff Y, Hudson M, Suissa S (2009) Combined oral contraceptive use and the risk of systemic lupus erythematosus. Arthritis Rheum 61: 476–481.
39. Berghöfer B, Frommer T, Haley G, Fink L, Bein G, et al. (2006) TLR7 ligands induce higher IFN-alpha production in females. J Immunol 177: 2088–2096.
40. Dai R, Phillips RA, Karpuzoglu E, Khan D, Ahmed SA (2009) Estrogen regulates transcription factors STAT-1 and NF-κB to promote inducible nitric oxide synthase and inflammatory responses. J Immunol 183: 6998–7005.
41. Smith-Bouvier DL, Divekar AA, Sasidhar M, Du S, Tiwari-Woodruff SK, et al. (2008) A role for sex chromosome complement in the female bias in autoimmune disease. J Exp Med 205: 1099–1108.

4

Antibodies Elicited in Response to EBNA-1 may Cross-React with dsDNA

Pragya Yadav[1,2], **Hoa Tran**[3], **Roland Ebegbe**[3], **Paul Gottlieb**[2,3,4], **Hui Wei**[4], **Rita H. Lewis**[3], **Alice Mumbey-Wafula**[4], **Atira Kaplan**[4], **Elina Kholdarova**[4], **Linda Spatz**[2,3,4]*

1 Department of Chemistry, The City College of New York and the Graduate Center of the City University of New York, New York, New York, United States of America, 2 The Ph.D. program in Biochemistry, The City College of New York and the Graduate Center of the City University of New York, New York, New York, United States of America, 3 The Graduate School of Biology, The City College of New York, New York, New York, United States of America, 4 Department of Microbiology and Immunology, Sophie Davis School of Biomedical Education, The City College of New York, New York, New York, United States of America

Abstract

Background: Several genetic and environmental factors have been linked to Systemic Lupus Erythematosus (SLE). One environmental trigger that has a strong association with SLE is the Epstein Barr Virus (EBV). Our laboratory previously demonstrated that BALB/c mice expressing the complete EBNA-1 protein can develop antibodies to double stranded DNA (dsDNA). The present study was undertaken to understand why anti-dsDNA antibodies arise during the immune response to EBNA-1.

Methodology/Principal Findings: In this study, we demonstrated that mouse antibodies elicited in response to EBNA-1 cross-react with dsDNA. First, we showed that adsorption of sera reactive with EBNA-1 and dsDNA, on dsDNA cellulose columns, diminished reactivity with EBNA-1. Next, we generated mononclonal antibodies (MAbs) to EBNA-1 and showed, by several methods, that they also reacted with dsDNA. Examination of two cross-reactive MAbs—3D4, generated in this laboratory, and 0211, a commercial MAb—revealed that 3D4 recognizes the carboxyl region of EBNA-1, while 0211 recognizes both the amino and carboxyl regions. In addition, 0211 binds moderately well to the ribonucleoprotein, Sm, which has been reported by others to elicit a cross-reactive response with EBNA-1, while 3D4 binds only weakly to Sm. This suggests that the epitope in the carboxyl region may be more important for cross-reactivity with dsDNA while the epitope in the amino region may be more important for cross-reactivity with Sm.

Conclusions/Significance: In conclusion, our results demonstrate that antibodies to the EBNA-1 protein cross-react with dsDNA. This study is significant because it demonstrates a direct link between the viral antigen and the development of anti-dsDNA antibodies, which are the hallmark of SLE. Furthermore, it illustrates the crucial need to identify the epitopes in EBNA-1 responsible for this cross-reactivity so that therapeutic strategies can be designed to mask these regions from the immune system following EBV exposure.

Editor: Paulo Lee Ho, Instituto Butantan, Brazil

Funding: This study was supported by grants SO6 GM 08168 from the National Institute of General Medical Sciences (NIGMS)/Support of Continuous Research Excellence (SCORE), NIH/NCRR/RCMI 5G12 RR03060 from the National Center for Research Resources Centers in Minority Institutions and the Professional Staff Congress at the City University of New York (PSC-CUNY) foundation. The funders had no role in study design, data collection and analysis, decision to publish, or preparation of the manuscript.

Competing Interests: The authors have declared that no competing interests exist.

* E-mail: lspatz@med.cuny.edu

Introduction

Systemic Lupus Erythematosus (SLE) is a chronic autoimmune disease characterized by the production of antibodies to double stranded DNA (dsDNA) and ribonucleoproteins. The etiology of SLE is unknown, although genetic and environmental causes have been implicated. Several viruses have been linked to SLE, however, the strongest association has been made with the Epstein-Barr virus (EBV). EBV is a lymphotropic, dsDNA herpes virus that infects 90–95% of adults in the United States [1]. Despite this high incidence of infection, only a small subset of infected individuals will develop SLE [2]. Epidemiological studies have demonstrated a higher incidence of EBV infection and higher titers of antibodies to EBV in both young and adult lupus patients relative to healthy individuals. James et al., observed seroconversion (development of IgG antibodies to EBV viral capsid antigen) in 99% of adolescent SLE patients compared to 70% of healthy adolescents and 72% of adolescents with other rheumatic diseases [3]. In addition, they observed by PCR analysis, the presence of EBV DNA in lymphocytes of 100% of SLE patients tested, compared to 72% of controls. McClain et.al. observed that antibodies to a major EBV nuclear antigen, EBNA-1, which is continuously expressed in latently infected B cells, arose in all pediatric SLE patients examined compared to only 69% of healthy pediatric controls [4].

EBNA-1 is a DNA binding protein that maintains replication of the EBV genome within infected cells. It is also required for maintaining viral latency. Several studies suggest that exposure to

EBNA-1 following EBV infection, can lead to an autoimmune response in some individuals, which may play a role in SLE disease etiology. It has been reported that antibodies to epitopes on EBNA-1 cross-react with epitopes on Sm, a ribonucleoprotein complex consisting of a core of polypeptides (B/B′, D, E, F, G) [5,6]. Sabbatini et al. demonstrated that antibodies to Sm D could be generated in mice immunized with a Gly-Arg rich peptide derived from the amino terminal end of EBNA-1 [7]. James et al revealed that antibodies to Sm B/B′ could be elicited in rabbits and mice following immunization with a proline rich peptide in the carboxyl end of EBNA-1 (PPPGRRP) that has homology to a proline rich region (PPPGMRPP) found in Sm [8]. In addition, they observed that some animals subsequently developed antibodies to dsDNA , which they hypothesized arose as a consequence of epitope spreading, although this was not proven. More recently, Poole et al showed that rabbits and mice injected with the proline rich peptide of EBNA-1, subsequently develop antibodies to U1 ribonucleoproteins, RNP A and RNP C as a consequence of epitope spreading [9].

Our laboratory previously reported, that BALB/c mice immunized with an EBNA-1 expression vector that expressed either the entire EBNA-1 protein or EBNA-1 lacking the Gly-Ala repeat, developed antibodies to dsDNA as well as to Sm [10]. It was assumed that the antibodies to Sm arose because of cross-reactivity with EBNA-1 as previously reported, however, the basis for the anti-dsDNA response was unknown. The present study was undertaken to address this issue. Our results strikingly reveal that many antibodies elicited in response to EBNA-1 actually cross-react with dsDNA.

Results

Mice injected with purified recombinant EBNA-1 protein develop antibodies to dsDNA

We were interested in determining how anti-dsDNA antibodies could arise in mice that develop anti-EBNA-1 antibodies upon exposure to EBNA-1 protein. In our previous study, we generated an anti-EBNA-1 response in mice by injecting them with an EBNA-1 expression vector. However, not all mice developed anti-EBNA-1 antibodies, presumably because they did not all express an adequate concentration of the EBNA-1 protein [10]. In the present study, in order to examine the EBNA-1 response, we decided to inject mice with purified recombinant EBNA-1 protein (rEBNA-1) rather than the EBNA-1 expression vector. EBNA-1 protein used for injections was prepared in our laboratory from a baculovirus vector obtained from Lori Frappier (McMaster University, Ontario, Canada). The rEBNA-1 protein encoded by this vector lacks most of the Gly-Ala repeat. It has been shown that the Gly-Ala repeat is not required for the replication, transactivation or segregation function of EBNA-1, although, it does enable EBNA-1 to escape detection by cytotoxic CD8$^+$ T cells [11,12]. The MW of the rEBNA-1 protein lacking the Gly-Ala repeat is approximately 52Kda.

Five, 6 week old, female, BALB/c mice were injected with 50 μg of rEBNA-1 protein in CFA and were boosted 2 times at weeks 3 and 9 with 25 μg of rEBNA-1 in IFA. Five age and sex matched control BALB/c mice were immunized with CFA alone and boosted with IFA and 5 mice were used as uninjected age matched controls. We observed that all 5 mice injected with rEBNA-1 developed IgG antibodies to EBNA-1 within the first 3 weeks (Figure 1A). In addition, mice developed antibodies to dsDNA, although, the kinetics of the anti-dsDNA response lagged behind that of the anti-EBNA-1 response suggesting that anti-dsDNA antibodies may have developed over time as a conse-

quence of epitope spreading or somatic mutation (Figure 1B). Some mice immunized with adjuvant only, also developed antibodies to dsDNA but with the exception of one mouse, their levels of anti-dsDNA antibody were never as high as that of mice injected with rEBNA-1 in adjuvant. Intraperitoneal delivery of CFA has been shown by others to elicit the production of autoantibodies in mice, including the production of anti-DNA antibodies [13]. It is extremely unlikely that the anti-dsDNA response in rEBNA-1 injected mice was due primarily to adjuvant, as our previous DNA based inoculation studies using EBNA-1 expression vectors in the absence of adjuvant, also elicited the production of anti-dsDNA antibodies [10].

Week 12 sera from all 5 rEBNA-1 injected mice were serially diluted and tested for binding to EBNA-1 (Figure 1C) and dsDNA (Figure 1D) by ELISA. All rEBNA-1 injected mice developed high titers of antibody to EBNA-1 and dsDNA. However, the anti-EBNA-1 titers were higher than the anti-dsDNA titers suggesting that either the concentration of antibodies to EBNA-1 were higher than the concentration of antibodies to dsDNA or the affinities of the antibodies to EBNA-1 were higher than for dsDNA. At a dilution of 1:6400, the anti-EBNA-1 response in all mice was greater than 3 standard deviations above the mean of similarly diluted uninjected control mice (dotted line). At a dilution of 1:800, the anti-dsDNA response was greater than 3 standard deviations above the mean of uninjected control mice (dotted line). No anti-dsDNA response was observed at a dilution of 1:6400.

To confirm the specificity of the anti-dsDNA response, week 12 sera from mice injected with rEBNA-1 were diluted 1:50 and used to immunostain Crithidia luciliae slides. The presence of antibody to dsDNA was indicated by binding to the kinetoplast (Figure 1E, left panel). In contrast, sera from adjuvant immunized mice did not reveal kinetoplast binding (Figure 1E, right panel) indicating that either the anti-DNA antibodies present in these mice were of lower affinity than the anti-dsDNA antibodies obtained from rEBNA-1 injected mice or they were not specific for dsDNA.

To determine whether any of the antibodies to EBNA-1generated in rEBNA-1 injected mice also cross-reacted with dsDNA, week 12 sera from all 5 EBNA-1 injected mice were adsorbed over dsDNA-cellulose beads to remove dsDNA reactive antibodies and then sera were tested by ELISA to determine if adsorbed sera showed reduced binding to EBNA-1. Loss of antibody in the sera due to non specific sticking to cellulose was determined by adsorbing sera to cellulose only beads. Figure 2, represents the OD 405 nm of anti-dsDNA (A) and anti-EBNA-1 antibody (B), pre and post adsorption onto dsDNA cellulose beads, after the value for non specific binding to cellulose was subtracted. We observed a significant decrease in anti-dsDNA antibody activity following adsorption on dsDNA cellulose beads, in mouse 1, 3, 4, and 5 (p<0.001) (Figure 2A). In a similar trend, we observed a significant decrease in anti-EBNA-1 activity in the sera from mouse 1, 3, 4, and 5, following adsorption on dsDNA cellulose (p<0.005) (Figure 2B). Mouse 2 showed a small decrease in anti-dsDNA and anti-EBNA-1 activity following adsorption on dsDNA cellulose although it was not significant. This is likely because mouse 2 developed a negligible response to dsDNA following injection with rEBNA-1 although the anti-EBNA-1 response was significant. The observation that a reduction of anti-dsDNA antibody on a dsDNA cellulose column, led to a parallel reduction of anti-EBNA-1 activity, suggests that anti-EBNA-1 antibody in the sera of some rEBNA-1 injected mice, cross-reacts with dsDNA.

Since week 4 rEBNA-1 injected mice displayed a significant delay in the development of a high titer anti-dsDNA but not anti-EBNA-1 response (Figure 1B), we wanted to examine whether

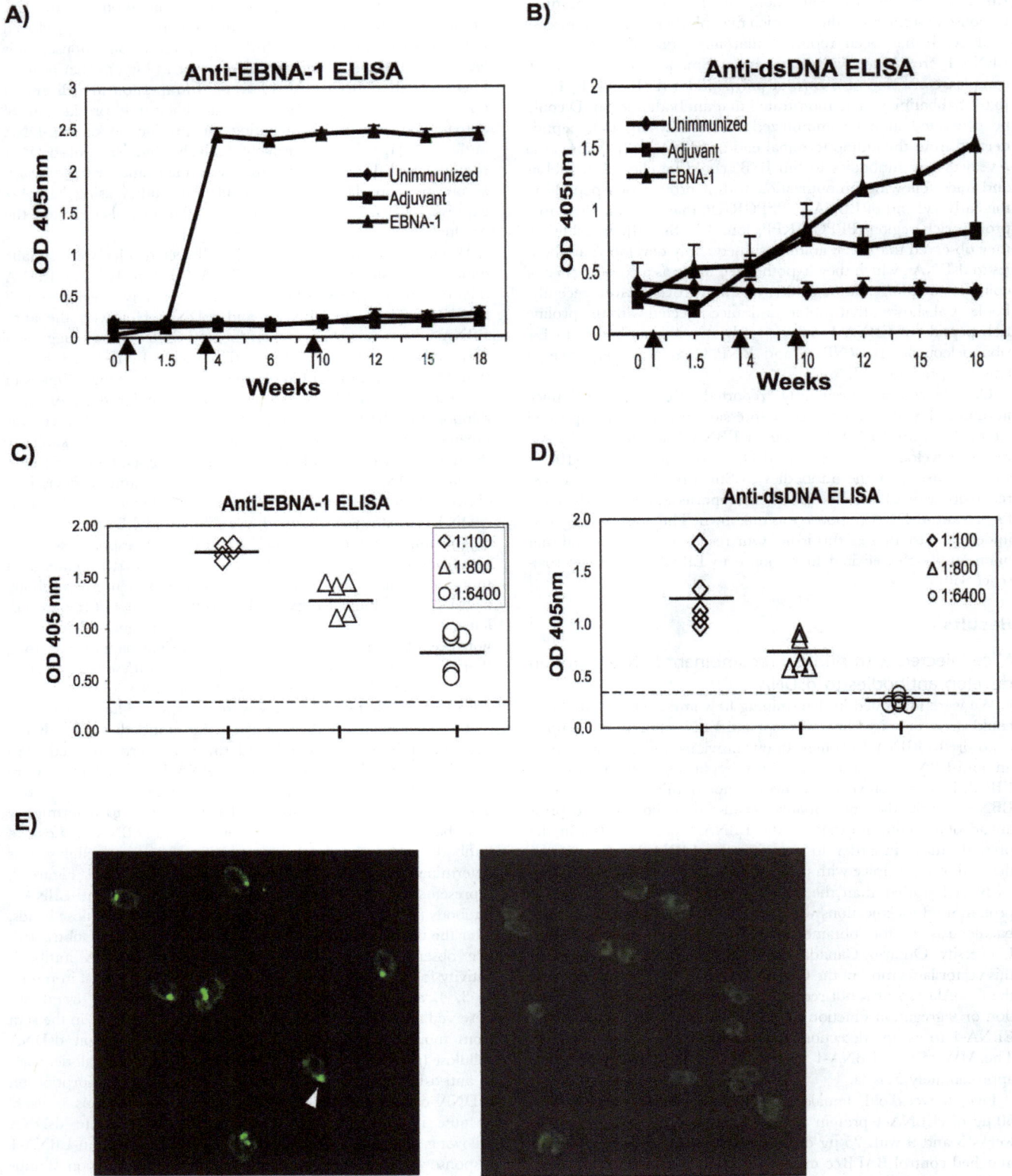

Figure 1. rEBNA-1 injected mice develop antibodies to EBNA-1 and dsDNA. Mice were unimmunized or injected ip with rEBNA-1 emulsified in CFA or CFA alone and boosted with rEBNA-1 emulsified in IFA or IFA alone (arrows indicate week of initial injection and boosts). Mice were bled at weeks 1.5, 4, 6, 10, 12, 15, and 18 and sera tested by ELISA for antibody to EBNA-1 (A) and dsDNA (B). Results are the average of 5 mice in each group. Standard deviations are indicated. (C and D) Eight fold serial dilutions of week 12 sera from all 5 rEBNA-1 injected mice were tested by ELISA for antibody titers to EBNA-1 (C) and dsDNA (D). Dotted line represents 3 standard deviations above the mean absorption of sera from week 12 uninjected control mice. (E) Serum from a week 12 mouse injected with rEBNA-1 (left panel) or adjuvant only (right panel) was diluted 1:50 and used

to immunostain Crithidia luciliae slides. Immunostaining of the dsDNA in the kinetoplast of Crithidia luciliae is observed (left panel) as indicated by arrow. Results are representative of 3 rEBNA-1 and 3 adjuvant only, injected mice.

there was any evidence of cross-reactivity to dsDNA in week 4 sera. We therefore adsorbed week 4 sera over dsDNA cellulose beads. Interestingly, we also observed some reduction in binding to dsDNA and EBNA-1 following adsorption on dsDNA cellulose (data not shown) suggesting that the cross-reactive response arose early. However, since the anti-dsDNA response was much weaker at week 4 than week 12, epitope spreading may have played a role in refining the cross-reactive response over time.

Generation of monoclonal antibodies to EBNA- 1 that cross-react with dsDNA

Although, adsorption studies suggested that antibodies to EBNA-1 generated in rEBNA-1 injected mice cross-creacted with dsDNA they did not prove this. To confirm these results, we therefore generated monoclonal anti-EBNA-1 antibodies from rEBNA-1 injected mice and tested these antibodies for binding to dsDNA by ELISA. To generate monoclonal antibodies to EBNA-1, splenocytes from rEBNA-1 injected BALB/c mice containing serum IgG antibodies to both EBNA-1 and dsDNA, were fused to NSO cells. Hybridoma supernatants were screened by ELISA for IgG antibodies to EBNA-1 and dsDNA. In an initial screen of one fusion, we observed that the majority of clones that tested positive for antibody reactivity to EBNA-1 were also positive for reactivity to dsDNA (10 out of 14 or 71%). Seven clones that were positive for antibodies to EBNA-1 were subcloned two times to insure clonality. Supernatants from these hybridomas were then tested for antibodies to EBNA-1 and dsDNA. In addition, they were tested for the presence of antibodies to the blocking agent Bovine Serum Albumin (BSA). One of the subclones, 3F3, secreted antibody specific for EBNA-1 only (Table 1). Three subclones, secreted monoclonal antibody that reacted strongly with both EBNA-1 and dsDNA and did not bind BSA. Subclone 3D4 is representative of this group (Table 1). Three other subclones, represented by 9G3, secreted antibody that bound not only to EBNA-1 and dsDNA but BSA as well (Table 1).

In the present study we chose to focus on 3D4 because it is an IgG antibody that binds strongly to dsDNA, which is characteristic

of many pathogenic IgG anti-dsDNA antibodies that arise in SLE. In addition, it's strong binding to both EBNA-1 and dsDNA made it a good candidate for studying the basis of this cross-reactive response. The other antibodies such as 9G3 that also reacted with BSA (and casein), were not further characterized in this study because of concern that this would lead to non specific binding in ELISAs and Western blots; assays which require these blocking reagents. In addition these antibodies displayed a much weaker affinity for EBNA-1 and dsDNA making them less desirable to use in our initial attempt to identify epitopes in EBNA-1 that play a role in cross-reactivity to dsDNA.

3D4 was isolated from hybridoma supernatant, on a protein G column. Following purification, 3D4 was shown to bind to EBNA-1 by ELISA even at concentrations as low as 0.125 µg/ml (Figure 3A). Specificity of this antibody was demonstrated by its lack of binding to a control viral antigen, cystovirus RNA polymerase, P2, isolated by Gottlieb et al [14] and BSA (Figure 3A).

Purified 3D4 was also shown to cross-react with dsDNA by ELISA (Figure 3B). 3D4 was shown by ELISA to be of the IgG1 isotype (Figure 3C). Reactivity of 3D4 with dsDNA was confirmed by its ability to recognize the dsDNA containing kinetoplasts of Crithidia luciliae (Figure 3D, left panel). An IgG1 isotype control MAb failed to bind kinetoplasts (Figure 3D, right panel). Cross-reactivity of 3D4 was further demonstrated by adsorption of the purified MAb over dsDNA cellulose beads and then testing pre and post adsorbed antibody for binding to dsDNA and EBNA-1 by ELISA and Western blot (Figure 3E and F). Adsorption over dsDNA cellulose resulted in complete depletion of 3D4 as detected by anti-dsDNA and and anti-EBNA-1 ELISAs (Figure 3E). Post dsDNA-cellulose adsorbed 3D4 antibody also showed dramatically reduced binding to EBNA-1 compared to pre-adsorbed 3D4, by Western blot (Figure 3F, right panel, compare lanes 2 and 4). No binding of pre-adsorbed 3D4 antibody to BSA was observed (lane 3).

We were also interested in determining whether a monoclonal anti-EBNA-1antibody isolated from a completely different source

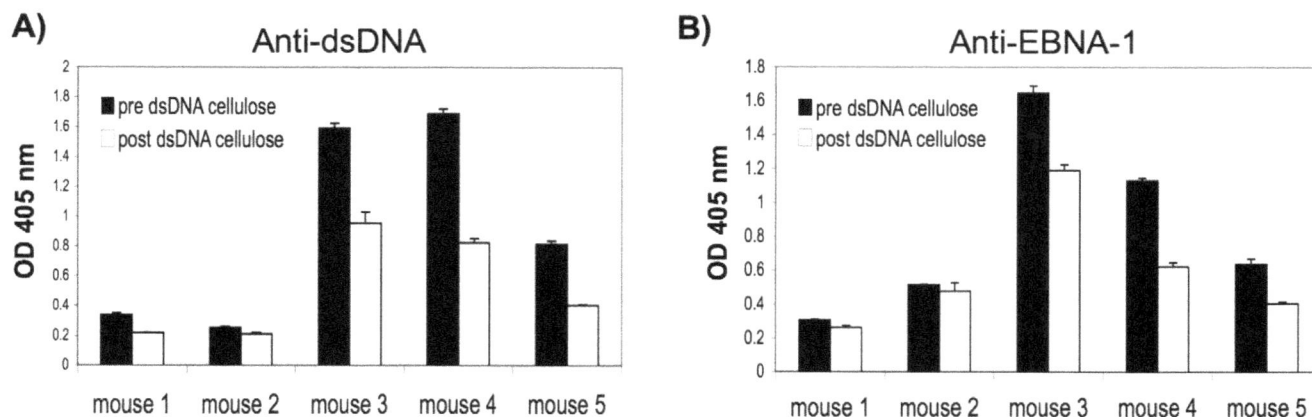

Figure 2. Sera from EBNA-1 injected mice display reduced binding to EBNA-1 following adsorption onto dsDNA cellulose beads.
Week 12 sera from all five rEBNA-1 injected mice were adsorbed onto dsDNA cellulose beads and pre and post adsorbed sera were tested by ELISA for binding to dsDNA (A) and EBNA-1 (B). Results represent OD 405 nm values after subtraction of non specific binding to cellulose only beads. Standard deviations of triplicate wells are indicated. Sera were diluted 1:5000 prior to adsorption. One tailed, unpaired t test was used to compare OD 405 nm before and after adsorption on dsDNA cellulose (t<0.001 for mouse 1,3, 4, and 5 in (A) and t<0 .005 for mouse 1, 3, 4, and 5 in (B)).

Table 1. Reactivity of representative monoclonal antibodies to EBNA-1, dsDNA, and BSA.

MAbs	anti-EBNA-1	anti-dsDNA	anti-BSA	Source
3D4	+++	+++	−	this study
9G3	+	+	+	this study
3F3	++	−	−	this study
0211	++	++	−	Commercial MAb Pierce, Rockford, IL

+++ strong binding.
++ moderate binding.
+ weak binding.

would have similar binding properties to the 3D4 MAb isolated in our laboratory. We therefore examined the ability of a commercially prepared monoclonal IgG1 anti-EBNA-1 antibody, 0211 (Thermo Fisher Scientific/Pierce, Rockford, IL) to cross-react with dsDNA. The only information known about 0211 is that it was generated in response to EBNA-1, however, the exact epitope that it recognizes has not yet been identified. We first confirmed by ELISA, that this antibody binds to EBNA-1 but not to BSA or P2 (Figure 4A). We next observed by ELISA that this antibody also cross-reacts with dsDNA (Figure 4B). Furthermore, adsorption of 0211 on a dsDNA cellulose column, resulted in complete depletion of the antibody as detected by anti-dsDNA and anti-EBNA-1 ELISAs (Figure 4C). A reduction in binding of post dsDNA cellulose adsorbed antibody to EBNA-1 was also demonstrated by Western blot (Figure 4D, right panel, compare lanes 2 and 4). No binding of pre-adsorbed 0211 antibody to BSA was observed (lane 3).

A comparison of MAbs 3D4 and 0211 revealed that although both antibodies bind strongly to EBNA-1, 3D4 has an even higher affinity for EBNA-1 than 0211 (Figure 5A). At a concentration of 0.1 μg/ml, 3D4 still bound robustly to EBNA-1 while binding by 0211 was negligible.

MAbs 3D4 and 0211 were examined for binding to Sm and a panel of antigens

MAbs 3D4 and 0211 were also examined for binding to Sm, lipopolysaccharide (LPS), BSA, and proteinase -3 (PR-3) which is the target autoantigen in Wegener's granulomatosis. Antibodies to PR-3 are a subgroup of classic anti-neutrophil cytoplasmic antibodies (cANCA). At 5 μg/ml, 3D4 displayed negligible binding to Sm relative to BSA (Figure 5B) while 0211 bound moderately well to Sm (Figure 5C). We also tested the binding of 3D4 and 0211 to LPS because it is negatively charged [15]. Since dsDNA is negatively charged, we wondered whether the MAbs would bind other negatively charged antigens. However, we observed that both 3D4 and 0211 failed to bind LPS.

MAbs 3D4 and 0211 display differences in reactivity to the amino and carboxyl regions of EBNA-1

To begin to understand whether MAbs 3D4 and 0211 recognize the same or different regions of EBNA-1, they were examined by ELISA for binding to three truncated recombinant EBNA-1 proteins, LS7, LS8, and LS9, isolated in this laboratory from E. coli. These truncated recombinant proteins are comprised of the amino or carboxyl regions of EBNA-1. The protein designated LS8, is comprised of the amino region of rEBNA-1, from the initial Met residue to aa 404 (Figure 6A). Like rEBNA-1 used in this study, it lacks most of the Gly-Ala repeat. It contains the PPPGRPP region in EBNA-1 (aa 398–404) that was shown by James et al to be

homologous to a proline rich epitope in Sm B/B' [8]. LS7 is identical to LS8 except that it terminates at aa 393 and therefore lacks the PPPGRPP epitope (Figure 6A). The rational for generating two amino fragments, one with and one without the proline rich epitope was to determine whether this epitope which is responsible for eliciting cross-reactivity with Sm is also involved in eliciting cross-reactivity with dsDNA. LS9 comprises the carboxyl region of the rEBNA-1 protein from aa 410 to the terminal aa 641 and lacks the proline epitope (Figure 6A). MAb 3D4 was observed to bind strongly to LS9 but not at all to LS7 or LS8 (Figure 6B). The kinetics of 3D4 binding to LS9 closely paralleled the kinetics of binding to the entire rEBNA-1 protein indicating that this carboxyl region (aa 410–641) is sufficient for optimal recognition by 3D4. Adsorption of 3D4 to dsDNA cellulose was also observed to remove all binding to the carboxyl fragment. Taken together these results suggest that the cross-reactive epitope recognized by 3D4, is configured within the carboxyl region.

MAb 0211 was observed to bind all three truncated proteins indicating that it recognizes epitopes in both the amino and carboxyl regions of EBNA-1, however the binding to the amino proteins, LS7 and LS8 is better than the binding to the carboxyl protein, LS9 (Figure 6C). Interestingly, 0211 binds more strongly to LS7 than LS8 and since LS7 does not contain the PPPGRPP epitope, this indicates that the proline epitope is not necessary for the binding of 0211 to EBNA-1. Furthermore, this proline rich region may structurally interfere with binding by 0211. It cannot be determined at this time whether the epitope in the amino or carboxyl region of EBNA-1 is responsible for MAb 0211's cross-reactivity with dsDNA.

Despite the fact that 3D4 and 0211 bind differently to the amino and carboxyl regions of EBNA-1, both antibodies still cross-react with dsDNA. Consequently there could be more than one EBNA-1 epitope that could be linear or conformational, that acts as a mimotope for dsDNA. Alternatively, the epitope (s) in the carboxyl region may be more important for cross-reactivity with dsDNA and since 0211 also binds Sm, the epitope in the amino region may be more important for cross-reactivity with Sm.

3D4 binds to a 148 aa core domain in the carboxyl region of EBNA-1 that lacks the negatively charged C-terminal amino acids

To begin to identify a smaller fragment in the carboxyl region of EBNA-1 that contains the epitope recognized by 3D4, we examined the binding of this MAb to three truncated carboxyl fragments; $EBNA_{452-641}$, $EBNA_{459-619}$, and $EBNA_{459-607}$ (Figure 7A). These fragments are expressed by plasmids kindly provided to us by Dr. Lori Frappier [16]. We observed that 3D4 bound all 3 fragments equally well and did not show diminished binding to these fragments relative to the entire carboxyl region ($EBNA_{410-641}$) (Figure 7B). In

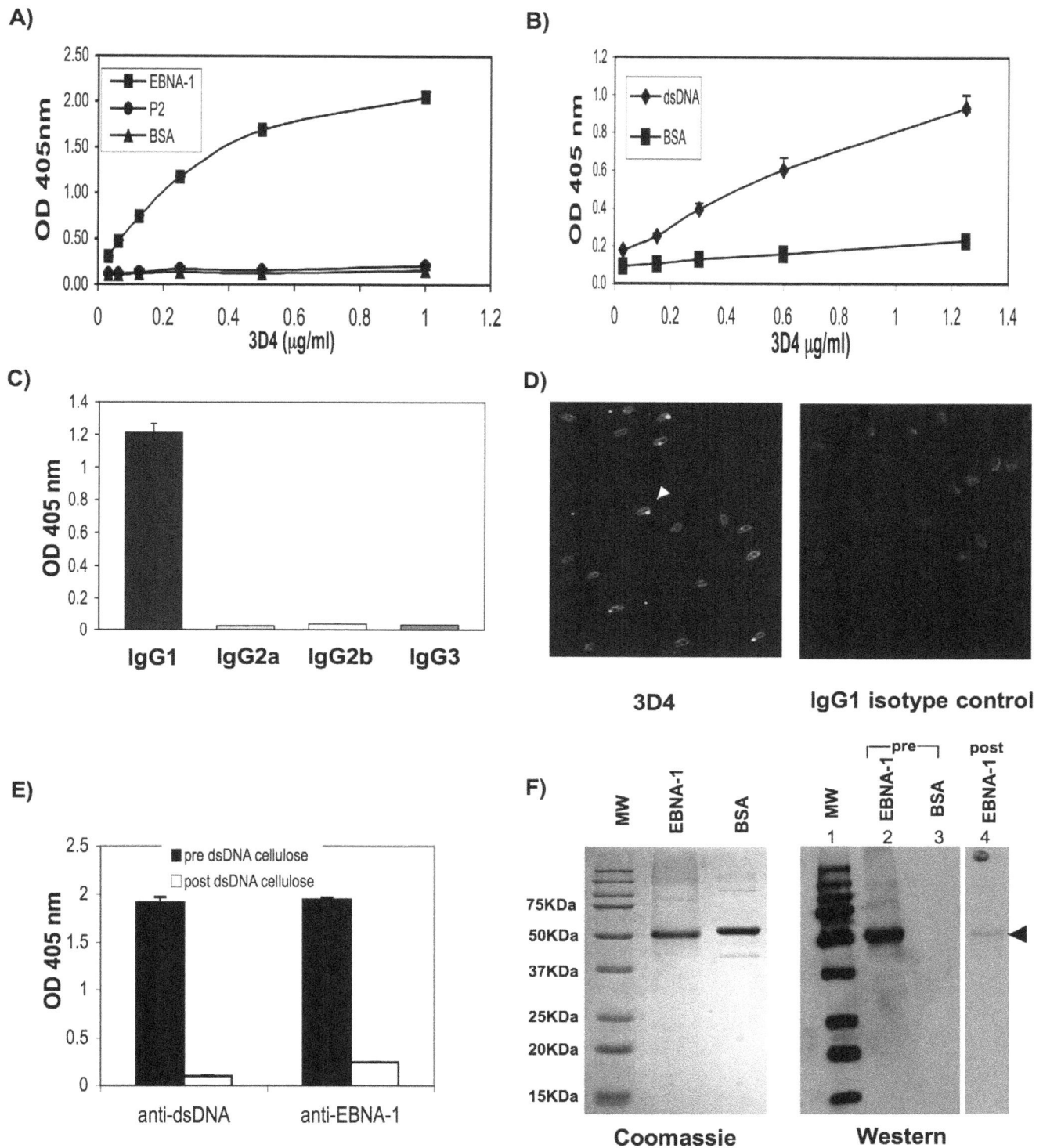

Figure 3. MAb, 3D4, is specific for both EBNA-1 and dsDNA. (A) Anti-EBNA-1 ELISA. 3D4 was tested by ELISA, at increasing concentrations, for binding to EBNA-1, BSA, and the cystovirus, polymerase protein, P2 (negative control) coated on Costar plates. Plates were read at 405 nm at 20 minutes. 3D4 shows specificity for EBNA-1 under these conditions. Results are the averages of triplicates and standard deviations are indicated. (B) 3D4 was tested by ELISA for binding to dsDNA coated on Immulon-2 plates. Plates were read at 405 nm at 1 hour. Results in A and B are the average of triplicates and standard deviations are indicated. (C) 3D4 antibody is of the IgG1 isotype. ELISA plates coated with unlabeled anti-IgG1, anti-IgG2a, anti-IgG2b, or anti-IgG3 were incubated with 1.5 µg/ml of 3D4 MAb followed by the respective polyclonal isotype specific antibodies conjugated to alkaline phosphatase. (D) Purified 3D4 at a concentration of 10 µg/ml was examined for binding to Crithidia luciliae slides. Left panel shows the binding of 3D4 to kinetoplasts of Crithidia luciliae (arrow). Right panel; IgG1 isotype control antibody, does not bind specifically to kinetoplasts. (E & F) 3D4 was adsorbed on a dsDNA cellulose column and pre and post adsorbed antibody were tested for binding to dsDNA and EBNA-1 by ELISA (E) and to EBNA-1 by Western blot (F). (E) 3D4 adsorbed on dsDNA cellulose beads was completely depleted of antibody with reactivity for dsDNA and

EBNA-1 as detected by ELISA. Results represent OD 405 nm values after subtraction of non specific binding to cellulose only beads. Standard deviations of triplicate wells are indicated. Anti-dsDNA and anti-EBNA-1 ELISAs were performed on Immulon-2 and Costar plates respectively and ELISAs were developed when ODs on each plate reached maximal values. (F) Post dsDNA cellulose adsorbed 3D4 shows reduced binding to EBNA-1 by Western blot. Left panel: Coomassie stained polyacrylamide gel. Right panel: Western blot: filters were immunostained with pre (lanes 2 and 3) or post dsDNA cellulose adsorbed 3D4 MAb (lane 4). Molecular weight markers used in Western blot were conjugated to *strep-tag* and were detected with Strep-Tactin-HRP.

fact 3D4 displayed optimal binding to the smallest fragment, EBNA$_{459-607}$ suggesting that the cross-reactive epitope lies within this 148 aa region. The carboxyl region of EBNA-1 has a net negative charge due to the high frequency of negatively charged amino acids at the C-terminus (aa 619–641). Twelve out of 22 of the C terminal amino acids are either glutamic or aspartic acid. Both, EBNA$_{459-619}$, and EBNA$_{459-607}$ lack these negatively charged amino acids. Since removal of these negatively charged amino acids did not diminish recognition by 3D4, this suggests that charge

interaction is not the basis for 3D4's binding to EBNA-1. MAb, 0211 displays a similar binding pattern to the truncated carboxyl fragments of EBNA-1 with maximal binding to the two smallest fragments EBNA$_{459-619}$ and EBNA$_{459-607}$ (data not shown).

Discussion

This study demonstrates for the first time, that some antibodies that arise in response to EBNA-1 cross-react with dsDNA. Our

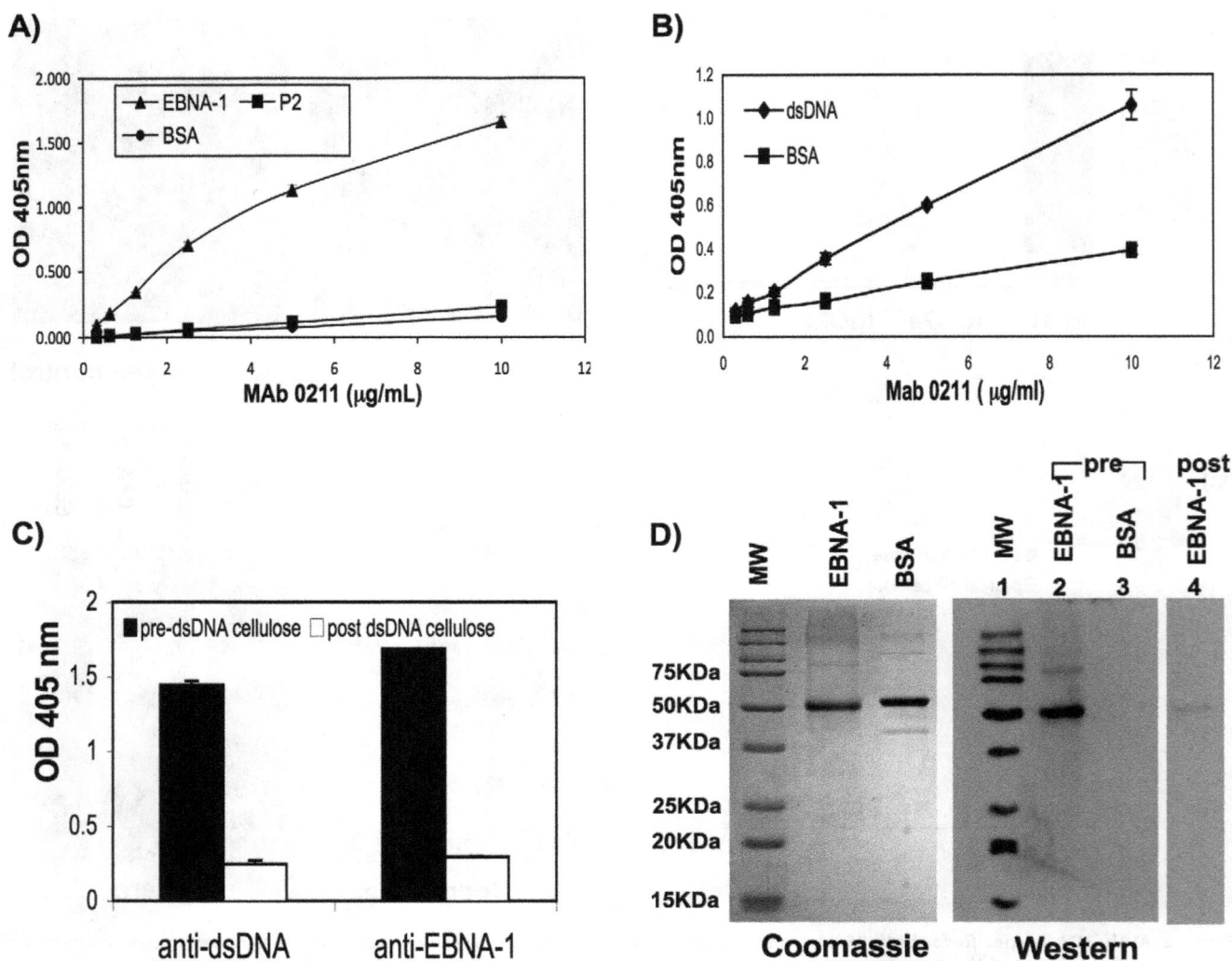

Figure 4. Commercial MAb, 0211 cross-reacts with dsDNA. (A) MAb 0211 binds to EBNA-1 as detected by ELISA but not P2, or BSA. (B) MAb 0211 binds to dsDNA as detected by ELISA. (C & D) MAb 0211 was adsorbed onto dsDNA cellulose beads and pre and post adsorbed antibody were tested for binding to dsDNA and EBNA-1 by ELISA. (C) MAb 0211 adsorbed on dsDNA cellulose beads, was completely depleted of antibody reactivity for dsDNA and EBNA-1. Anti-dsDNA and anti-EBNA-1 ELISAs were performed on separate ELISA plates and ELISAs were developed when ODs reached maximal values. Results represent OD 405 nm values after subtraction of non specific binding to cellulose only beads. (D) Post dsDNA cellulose adsorbed MAb 0211 shows reduced binding to rEBNA-1 by Western blot. Left panel: Coomassie stained polyacrylamide gel. Right panel: Western blot: filters were immunostained with pre (lanes 2 and 3) or post dsDNA cellulose adsorbed 0211 (lane 4) as indicated.

A)

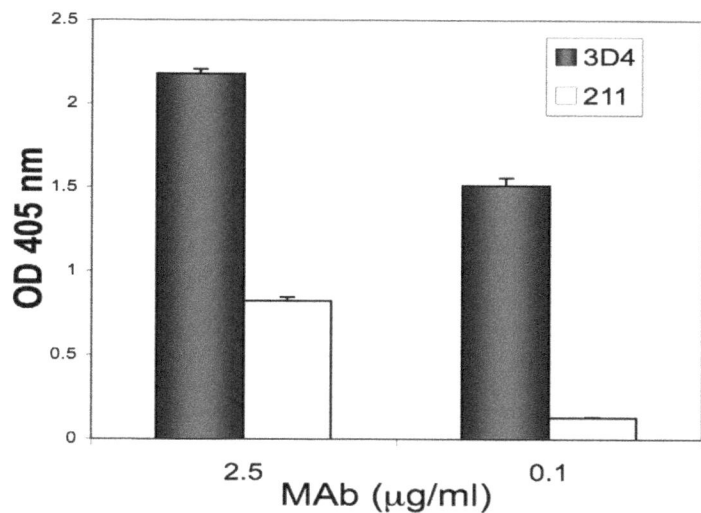

B)

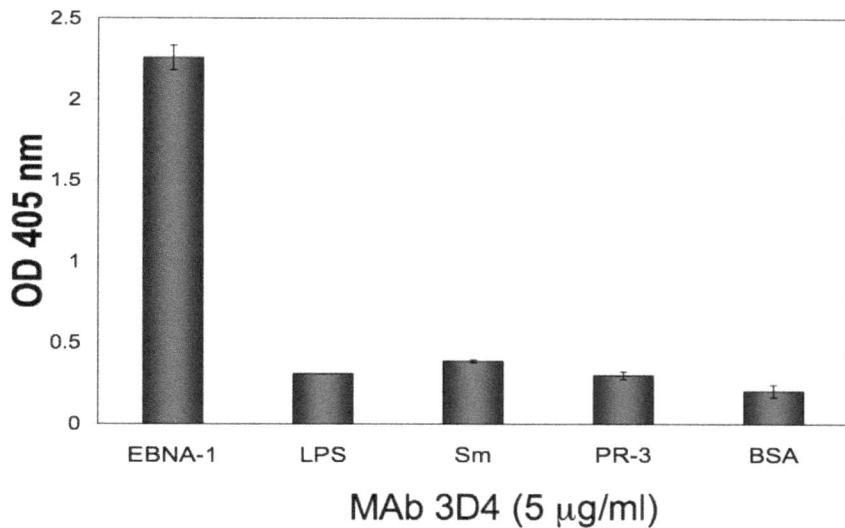

C)

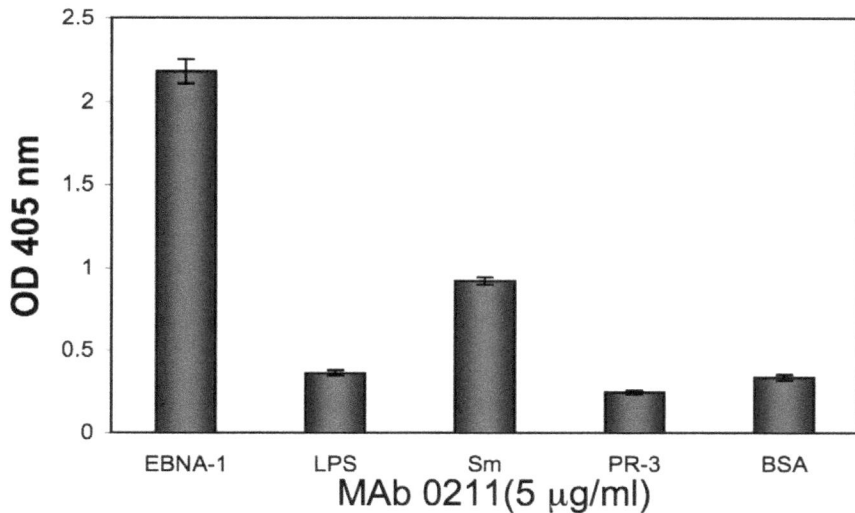

Figure 5. Comparison of the binding affinity and specificity of 3D4 and 0211. (A) Binding of 3D4 to EBNA-1 is compared to that of 0211 by ELISA at two different concentrations of MAbs. 3D4 binds more strongly to EBNA-1 than 0211. (B) Binding of 3D4 to several antigens is examined by ELISA. 3D4 does not show significant binding to other antigens tested. (C) Binding of 0211 to several antigens is examined by ELISA. 0211 binds moderately to Sm but not to the other antigens tested.

laboratory previously demonstrated that EBNA-1 expression could elicit an anti-dsDNA response, however, it was not known at the time whether the antibodies to dsDNA were distinct from the anti-EBNA-1 antibodies or whether the same antibodies that bound EBNA-1 were also able to recognize dsDNA. The demonstration that purified monoclonal IgG antibodies to EBNA-1 also bind dsDNA and that adsorption of these antibodies on a dsDNA cellulose column, removes EBNA-1 reactivity, confirms the cross-reactive nature of these antibodies. However, this does not exclude the potential role of epitope spreading in the development of the cross-reactive response. The delay in the development of a strong anti-dsDNA response relative to the anti-EBNA-1 response suggests that cross-reactivity continues to develop over time. It may be that early in the response to EBNA-1, the epitopes that are targeted, elicit only a weakly cross-reactive response to dsDNA. Later in the response, other epitopes may be targeted as a result of intra-molecular epitope spreading and these latter epitopes may be the ones that are responsible for cross-reactivity with dsDNA. Alternatively, antibodies that cross-react more strongly with dsDNA may arise later in the immune response as a consequence of somatic mutation. A specific mutation in the variable heavy and/or light chain regions of an anti-EBNA-1 antibody may alter its specificity from one that only recognizes EBNA-1 to one that recognizes EBNA-1 as well as dsDNA.

While all mice injected with EBNA-1 developed antibodies to dsDNA, we did not consistently observe features of clinical lupus in these mice. Two out of 5 injected mice had significant levels of protein but no blood in their urine relative to uninjected mice. The kidney of 1 out of 3 mice examined at 3 months post injection, had evidence of some IgG immune complex deposition, however, none of the kidneys examined showed signs of lupus histopathology (data not shown). Future studies will include examining a larger cohort of mice for evidence of glomerulonephritis and investigating whether 3D4 and 0211 can deposit in the kidney.

Antibodies to a variety of self proteins have been reported to cross-react with dsDNA, such as antibodies to extracellular matrix protein, HP8, ribosomal P protein, elongation factor-2 (EF-2), α-actinin, the NMDA receptor and Sm D [17,18,19,20,21,22]. Antibodies targeting peptide mimotopes of dsDNA such as DWEYSVWLSN and RLTSSLRYNP have also been reported [23,24]. In addition, antibodies to microbial antigens such as glycolipid components of the cell wall of Mycobacterium tuberculosis, phosphorylcholine in the cell wall of Streptococcus pneumoniae or proteins in Burkholderia fungorum have been observed to cross-react with dsDNA [25,26,27,28]. It is unclear how these antigens act as molecular mimics to dsDNA, but it may be due to similarities in the 3 dimensional structures of these antigens and dsDNA. Evidence from some studies suggest that conformational epitopes are the targets of antibodies that cross-react with dsDNA and self proteins [29,30].

Most of the monoclonal anti-EBNA-1 antibodies generated in this study were found to cross-react with dsDNA. Very few of them were found to recognize EBNA-1 only. This may be because mice that were selected for fusion had already developed maximal levels of cross-reactive antibodies either due to epitope spreading or somatic mutation. In addition, the rEBNA-1 protein used in our injection studies, lacks the Gly-Ala repeat which has been shown to be a major epitope that elicits anti-EBNA-1 antibodies in normal

individuals [31]. It may be that in the absence of the Gly-Ala repeat, the response is biased towards other epitopes some of which happen to elicit antibodies that also cross-react with dsDNA. It was previously demonstrated that patients with lupus tend to mount an immune response to different epitopes on EBNA-1 than healthy individuals [4,31,32]. While sera from healthy individuals, preferentially react with the Gly-Ala repeat, sera from lupus patients tend to recognize epitopes in the amino and carboxyl terminal regions of EBNA-1 that are more likely to be cross-reactive with nuclear autoantigens. It is not clear whether lupus patients are genetically predisposed to developing cross-reactive antibodies or whether they have a defect in B cell tolerance leading to failed regulation of the autoreactive B cells producing these antibodies.

The two MAbs that were extensively characterized in this study, 3D4 and 0211, bind to EBNA-1 and dsDNA, yet 3D4 recognizes only the carboxyl region in EBNA-1, while 0211 recognizes both the amino and carboxyl regions. A homology search failed to find any region in EBNA-1 that is homologous to two previously described peptide mimotopes for dsDNA; DWEYSVWLSN and RLTSSLRYNP. It is not yet known whether 3D4 and 0211 recognize a homologous epitope in the carboxyl region, however the C-terminal negatively charged amino acids do not appear to be necessary for the binding of either of these MAbs to the carboxyl region.

MAb 0211 binds moderately well to Sm while 3D4 displays negligible binding to Sm. The basis for the cross-reactivity of 0211 with Sm does not seem to be dependent on the proline rich epitope described by James et al, since 0211 binds even stronger to a truncated amino fragment of EBNA-1 lacking this determinant [8]. It is not yet clear whether the epitopes in the amino and carboxyl region recognized by 0211 share homology. However, the observation that 0211 binds to both Sm and the amino fragment, while 3D4 binds to the carboxyl region only, suggests that an epitope in the amino fragment may be more important for cross-reactivity with Sm while an epitope in the carboxyl region may be important for cross-reactivity with dsDNA. In a preliminary study that is consistent with this, we recently identified a monoclonal IgM antibody that reacts strongly with EBNA-1 and dsDNA but not Sm and only recognizes the carboxyl region of EBNA-1. In addition, recent studies reveal that the MAb, 9G3 (Table 1) that recognizes BSA, also cross-reacts with Sm, and binds to both the amino and carboxyl fragments of EBNA-1 (preliminary data). The polyreactive nature of this antibody, which will be examined in more depth in future studies, is potentially important since polyreactive antibodies have been shown to be the precursors of more pathogenic antibodies in lupus [33].

As previously mentioned, the basis for antibody cross-reactivity with EBNA-1 and dsDNA does not appear to be charge interactions since removal of the negatively charged amino acids from the carboxyl region of EBNA-1 does not diminish binding to this region (Figure 7). Furthermore, neither 3D4 nor 0211 recognize LPS which is negatively charged (Figure 5). It is possible that the epitopes in EBNA-1 that cross-react with dsDNA are structural. The X-ray structure of the crystallized VBS/DNA binding region of EBNA-1 has been determined and reveals two distinct domains; a core domain that mediates protein dimerization and a flanking domain that mediates base contact with

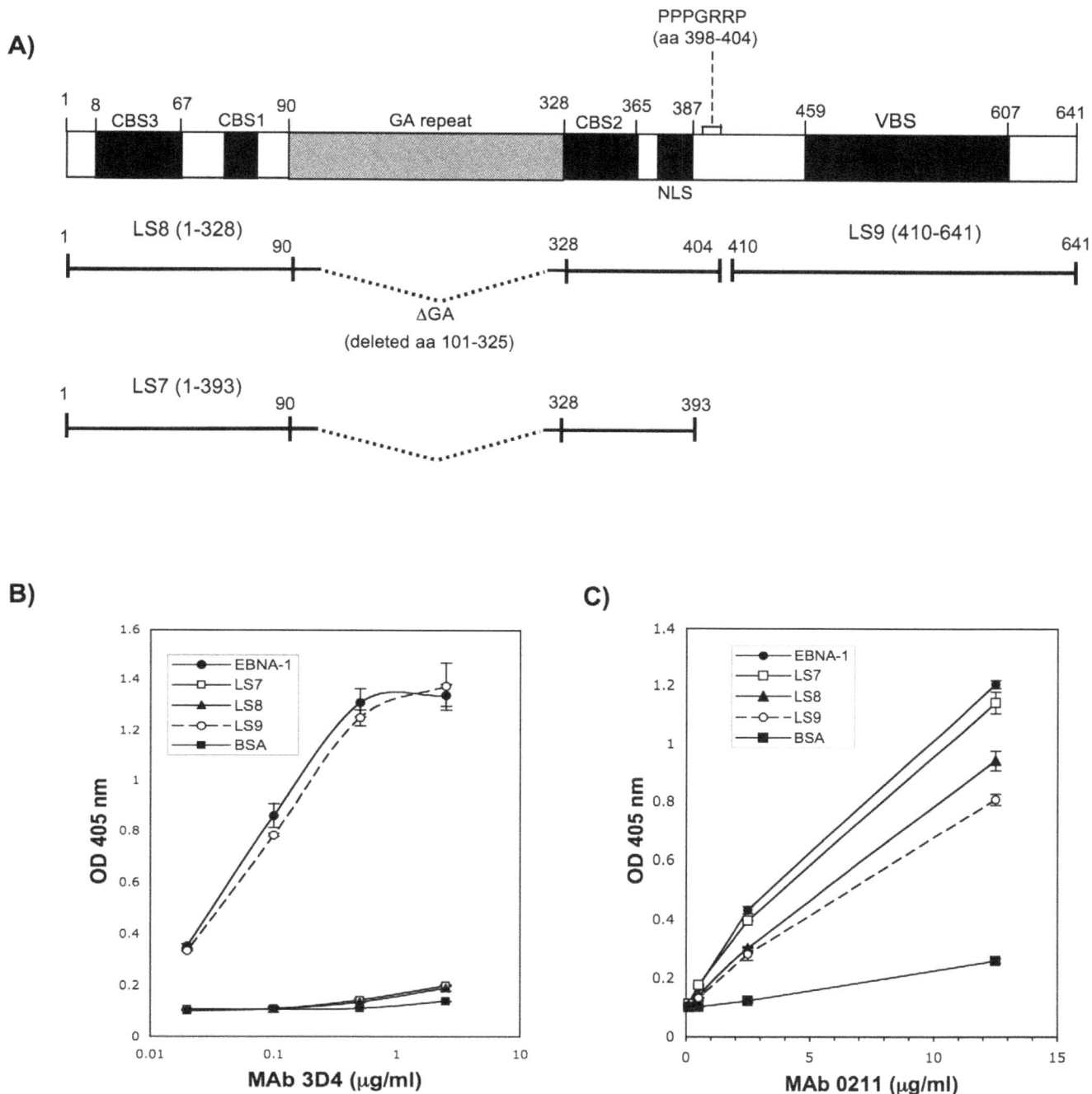

Figure 6. 3D4 binds to the carboxyl region while 0211 binds to both the carboxyl and amino regions of EBNA-1. (A) Functional map of the complete EBNA-1 protein containing the Gly-Ala repeat region (GA). CBS 1,2,3; chromatin binding sites, NLS; nuclear localization site, VBS: viral binding site. LS8 denotes the amino fragment (aa 1–404) lacking most of the GA repeat. LS7 denotes the amino fragment (aa 1–393) lacking the GA repeat and lacking PPPGRRP. LS9 denotes the carboxyl fragment (aa 410–641). (B) MAb 3D4 is strongly reactive with LS9 but not LS8 or LS7 as detected by ELISA. (C) MAb 0211 is reactive with LS7, LS8 and LS9 as detected by ELISA. Results in B and C are the average of triplicate wells.

dsDNA [34]. These domains possess much secondary structure, which may serve as targets for antibodies that cross-react with dsDNA. The core domain (aa 504–607) contains a ß sheet, an α helix and a proline loop and the flanking domain (aa 470–503) contains α helixes. Potentially, the cross-reactive antibodies may recognize a portion of the α helix that mimics the α helix in dsDNA. The X-ray crystal structure of the N-terminus has not yet been resolved. However, this region appears to be less structured than the carboxyl region and could be flexible enough to fold onto itself or the carboxyl region providing multiple opportunities for antibody interaction.

It will be important in future studies to map the epitopes in EBNA-1 that lead to the cross-reactivity with dsDNA and determine whether or not these epitopes are conformational. Identifying these epitopes and individuals who preferentially produce antibody responses to them, may be useful for

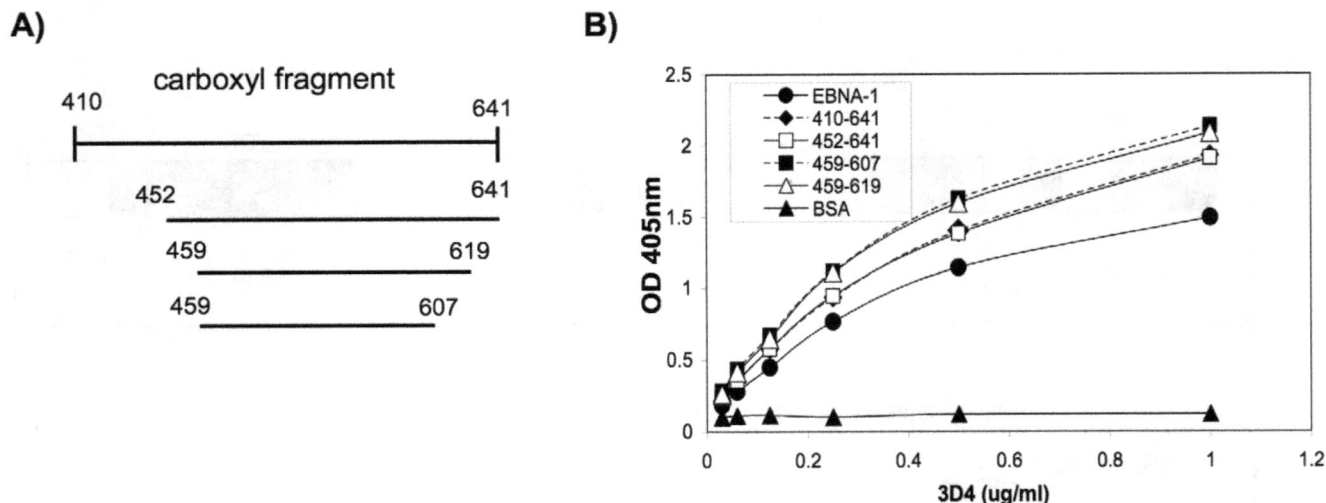

Figure 7. 3D4 recognizes a 148 aa core domain in the carboxyl region of EBNA-1. (A) Map of the carboxyl region of EBNA-1 and 3 truncated carboxyl fragments. (B) 3D4 was tested by ELISA for binding to the 3 truncated fragments of EBNA-1. 3D4 binds strongly to all 3 fragments, the smallest being EBNA$_{459-607}$.

determining those who are at risk of developing lupus so that early treatment strategies can be initiated. In addition, knowledge of these epitopes may help in the design of therapeutic strategies that can mask these epitopes thereby preventing the immune system from mounting a cross-reactive response to them.

Materials and Methods

All animals were handled in strict accordance with good animal practice as defined by federal and state policies set forth by The Public Health Service Policy on the Humane Care and Use of Laboratory Animals (PHS 1986), The Guide for the Care and Use of Laboratory Animals (ILAR 1996), and The USDA Animal Welfare Act (CFR 1985). All work done with animals in this study, was approved by The Institutional Animal Care and Use Committee (IACUC) at The City College of New York, (approval numbers 626 and 828).

Extraction, Purification and Characterization of rEBNA-1 lacking the Gly-Ala repeat

The EBNA-1 baculovirus expression vector used in this study was a generous gift from Dr. Lori Frappier (McMaster University, Ontario, Canada). Recombinant EBNA-1 protein (rEBNA-1) was isolated from this baculovirus expression vector according to Lori Frappier (personal communication and modifications of Frappier and O'Donnell) [35]. This vector encodes an EBNA-1 protein that has a deletion of most of the Gly-Ala repeat and has a 6× His tag on the N-terminus, which allows for the protein's isolation on a Ni^{2+} metal affinity column. Briefly, SF9 cells were grown in serum-free insect cell culture medium, Sf-900 II SFM (Invitrogen, Carlsbad, CA) at 27°C. Cells were resuspended at a concentration of 1×10^6 cells per ml and 100 ml of cells (100×10^6 cells total) were infected with 500 µl of high titer recombinant EBNA-1 baculovirus and grown in 500 ml Erlenmeyer flasks (Corning, Acton, MA) at 27°C in an air shaker for 60 hours. The cells were then harvested by centrifuging at 2000 rpm at 4°C for 10 minutes. The cell pellets were resuspended in 25 ml of a hypotonic buffer (20 mM HEPES pH 7.8, 1 mM MgCl$_2$, 1 mM PMSF and 10 µM

leupeptin) and allowed to swell on ice for 10 minutes. Cells were then dounced 20 times on ice and centrifuged at 4°C at 3000 rpm for 10 minutes. Supernatant was discarded. The pellet containing intact nuclei was resuspended in 25 ml of hypotonic buffer containing 2.7 ml of 5 M NaCl. After douncing on ice to open the nuclear envelope, the fraction was centrifuged at 18,000 rpm for 20 minutes and the supernatant containing rEBNA-1 protein was collected. Further purification of rEBNA-1 was performed employing a nickel agarose (Ni^{2+}-NTA) (QIAGEN, Valencia, CA) column according to modifications of Ceccarelli and Frappier [12]. Ni^{2+}-NTA agarose (1ml) was equilibrated in column buffer (0.2 M Hepes pH 7.8, 0.5 M NaCl, 10% glycerol) containing 5 mM imidazole, at room temperature. The nuclear extract was incubated with pre-equilibrated Ni^{2+}-NTA at room temperature for 2 hours, with rocking. After incubation, a column was packed with the nuclear extract/Ni^{2+}-NTA slurry. The column was washed slowly with column buffer containing 5 mM imidazole followed by column buffer containing 25 mM imidazole. Next, the EBNA-1 protein was eluted with column buffer containing 300 mM imidazole. The protein was then concentrated and the buffer exchanged with PBS, 250 mM NaCl using an Amicon Centrifugal filter (10,000 molecular weight cut off) (Millipore, Billerica, MA). The protein was then resolved by 12% SDS-PAGE followed by a Western blot and immunostaining with a monoclonal antibody to EBNA-1.

Injection of mice with rEBNA-1 protein

Fifteen, six week old, female BALB/c mice were used for injection studies. Five mice were injected intraperitoneally (ip) with 50 µg of rEBNA-1 protein in complete Freund's adjuvant (CFA) (Sigma, St Louis, MO) in a 1:1 (v/v) ratio and boosted twice (at weeks 3 and 9) with 25 µg of rEBNA-1 in incomplete Freund's adjuvant (IFA). Five mice were injected with CFA only and boosted with IFA and 5 age-matched control mice remained uninjected throughout the study. The mice were bled immediately before injection and at weeks 1.5, 4, 6, 10, 12, 15 and 18. The sera obtained, from these mice were tested for anti-EBNA-1 and anti-dsDNA antibodies by ELISA.

Construction of plasmids encoding the amino and carboxyl regions of EBNA-1

Truncated EBNA-1 proteins were isolated from plasmid transformed E. coli cells. The pLS8 expression plasmid carries the encoding sequence for the amino terminus of the EBNA-1 antigen, from the initial Met residue to amino acid position 404 and lacks virtually all of the Gly-Ala repeat. It was prepared by PCR amplification of the EBNA-1 gene from pMRC72 [10] which contains the EBNA-1 coding sequence, but lacks the Gly-Ala repeat, using the following primer pair; EBV7, 5-CATATGTCTGACGAGGGGC CAGGT-3′ (forward primer) and EBV6, 5′-CTCGAGTTATGGCCTTCTACCTGG-3′ (reverse primer). The pLS7 expression plasmid also carries the encoding sequence for the amino terminus of the EBNA-1 protein, from the initial Met residue but it terminates at amino acid position 393. Like pLS8, it lacks most of the Gly-Ala repeat. However, unlike pLS8, it is missing the PPPGRRP epitope (aa 398–404). It was prepared from pMRC72 using the following primer pair; EBV7 (see above) and EBV5, 5′ CTCGAGTTAA-GACCCGGAT GATGA 3′ (reverse primer). The pLS9 expression plasmid carries the EBNA-1 encoding sequence for the carboxyl terminus of EBNA-1 from amino acids 410 to 641. It was also prepared by PCR amplification of the EBNA-1 gene from pMRC72 using the following primer pair; EBV3, 5′-CAT-ATGGGGGAA GCCGATTA TTTTGAAT-3′ (forward primer) and EBV 4, 5′-CTCGAGTTACTCCTGCCCTTCCTC-3′ (reverse primer). The PCR amplifications were performed for 30 cycles. The amino and carboxyl PCR fragments were digested with Nde1 and Xho1 and inserted into the pET28A expression vector (Novagen, San Diego, CA) which contains an N-terminal $6 \times$ His tag.

Isolation of truncated recombinant EBNA-1 proteins

E. coli colonies transformed with pLS7, pLS8, or pLS9 (see above) were selected on LB ampicillin plates and grown at 37°C in 50 ml of LB media containing 1% glucose. Cultures were diluted in 490 ml LB with 0.1 mM IPTG and grown for several hours at 20°C to a final OD_{600} of approximately 0.6. Cultures were harvested and re-suspended in lysis buffer (50 mM Tris-Hcl, pH 7.8, 250 mM NaCl) containing 1.0 mM PMSF. Cells were sonicated for 15 minutes on ice with a 4 second on pulse, 6 seconds off at a 30% amplitude. The cell lysate was cleared by centrifugation at 10,000 rpm for 30 minutes at 4°C and filtered through a 45 μM filter. Five mls of Ni^{2+}-NTA beads equilibrated with lysis buffer were added to the cleared supernatant and incubated with gentle rocking at room temperature. The beads (bound to the recombinant protein) were separated from the supernatant by low- speed centrifugation. They were then washed 6 times with wash buffer (50 mM Tris-HCl, ph 7.8, 250 mM Nacl, 60 mM imidazol, and 10% glycerol). Two ml of elution buffer (50 mM Tris-Hcl, pH 7.8, 250 mM NaCl, 250 mM imidazol, 10% glycerol) were added to the beads and beads were rocked for 15 minutes. The beads were removed from the reaction by low-speed centrifugation. Supernatants containing the recombinant protein were concentrated and the buffer was exchanged with PBS, 250 mM NaCl using an Amicon Centrifugal filter. Proteins were analyzed by SDS-PAGE and Western Blot.

Plasmids (vector pET15b) expressing the following EBNA-1 amino acid sequences; $EBNA_{452-641}$, $EBNA_{459-607}$, and $EBNA_{459-619}$ were gifts from Dr. Lori Frappier [16]. Soluble truncated EBNA-1 proteins were produced in Escherichia coli strain BL21 (DE3) and isolated from cell-lysates. Proteins were then purified over a Ni-NTA agarose column as described above. Proteins were analyzed by SDS-PAGE and Western Blot.

ELISAs

Detection of antibodies to EBNA-1, dsDNA, Sm, LPS, Proteinase 3 and BSA. Diluted serum samples from EBNA-1 injected mice, hybridoma supernatants, or purified monoclonal antibodies were tested for binding to EBNA-1, dsDNA, Sm, LPS, or PR-3 by ELISA as previously described [10,36]. For the detection of antibodies to EBNA-1, LPS, Proteinase 3, and BSA, Costar plates (Corning Incorporated, Corning, NY) were coated in PBS with 2.0–5.0 μg/ml of antigen. Costar plates were coated overnight with 5.0 μg/ml of Sm (Immunovision, Springdale, AR) in 0.1M carbonate buffer for the detection of antibodies to Sm. For the detection of antibodies to dsDNA, Immulon-2 plates (Dynatech Laboratories, Inc., Chantilly, VA) were coated with 100 μg/ml of calf thymus dsDNA.

Detection of antibody binding to truncated amino or carboxyl fragments of EBNA-1. Purified monoclonal antibodies were tested for binding to truncated amino (LS7 and LS8) and carboxyl regions (LS9, $EBNA_{452-641}$, $EBNA_{459-619}$, and $EBNA_{459-607}$) of EBNA-1. ELISA plates were coated with 2.0 μg/ml of the purified, truncated recombinant proteins isolated in this laboratory. Subsequent steps in the ELISA were performed according to Sundar et al [10].

Isotype ELISA. ELISA plates were coated with 50 μl of a 1:1000 dilution of either unlabeled goat anti-mouse IgG1, IgG2a, IgG2b or IgG3 (Southern Biotech, Birmingham, Alabama) and incubated at 37°C for one hour and overnight at 4°C. Monoclonal 3D4 antibody was diluted to 1.5 μg/ml and incubated on the plate for one hour at 37°C. Next, 50 μl of a 1:1000 dilution of goat anti-mouse IgG1 conjugated to alkaline phosphatase (AP), anti-IgG2a-AP, anti-IgG2b-AP, or anti-IgG3-AP (Southern Biotech) was added to wells coated with unlabeled anti-IgG1, anti-IgG2a, anti-IgG2b, or anti- IgG3 respectively. Color development was measured following the addition of 4-nitrophenyl-phosphate disodium salt as substrate and plates were read at 405 nm on a Titertek Multiscan ELISA plate reader.

Quantitative ELISA. A quantitative ELISA was performed, as previously described, to determine the concentration of purified monoclonal IgG antibodies in hybridoma supernatants [36]. Briefly, ELISA plates were coated overnight with 1.0 μg/well of goat anti-mouse IgG antibody (Southern Biotechnology). A commercial mouse monoclonal IgG antibody (Sigma) was serially diluted, beginning at a concentration of 200 ng/ml and used to generate a standard curve. Serial dilutions of monoclonal antibody purified in this laboratory were applied to the anti-IgG coated wells and the concentration of antibody was extrapolated from the standard curve. Monoclonal antibodies were detected with goat anti-mouse IgG antibody conjugated to AP followed by the addition of 4-nitrophenyl-phosphate disodium salt as substrate.

Crithidia Assay

Ready to use Crithidia slides from the CrithiDNA Anti-nDNA Antibody Test Kit from Antibodies Inc. (Davis, CA), were immunostained either with mouse sera from EBNA-1 injected mice, diluted 1/50 or with purified monoclonal antibody diluted to 10 μg/ml. Slides were incubated in a moist, dark chamber for 30 minutes at room temperature (RT). A positive control anti-dsDNA antibody was provided with the kit. A nonspecific monoclonal mouse IgG1 antibody was used as an isotype control (Sigma). Next, the slides were extensively washed with PBS and immunostained for 30 minutes at RT with a 1:250 dilution of biotinylated goat anti mouse IgG (Southern Biotech). This was followed by 20 μl of a 1:500 dilution of Streptavidin-FITC (Southern Biotech) for 30 minutes at RT. Slides were washed again and Prolong Gold Antifade, (Invitrogen, Carlsbad, CA) was added prior to examination by fluorescence microscopy using a Nikon Eclipse microscope, model, TE 2000-S at a magnification of 400×.

Western Blot

Proteins were analyzed by SDS-PAGE on a 12% gel and transferred to a nitrocellulose membrane using a Bio-Rad wet transfer apparatus (BioRad, Hercules, CA). After transfer, the membranes were blocked with 3% Milk-PBS for one hour at RT with shaking. The blot was incubated overnight at 4°C with a MAb generated in our laboratory (3D4), diluted to 1 μg/ml or a commercially prepared MAb, 0211 (Thermo Fisher Scientific/ Pierce, Rockford, IL) diluted to 10 μg/ml according to the manufacturers protocol. The membrane was washed 6 times in wash buffer (PBS, 0.05% Tween-20). Bound MAbs antibodies were detected with HRP-conjugated goat anti mouse IgG (Southern Biotech) diluted 1:20,000, followed by chemiluminescence using the Pierce ECL kit according to the manufacturers protocol (Pierce, Rockford, IL). Molecular weight markers conjugated to *strep-tag* (Precision plus protein WesternC) (Biorad, Hercules, CA) were detected with a 1:20,000 dilution of Strep-Tactin-HRP (Biorad).

Somatic Cell Fusion

BALB/c mice were immunized intraperitoneally (ip) with 50 μg/ml of rEBNA-1 in CFA and then boosted at 3, 7, and 12 weeks with 25 μg/ml of rEBNA-1 in IFA. Three to four days following the third boost, splenocytes were fused with NSO cells according to Iliev et al [37]. They were grown in complete HAT media supplemented with 20% FBS, 10% NCTC, 1% Penicillin-Streptomycin, 1% non-essential amino acids and 1% L-glutamine. Supernatants from hybridomas were tested for IgG anti-EBNA-1 and anti-dsDNA antibodies by ELISAs as described above.

Purification of Monoclonal Antibodies

Hybridomas producing a MAb to EBNA-1 were grown in serum free media (Hyclone, Logan, Utah) and 400 ml of

supernatant were collected for IgG purification. Antibody was purified from the supernatant by eluting it off a protein G Sepharose column (Gamma Bind™ Plus Sepharose ™ gel beads, Amersham Pharmacia, Uppsala, Sweden) with 0.1M glycine pH 2.5, according to the manufacturer's protocol. Column eluate was neutralized with 1M Tris-HCl. The purified antibody was dialyzed overnight with PBS and antibody concentration was determined by a quantitative ELISA (above).

Antibody adsorption on dsDNA-cellulose columns

Columns were packed with 0.5ml of calf thymus dsDNA-cellulose or cellulose beads (Sigma, St.Louis, MO) according to the manufacturer's protocol. The columns were washed with 10 mM Tris buffer pH 7.9 containing 1 mM EDTA. Columns were then blocked with 5% FBS-PBS overnight at 4°C. A 1/1,000 dilution of week 4 and a 1/5000 dilution of week 12, rEBNA-1 injected mouse sera or 5 μg/ml of MAbs, 3D4 or 0211 were slowly loaded onto cellulose and dsDNA cellulose columns and allowed to sit for 1 hour at 4°C. The flow through was collected and pre and post adsorbed sera or monoclonal antibody were tested for binding to dsDNA and EBNA-1 by ELISA and Western blot as described above.

Acknowledgments

We wish to thank Dr. Lori Frappier for supplying us with the recombinant EBNA-1 baculovirus. We also wish to thank Dr. David Fox Schechter for his advice and assistance in the isolation of the recombinant EBNA-1 protein.

Author Contributions

Conceived and designed the experiments: PY PG LAS. Performed the experiments: PY HT RE HW AMW AK EK. Analyzed the data: PY HT RE LAS. Contributed reagents/materials/analysis tools: PG. Wrote the paper: PY PG LAS. Assisted teaching students how to perform somatic cell fusions: RHL.

References

1. Evans AS, Niederman JC (1989) Epstein Barr virus. In ASEvans, ed. Viral Infections of Humans, Epidemiology and Control. New York: Plenum Publishing Corp. pp 265–292.
2. James JA, Neas BR, Moser KL, Bruner GR, Sestak AL, et al. (2001) Systemic lupus erythematosus in adults is associated with previous Epstein-Barr virus exposure. Arthr Rheum 44: 1122–1126.
3. James JA, Kaufman KM, Farris AD, Taylor-Albert E, Lehman TJA, et al. (1997) An increased prevalence of Epstein-Barr virus infection in young patients suggests a possible etiology for Systemic Lupus Erythematosus. J Clin Invest 100: 3019–3026.
4. McClain MT, Poole BD, Bruner BF, Kaufman KM, Harley JB, et al. (2006) An altered immune response to Epstein-B nuclear antigen 1 in pediatric Systemic Lupus Erythematosus. Arthritis & Rheumatism 54: 360–368.
5. Poole BD, Templeton AK, Guthridge JM, Brown EJ, Harley JB, et al. (2009) Aberrant Epstein-Barr viral infection in Systemic Lupus Erythematosus. Autoimmunity Rev 8: 337–342.
6. Harley J, Scofield RH, James JA (2000) Peptide induction of Systemic Lupus autoimmunity. In: MWCunningham, RSFujinami, eds. Molecular Mimicry, Microbes and Autoimmunity ASM Press. pp 109–126.
7. Sabbatini A, Bombardiera S, Migliorini P (1993) Autoantibodies from patients with systemic lupus erythematosus bind a shared sequence of SmD and Epstein-Barr virus-encoded nuclear antigen EBNA 1. Eur J Immunol 23: 1146–1152.
8. James JA, Scofield RH, Harley JB (1997b) Lupus humoral autoimmunity after short peptide immunization. Ann NY Acad Sci 815: 124–127.
9. Poole BD, Gross T, Maier S, Harley JB, James JA (2008) Lupus-like autoantibody development in rabbits and mice after immunization with EBNA-1 fragments. J Autoimmun 31: 362–371.
10. Sundar K, Jacques S, Gottlieb P, Villars R, Benito M-E, et al. (2004) Expression of the Epstein-Barr virus nuclear antigen-1 (EBNA-1) in the mouse can elicit the production of anti-dsDNA and anti-Sm antibodies. J Autoimmun 23: 127–140.

11. Levitskaya J, Coram M, Levisky V, Imreh S, Steigerwald-Mullen PM, et al. (1995) Inhibition of antigen processing by the internal repeat region of the Epstein-Barr virus nuclear antigen-1. Nature 375: 685–688.
12. Ceccarelli DFJ, Frappier L (2000) Functiional analyses of the EBNA-1 origin DNA binding protein of Epstein-Barr virus. J Virol 74: 4939–4948.
13. Fawcett PT, Dubbs SB, Fawcett LB, Doughty RA (1990) Induction of humoral manifestations of autoimmunity following intraperitoneal injection of complete Freund's adjuvant in mice. Autoimmunity 6: 249–256.
14. Gottlieb P, Potgieter C, Wei H, Toporovsky I (2002) Characterization of ø12, a bacteriophage related to ø6: nucleotide sequence of the large double-stranded RNA (dsRNA). Virology 295: 266–271.
15. Rana FR, Sultany CM, Blazyk J (1990) Interactions between Salmonella typhimurium lipopolysaccharide and the antimicrobial peptide magainin 2 amide. FEBS Lett 261: 464–467.
16. Summers H, Barwell JA, Pfuetzner RA, Edwards AM, Frappier L (1996) Cooperative assembly of EBNA1 on the Epstein-Barr virus latent origin of replication. J Virol 70: 1228–1231.
17. Zack DJ, Yamamoto K, Wong AL, Stempniak M, French C, et al. (1995) DNA mimics a self-protein that may be a target for some anti-DNA antibodies in systemic lupus erythematosus. J Immunol 154: 1987–1994.
18. Takeda I, Ravno K, Wolfson-Reichlin M, Reichlin M (1999) Heterogeneity of anti-dsDNA antibodies in their cross-reaction with ribosomal P protein. J Autoimmun 13: 423–428.
19. Deocharan B, Qing X, Lichauco J, Putterman C (2002) α-actinin is a cross-reactive renal target for pathogenic anti-DNA antibodies. J Immunol 168: 3072–3078.
20. DeGiorgio LA, Konstantinov KN, Lee SC, Hardin JA, Volpe BT, et al. (2001) A subset of lupus anti-DNA antibodies cross-reacts with the NR2 glutamate receptor in systemic lupus erythematosus. Nature Medicine 7: 1189–1193.

21. Alberdi F, Dadone J, Ryazanov A, Isenberg DA, Ravirajan C, et al. (2001) Cross-reaction of lupus anti-dsDNA antibodies with protein translation factor EF-2. Clin Immunol 98: 293–300.
22. Jiang C, Deshmukh US, Gaskin F, Bagavant H, Hanson J, et al. (2010) Differential responses to Smith D autoantigen by mice with HLA-DR and HLA-DQ transgenes: dominant responses by HLA-DR3 transgenic mice with diversification of autoantibodies to small nuclear ribonucleoprotein, double-stranded DNA, and nuclear antigens. J Immunol 184: 1085–1091.
23. Sun Y, Fong KY, Chung MC, Yao ZJ (2001) Peptide mimicking antigenic and immunogenic epitope of double-stranded DNA in systemic lupus erythematosus. Int Immunol 13: 223–232.
24. Gaynor B, Putterman C, Valadon P, Spatz L, Scharff MD, et al. (1997) Peptide inhibition of glomerular deposition of an anti-DNA antibody. Proc Natl Acad Sci USA 94: 1955–1960.
25. Zhang W, Reichlin M (2008) A possible link between infection with Burkholderia bacteria and systemic lupus erythematosus based on epitope mimicry. Clin Develop Immunol 2008: 1–7.
26. Shoenfeld Y, Vilner Y, Coates ARM, Rauch J, Lavie G, et al. (1986) Monoclonal anti-tuberculosis antibodies react with DNA and monoclonal anti-DNA antibodies react with Mycobacterium tuberculosis. Clin Exp Immunol 66: 255–261.
27. Sharma A, Isenberg DA, Diamnod B (2001) Crossreactivity of human anti-dsDNA antibodies to phosphorylcholine: clues to their origin. J Autoimmun 16: 479–484.
28. Limpanasithikul W, Ray S, Diamond B (1995) Cross-reactive antibodies have both protective and pathogenic potential. J Immunol 155: 967–973.
29. Riemekasten G, Marell J, Trebeljahr G, Klein R, Hausdorf G, et al. (1998) A novel epitope on the C-terminus of SmD1 is recognized by the majority of sera from patients with systemic lupus erythematosus. J Clin Invest 102: 754–763.
30. Workman CJ, Pfund WP, Voss EWJ (1998) Two dual specific (anti-IgG and anti-dsDNA) monoclonal autoantibodies derived from the NZB/NZW F1 recognize an epitope in the hinge region. J Protein Chem 17: 599–606.
31. Petersen J, Rhodes G, Roudier J, Vaughan JH (1990) Altered immune response to glycine-rich sequences of Epstein-Barr nuclear antigen-1 in patients with Rheumatoid Arthritis and Systemic Lupus Erytematosus. Arthr Rheum 33: 993–1000.
32. Marchini B, Dolcher MP, Sabbatini A, Klein G, Migliorini P (1994) Immune response to different sequences of the EBNA1 molecule in Epstein-Barr Virus-related disorders and in autoimmune diseases. J Autoimmun 7: 179–191.
33. Zhang J, Jacobi AM, Wang T, Berlin R, Volpe BT, et al. (2009) Polyreactive autoantibodies in systemic lupus erythematosus have pathogenic potential. J Autoimmun 2009: 270–274.
34. Bochkarev A, Barwell JA, Pfuetzner E, Bochkarev E, Frappier L, et al. (1996) Crystal structure of the DNA-binding domain of the Epstein-Barr virus origin-binding protein, EBNA-1, bound to DNA. Cell 84: 791–800.
35. Frappier L, O'Donnell M (1991) Overproduction, purification, and characterization of EBNA-1, the origin binding protein of Epstein-Barr V\virus. J Biol Chem 266: 7819–7826.
36. Taylor DK, Ito E, Thorn M, Sundar K, Tedder T, et al. (2006) Loss of tolerance of anti-dsDNA B cells in mice overexpressing CD19. Molec Immunol 43: 1776–1790.
37. Iliev A, Spatz L, Ray S, Diamond B (1994) Lack of allelic exclusion permits autoreactive B cells to escape deletion. J Immunol 153: 3551–3556.

5

Pregnancy and the Risk of Autoimmune Disease

Ali S. Khashan[1], Louise C. Kenny[1], Thomas M. Laursen[2], Uzma Mahmood[1], Preben B. Mortensen[2], Tine B. Henriksen[3], Keelin O'Donoghue[1]*

1 Anu Research Centre, Department of Obstetrics and Gynaecology, Cork University Maternity Hospital, University College Cork, Wilton, Cork, Republic of Ireland, 2 National Centre for Register-Based Research, University of Aarhus, Aarhus, Denmark, 3 Perinatal Epidemiology Research Unit, Department of Paediatrics, Aarhus University Hospital, Aarhus, Denmark

Abstract

Autoimmune diseases (AID) predominantly affect women of reproductive age. While basic molecular studies have implicated persisting fetal cells in the mother in some AID, supportive epidemiological evidence is limited. We investigated the effect of vaginal delivery, caesarean section (CS) and induced abortion on the risk of subsequent maternal AID. Using the Danish Civil Registration System (CRS) we identified women who were born between 1960 and 1992. We performed data linkage between the CRS other Danish national registers to identify women who had a pregnancy and those who developed AID. Women were categorised into 4 groups; nulligravida (control group), women who had 1st child by vaginal delivery, whose 1st delivery was by CS and who had abortions. Log-linear Poisson regression with person-years was used for data analysis adjusting for several potential confounders. There were 1,035,639 women aged >14 years and 25,570 developed AID: 43.4% nulligravida, 44.3% had their first pregnancy delivered vaginally, 7.6% CS and 4.1% abortions. The risk of AID was significantly higher in the 1st year after vaginal delivery (RR = 1.1[1.0, 1.2]) and CS (RR = 1.3[1.1, 1.5]) but significantly lower in the 1st year following abortion (RR = 0.7[0.6, 0.9]). These results suggest an association between pregnancy and the risk of subsequent maternal AID. Increased risks of AID after CS may be explained by amplified fetal cell traffic at delivery, while decreased risks after abortion may be due to the transfer of more primitive fetal stem cells. The increased risk of AID in the first year after delivery may also be related to greater testing during pregnancy.

Editor: Pablo Villoslada, Institute Biomedical Research August Pi Sunyer (IDIBAPS) - Hospital Clinic of Barcelona, Spain

Funding: The study was funded by Science Foundation Ireland. The funders had no role in study design, data collection and analysis, decision to publish, or preparation of the manuscript.

Competing Interests: The authors have declared that no competing interests exist.

* E-mail: k.odonoghue@ucc.ie

Introduction

Autoimmune diseases (AID) are most common among women and increase in incidence following their reproductive years [1]. AID are caused by an immune reaction against self–antigens due to disturbances in T or B cell regulation or function, and autoimmunity may occur in a genetically susceptible individual if an antigen is inadvertently targeted by T or B cells potentially due to environmental or other factors triggering a break in tolerance [2]. Those autoimmune diseases more common in women include systemic lupus erythematosus (SLE; 9:1), autoimmune thyroid disease (8:1), scleroderma (5:1), rheumatoid arthritis (4:1) and multiple sclerosis (3:1), while type 1 diabetes and inflammatory bowel diseases have almost the same female to male ratios of 1:1 and primary sclerosing cholangitis is more prevalent in men.

The human immune system shows some degree of sexual dimorphism. In general, women have higher CD4 cell counts than men, which contributes to an increased CD4/CD8 ratio [3], higher levels of plasma IgM and greater Th1 cytokine production [4]. Sex hormones have been implicated in autoimmunity due to their capacity to modulate the immune response via androgen and estrogen receptors [2]. Dramatic changes in the levels of estrogens, progesterone and other hormones such as cortisol also occur during pregnancy [1]. However, it is unlikely that the difference in sex hormones between women and men alone explains the preponderance of AID in women; most AID occur after reproductive years and administration of sex steroids does not have disease-altering effects [2].

Whether pregnancy or parity influence the development of AID remains a subject of much debate [1,2]. Since pregnancy involves complex interactions between hormonal and immunological factors, it is plausible that it could have differing effects on the development of AID [1]. While results of published studies on the association between pregnancy and SLE are contradictory [5,6], evidence suggests that the risk of multiple sclerosis onset is reduced during gestation and increased in the first 6 months after pregnancy [7,8]. It is unclear, despite much investigation, whether there is an association between parity and the risk of rheumatoid arthritis [9–11]. The currently available data do not provide convincing evidence that parity provides an explanation for the female predominance in the majority of autoimmune conditions.

Trafficking of fetal cells into the maternal circulation begins very early in the pregnancy and the effects of this cell traffic are long lasting [12,13]. All types of fetal cells, including stem cells, cross the placenta during normal pregnancy to enter the maternal blood and tissues, where they may be located decades after pregnancy [14–16]. Fetal microchimerism is defined as low levels of fetal cells persisting in maternal tissues during and after pregnancy. The connection between fetal microchimerism and human disease was first made by Nelson, who speculated that microchimerism might be the underlying basis for the higher prevalence of autoimmune disease in women [17]. This hypothesis is supported by the similarities of chronic graft versus host disease (GVHD) to some autoimmune conditions, the prevalence of these diseases in women, their increased incidence after reproductive years, and the fact that GVHD increases with HLA incompatibility of the donor [18–20].

Fetal microchimerism has now been investigated in many candidate AID, with some results supporting a role in disease pathogenesis [16,20,21]. However, no direct association has been shown between the presence of microchimeric cells and the progression of AID. Reports now suggest that most autoimmune conditions are not significantly associated with more microchimeric cells in blood or tissues when correctly compared to controls. In addition, although fetal cells do appear to accumulate in clinically affected organs, there is no conclusive evidence that fetal cells cause autoimmune disease [20,22]. Some authors suggest that an explanation for the conflicting results in studies relating fetal microchimerism and autoimmune disease is the migration of fetal cells preferentially into target organs of the disease rather than the circulation. Other explanations for the discrepancies in microchimerism results are differences in experimental designs and the sensitivity and specificity of the techniques used by different investigators [18]. Disease severity might also be a factor, and it may be the tissue damage of AID that leads to recruitment to and colonisation of injury sites by fetal cells, rather than autoimmunity itself [16].

Factors predisposing to the development of fetal microchimerism are much debated. There is more fetomaternal cell trafficking where the placenta is abnormal and in certain complications of the pregnancy such as fetal aneuploidy, pregnancy loss and pre-eclampsia [20,23,24]. However, early fetal loss seems the only pregnancy complication significantly influencing the development of microchimerism, and it has been speculated that miscarriage allows more primitive types of fetal cells with the greater capacity to differentiate to enter the maternal circulation [25]. Fetomaternal haemorrhage as a result of first trimester termination of pregnancy has been shown to cause an 80-fold increase in the number of fetal cells in maternal blood [26]. Fetomaternal haemorrhage is also likely to be greater after operative when compared to normal vaginal delivery and thus more microchimerism should be established after caesarean section delivery. It is accepted that even short-term microchimerism can lead to autoimmune disease and the higher amount of trafficking at caesarean section might increase the exposure of these mothers and facilitate the development of autoimmune disease.

The objective of this study was to find out whether risk of new onset autoimmune disease is higher after delivery by caesarean section compared to vaginal delivery and we also aimed to quantify the risk of autoimmune disease after abortion. We investigated the effect of vaginal delivery, caesarean section (CS) and abortion on the risk of subsequent maternal AID using data from the Danish National Registers.

Methods

Study cohort

The study cohort consisted of all women born in Denmark between January 1, 1962 and December 31, 1992. The data were obtained by linking the Danish Civil Registration System [27], the Danish National Hospital Register [28] and the Danish Medical Birth Register [29]. The linkage process was performed using the unique personal identification number (CPR-number), which is used in all national registers and enables accurate linkage between all registers [27]. The linkage process enabled us to identify the firstborn children for those women with children, mother and

infant place of birth, date of delivery, infant sex, date of migration of any woman who left the country and the woman's date of death if the woman died. From the Medical Birth Register, we obtained data on mode of delivery, induced abortion and date of abortion, single or multiple gestations. From the National Hospital Register we obtained information on AID diagnoses, together with inpatient or outpatient hospital contact. The National Hospital Register includes details of inpatient hospitalization from 1977 and inpatient and outpatient contact from 1995 onward. Date of onset of AID was defined as the date of the first contact with the hospital that led to the diagnosis.

Methods

Women were grouped in four exposure categories based on their first pregnancy only: 1) Women who had no previous pregnancy; 2) women who had a vaginal delivery; 3) women who had a CS, and 4) women who had an abortion. Abortion was defined as induced abortion before 20 weeks gestation based on International Classification of Disease revisions 8 and 10 (ICD-8: 640, 641, 642 & ICD-10: DO04) [30,31]. Thirty AID were identified according to ICD-8 and ICD-10 and are listed in Table 1. More details on AID in Denmark are available from recent publications [32].

The AID follow-up period was divided into 1) during pregnancy (this category was included for completeness), 2) first year following pregnancy, 3) second year following delivery, 4) third year following delivery, 5) more than three years but less than 10 years following delivery and 6) 10 years or more. This was also applied to the follow-up period following abortion. The follow-up period started in January 1, 1994 and ended in December 31, 2006. Women were followed-up for AID from their 14th birthday until their deaths, migration, onset of AID or end of study period, whichever came first. Women with a diagnosis of AID that included diabetes before the start of the follow-up period were excluded from the study cohort; as diabetes is generally accepted to have a different aetiology than other AID and its onset usually precedes the childbearing years.

Statistical analysis

Log-linear Poisson regression with aggregated person-years data was used to estimate the relative risk of AID in relation to vaginal delivery, CS and abortions [33]. The models of AID in relation to vaginal delivery and CS were adjusted for age (14–15, 16–17, and in 2 years categories thereafter), calendar year (94–95, 96–97, 98–99, 2000–2001, 2002–2003, 2004–2005, 2006), infant sex (male, female, multiple gestation, no pregnancy) and place of birth (capital city, capital city suburbs, large city, small city, rural area). Models of AID in relation to abortion were adjusted for age, calendar year and place of birth since we had no information on fetal sex in abortions. Age and calendar year were generated as time dependent variables and the other variables were time fixed.

The Poisson models were run separately for vaginal delivery, CS and abortion. The reference group in all the models consisted of women who had no records of pregnancy including abortion. Sensitivity analyses were performed to examine whether age, infant sex or multiple gestation had an effect on association between risk of AID and mode of delivery.

This study was conducted according to the principles expressed in the Declaration of Helsinki. The study was approved by the Danish Data Protection Agency and the Danish National Board of Health. The study was based on secondary data and no individuals were approached, nor did we have access to any other information from the participants. Thus it was not necessary to seek written consent.

Table 1. International classification of disease: autoimmune disease.

Autoimmune Disease	Categorization		Prevalence per 1000	
	ICD8	ICD10	ICD8/ICD10	ICD10 ONLY
Pernicious Anemia	281.0	D51.0	0.54	0.42
Autoimmune Hemolytic Anemia	283.90–91	D59.1	0.14	0.12
Idiopathic Thrombocytopenic Purpura	446.49	D69.3	0.49	0.48
Thyrotoxicosis	242.00	E05.0	4.99	4.82
Autoimmune Thyroiditis	245.03	E06.3	0.63	0.57
Type 1 Diabetes	249	E10	9.75	9.58
Primary Adrenocortical Insufficiency	255.1	E27.1	0.23	0.20
Multiple Sclerosis	340	G35	2.17	2.04
Guillain Barre Syndrome	354	G61.0	0.60	0.27
Iridocyclitis	364	H20	2.17	1.94
Crohn's Disease	563.01	K50	2.78	2.63
Ulcerative Colitis	563.19	K51	5.65	5.25
Autoimmune Hepatitis	571.93	K73	0.51	0.39
Primary Biliary Cirrhosis	571.90	K74.3	0.16	0.13
Coeliac Disease	269.00	K90.0	0.76	0.70
Pemphigus	694 (×694.05)	L10	0.08	0.07
Pemphigoid	694.05	L12	0.14	0.14
Psoriasis vulgaris	696.09–10, 696.19	L40 (xL40.4)	3.43	2.94
Alopecia Areata	704.00	L63	0.34	0.30
Vitiligo	709.01	L80.9	0.24	0.21
Seropositive Rheumatoid Arthritis	712.19, 712.39, 712.59	M05–M06	6.20	5.82
Juvenile Arthritis	712.09	M08	0.86	0.71
Wegener's Granulomatosis	446.29	M31.3	0.18	0.18
Dermatopolymyositis	716	M33	0.21	0.17
Polymyalgia Rheumatica	446.30–31, 446.39	M31.5–6, M35.3	3.02	2.78
Myasthenia Gravis	733.09	G70.0	0.22	0.19
Systemic Sclerosis	734.0	M34	0.30	0.28
Systemic Lupus Erythematosus	734.19	M32.1, M32.9	0.59	0.53
Sjogren's Syndrome	734.90	M35.0	0.78	0.75
Ankylosing Spondylitis	712.49	M45.9	0.85	0.75

Results

During the study period there were 1,035,639 women in Denmark aged 14 years or more. Of those women 25,570 (2.4%) had a diagnosis of AID during 10,786,229 person-years of follow-up. 459,049 women had their first pregnancy delivered vaginally and 11,439 (2.5%) had an AID. 78,694 women had their first pregnancy delivered by CS, of which 1,787 (2.3%) had an AID, and 186,220 had an abortion in their first pregnancy, of which 4,723 (2.5%) had an AID. 455,214 women had no record of a pregnancy during the study period, of which 11,165 (2.4%) had an AID diagnosis. Of the 186,220 women who had abortions, only 42,682 had no records of other pregnancies, thus the numbers do not add up to 1,035,639. When we excluded women who had records of childbirth and abortions in the study cohort, we had 334,205 women with a normal delivery and 60,000 delivered by CS, while 42,682 had abortions, 455,214 had no pregnancy, and 143,538 had abortions and delivery.

Table 2 presents the incidence of AID in relation to age, calendar year, infant sex, multiple gestation and place of birth. It

appears that women who were pregnant had a higher incidence of AID than those who had no pregnancy records and women who had singletons had slightly higher incidence of AID than those who had multiple gestation. It also appeared that the incidence of AID increased with age and with the size of the place of birth.

Table 3 presents the relative risk (RR) estimates of AID in relation to normal delivery, CS and abortion. There was no evidence to support an association between risk of AID and vaginal delivery (RR = 0.91, [95% CI: 0.84, 0.99]), CS (RR = 1.02, [95% CI: 0.94, 1.11]) or abortion (RR = 0.97, [95% CI: 0.92, 1.04]) for all follow-up period after delivery. The estimates show that the risk of AID during pregnancy was significantly reduced in relation to vaginal delivery (RR = 0.76, [95% CI: 0.63, 0.93]) and significantly increased in relation to CS (RR = 1.82, [95% CI: 1.39, 2.38]). In contrast, the RR of AID during pregnancy in relation to abortion was close to one and not significantly changed (RR = 0.92, [95% CI: 0.62, 1.37]).

The risk of AID appeared to be moderately increased in the first year following a pregnancy that ended in vaginal delivery

Table 2. Distribution of 25,570 women with autoimmune disease and 10.8 million person-years of follow-up in a cohort of 1 million women residing in Denmark.

Variable	Cases	Person years	Incidence per 100,000 person years
Infant Sex			
Female	6289	2300317	273.2
Male	6572	2423568	271.2
Multiple gestation	185	72368	255.6
No children	12524	5989845	209.1
Age			
14–19	3007	2100277	143.2
20–25	5021	2295805	218.7
26–29	4377	1694776	258.3
30–35	7188	2612313	275.2
36–41	4816	1669130	288.5
42+	1161	413795.5	280.6
Calendar year			
94–95	2941	1413014	208.1
96–97	3258	1502817	216.8
98–99	3723	1588335	234.4
2000–2001	4111	1676766	245.2
2002–2003	4654	1768593	263.1
2004–2005	4760	1866601	255.0
2006	2123	969972	218.9
Place of birth (mother)			
Capital city	4585	1728824	265.2
Capital city suburbs	2553	1084167	235.5
Large city	3500	1399005	250.2
Small city	9156	3871445	236.5
Rural area	5776	2702656	213.7

a 'No children' includes abortions.

(RR = 1.15, [95% CI: 1.03, 1.28]), and CS (RR = 1.30, [95% CI: 1.10, 1.55]) and moderately reduced in the first year following abortion (RR = 0.70, [95% CI: 0.56, 0.88]). However, the risk of AID was not significantly changed after the first year following delivery apart from a reduction of the risk between year three and year 10 following normal delivery (Table 3).

Table 3. Adjusted relative risk estimates of maternal autoimmune disease in relation to pregnancy.

Follow-up period	AID and vaginal delivery (N)	Vaginal delivery adjusted RR (95% CI	AID and CS (N)	CS Adjusted RR (95% CI)	AID and abortions (N)	Abortion Adjusted RR (95% CI)
No pregnancy	11165	Reference	11165	Reference	11165	Reference
During first pregnancy	105	0.76(0.63, 0.93)	54	1.82(1.39, 2.38)	25	0.92(0.62, 1.37)
All follow-up period	8206	0.91(0.84, 0.99)	1317	1.02(0.94, 1.11)	1154	0.97(0.92, 1.04)
0 to 11 months	673	1.15(1.03, 1.28)	155	1.30(1.10, 1.55)	78	0.70(0.56, 0.88)
12 to 23	539	0.91(0.81, 1.02)	111	0.99(0.81, 1.20)	104	0.96(0.79, 1.16)
24 to 35	544	0.90(0.81, 1.01)	114	1.08(0.89, 1.31)	93	0.90(0.74, 1.11)
36 to 119	3425	0.84(0.78, 0.92)	546	0.97(0.87, 1.07)	566	1.02(0.94, 1.11
120+	3025	0.95(0.88, 1.04)	391	1.01(0.89, 1.13)	313	1.02(0.91, 1.15)

Vaginal delivery and CS models were adjusted for age, calendar year, infant sex and place of birth. Abortion models were adjusted for age, calendar year and infant place of birth. We had no information about fetal sex or number of babies in abortions. Repeating vaginal delivery and CS models for singletons only did not change the estimates. Negative binomial regression models showed that the Poisson models were not over dispersed.

Table 4. Adjusted relative risk estimates of maternal Seropositive Rheumatoid Arthritis in relation to pregnancy.

Follow-up period	Cases in vaginal delivery	Vaginal delivery adjusted RR (95% CI)	Cases in CS	CS Adjusted RR (95% CI)	Cases in abortions	Abortion Adjusted RR (95% CI)
No pregnancy (reference)	721	Reference	721	Reference	721	Reference
During pregnancy	6	0.64(0.28 1.43)	1	0.49(0.07, 3.46)	1	0.57(0.09, 4.08)
All follow-up period	758	0.72(0.55, 0.96)	143	1.17(0.88, 1.55)	79	0.93(0.74, 1.18)
0 to 11 months	50	0.82(0.55, 1.21)	10	1.01(0.58, 1.95)	2	0.28(0.07, 1.12)
12 to 23	26	0.41(0.26, 0.67)	12	1.25(0.68, 2.32)	7	0.99(0.47, 2.09)
24 to 35	45	0.70(0.47, 1.05)	10	1.09(0.56, 2.12)	4	0.60(0.22, 1.59)
36 to 119	293	0.64(0.48, 0.87)	59	1.12(0.79, 1.59)	37	0.97(0.69, 1.35)
120+	344	0.86(0.64, 1.16)	52	1.26(0.88, 1.81)	29	1.16(0.79, 1.70)

Vaginal delivery and CS models were adjusted for age, calendar year, infant sex and place of birth. Abortion models were adjusted for age, calendar year, infant place of birth. We had no information about fetal sex or number of babies in abortions.

To examine the effect of age on the observed associations we repeated the Poisson models as described earlier for three age groups: 1) <24 years; 2) ≥24 and <35 years; 3) ≥35 years. The RR estimates of AID were similar in the three age groups following vaginal delivery and abortion. In contrast, the RR of AID in the first year following CS appeared to be higher in the younger (RR = 1.62; [95% CI: 1.03, 2.57]) and older women (RR = 1.61, [95% CI: 0.97, 2.68]). Also, there was a non-significant increase in risk of AID in the second year following CS in the older women (RR = 1.42, [95% CI: 0.87, 2.33]).

We also examined the effect of fetal sex and multiple gestations on the observed estimates. Separate analyses for males, females and singleton pregnancies did not change the results materially.

Tables 4, 5, 6, 7 present the relative risk estimates of specific AID types in relation to vaginal delivery, CS and abortion. There was little evidence to support an association between risk of rheumatoid arthritis (RA) and vaginal delivery (RR = 0.72, [95% CI: 0.55, 0.96]), CS (RR = 1.17, [95% CI: 0.88, 1.55]) or abortion (RR = 0.93, [95% CI: 0.74, 1.18]) during the follow-up period after delivery. A reduction of the risk of RA three to 10 years after vaginal delivery was observed (Table 4). No association was observed between the mode of delivery and Multiple Sclerosis (Table 5). The risk of thyrotoxicosis was increased in the first year after both vaginal delivery (RR 2.15, [95% CI: 172, 2.68]) and CS

(RR 1.87, [85% CI: 1.33, 2.64]), but not when the first pregnancy resulted in an abortion (Table 6). Finally the risk of inflammatory bowel disease appeared to be reduced following abortion (RR = 0.86, [95% CI: 0.76, 0.97]), but was not significantly changed after vaginal delivery or CS in the same follow up period (Table 7).

Discussion

In this study we report the risk of autoimmune disease during and after pregnancy. Overall the risk of AID in women was significantly higher in the first year following vaginal delivery or CS, but was lower in the first year following abortion. While the risk of AID was reduced between the 3rd and 10th year following vaginal delivery, there was no evidence of a change in the risk of AID beyond the first year following CS or abortion. However, women who were pregnant had a higher incidence of AID than those who had no pregnancy records.

Pregnancy has both short and long term effects on the woman's immune system [2]. Fetal microchimerism, or low levels of fetal cells persisting in the mother, is implicated in the pathogenesis of autoimmune diseases, which have a predilection for women after childbearing [18]. While basic molecular studies have implicated persisting fetal cells in the mother in some AID, supportive

Table 5. Adjusted relative risk estimates of maternal Multiple Sclerosis in relation to pregnancy.

Follow-up period	Cases in vaginal delivery	Vaginal delivery adjusted RR (95% CI)	Cases in CS	CS Adjusted RR (95% CI)	Cases in abortion	Abortion Adjusted RR (95% CI)
No pregnancy (reference)	865	Reference	865	Reference	865	Reference
During pregnancy	8	0.58(0.29, 1.17)	4	1.31(0.49, 3.50)	3	1.51(0.48, 4.68)
All follow-up period	756	1.06(0.82, 1.38)	109	0.93(0.71, 1.22)	118	0.99(0.81, 1.20)
0 to 11 months	47	1.14(0.78, 1.68)	12	1.26(0.69, 2.29)	8	0.94(0.47, 1.88)
12 to 23	25	0.58(0.36, 0.93)	7	0.75(0.35, 1.63)	9	1.01(0.52, 1.95)
24 to 35	46	1.03(0.70, 1.52)	5	0.56(0.23, 1.38)	8	0.90(0.45, 1.81)
36 to 119	333	1.03(0.78, 1.36)	51	0.99(0.71, 1.40)	52	0.94(0.71, 1.24)
120+	305	1.18(0.89, 1.57)	34	0.89(0.60, 1.32)	41	1.08(0.79, 1.50)

Vaginal delivery and CS models were adjusted for age, calendar year, infant sex and place of birth. Abortion models were adjusted for age, calendar year, infant place of birth. We had no information about fetal sex or number of babies in abortions.

Table 6. Adjusted relative risk estimates of maternal Thyrotoxicosis in relation to pregnancy.

Follow-up period	Cases in vaginal delivery	Vaginal delivery adjusted RR (95% CI)	Cases in CS	CS Adjusted RR (95% CI)	Cases in abortions	Abortion Adjusted RR (95% CI)
No pregnancy (reference)	1545	Reference	1545	Reference	1545	Reference
During pregnancy	27	1.17(0.80, 1.72)	11	2.14(1.18, 3.88)	3	0.86(0.28, 2.67)
All follow-up period	1843	1.18(0.99, 1.41)	278	1.18(0.99, 1.42)	226	1.19(1.03, 1.37)
0 to 11 months	204	2.15(1.72, 2.68)	40	1.87(1.33, 2.64)	11	0.75(0.41, 1.35)
12 to 23	149	1.51(1.19, 1.92)	27	1.33(0.89, 1.98)	15	0.99(0.60, 1.65)
24 to 35	121	1.19(0.93, 1.53)	20	1.04(0.66, 1.65)	21	1.40(0.91, 2.17)
36 to 119	721	1.01(0.83, 1.21)	107	1.04(0.82, 1.31)	113	1.23(1.02, 1.49)
120+	648	1.14(0.94, 1.39)	84	1.19(0.92, 1.54)	66	1.23(0.95, 1.58)

Vaginal delivery and CS models were adjusted for age, calendar year, infant sex and place of birth. Abortion models were adjusted for age, calendar year, infant place of birth. We had no information about fetal sex or number of babies in abortions.

epidemiological evidence is limited. To our knowledge, this is the first epidemiological study on the risk of AID following pregnancy. The main strength of the paper is the large cohort used and the fact that it is population based, which avoids the problem of selection bias.

We hypothesized that the risk of AID is increased following pregnancy. Further, if fetomaternal cell trafficking is implicated in the etiology of AID after pregnancy, we expected the highest increase in AID diagnosis following (i) CS, due to increased fetomaternal hemorrhage, and (ii) abortion, as fetal loss has been shown to be the only pregnancy complication significantly influencing microchimerism. The first year after pregnancy should be relevant, being the time period closest to the fetomaternal hemorrhage occurring at delivery. Our results confirm an increase in AID in the first year after CS. The unexpected finding of a reduction in AID risk after abortion may be explained by the premise that early fetal loss allows a higher number of fetal stem or progenitor cells to enter maternal blood, and that these cell types are more likely to engraft maternal tissues long-term, and be beneficial in their role [13,20,25].

As pregnancy involves complicated and dynamic interactions between the endocrine and immune systems, it is possible that it could have differential effects on the development of an autoimmune disease depending on its timing or even complexity relative to

the events that are likely to precede obvious clinical disease [1]. This may explain our findings during and following pregnancy, and the variation between mode of delivery or length of pregnancy.

There were several limitations to our approach. First, since we included data on the first pregnancy only, we did not account for the effect of subsequent pregnancies on the risk of AID. However, the effect we observed on risk of AID was manifest in the first year after pregnancy, which precludes subsequent pregnancies being responsible in the vast majority of women. We accept that in some cases another pregnancy may have occurred in the year follow-up period after a first trimester abortion and that this instead may influence the reduction in AID found. Other studies have previously failed to show an association with parity and the development of AID [1].

Second, it is possible that the increased risk of AID that we observed is linked to the increased risk of AID presenting during pregnancy. Women may be more likely to be tested for AID (along with other diseases) during pregnancy, and it is also possible that some of these diagnoses were not confirmed until after pregnancy. Further, women with symptoms related to AID may experience a complicated pregnancy and thus require delivery by CS. If that is the case then the association that we describe could be related to more testing during pregnancy rather than effects of fetomaternal cell trafficking.

Table 7. Adjusted relative risk estimates of maternal IBD (Colitis and Crohn's disease) in relation to pregnancy.

Follow-up period	Cases in normal delivery	Normal delivery RR (95% CI)	Cases in CS	CS Adjusted RR (95% CI)	Cases in abortions	Abortion Adjusted RR (95% CI)
No pregnancy (reference)	3442	Reference	3442	Reference	3442	Reference
During pregnancy	26	0.68(0.46, 1.00)	17	2.16(1.34, 3.49)	5	0.56(0.23, 1.35)
All follow-up period	1823	0.91(0.77, 1.07)	263	0.85(0.71, 1.01)	279	0.86(0.76, 0.97)
0 to 11 months	167	1.02(0.82, 1.27)	33	0.98(0.68, 1.41)	16	0.44(0.27, 0.72)
12 to 23	144	0.90(0.71, 1.13)	27	0.87(0.59, 1.30)	26	0.74(0.50, 1.09)
24 to 35	129	0.83(0.65, 1.05)	30	1.06(0.73, 1.55)	31	0.95(0.67, 1.36)
36 to 119	802	0.86(0.72, 1.03)	109	0.79(0.63, 0.99)	156	1.00(0.85, 1.18)
120+	581	0.97(0.81, 1.17)	64	0.81(0.61, 1.07)	50	0.78(0.58, 1.03)

Vaginal delivery and CS models were adjusted for age, calendar year, infant sex and place of birth. Abortion models were adjusted for age, calendar year, infant place of birth. We had no information about fetal sex or number of babies in abortions.

Third, another limitation of the study was the inability to report the risk of AID after spontaneous abortion. This would be relevant as not only are the risks of spontaneous abortion increased with some AID, but also microchimerism is more likely to be established after induced abortion. We were only able to obtain data on induced abortion from the Danish Medical Birth Register.

Finally, we report limited details on the increased risk of each individual AID, as small numbers of affected women in some disease categories during the follow-up period prevents accurate statistical analysis in all groups. Nonetheless we believe these data are important to report, as they show the relationship between pregnancy and maternal AID in a large population-based cohort over a detailed follow-up period.

We suggest an association between pregnancy and the risk of subsequent maternal AID, with a significant impact on the first year after delivery. However, given the number of unanswered questions and the available data, conclusions on the role of fetal microchimerism in the development of autoimmune diseases cannot be drawn.

Acknowledgments

We thank Marianne G. Pedersen, MSc, National Centre for Register-based Research, University of Aarhus, Denmark, for her assistance with the study design. We thank Professor William Eaton, Department of Mental Health, Johns Hopkins Bloomberg School of Public Health, for his contribution to the database used in the present study.

Author Contributions

Conceived and designed the experiments: ASK LCK UM TML KOD. Performed the experiments: ASK TML TBH KOD. Analyzed the data: ASK TML TBH PBM KOD. Contributed reagents/materials/analysis tools: LCK TML TBH PBM. Wrote the paper: ASK LCK TML UM KOD.

References

1. Borchers AT, Naguwa SM, Keen CL, Gershwin ME (2010) The implications of autoimmunity and pregnancy. J Autoimmun 34(3): J287–99.
2. Adams Waldorf KM, Nelson JL (2008) Autoimmune disease during pregnancy and the microchimerism legacy of pregnancy. Immunol Invest 37(5): 631–44.
3. Amadori A, Zamarchi R, De Silvestro G, Forza G, Cavatton G, et al. (1995) Genetic control of the CD4/CD8 T-cell ratio in humans. Nat Med (12): 1279–83.
4. Butterworth M, McClellan B, Allansmith M (1967) Influence of sex in immunoglobulin levels. Nature 214(5094): 1224–5.
5. Ulff-Moller CJ, Jorgensen KT, Pedersen BV, Nielsen NM, Frisch M (2009) Reproductive factors and risk of systemic lupus erythematosus: nationwide cohort study in Denmark. J Rheumatol 36(9): 1903–9.
6. Cooper GS, Dooley MA, Treadwell EL, St Clair EW, Gilkeson GS (2002) Hormonal and reproductive risk factors for development of systemic lupus erythematosus: results of a population-based, case-control study. Arthritis Rheum 46(7): 1830–9.
7. Runmarker B, Andersen O (1995) Pregnancy is associated with a lower risk of onset and a better prognosis in multiple sclerosis. Brain 118(Pt 1): 253–61.
8. Alonso A, Clark CJ (2009) Oral contraceptives and the risk of multiple sclerosis: a review of the epidemiologic evidence. J Neurol Sci 286(1–2): 73–5.
9. Jorgensen KT, Pedersen BV, Jacobsen S, Biggar RJ, Frisch M (2010) National cohort study of reproductive risk factors for rheumatoid arthritis in Denmark: a role for hyperemesis, gestational hypertension and pre-eclampsia? Ann Rheum Dis 69(2): 358–63.
10. Ostensen M, Villiger PM (2007) The remission of rheumatoid arthritis during pregnancy. Semin Immunopathol 29(2): 185–91.
11. Heliovaara M, Aho K, Reunanen A, Knekt P, Aromaa A (1995) Parity and risk of rheumatoid arthritis in Finnish women. Br J Rheumatol 34(7): 625–8.
12. Lissauer DM, Piper KP, Moss PA, Kilby MD (2009) Fetal microchimerism: the cellular and immunological legacy of pregnancy. Expert Rev Mol Med 11: e33.
13. O'Donoghue K (2006) Implications of fetal stem cell trafficking in pregnancy. Reviews in Gynaecological and Perinatal Practice 6: 87–98.
14. Bianchi DW, Zickwolf GK, Weil GJ, Sylvester S, DeMaria MA (1996) Male fetal progenitor cells persist in maternal blood for as long as 27 years postpartum. Proc Natl Acad Sci U S A 93(2): 705–8.
15. O'Donoghue K, Chan J, de la Fuente J, Kennea N, Sandison A, et al. (2004) Microchimerism in female bone marrow and bone decades after fetal mesenchymal stem-cell trafficking of pregnancy. Lancet 364(9429): 179–82.
16. Klonisch T, Drouin R (2009) Fetal-maternal exchange of multipotent stem/progenitor cells: microchimerism in diagnosis and disease. Trends Mol Med 15(11): 510–8.
17. Nelson JL, Furst DE, Maloney S, Gooley T, Evans PC, et al. (1998) Microchimerism and HLA-compatible relationships of pregnancy in scleroderma. Lancet 351(9102): 559–62.
18. Nelson JL (1998) Microchimerism and the pathogenesis of systemic sclerosis. Curr Opin Rheumatol 10(6): 564–71.
19. Nelson JL (1996) Maternal-fetal immunology and autoimmune disease: is some autoimmune disease auto-alloimmune or allo-autoimmune? Arthritis Rheum 39(2): 191–4.
20. Miech RP (2010) The role of fetal microchimerism in autoimmune disease. Int J Clin Exp Med 3(2): 164–8.
21. Nelson JL (2002) Pregnancy and Microchimerism in Autoimmune Disease: Protector or Insurgent? Arthritis Rheum 46(2): 291–297.
22. Lambert N, Nelson JL (2003) Microchimerism in autoimmune disease: more questions than answers? Autoimmun Rev 2(3): 133–9.
23. Bianchi DW, Williams JM, Sullivan LM, Hanson FW, Klinger KW, et al. (1997) PCR quantitation of fetal cells in maternal blood in normal and aneuploid pregnancies. Am J Hum Genet 61(4): 822–9.
24. Jansen MW, Korver-Hakkennes K, van Leenen D, Visser W, in 't Veld PA, et al. (2001) Significantly higher number of fetal cells in the maternal circulation of women with pre-eclampsia. Prenat Diagn 21(12): 1022–6.
25. Khosrotehrani K, Johnson KL, Lau J, Dupuy A, Cha DH, et al. (2003) The influence of fetal loss on the presence of fetal cell microchimerism: a systematic review. Arthritis Rheum 48(11): 3237–41.
26. Bianchi DW, Farina A, Weber W, Delli-Bovi LC, Deriso M, et al. (2001) Significant fetal-maternal hemorrhage after termination of pregnancy: implications for development of fetal cell microchimerism. Am J Obstet Gynecol 184(4): 703–6.
27. Pedersen CB, Gotzsche H, Moller JO, Mortensen PB (2006) The Danish Civil Registration System. A cohort of eight million persons. Dan Med Bull 53(4): 441–9.
28. Andersen TF, Madsen M, Jorgensen J, Mellemkjoer L, Olsen JH (1999) The Danish National Hospital Register. A valuable source of data for modern health sciences. Dan Med Bull 46(3): 263–8.
29. Knudsen LB, Olsen J (1998) The Danish Medical Birth Registry. Dan Med Bull 45(3): 320–3.
30. Manual of the International Classification of Disease (ICD8). Geneva, Switzerland: World Health Organization.
31. The ICD-10 Classification of Mental and Behavioral Disorders. Geneva, Switzerland: World Health Organization.
32. Eaton WW, Rose NR, Kalaydjian A, Pedersen MG, Mortensen PB (2007) Epidemiology of autoimmune diseases in Denmark. J Autoimmun 29(1): 1–9.
33. Breslow NE, Day NE (1987) Statistical methods in cancer research: The design and analysis of cohort studies. Lyon: International agency for research on cancer.

6

Identification of Unique MicroRNA Signature Associated with Lupus Nephritis

Jeannie L. Te[1], Igor M. Dozmorov[1], Joel M. Guthridge[2], Kim L. Nguyen[1], Joshua W. Cavett[1], Jennifer A. Kelly[1], Gail R. Bruner[1], John B. Harley[1,3,4], Joshua O. Ojwang[1]*

1 Department of Arthritis and Immunology, Oklahoma Medical Research Foundation, Oklahoma City, Oklahoma, United States of America, 2 Department of Clinical Immunology, Oklahoma Medical Research Foundation, Oklahoma City, Oklahoma, United States of America, 3 Department of Medicine, University of Oklahoma Health Sciences Center, Oklahoma City, Oklahoma, United States of America, 4 United States Department of Veterans Affairs Medical Center, Oklahoma City, Oklahoma, United States of America

Abstract

MicroRNAs (miRNA) have emerged as an important new class of modulators of gene expression. In this study we investigated miRNA that are differentially expressed in lupus nephritis. Microarray technology was used to investigate differentially expressed miRNA in peripheral blood mononuclear cells (PBMCs) and Epstein-Barr Virus (EBV)-transformed cell lines obtained from lupus nephritis affected patients and unaffected controls. TaqMan-based stem-loop real-time polymerase chain reaction was used for validation. Microarray analysis of miRNA expressed in both African American (AA) and European American (EA) derived lupus nephritis samples revealed 29 and 50 differentially expressed miRNA, respectively, of 850 tested. There were 18 miRNA that were differentially expressed in both racial groups. When samples from both racial groups and different specimen types were considered, there were 5 primary miRNA that were differentially expressed. We have identified 5 miRNA; hsa-miR-371-5P, hsa-miR-423-5P, hsa-miR-638, hsa-miR-1224-3P and hsa-miR-663 that were differentially expressed in lupus nephritis across different racial groups and all specimen types tested. Hsa-miR-371-5P, hsa-miR-1224-3P and hsa-miR-423-5P, are reported here for the first time to be associated with lupus nephritis. Our work establishes EBV-transformed B cell lines as a useful model for the discovery of miRNA as biomarkers for SLE. Based on these findings, we postulate that these differentially expressed miRNA may be potential novel biomarkers for SLE as well as help elucidate pathogenic mechanisms of lupus nephritis. The investigation of miRNA profiles in SLE may lead to the discovery and development of novel methods to diagnosis, treat and prevent SLE.

Editor: Terry Means, Massachusetts General Hospital/Harvard University, United States of America

Funding: This work was supported in part by National Institutes of Health (Centers of Biomedical Research Excellence (COBRE) Pilot Grant 0169-04-12-4, NO1-AR62277, PO1-AI 083194, R37-AI 24717, RO1-AR42460, PO1-AR049084, P20 RR020143, R01 AI045050, P30 AR053483, GORDRCC AR053483), the United States Department of Veteran Affairs, the Alliance for Lupus Research, Lupus Family Registry and Repository (LFRR), and the American Cancer Society (IRG-05-066-04). The funders had no role in study design, data collection and analysis, decision to publish, or preparation of the manuscript.

Competing Interests: The authors have declared that no competing interests exist.

* E-mail: Joshua-ojwang@omrf.org

Introduction

Systemic Lupus Erythematosus (SLE) is a complex autoimmune disease. The immunological hallmark of SLE is the production of a range of autoantibodies directed at ubiquitous nuclear components. It is characterized by immune-mediated damage to multiple organ systems with a corresponding diverse array of systemic symptoms. The etiology of SLE is still undetermined, but it is known to involve a complex interaction of genetic and environmental factors [1][2]. SLE has a prevalence of ~40 cases per 100,000 individuals with onset typically occurring in women of childbearing age (F:M ratio 9:1) [3]. There is a diverse variation in disease prevalence in different ethnic populations with a 3–4 times increased prevalence in African American (AA) [3,4], and an elevated rate of nephritis relative to European Americans (EA). AA lupus has an earlier age of onset and a clinically more severe phenotype [5]. Nephritis is often a severe manifestation of SLE [6,7] and is frequently linked to a poor long-term prognosis with a greater than four-fold increase in mortality [8].

Current aggressive immunosuppression therapies are effective in controlling renal lupus flares and have improved disease outcomes, but side effects such as infection, malignancy, metabolic disturbances, and infertility make this treatment option unsatisfactory. Potential contributions of microRNA to the pathogenesis and mechanisms of damage to kidneys in SLE-associated nephritis may allow development of more specific, effective, and less toxic therapies. In addition, conventional immunosuppressive drugs for treatment of SLE associated nephritis, such as corticosteroids, cyclophosphamide, and azathioprine, could be used more effectively and with fewer side effects if clinicians could accurately predict SLE-associated nephritis or renal flare and response to treatment [9]. The use of unique miRNA expression signatures could be an important and cost-effective means to monitor predisposition to lupus nephritis or its pathogenesis.

Small non-coding RNA molecules (microRNA or miRNA) are a gene expression and protein synthesis modulating mechanism that has been recently identified in several species including humans. These miRNA are single-stranded RNA molecules of about 20–25 nucleotides (nt) encoded by nuclear genes (70–150 nt) and are highly conserved among species. These genes are not translated into proteins but are processed from primary transcripts (called pri-miRNA) to short stem-loop structures called pre-miRNA and finally to functional miRNA. The expression pattern of miRNA varies over time and between tissues. These mature miRNA molecules are partially complementary to one or more mRNA sequences and they function through sequence-specific down-regulation of their target mRNA via mRNA degradation or inhibition of translation [10]. In the public miRNA database (miRBase) there are over 700 proposed human miRNA.

MiRNA are now recognized as one of the most highly abundant agents of gene regulation at the post-transcriptional level in higher eukaryotes [11,12]. It is estimated that miRNAs account for 1–5% of expressed genes in the animal genome and about 20–30% of all human mRNA are known to be miRNA targets. Because miRNA function as managers in gene regulatory networks, they are distinct from other biomarkers because they may have an upstream and potentially pathogenic role in the disease process. Quantitation of miRNA gene expression levels has become an essential step in understanding mechanisms for cellular processes such as cell differentiation, cell proliferation and cell death, and has shown great promise in identifying effective biomarkers that correlate with human diseases [13].

Although dysregulation of miRNA expression has been characterized mostly in cancer, it has recently been studied in many other diseases. Specifically, miRNA have been proposed as a regulator of immune cell development [14], playing a role in the inflammatory response [15] and as a key player in the pathogenesis of neurodegenerative diseases [16]. The relationship between SLE and miRNA was first reported by Dai et al who studied the relationship in PBMCs [17] and renal biopsies [9] obtained from Chinese SLE patients. The role miRNA play in autoimmune diseases is incomplete or only beginning to be characterized especially with regard to miRNA. However, the importance of miRNA on post-transcriptional regulation of gene expression in SLE is emerging with some surprising results. In one relevant example a mouse model of SLE with defects in miRNA regulation of mRNA induced disease. Here miRNA101 suppresses expression of the ICOS (a costimilatory molecule on T cells), which is defective in sanroque model of lupus, leading to stimulation of autoreactive B cells and a lupus-like illness [18]. Understanding the role of miRNA in SLE may have important implications for disease pathology.

We evaluated miRNA expression by microarray technology in samples obtained from lupus nephritis patients and unaffected controls. In these samples we identified changes in miRNA expression that correlate with lupus. Five miRNA (hsa-miR-371-5P, hsa-miR-423-5P, hsa-miR-638, hsa-miR-1224-3P and hsa-miR-663) were differentially expressed across different racial groups and in all specimen types tested. Three of these miRNA (hsa-miR-371-5P, hsa-miR-1224-3P and hsa-miR-423-5P) were associated with lupus nephritis and are reported here for the first time. These miRNA may be potential novel biomarkers or may help to elucidate pathogenic mechanisms of lupus nephritis.

Results

MiRNA expression profiles in EBV-transformed B-cell lines derived from SLE African American samples

In the initial effort to use lupus study participants derived EBV-transformed B-cell lines to identify differentially expressed miRNA in lupus patients, we performed microarray analysis of miRNA expression profiles in EBV-transformed cells from 10 AA SLE

patients with nephritis as well as from unaffected controls. Patients were matched by gender, age and race.

We observed a total of 29 miRNAs that were differentially expressed in SLE-affected patients compared to unaffected controls (**Table 1**). Twenty four were up-regulated and 5 were down-regulated in these SLE samples.

Validation of the miRNA expression

To validate microarray results, three miRNA—has-miR-148A, has-miR-423-5P and has-miR-371-5P—were randomly selected for quantitative real-time PCR (QRT-PCR) verification using stem-loop real-time PCR. In this study a new set of RNA isolated from another culture of EBV-transformed B-cell lines was used as described in Material and Methods. The RNA used in these experiments was extracted at a different time from the EBV-transformed cell lines obtained from 3 SLE patients and a control pool (2 unaffected donors). The QRT-PCR results obtained here validated the microarray data (data not shown) because the ratios (see Materials and Method Section) in both experiments were very similar. For example, the ratios of has-miR-148A, has-miR-423-5P and has-miR-

Table 1. MiRNAs differentially expressed in SLE African American samples derived cell lines.

Differential Expression Type	MiRNA Name	Mean Ratio
Up-regulated	hsa-miR-886-3P	4.87±1.43
	hsa-miR-142-3P	2.84±0.45
	hsa-miR-23A	2.62±0.89
	hsa-miR-602	2.51±0.71
	hsa-miR-371-5P	2.44±1.20
	hsa-miR-125A-3P	2.34±1.12
	hsa-miR-720	2.33±0.67
	hsa-miR-148A	2.32±0.66
	hsa-miR-142-5P	2.23±0.65
	hsa-let-7I	2.20±0.80
	hsa-miR-27A	2.09±0.45
	hsa-miR-92B*	2.09±0.35
	hsa-miR-487B	2.07±0.55
	hsa-miR-26A	2.02±0.04
	hsa-miR-373*	2.02±0.44
	hsa-miR-181A	2.01±1.27
	hsa-miR-663	1.86±0.25
	hsa-miR-27B	1.80±0.17
	hsa-miR-23B	1.80±0.28
	hsa-miR-30C	1.80±0.08
	hsa-miR-191	1.73±0.30
	hsa-miR-638	1.62±0.12
	hsa-miR-24	1.59±1.00
	hsa-miR-423-5P	1.53±1.29
Down-regulated	hsa-miR-342-3P	0.60±0.03
	hsa-miR-328-5P	0.51±0.15
	hsa-miR-1224-3P	0.48±0.06
	hsa-miR-1228*	0.38±0.10
	hsa-miR-149*	0.35±0.14

371-5P in microarray test are 2.32, 1.53 and 2.44, respectively; while in QRT-PCR test they were 2.54, 1.63 and 2.72.

MiRNAs expression profile in PBMCs derived from SLE African American samples

The hypothesis guiding our study is that a distinct profile of miRNA expression alters gene expression to contribute to SLE, and more specifically that this profile is evident in B cells and is retained and faithfully represented in these transformed cell lines. To investigate the authenticity of EBV-miRNAs association with SLE, RNA extracted from frozen PBMCs obtained from the LFRR of AA SLE-affected patients and unaffected matched controls were used. In this study miRNA profiles were obtained by comparing the pool of SLE patients (5 AA in the SLE pool) and the pool of control (5 AA in the control pool) samples. The individual RNA of appropriate samples was added into each pool after RNA extraction.

As shown in **Table 2**, a total of 21 miRNA were differentially expressed in the SLE-affected samples compared to the unaffected matched controls. Twenty miRNA were up-regulated and one was down-regulated. The study also revealed that the 6 miRNA; hsa-miR-342-3P, hsa-miR-27B, hsa-miR-371-5P, hsa-miR-423-5P, hsa-miR-638 and hsa-miR-663, were differentially expressed in both experiments using EBV-transformed B-cell lines (Table 1) and PBMCs. This indicates that EBV-transformed B-cell lines derived from SLE-affected patients and unaffected controls can be used to develop a miRNA signature associated with SLE. The use of EBV-transformed B-cells in these types of studies has advantages because the cell lines are assumed to be cultured in a uniform environment independent of the consequences of the

Table 2. MiRNAs differentially expressed in SLE African American samples derived PBMCs.

Differential Expression Type	MiRNA Name	Mean Ratio
Up-regulated	hsa-miR-675	3.96
	hsa-miR-199A-3P-199B-3P	3.34
	hsa-miR-371-5P	2.80
	hsa-miR-18A	2.74
	hsa-miR-199A-5P	2.53
	hsa-miR-150*	2.47
	hsa-miR-185	2.33
	hsa-miR-20B	2.13
	hsa-miR-223	1.97
	hsa-miR-663	1.94
	hsa-miR-25	1.88
	hsa-miR-423-3P	1.86
	hsa-miR-93	1.79
	hsa-miR-638	1.69
	hsa-miR-301A	1.64
	hsa-miR-27B	1.61
	hsa-miR-361-3P	1.55
	hsa-miR-92A	1.53
	hsa-miR-155	1.53
	hsa-miR-145	1.51
Down-regulated	hsa-miR-342-3P	0.63

disease and pathogenesis of SLE can be studied in a patient population that may not be accessible or are no longer living.

MiRNAs expression profile in SLE European American samples

The preceding experiments performed with AA samples established the utility of the EBV-transformed B- cell lines obtained from SLE-affected patients as suitable reagents for evaluating miRNA association with lupus. Therefore, to extend the study to another ancestry, we used EBV-transformed B-cell lines obtained from 10 SLE-affected patients and 10 matched unaffected controls to investigate differential miRNA expression in EA.

A total of 50 miRNA (**Table 3**) were differentially expressed in the EA SLE-affected samples compared to the unaffected matched controls. Forty-two were up-regulated and 8 were down-regulated. In this study 17 and 7 miRNA that were previously differentially expressed in AA SLE derived B-cell lines and PBMCs, respectively, (Tables 1 and 2) were also differentially expressed in these EA samples. These results suggest that specific miRNAs differentially expressed across racial groups may be SLE disease specific.

MiRNAs expression profiles in SLE discordant identical twins

The evidence for a strong genetic component to SLE comes from the many genes shown to be associated with SLE as well as the observations that SLE disease concordance rate is 24–58% for monozygotic twins compared to 2–5% for dizygotic twins and other siblings is a 10-fold difference [1]. To examine the miRNA profile in AA SLE discordant identical twins, we used EBV-transformed B-cell lines obtained from a SLE-affected twin and an unaffected monozygotic twin as control. The SLE twin was both anti-dsDNA and renal-disorder negative.

In this study a total of 31 miRNAs (**Table 4**) were differentially expressed in SLE-affected twin compared to the unaffected monozygotic twin controls. Twenty-nine were up-regulated and 2 were down-regulated. Of these, 9, 15 and 18 were previously shown to be differentially expressed in PBMCs, AA cell lines and EA cell lines, respectively.

Discussion

The experiments reported here were performed primarily using EBV-transformed B cell lines obtained from SLE-affected patients and unaffected controls. Our results suggest EBV-transformed B cell lines are a useful reagent for discovery of miRNA as biomarkers for SLE. The use of EBV-transformed B-cells in these studies has several advantages; i) The Lupus Family Registry and Repository (LFRR) at Oklahoma Medical Research Foundation (OMRF) has a substantial number of EBV-transformed cell lines obtained from SLE cases and controls, which are readily available for study. ii) The cell lines are 100% B-cells and therefore eliminate cell population variations. iii) The cells allow the identification and characterization of B-cell specific miRNAs that are associated with SLE. Therefore, the mechanism by which SLE differentially-expressed miRNAs affects a subset of target genes can be investigated by focusing on the pathway that leads to B-cell activation.

Here, we investigated the association of miRNA with SLE. Using miRNA microarray analysis, we isolated and analyzed miRNA in EBV-transformed B-cell lines and frozen PMBCs obtained from SLE-affected patients with nephritis as well as unaffected controls. The study identified 5 miRNA—hsa-miR-371-5P, hsa-miR-423-5P, hsa-miR-638, hsa-miR-1224-3P and

Table 3. MiRNAs differentially expressed in SLE European American samples derived cell lines.

Differential Expression Type	MiRNA Name	Mean Ratio
Up-regulated	hsa-miR-638	6.90±1.33
	hsa-miR-328-5P	6.45±1.50
	hsa-miR-1228*	5.86±3.56
	hsa-miR-663	5.34±0.75
	hsa-miR-92B*	5.07±3.91
	hsa-miR-371-5P	4.92±1.20
	hsa-miR-675	4.88±2.00
	hsa-miR-125A-3P	4.71±2.56
	hsa-miR-483-5P	4.60±1.51
	hsa-miR-665	4.44±2.90
	hsa-miR-602	4.37±3.98
	hsa-miR-187*	4.33±2.75
	hsa-miR-423-3P	4.23±1.17
	hsa-miR-583	4.01±1.50
	hsa-miR-654-5P	3.73±1.98
	hsa-miR-150*	3.63±0.95
	hsa-miR-933	3.50±1.17
	hsa-miR-149*	3.47±1.54
	hsa-miR-744	3.40±1.29
	hsa-miR-516A-5P	3.31±0.65
	hsa-miR-373*	3.25±1.01
	hsa-miR-550	3.15±1.50
	hsa-miR-92B	3.05±0.91
	hsa-miR-181A	3.03±1.98
	hsa-miR-320A	2.82±1.47
	hsa-miR-30C-1*	2.78±0.90
	hsa-miR-378	2.69±0.86
	hsa-miR-30B	2.66±0.37
	hsa-miR-30D	2.59±0.89
	hsa-miR-198	2.42±0.46
	hsa-miR-298	2.29±0.18
	hsa-miR-874	2.28±0.67
	hsa-miR-135A*	2.14±0.64
	hsa-miR-765	2.03±0.57
	hsa-miR-659	1.98±0.53
	hsa-miR-193B	1.95±0.30
	hsa-miR-494	1.83±1.54
	hsa-miR-222	1.75±0.81
	hsa-miR-142-3P	1.74±1.45
	hsa-miR-29C	1.66±0.15
	hsa-miR-140-3P	1.61±0.68
	hsa-miR-148A	1.61±1.31
Down-regulated	hsa-miR-20A	0.58±0.07
	hsa-miR-26A	0.53±0.09
	hsa-miR-768-3P	0.50±0.11
	hsa-miR-1224-3P	0.50±0.10
	hsa-miR-886-3P	0.49±0.12
	hsa-miR-720	0.48±0.08

Table 3. Cont.

Differential Expression Type	MiRNA Name	Mean Ratio
	hsa-miR-155	0.46±0.11

hsa-miR-663—that were differentially expressed across different ancestries and all specimen types tested. The miRNA, hsa-miR-371-5P, hsa-miR-1224-3P and hsa-miR-423-5P, are associated with lupus nephritis and are reported here for the first time. The other two miRNA we detected in this study, hsa-miR-638 and hsa-miR-663, have previously been reported [9] to be associated with lupus nephritis in Chinese renal biopsies samples. The three miRNA—hsa-miR-181, hsa-miR-186, and hsa-miR-590-3p—together predicted to target a number of lupus genes [19], only

Table 4. MiRNAs profile from monozygotic discordant twins.

Differential Expression Type	MiRNA Name	Mean Ratio
Up-regulated	hsa-miR-638	13.82
	hsa-miR-149*	6.64
	hsa-miR-1228*	5.48
	hsa-miR-146A	5.05
	hsa-miR-328-5P	4.86
	hsa-miR-146B-5P	3.74
	hsa-miR-423-3P	3.65
	hsa-miR-34A	3.42
	hsa-miR-29A	3.05
	hsa-miR-675	2.94
	hsa-miR-24	2.84
	hsa-miR-663	2.84
	hsa-miR-222	2.83
	hsa-miR-371-5P	2.65
	hsa-miR-21	2.47
	hsa-miR-92B*	2.47
	hsa-miR-221	2.37
	hsa-miR-30D	2.09
	hsa-miR-23A	2.01
	hsa-miR-342-3P	2.00
	hsa-Let-7I	1.93
	hsa-Let-7G	1.92
	hsa-miR-92A	1.85
	hsa-miR-150*	1.83
	hsa-Let-7C	1.80
	hsa-miR-125A-3P	1.80
	hsa-Let-7F	1.66
	hsa-miR-483-3P	1.64
	hsa-miR-373*	1.57
Down-regulated	hsa-miR-720	0.50
	hsa-miR-155	0.47

hsa-miRNA 181 was found to be differentially expressed in RNA isolated from EBV-transformed B-cell lines obtained both AA and EA SLE affected patients. The miRNA reported here may serve as SLE-specific signature miRNA and could be used as a biomarker for the diagnosis of at least lupus nephritis.

Lupus nephritis is severe and the available treatment regimens are effective; however, because of the side effects, treatments are associated with significant morbidity and mortality [9]. The discovery and development of new biomarkers such as the miRNA detected in this study of lupus nephritis could help in mitigating the side effects of the treatments by predicting the onset, severity and response of renal flares and thus allowing for the adjustment of therapy with the disease stage.

Our miRNA microarray analysis also revealed additional 7 miRNA—hsa-miR-1228*, hsa-miR-125A-3P, hsa-miR-149*, hsa-miR-328-5P, hsa-miR-373*, hsa-miR-720 and hsa-miR-92B*—that were differentially expressed in cell lines but not in frozen PBMC samples. This may be due to fact that the PMBC experiment was done on pooled samples or due to a difference in specimen types. The miRNA hsa-miR-342-3P was differentially expressed in AA samples only. The 10 miRNA reported here have also been reported elsewhere [9] further confirming the utility of EBV-transformed cell lines. As has been reported in previous studies [9] our study also did not reproduce most of the miRNA profile reported by Tang et al. [20], In fact the primary miRNA, has-miR-146a, they determined to be associated with lupus, was only shown to be differentially expressed in discordant identical twins microarray analysis. This could be attributable to differences in the methodology used, and/or major SLE phenotype studied in each case because the SLE identical twin was one of the two patients that was negative for both renal-disorder and anti-dsDNA (**Table 5**). This observation might be anticipated because SLE is a complex disease and therefore, each major SLE phenotype might have different miRNA profiles and from this study we can speculate that has-miR-146a may be differentially expressed in SLE patients who are negative for renal-disorder or anti-dsDNA or both.

In the effort to explore the possible molecular mechanisms of the regulation by the 5 major miRNA identified above, we used bioinformatics prediction tools such as miRBase at http://www.mirbase.org/to search for the potential molecular targets among the genes that have been reported to associate with SLE pathogenesis [21–25]. This bioinformatics investigation revealed the potential gene targets for the primary miRNA identified in this study (**Table 6**) and most of these genes products are important mediators of IFN signaling. These encouraging and interesting observations link these miRNA to multiple components in the IFN pathway.

Because miRNAs function as managers in gene regulatory networks, they may provide quantitative regulation of genes instead of on and off switch signals; therefore, they can be considered as molecules that optimize a cell's response to external stimuli [26]. The work we present here, taken together with studies reported previously on Chinese patients with lupus [17] [20] indicate that there is good reason to further investigate the connections between specific miRNAs and lupus. We and others have identified novel miRNA associated with lupus nephritis, and these molecules are potentially important diagnostic biomarkers and may be involved in the pathogenesis of lupus nephritis.

Materials and Methods

Ethics

The study we describe was approved by the OMRF Institutional Review Board (IRB) and all samples were obtained with the written informed consents of the subjects.

Study subjects

Samples for these studies were obtained from the SLE patients and controls recruited by the Oklahoma Medical Research Foundation (OMRF) Lupus Family Registry and Repository (LFRR). The LFRR is a unique SLE research resource. The repository contains blood products from SLE patients and unaffected controls from across the United States, Canada, Puerto Rico, and the US Virgin Islands. In addition, the permanent B-cell lines have been established for most of the peripheral blood lymphocytes from both SLE patients and healthy donors. Finally, the LFRR also store frozen peripheral blood mononuclear cells (PBMCs) obtained from some SLE patients and unaffected controls. A total of 52 samples were used in this study. These included 26 SLE affected and 26 unaffected controls. Of these, 32 were from African American (AA) and 20 from European American (EA) racial groups. The 52 samples were made up of 42 Epstein-Barr virus (EBV)-transformed cell lines and 10 PBMCs. All SLE patients fulfilled at least four out of 11 of the American

Table 5. Clinical features of the subjects in the study.

Characteristics	SLE Affected Patients (n = 26)	Unaffected Controls (n = 26)
Gender, no. Male/Female	1/25	1/25
Ethnicity, no. AA/EA	16/10	16/10
Year of birth, mean±SD	1962.31±11.01	1962.85±12.51
Age at sample, mean±SD	40.69±11.10	39.73±12.90
Age at onset, mean±SD	31.88±11.25	NA
Anti-dsDNA, no. positive/negative	24/2	0/26
Renal Disorder, no. positive/negative	24/2	0/26
Proteinuria, no. positive/negative	24/2	0/26
Malar Rash, no. positive/negative	16/10	0/26
Discoid Rash, no. positive/negative	11/15	0/26
Photosensitivity, no. positive/negative	13/13	0/26
Oral Ulcer, no. positive/negative	12/14	0/26
Arthritis, no. positive/negative	26/0	0/26
Serositis, no. positive/negative	20/6	0/26
Neuro Disorder, no. positive/negative	5/21	0/26
Hemolytic Anemia, no. positive/negative	5/21	0/26
Medications (Steroids or/and others)	26/26	NA

Table 6. The potential gene target for the primary differentially expressed miRNA.

Major miRNA identified	Potential molecular Targets
hsa-miR-371-5P	IL32, IFIT3, IFIT2, FGR, IRF5, CD40, PTTG1
hsa-miR-423-5P	SLC2A4, VGF, SOX12
hsa-miR-638	CD79B, LY6E, ZNF330
hsa-miR-663	IL32, IFI35, CENTA1, LY6E, ZNF330
hsa-miR-1224-3P	GPDH, PMVK, BSG

College of Rheumatology (ACR) criterion classifications [27], and at least 24 of these patients met the ACR criteria for lupus nephritis. These cases were in general being actively treated. All of them had been given or were taking prednisone or a comparable corticosteroid. Of the 26, hydroxychloroquine or cloroquine (n = 1) had been used in 16. Azathiaprine was used in 18, cyslophos[phamied in 9 and one each for cyclosporine and mycophenolate mofetil. Nonsteriodal anti-inflammatory drugs has been used in 21 of the cases. We had no therapeutic history from the controls. Additional clinical information on the participants is given in Table 5.

Preparation of EBV-transformed B-cell lines

Epstein-Barr virus-transformed cell lines of the SLE patients and controls were obtained from the LFRR. The permanent B-cell lines were established by EBV transformation of peripheral blood lymphocytes from both SLE patients and apparently healthy donors as described elsewhere [28]. At the time of experiment, the selected EBV-transformed B cell lines were thawed and after overnight incubation at $37°C$ in a humid atmosphere with 5% CO_2, the culture media was transferred to 15 ml conical tubes and centrifuged for 10 minutes at $300×g$. The cell pellet resuspended in fresh complete RPMI media in T-25 flasks and expanded. One million subconfluent cells was transferred to 50 ml conical tubes and centrifugation step above repeated. Cells were washed twice with 5 ml 1X PBS and pellets were flash frozen in liquid nitrogen for 20–30 seconds and stored at $−80°C$ until they were used for preparation of total RNA.

Preparation of Frozen PBMCs

PBMCs (stored in liquid nitrogen) were obtained from the LFRR. Vials containing approximately one million cells were thawed in a water bath at $37°C$ and transferred into 50 ml conical tubes containing 10 ml of complete media previously warmed at $37°C$. The 50 ml conical tubes were centrifuged for 10 minutes at $300×g$ and the supernatants decanted. The cells were washed twice with 5 ml 1X PBS and the pellets flash frozen in liquid nitrogen for 20–30 seconds followed by storage at $−80°C$ until isolation of total RNA.

miRNA isolation

Two to 10 micrograms of total RNA were isolated from cell suspensions of approximately 10^6 EBV-transformed B cells from individual cell lines using a Trizol-based (Tri Reagent® [Sigma-Aldrich, #T9424] or Trizol® [Invitrogen, #15596-026]) approach. This method captures small miRNAs that are lost by silica-based isolation methods.

Cells were centrifuged and cell pellets lysed in Trizol reagent followed by processing according to the manufacturer's protocol. Briefly, the aqueous phase of the cell lysate for each cell line was transferred to a fresh tube and 0.5 ml of isopropanol per ml of Trizol reagent used in the cell preparation was added to precipitate RNA. The samples were incubated at room temperature for 5–10 minutes and then centrifuged at $12,000×g$ for 10 minutes at $4°C$. The RNA precipitate formed a pellet on the side and bottom of the tube. The supernatant was removed from each tube and the RNA pellets washed by adding 1 ml of 75% ethanol per ml of Trizol reagent used in the cell preparation; the tubes were mixed by vortexing and then centrifuged at $7,500×g$ for 5 minutes at $4°C$. RNA pellets were briefly dried by air-drying or under vacuum. RNA pellets were then dissolved by adding appropriate volume of formamide, water or 0.5% SDS solution. To facilitate dissolution, the RNA samples were mixed by repeat pipetting with micropipetting at $55–60°C$ for 10–15 minutes. The

concentration and quantity of RNA were measured by UV absorbance at 260 and 280 nm (A260/280 ratio) and checked by gel electrophoresis. RNA samples were quality checked via the Agilent 2100 Bioanalyzer platform (Agilent Technologies). The results of the Bioanalyzer run were visualized in a gel image and an electropherogram. The yields were 8–15 µg and RNA Integrity Number (RIN) was between 7.2 and 10. According to published data, RNA with a RIN number >6 is of sufficient quality for gene expression profiling experiments as well as miRNA microarray experiments [29,30].

MiRNA microarray analysis

miRNAs were labeled using 2 µg of total RNA and an Exiqon miRCURY™ Labeling Kit (#208032) or Exiqon Power Labeling kit (208032-A) according to manufacturer's specifications. These kits use total RNA and enrichment of small RNA is not necessary. The miRNA analysis was performed at Miltenyi Biotec Inc using miRXplore Microarray product (Miltenyi Biotec Inc; Auburn, CA). The microarray kit contains gene-specific oligonucleotide probes generated from 850 human, 584 mouse, 426 rat and 122 viral precursor miRNAs. MiRXplore Microarrays carry DNA oligonucleotides with a reverse-complementary sequence of mature miRNAs. RNA samples to be analyzed were directly labeled. After fluorescent labeling of miRNAs, the sample was hybridized to the miRXplore Microarray. The fluorescence signals generated by hybridization of miRNAs to array complementary DNAs were detected and quantified using an Agilent laser scanner (Agilent Technologies).

The miRNA labeling by manufacturer's protocol employed monoreactive Cy5 dye (Amersham Pharmacia Biotech, LTD) for dyeing. The fluorescently labeled samples were hybridized overnight to topic defined PIQOR™ miRXplore Microarrays using the a-Hyb™ Hybridization Station. In general, control samples are labeled with Hy3 and experimental samples are labeled with Hy5. The fluorescent probes were lyophilized, resuspended in 15 µl of diethyl pyrocarbonate (DEPC) water and 5 µl of 4× hybridization buffer, denatured by heating for 5 minutes at $70°C$ and then snap-cooled on ice for 15 minutes. The fluorescent probes were hybridized for 20 hours at $42°C$ in a rotating hybridization oven and 0.25–1 µg of total RNA was used per labeling reaction per slide hybridization. After hybridization, slides were washed and then scanned (Agilent Technologies).

Image and Data Analysis

Mean signal and mean local background intensities were obtained for each spot of the microarray images using the ImaGene software (Biodiscovery). Low-quality spots were flagged and excluded from data analysis. Unflagged spots were analyzed with the PIQOR™ Analyzer software. The PIQOR Analyzer allows automated data processing of the raw data text files derived from the ImaGene software. This includes background subtraction to obtain the net signal intensity, data normalization, and calculation of the Hy5/Hy3 ratios for the species of interest. As an additional quality filtering step, only spots/genes are used for the calculation of the Hy5/Hy3 ratio. Signals that are equal to or higher than the 50% percentile of the background signal intensities is used to generate a double-log scatter plot.

MiRNA ratio calculation

The PIQOR™ Analyzer calculates all normalized mean Hy5/Hy3 ratios of the four replicates per gene. MiRNAs that are >1.5-fold up- or down-regulated represent putative candidate miRNAs and are highlighted by green and red colors in the miRNA re-ratio list. Green color indicates a <0.66-fold down-regulation, corresponding to a fold change < -1.5 of a certain miRNA in comparison to the control sample. Red color indicates a more than 1.5-fold induction of the respective miRNA in comparison to the control.

The entire microarray data are MIAME compliant and the raw data have been deposited in a MIAME compliant database (GEO) and the accession number is GSE21384.

Quantitative real-time PCR verification of microarray results

Quantitative reverse transcription-PCR (RT-PCR) assays were performed using a TaqMan miRNA assay kit (Applied Biosystems, Foster City, CA) for the mature miRNA. The miR-148A, miR-423-5P and miR-371-5p were randomly selected miRNAs for this assay. Reverse transcription (RT) was performed using TaqMan MicroRNA RT kit (Applied Biosystems). In this reaction of mature miRNA 2 ng/μl of total RNA, 1× target-specific stem-loop RT primer, 3.33 U/μl reverse transcriptase, 0.25 U/μl RNase inhibitor, 0.25 mM dNTPs, and 1× reaction buffer were run in a total reaction volume of 15 μl and incubated at 16°C for 30 min, 42°C for 30 min, and 85°C for 5 minutes in a thermocycler (Applied Biosystems).

Real-time PCR was performed using an Applied Biosystems 7900HT Sequence Detection System in a 10-μl PCR mixture containing 1.33 μl of RT product, 2× TaqMan Universal PCR Master Mix, 0.2 μM TaqMan probe, 15 μM forward primer, and 0.7 μM reverse primer. Each SYBR Green reaction was performed with 1.0 μl of template cDNA, 10 μL of SYBR Green

mixture, 1.5 μM primer, and water to adjust the final volume to 20 μl.

The forward primer sequences for selected miRNAs and U6 were purchased from Applied Biosystems and used for real-time PCR validation. These primers are: miR-148A: 5′-TCAGTG-CACTACAGAACTTTGT-3′, miR-423-5P: 5′-TGAGGGGCA-GAGAGCGAGACTTT-3′ and miR-371-5p: 5′ ACTCAAACT-GTGGGGGCACT-3′. All reactions were incubated in a 96-well plate at 95°C for 10 minutes, followed by 40 cycles of 95°C for 15 seconds, and 60°C for 1 minute; all were performed in triplicate. The U6 gene was used as a control to normalize differences in total RNA levels in each sample. The relative amount of each miRNA to U6 RNA was expressed using equation $2^{-\Delta\Delta C_t}$, where $\Delta\Delta C_t = (C_{t\ miRNA} - C_{t\ U6})$. The value of each control sample was set at 1 and was used to calculate the fold change in target genes.

Acknowledgments

We thank Dr. John Knight and Ellen Goodmon for the editorial help during the preparation of this manuscript.

Author Contributions

Conceived and designed the experiments: JMG JBH JOO. Performed the experiments: JLT KLN JWC JOO. Analyzed the data: ID JOO. Contributed reagents/materials/analysis tools: JAK GB. Wrote the paper: JOO.

References

1. Deapen D, Escalante A, Weinrib L, Horwitz D, Bachman B, et al. (1992) A revised estimate of twin concordance in systemic lupus erythematosus. Arthritis Rheum 35: 311–318.
2. Alarcon-Segovia D, Alarcon-Riquelme ME, Cardiel MH, Caeiro F, Massardo L, et al. (2005) Familial aggregation of systemic lupus erythematosus, rheumatoid arthritis, and other autoimmune diseases in 1,177 lupus patients from the GLADEL cohort. Arthritis Rheum 52: 1138–1147.
3. McCarty DJ, Manzi S, Medsger TA, Jr., Ramsey-Goldman R, LaPorte RE, et al. (1995) Incidence of systemic lupus erythematosus. Race and gender differences. Arthritis Rheum 38: 1260–1270.
4. Johnson AE, Gordon C, Palmer RG, Bacon PA (1995) The prevalence and incidence of systemic lupus erythematosus in Birmingham, England. Relationship to ethnicity and country of birth. Arthritis Rheum 38: 551–558.
5. Fessel WJ (1974) Systemic lupus erythematosus in the community. Incidence, prevalence, outcome, and first symptoms; the high prevalence in black women. Arch Intern Med 134: 1027–1035.
6. Nossent JC, Bronsveld W, Swaak AJ (1989) Systemic lupus erythematosus. III. Observations on clinical renal involvement and follow up of renal function: Dutch experience with 110 patients studied prospectively. Ann Rheum Dis 48: 810–816.
7. Mak A, Mok CC, Chu WP, To CH, Wong SN, et al. (2007) Renal damage in systemic lupus erythematosus: a comparative analysis of different age groups. Lupus 16: 28–34.
8. Bernatsky S, Boivin JF, Joseph L, Manzi S, Ginzler E, et al. (2006) Mortality in systemic lupus erythematosus. Arthritis Rheum 54: 2550–2557.
9. Dai Y, Sui W, Lan H, Yan Q, Huang H, et al. (2009) Comprehensive analysis of microRNA expression patterns in renal biopsies of lupus nephritis patients. Rheumatol Int 29: 749–754.
10. Bartel DP (2004) MicroRNAs: genomics, biogenesis, mechanism, and function. Cell 116: 281–297.
11. Bentwich I, Avniel A, Karov Y, Aharonov R, Gilad S, et al. (2005) Identification of hundreds of conserved and nonconserved human microRNAs. Nat Genet 37: 766–770.
12. Berezikov E, Guryev V, van de BJ, Wienholds E, Plasterk RH, et al. (2005) Phylogenetic shadowing and computational identification of human microRNA genes. Cell 120: 21–24.
13. Calin GA, Croce CM (2006) Genomics of chronic lymphocytic leukemia microRNAs as new players with clinical significance. Semin Oncol 33: 167–173.
14. Baltimore D, Boldin MP, O'Connell RM, Rao DS, Taganov KD (2008) MicroRNAs: new regulators of immune cell development and function. Nat Immunol 9: 839–845.
15. O'Connell RM, Rao DS, Chaudhuri AA, Boldin MP, Taganov KD, et al. (2008) Sustained expression of microRNA-155 in hematopoietic stem cells causes a myeloproliferative disorder. J Exp Med 205: 585–594.

16. Nelson PT, Wang WX, Rajeev BW (2008) MicroRNAs (miRNAs) in neurodegenerative diseases. Brain Pathol 18: 130–138.
17. Dai Y, Huang YS, Tang M, Lv TY, Hu CX, et al. (2007) Microarray analysis of microRNA expression in peripheral blood cells of systemic lupus erythematosus patients. Lupus 16: 939–946.
18. Miller DT, Shen Y, Weiss LA, Korn J, Anselm I, et al. (2008) Microdeletion/duplication at 15q13.2q13.3 among individuals with features of autism and other neuropsychiatirc disorders. J Med Genet doi:10.1136/jmg.2008.059907.
19. Vinuesa CG, Rigby RJ, Yu D (2009) Logic and extent of miRNA-mediated control of autoimmune gene expression. Int Rev Immunol 28: 112–138.
20. Tang Y, Luo X, Cui H, Ni X, Yuan M, et al. (2009) MicroRNA-146A contributes to abnormal activation of the type i interferon pathway in human lupus by targeting the key signaling proteins. Arthritis Rheum 60: 1065–1075.
21. Huang X, Shen N, Bao C, Gu Y, Wu L, et al. (2008) Interferon-induced protein IFIT4 is associated with systemic lupus erythematosus and promotes differentiation of monocytes into dendritic cell-like cells. Arthritis Res Ther 10: R91.
22. Tang J, Gu Y, Zhang M, Ye S, Chen X, et al. (2008) Increased expression of the type I interferon-inducible gene, lymphocyte antigen 6 complex locus E, in peripheral blood cells is predictive of lupus activity in a large cohort of Chinese lupus patients. Lupus 17: 805–813.
23. Feng X, Wu H, Grossman JM, Hanivadhanakul P, FitzGerald JD, et al. (2006) Association of increased interferon-inducible gene expression with disease activity and lupus nephritis in patients with systemic lupus erythematosus. Arthritis Rheum 54: 2951–2962.
24. Kirou KA, Lee C, George S, Louca K, Peterson MG, et al. (2005) Activation of the interferon-alpha pathway identifies a subgroup of systemic lupus erythematosus patients with distinct serologic features and active disease. Arthritis Rheum 52: 1491–1503.
25. Karonitsch T, Feierl E, Steiner CW, Dalwigk K, Korb A, et al. (2009) Activation of the interferon-gamma signaling pathway in systemic lupus erythematosus peripheral blood mononuclear cells. Arthritis Rheum 60: 1463–1471.
26. Taganov KD, Boldin MP, Baltimore D (2007) MicroRNAs and immunity: tiny players in a big field. Immunity 26: 133–137.
27. Tan EM, Cohen AS, Fries JF, Masi AT, McShane DJ, et al. (1982) The 1982 revised criteria for the classification of systemic lupus erythematosus. Arthritis Rheum 25: 1271–1277.
28. Compton LJ, Steinberg AD, Sano H (1984) Nuclear DNA degradation in lymphocytes of patients with systemic lupus erythematosus. J Immunol 133: 213–216.
29. Fleige S, Walf V, Huch S, Prgomet C, Sehm J, et al. (2006) Comparison of relative mRNA quantification models and the impact of RNA integrity in quantitative real-time RT-PCR. Biotechnol Lett 28: 1601–1613.
30. Fleige S, Pfaffl MW (2006) RNA integrity and the effect on the real-time qRT-PCR performance. Mol Aspects Med 27: 126–139.

7

Importance of Correlation between Gene Expression Levels: Application to the Type I Interferon Signature in Rheumatoid Arthritis

Frédéric Reynier[1], Fabien Petit[1], Malick Paye[1], Fanny Turrel-Davin[1], Pierre-Emmanuel Imbert[1], Arnaud Hot[1], Bruno Mougin[1], Pierre Miossec[1,2]*

1 Joint Unit Hospices Civils de Lyon - bioMérieux, Hôpital Edouard Herriot, Lyon, France, 2 Department of Clinical Immunology and Rheumatology, and immunogenomics and Inflammation Research Unit EA 4130, University of Lyon, Hôpital Edouard Herriot, Lyon, France

Abstract

Background: The analysis of gene expression data shows that many genes display similarity in their expression profiles suggesting some co-regulation. Here, we investigated the co-expression patterns in gene expression data and proposed a correlation-based research method to stratify individuals.

Methodology/Principal Findings: Using blood from rheumatoid arthritis (RA) patients, we investigated the gene expression profiles from whole blood using Affymetrix microarray technology. Co-expressed genes were analyzed by a biclustering method, followed by gene ontology analysis of the relevant biclusters. Taking the type I interferon (IFN) pathway as an example, a classification algorithm was developed from the 102 RA patients and extended to 10 systemic lupus erythematosus (SLE) patients and 100 healthy volunteers to further characterize individuals. We developed a correlation-based algorithm referred to as Classification Algorithm Based on a Biological Signature (CABS), an alternative to other approaches focused specifically on the expression levels. This algorithm applied to the expression of 35 IFN-related genes showed that the IFN signature presented a heterogeneous expression between RA, SLE and healthy controls which could reflect the level of global IFN signature activation. Moreover, the monitoring of the IFN-related genes during the anti-TNF treatment identified changes in type I IFN gene activity induced in RA patients.

Conclusions: In conclusion, we have proposed an original method to analyze genes sharing an expression pattern and a biological function showing that the activation levels of a biological signature could be characterized by its overall state of correlation.

Editor: Pierre Bobé, Institut Jacques Monod, France

Funding: There are no current external funding sources for this study. This work was supported by both bioMérieux and Hospices Civils de Lyon, with a 50/50 shared contribution. This support goes to a mixed research unit of which Professor Miossec is the director. The funders had no role in study design, data collection and analysis, decision to publish, or preparation of the manuscript.

Competing Interests: The authors have the following competing interests: Some authors are employed by the diagnostic company bioMérieux. There are no patents, products in development or marketed products to declare.

* E-mail: pierre.miossec@univ-lyon1.fr

Introduction

A wide range of methods for microarray data analysis have evolved, ranging from simple fold-change approaches to many complex and computationally demanding techniques [1]. Gene expression profiling by microarray technology has become a widely used strategy for investigating the molecular mechanisms underlying many complex diseases [2]. However, the analysis is further complicated by the biological heterogeneity encountered in most of the diseases.

A common observation in the analysis of gene expression is that many genes show similar expression patterns [3] which may share biological functions under common regulatory control. Moreover, these co-expressed genes are frequently clustered according to their expression patterns in subset of experimental conditions [4]. Thus, gene co-expression instead of differential expression could

be informative as well. Bi-clustering methods seek gene similarity in subsets of available conditions, which is more appropriate for functionally heterogeneous data [5,6].

We have further explored this approach to study the heterogeneity of rheumatoid arthritis (RA) patients regarding their mRNA profiles in whole blood samples. In the context of RA, the clinical presentation of patients shows a high degree of heterogeneity, ranging from mild cases with a benign course to severe and erosive disease. In RA, gene expression profiling has been used to stratify patients based on molecular criteria using synovial tissue [7,8] and more recently from peripheral blood cells [9].

Here, we took the signature of interferon (IFN)-related genes as an example to study correlation levels between genes composing that signature. A biclustering algorithm was applied to study a large gene expression dataset from peripheral whole blood of 102 RA patients. A correlation-based search algorithm referred to as

Classification Algorithm Based on a Biological Signature (CABS) was developed to characterize patients based on their IFN signature. In RA patients with an activated IFN signature, gene expression levels were highly correlated and this was linked to the level of global IFN signature activation.

Results

Analysis of heterogeneity in RA with the biclustering method

Based on 102 RA patients, the study of biological data heterogeneity was conducted with a biclustering approach. This method using the SAMBA algorithm performs clustering on genes and conditions simultaneously in order to identify subsets of genes that show similar expression patterns across specific subsets of patients and vice versa. After data filtering, 121 biclusters were identified from 9,856 selected probe sets. To draw a clear picture of these co-expressed gene groups, the TANGO algorithm was used for GO functional enrichment analysis. The details of the results are given in table S1. Among them, these results have highlighted the importance of immune regulation across the "immune response" and "response to virus" ontology groups (biclusters 4, 21, 34, 35 and 39; see Table S1 as supplement information). Subsequently, we focused on bicluster 4 which represents the largest number of genes in these two GO categories.

Ingenuity pathway analysis of IFN signature

To further elucidate the importance of immune regulation, we conducted pathway analyses on bicluster 4 (n = 37 genes). To summarize, a pathway corresponding to interferon signaling (*IFI35, IFIT1, IFIT3, IFITM1, IRF9, MX1, OAS1, STAT2*) was prominently represented (B-H p-value = 1.86E-13). Moreover, a literature review showed that 35 genes among the 37 appeared directly or indirectly related to interferon. Thereafter, IPA was conducted on the 35 genes which composed the IFN signature. IPA can not only build associations of genes identified in our analysis ("focus" genes), but also predict the involvement of additional molecules not associated in the main gene list. Out of the list, 32 genes were found in the IPA knowledge database, and are labelled "focus genes". Based on these focus genes, IPA generated a biological network (score 85, focus genes 32) providing evidence that type I IFN represented by the *IFNα* and *IFNβ* genes is responsible for the activation of IFN-related genes (Figure 1). The list of these 35 genes is presented in the right column of figure 2.

Activation of IFN pathway in a sub-group of RA patients

To visualize the expression profiles of the 35 IFN-response genes among all RA patients and to investigate their interactions, a hierarchical clustering was performed with the Spotfire Decision Site 8.2.1. This clustering separated the samples into two main groups, one of patients with RA (n = 26/102, 25.5%) with high expression (Figure 2, blue dendrogram) of this set of IFN-related genes (IFN^{high}) and another (n = 76/102, 74.5%) with lower expression (Figure 2, purple dendrogram) (IFN^{low}).

Characterization of the IFN signature based on a correlation approach

The expression pattern of 35 IFN-response genes was defined as the "IFN signature". To go further in the description of the IFN-related genes, the correlation levels between the co-expressed genes were assessed in the two groups of RA patients. Interestingly, the analysis revealed disparities between correlation

levels. The group associated with high IFN expression level showed a better correlation ($R_{median} = 0.63$) than the other one ($R_{median} = 0.33$), with a significant difference (p = 8.46E-13), suggesting a functional difference in the activated state of these genes. A classification algorithm was applied to obtain a better characterization of the IFN signature based on the correlation of the 35 gene expression levels. The results showed that the IFN signature presented a large variation between individuals (Figure 3). 15/100 HC (15%), 22/102 RA patients (22%) and 10/10 SLE patients (100%) with a decision variable ≥ 1 for the high signature (IFN^{high}) were identified, while the remainder of individuals, with a decision variable < 1, were defined as IFN^{low}. From the sub-groups identified by the CABS, the comparison of the correlation profiles showed heterogeneous distributions (Figure 4). Two groups were observed, first with RA and SLE patients with a high IFN signature and a median correlation of 0.63 and 0.68 respectively; second with RA patients and HC IFN^{low} and a median correlation of 0.33 and 0.27 respectively. However, the shape of the curve for the HC IFN^{high} ($R_{median} = 0.44$; Figure 4, blue line) is very different from that seen for the IFN high RA or SLE patients and for the IFN low RA or controls. This suggests a very heterogeneous activation status of genes in this group of controls.

Comparison of characterization methods of IFN signature

A comparative analysis between correlation-based approach (CABS) and the classical "IFN score" based on the average values of gene expression was performed (Figure 5). First, this figure showed a correlation between the decision variable (correlation value) and the average values of gene expression (Spearman correlation test, r = 0.65, p-value<0.0001). Second, based on the respective thresholds, this comparison revealed differences between both approaches (9%). Individuals (black triangles) with a high average expression value of IFN-related genes were associated with a low level of correlation and vice versa with individuals represented by a black square.

Effect of TNF inhibition on IFN pathway activation

The functional relationship between TNF inhibition and possible changes in IFN pathway activation was studied. CABS was used to assess the correlation levels in RA patients before and after anti-TNFα treatment. Out of the subgroup of 43 RA patients treated with anti-TNF, 22 RA patients (11 RA IFN^{high} and 11 RA IFN^{low}; infliximab n = 6, etanercept n = 10 and adalimumab n = 6) were evaluated at 6 months for treatment response using the DAS28 criteria. Although the values appeared quite heterogeneous, a statistical significant decrease (p = 0.0186) of the correlation level was observed in patients associated with high IFN signature (Figure 6A). In contrast, a statistical significant increase (p = 0.002) of correlation levels was seen in RA patients with low IFN signature before treatment (Figure 6B). Despite a significant increase, the majority of these RA patients IFN^{low} did not reach the threshold of positivity. No statistical association was observed between the molecular stratification of RA patients (IFN^{high}/IFN^{low}) and the clinical characteristics presented in table 1 or the response to treatment at 6 months.

Discussion

In this study, the heterogeneous nature of RA was addressed at a molecular level and the data showed that disease characteristics could be reflected by gene expression levels in whole blood. Using microarray technology, RA patients could be categorized into 121 biclusters, sub-groups of patients sharing a same profile for a group

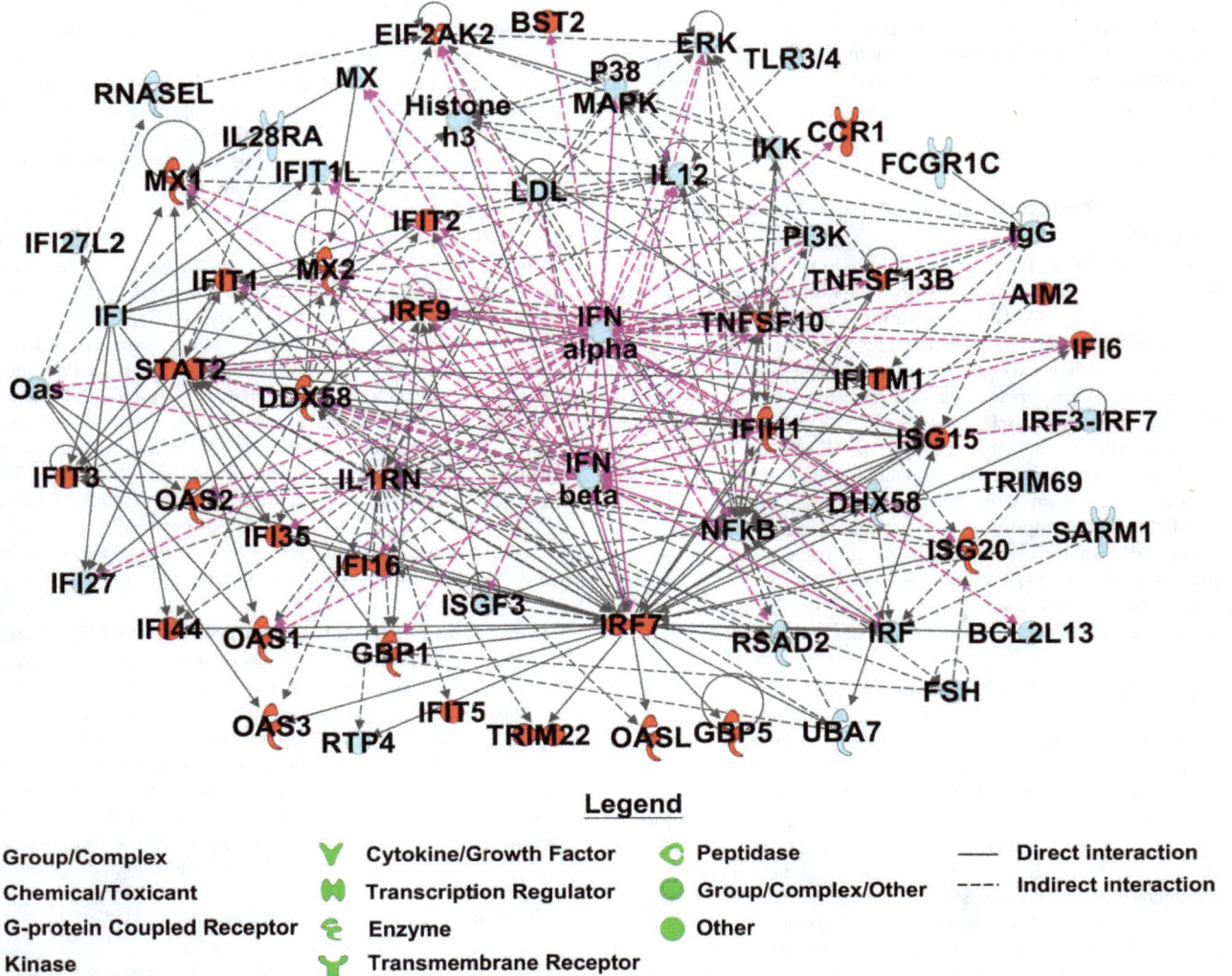

Figure 1. The network derived from the 35 genes which composed the IFN signature using Ingenuity Pathway Analysis (IPA) software. Edges (gene relationships) are displayed with labels that describe the nature of the relationship between nodes (genes). Nodes are displayed using various shapes that represent the functional class of the gene product. Genes in red belong to the list of the 35 IFN-related genes. Genes in blue were integrated into the computationally generated networks on the basis of the evidence stored in the IPA knowledge memory indicating a relevance to this network. The network showed central connection represented by the type I interferon. The pink arrows represent the direct and indirect interactions for genes of type I family of interferons (IFN-α, IFN-β).

of genes. With the type I IFN signature as an example, we showed a variation of the correlation level within 102 RA patients representative to the RA population. Each patient can be characterized by a single correlation value of the expression observed for the 35 IFN-related genes. Interestingly, our results revealed a heterogeneous IFN expression (Figure 2) characterized by a correlation level of the gene expression which may reflect the global IFN signature activation. This method allowed us to define two well separated groups (IFN^{low} vs. IFN^{high}; p = 8.46E-13) based on the correlation levels with the IFN^{high} corresponding to 22% of our RA patients cohort. In fact, it was shown that genes with similar functions usually are co-expressed under certain experimental conditions only [4]. The sample profiles can resemble to the physiological relationships expected between the studied samples [10]. Prieto C. et al. demonstrated that studies of heterogeneous datasets, mixing many case samples from pathological or altered states with "normal" samples disturb gene co-expression analysis. In the context of these observations, our

results suggest that the co-expressed gene clusters, defining functional groups, depend on the activation status.

The method commonly used in the literature does not take into account the activation status of the biological signature, which could generate some misclassification. Indeed, the increase of IFN regulated genes has been reported in different diseases like SLE [11], systemic sclerosis [12], multiple sclerosis [13] and in tissues from patients with Sjögren's syndrome [14], type I diabetes [15,16] and dermatomyositis [17,18]. To characterize the IFN signature, an IFN "score" is calculated for each patient and control based on the average expression of genes which composed the signature [9,11,15,18,19,20]. However, this approach does not take into account the co-regulation of these IFN-related genes. When genes are co-regulated under various biological conditions, the corresponding expression profiles may display relative similarity or co-expression [21]. Our method offers an alternative with which the IFN signature could be characterized by the level of global correlation (Figures 3 and 4) and not solely by the

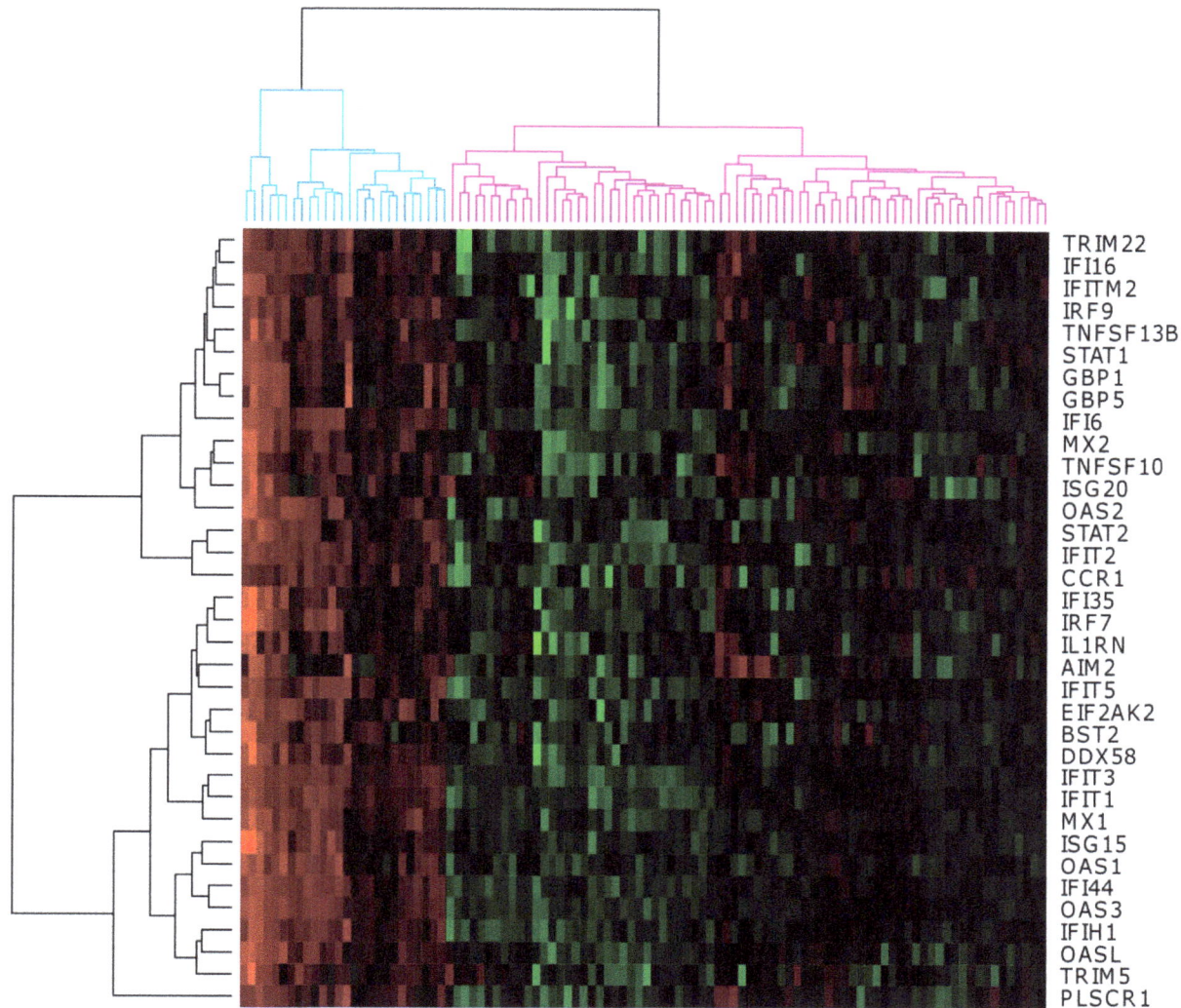

Figure 2. Gene expression profiles from the IFN signature. Unsupervised hierarchical clustering of 35 IFN-related genes that distinguish rheumatoid arthritis (RA) patients IFN^high (blue dendrogram) from RA patients IFN^low (purple dendrogram). Each row represents a gene; each column shows the expression for 35 IFN-related genes expressed by each patients. Red indicates genes that are expressed at higher levels and green indicates genes that are expressed at lower levels.

expression levels. In fact, analyses of our results based on the mean expression of the IFN-related genes showed disparities in the classification of HC and RA patients (9%, Figure 5). These differences between gene expression and correlation levels in the IFN signature could be explained by different factors. Studies showed that IFN-related genes could be regulated by several independent pathways on IFN signaling [22,23]. Their expression could be also controlled by the polymorphic sequences which mainly composed the promoter regions of theses genes [24,25]. These different factors could explain the presence of individual heterogeneity in the expression of these genes and thus the discrepancies observed between the two approaches.

To better understand differences between disease and healthy status, different approaches like transcriptomics or proteomics analyses allow the study of molecular networks and signaling pathways, with the major challenge of integrating this information into a systems approach [15]. Our method permits to identify truly active biological networks associating only with high levels of correlation of biological signature components. Indeed, taking into

account this new correlation aspect for the interpretation of biological networks should allow capturing the actually activated mechanisms at the cellular level.

Interestingly, such correlation-based approach can be advantageously applied to investigate the dynamics of evolution of cellular mechanisms like response to treatment. As an example, in the context of RA, we have applied this method to monitor patients treated by anti-TNF therapy. Although the cross-regulation of *TNFα* and *IFNα* has been previously described [26], the effects of anti-TNF treatment on the expression of IFN-related genes had never been shown by such approach. The results showed that a high IFN signature was conserved after anti-TNF treatment (Figure 6A), while a significant increase was observed in RA IFN^low six months after treatment (Figure 6B). However, the level of positivity has never reached the one observed in SLE patients, known to strongly express the IFN signature. This observation could explain that RA patients treated with anti-TNF develop rather benign clinical symptoms of SLE that are reversible after discontinuation of therapy [27,28]. Contrary to a recent

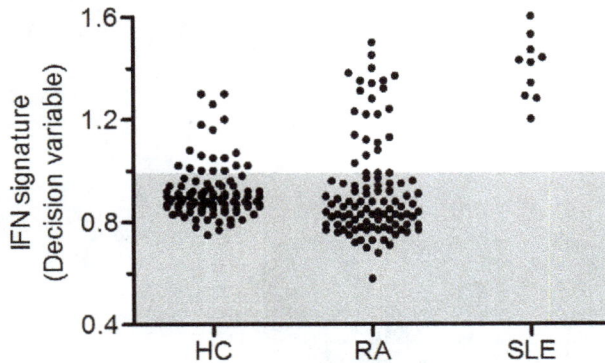

Figure 3. Stratification of individuals according to the IFN signature. Each point represents a single individual with the decision variable calculated from the Classification Algorithm based on a Biological Signature (CABS). The shaded box indicates the normal range according to the rule of the CABS: If $D_{high\_low} \geq 1$, the signature is defined as "high signature" and If $D_{high\_low} < 1$, the signature is defined as "low signature" knowing that $D_{high\_low} = COR_{high}/COR_{low}$.

publication [29], we did not find clinical relevance associated to this IFN signature. The authors showed that an increased IFN-response gene activity after anti-TNF treatment was linked to a poor clinical outcome. In our results, only a trend was observed according to the delta DAS28 score (p = 0.07, data not shown). Besides the difference in method used or the sample size which may explain the discrepancies, our study presented RA patients with a large panel of anti-TNF treatments (infliximab, etanercept and adalimumab). Indeed, several studies suggest differential

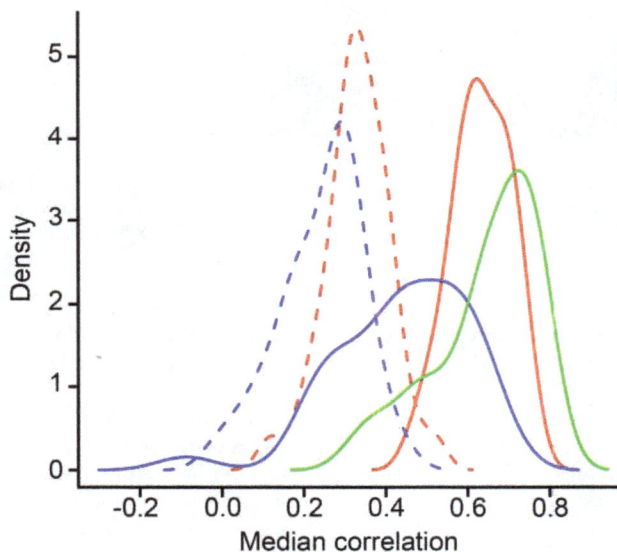

Figure 4. Correlation profiles from the different groups. A correlation index was defined for each gene of the IFN signature as the median of its correlations with the remaining genes. Thus, the correlation profiles for the different groups: healthy controls (HC) IFN[low] (blue dotted), HC IFN[high] (blue line), rheumatoid arthritis patients (RA) IFN[low] (red dotted) and RA IFN[high] (red line) and systemic lupus erythematosus patients (SLE) IFN[high] (green line), are represented using the 35 calculated correlation indexes from the IFN signature genes. The median values of the correlation indexes obtained for the different groups are 0.27, 0.44, 0.33, 0.63 and 0.68, respectively.

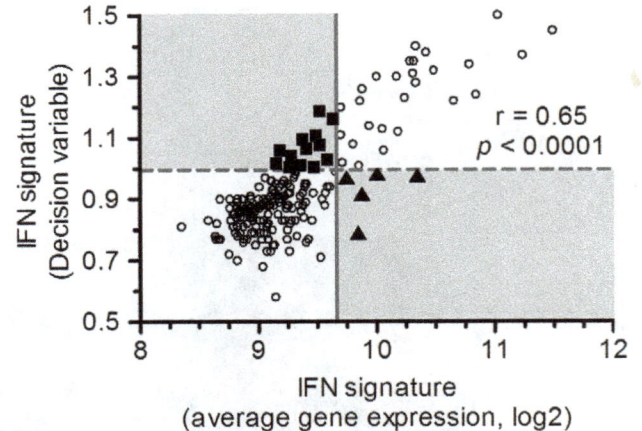

Figure 5. Comparative analysis of characterization methods of IFN signature. Each dot represents a single individual. The y-axis represents the decision variable of the IFN signature calculated from CABS. The grey dotted line indicates the threshold according to the rule of the CABS: If $D_{high\_low} \geq 1$, the signature is defined as "high signature" and If $D_{high\_low} < 1$, the signature is defined as "low signature" knowing that $D_{high\_low} = COR_{high}/COR_{low}$. The x-axis represents the average values of gene expression of the IFN signature. The solid grey line indicates the threshold of IFN response, by calculating the 95% limits of the HC (normal values, defined as the mean (SD) expression of the 35 IFN-related genes, ±1.96 SD). If the average gene expression is ≥9.68, the signature is defined as "high signature" and if average gene expression ratio is <9.68, the signature is defined as "low signature". The shaded boxes show the divergence observed between both methods. The black triangles represent individuals with high average values of gene expression and low decision variable. The black squares represent individuals with low average values of gene expression and high decision variable.

effects of anti-TNF treatments on IFN-response activity which could explain the lack of specificity in our study [29].

Interestingly, our method using CABS allowed us to pinpoint type I IFN signaling as a means to stratify RA patients even starting with whole blood transcriptomics analysis from samples collected in PAXgene tubes. Similar analyses can be performed for the other identified biclusters, highlighting the obvious advantage of whole blood transcriptomics. Using the example of the IFN signature, the use of correlations showed interest in the characterization of the genes sharing both an expression pattern and a biological function. The use of expression correlations may be a better way to obtain a global picture of an activated signature in various disease conditions.

Methods

Ethics statement

All subjects provided written informed consent and the study was approved by the local Ethical Committee for clinical research of the University hospitals of Lyon.

Patients and controls

102 RA patients fulfilling the revised American College of Rheumatology 1987 criteria for RA [30] were enrolled. Their clinical characteristics are shown in table 1. Among the 102 RA patients, a subgroup of RA patients treated for 6 months with anti-TNF, 22 RA patients characterized as IFN[high] (n = 11) and IFN[low] (n = 11), were included (IFN[high] group: infliximab n = 4, etanercept n = 3 and adalimumab n = 4; IFN[low] group: infliximab n = 2,

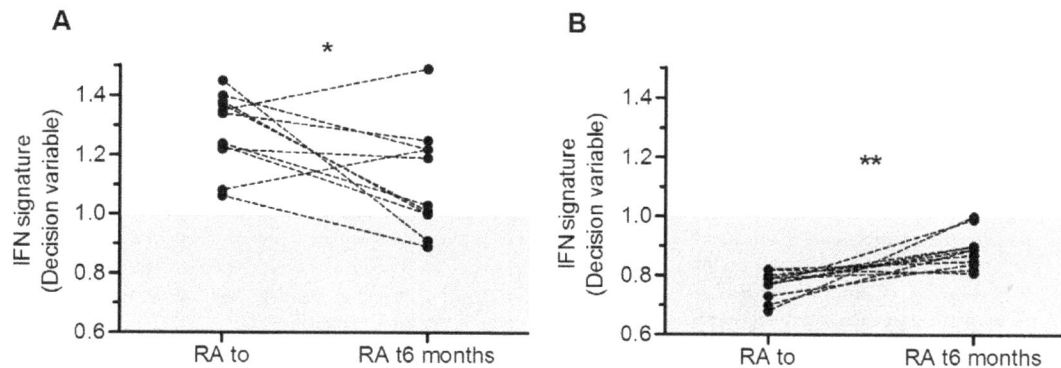

Figure 6. Follow-up the IFN signature in patients with rheumatoid arthritis (RA) treated with anti-TNF. Each point represents a single individual with the decision variable calculated from the Classification Algorithm based on a Biological Signature (CABS). The shaded box indicates the normal range according to the rule of the CABS: If $D_{high\_low} \geq 1$, the signature is defined as "high *signature*" and If $D_{high\_low} < 1$, the signature is defined as "low signature" knowing that $D_{high\_low} = COR_{high}/COR_{low}$. The Wilcoxon signed rank test was used to evaluate the statistical significance between patients before and after anti-TNF treatment **A**) (*$p = 0.0186$) **B**) (**$p = 0.002$).

etanercept n = 7 and adalimumab n = 2). As an IFN positive control group (IFN[high]), 10 systemic lupus erythematosus patients (SLE) fulfilling the American College of Rheumatology criteria for the SLE [31] were studied. In addition, 100 age- and sex-matched healthy control subjects (HC) without any familial history of RA, autoimmune disease and concomitant medication were also recruited.

Sample collection, processing and microarray hybridization

Peripheral blood samples were collected in PAXgene™ Blood RNA tubes (PreAnalytix, Hilden, Germany) in order to stabilize mRNA [32]. Blood samples were incubated at room temperature for 2 h, and then stored at −20°C until RNA extraction according to the manufacturer's instructions. Briefly, RNA was isolated using the PAXgene™ Blood RNA kit (PreAnalytix). Following cell lysis, nucleic acids were pelleted and treated with a buffer containing

Table 1. Demographic and clinical characteristics of the patients and control subjects.

	RA (n = 102)	SLE (n = 10)	C (n = 100)
Demographic data			
Age[a]	50 (40,3–60)	37 (34–44)	57 (52–63)
Sex: Female, Male	79F, 23M	10F	86F, 14M
Disease characteristics			
ESR[a]	18 (8–44)	NA	NA
Rheumatoid Factor pos.(%)	70 (68,6)	NA	NA
Disease duration (years)[a]	5 (2–9)	4 (3–6)	NA
Disease activity	4,2 (3,3–5,2)[b]	13 (12–17.5)[c]	NA
Medication			
MTX (%)	87 (85,3)	NA	NA
MTX dose[a]	15 (15–20)	NA	NA

[a]Median (Q1–Q3).
[b]DAS28: Disease Activity Score.
[c]SLEDAI: Systemic Lupus Erythematosus Disease Activity Index.
ESR: Erythrocyte Sedimentation Rate; MTX: Methotrexate.

proteinase K. After digestion with a RNase-free DNase (Qiagen, Valencia, CA, USA), RNA was subsequently purified on PAXgen-e™ spin columns and eluted in 80 μl of elution buffer. The quality of RNA was determined with the Bioanalyzer® 2100 (Agilent Technologies, Waldbronn, Germany), following the manufacturer's protocol. cDNA was synthesized from 50 ng of total RNA using the WT-Ovation™ System (NuGEN, San Carlos, CA, USA) powered by Ribo-SPIA™ technology. Fragmented cDNA was end labeled with a biotin-conjugated nucleotide analog (DLR-1a; Affymetrix, Santa Clara, CA, USA) using terminal transferase (Roche Diagnostics, Mannheim, Germany). Fragmented and labeled cDNA was hybridized for 18 h at 50°C in a hybridization solution containing 7% DMSO. Hybridization was performed using GeneChip® Human Genome U133 Plus 2.0 arrays (Affymetrix), containing 54,675 probe sets corresponding to 38,500 identified genes. After washing, chips were stained with streptavidin-phycoerythrin according to Affymetrix EukGE-WS2v4 protocol using the Fluidic FS450 station. The microarrays were read with the GeneChip® Scanner 3000 (Affymetrix). Affymetrix GeneChip Operating Software version 1.4 (GCOS) was used to manage Affymetrix GeneChip array data and to automate the control of GeneChip fluidics stations and scanners.

Data analysis

Data processing. Expression data were generated using the Robust Multi-array Average (RMA) method [33] implemented in the Affy package of the Bioconductor microarray analysis environment (http://www.bioconductor.org). The RMA method consists of three steps: background adjustment, quantile normalization [34] and probe set summary of the log-normalized data applying a median polishing procedure. Before the analysis of heterogeneity, two filters were applied based on expression level and variability to lower the dimensionality of the data and to avoid false discoveries. First, genes with a median expression value below a given threshold were eliminated. This threshold was set to 6 in log base 2 corresponding to twice the average background level. The second filter eliminated genes with a low variation. Thus, the Median Absolute Deviation (MAD) for the remaining genes was calculated and those with a MAD lower than the median of the MAD calculated over the remaining genes after intensity based filtering were eliminated.

Biclustering and functional enrichment analyses. The SAMBA algorithm (Statistical-Algorithmic Method for Bicluster

Analysis) implemented in EXPANDER 4.0.3 (EXPression ANalyzer and DisplayER) was used for the biclustering [35]. This algorithm uses probabilistic modeling of the data and theoretical graph techniques to identify such subsets of genes that behave similarly across a subset of patients [36].

The TANGO algorithm (Tool for Analysis of GO enrichment), implemented in EXPANDER 4.0.3, was used to identify the biological significance of these biclusters [35].

Interferon molecular pathway analysis. Canonical pathway analyses was performed to define overrepresentation of canonical pathways of the selected genes. Canonical pathway analyses of specific genes coming from statistical analysis were performed using Ingenuity Pathway Analysis (IPA), (www. ingenuity.com). B-H multiple testing correction p-value test was used to calculate the p-value for determining the probability that each canonical pathway assigned to the dataset was due to chance alone. P-value<0.01 was applied in calculations and the Human Genome U133 Plus 2.0 array was used as the reference when ranking the statistical significance of canonical pathways.

Networks of the IFN genes were constructed using Ingenuity Pathway Analysis (IPA), (www.ingenuity.com). Genes were found in the IPA knowledge database are labeled "focus" genes. Based on the focus genes, IPA generated a set of molecular networks with a cutoff of 70 genes for each network based on interactions between uploaded genes and all other genes/proteins stored in the knowledge base. Each network is assigned a score according to the number of focus genes in our dataset. These scores are derived from negative logarithm of the P and are indicators of the degree of significance. Scores of 4 or higher have 99.9% confidence level of significance as defined in detail elsewhere [37].

Classification Algorithm based on a Biological Signature (CABS). Taking the example of the IFN-related genes, a classification algorithm was developed to identify individuals with or without this biological signature. Applied to the IFN-related genes, the CABS is divided into three steps.

Step 1 Prototype construction: Two groups of RA patients (IFN^{high}; IFN^{low}) were identified from the hierarchical clustering representing the 35 IFN-related genes which characterized the IFN signature (Figure 2). The prototype was defined from these two groups. Median expression values was calculated in the two groups. Prototype Pi was defined from group i; the vector

$(Gi_1,...,Gi_M)$ represents the expression of the prototype Pi, where i is high or low, Gij is the median expression of gene j in group i, M is the size of the IFN signature.

Step 2 Decision Variable Calculation: Given the definition of the prototypes described above, a criteria was needed to assess the similarity of a given individual to those prototypes. For a given individual, the IFN signature profile was defined as the vector corresponding to the expression level of the 35 genes constituting the signature. The similarity of this profile with both prototypes was calculated using the Pearson correlation coefficient and noted COR_{high} et COR_{low}. The decision variable calculation was given by the ratio between these two correlations: $D_{high\_low} = COR_{high}/COR_{low}$ indicating proximity to one or other of the prototypes.

Step 3 : Decision Making: Given the decision variable describe above, an individual was assigned High IFN if the ratio $D_{high\_low} \geq 1$ meaning that $COR_{high} \geq COR_{low}$. Inversely, an individual was assigned low IFN if the ratio $D_{high\_low} < 1$ meaning that $COR_{high} < COR_{low}$.

Supporting Information

Table S1 Ontological analysis of the 121 biclusters obtained from the 102 RA patients. The TANGO algorithm (Tool for Analysis of GO enrichment) was used to identify the biological significance of 121 biclusters from 9,856 selected probe sets (see material and methods for details). Among them, these results have highlighted the importance of immune regulation across the "immune response" and "response to virus" ontology groups (biclusters 4, 21, 34, 35 and 39. Processes with corrected p value<0.05 were considered significant [36].

Acknowledgments

The authors wish to thank Prof. Charles Auffray and Dr. François Mallet for their critical comments.

Author Contributions

Conceived and designed the experiments: FP BM PM. Performed the experiments: FR FP FT. Analyzed the data: FR MP. Contributed reagents/materials/analysis tools: PI AH. Wrote the paper: FR PM.

References

1. Kerr MK (2003) Design considerations for efficient and effective microarray studies. Biometrics 59: 822–828.
2. Wheelan SJ, Martinez Murillo F, Boeke JD (2008) The incredible shrinking world of DNA microarrays. Mol Biosyst 4: 726–732.
3. Eisen MB, Spellman PT, Brown PO, Botstein D (1998) Cluster analysis and display of genome-wide expression patterns. Proc Natl Acad Sci U S A 95: 14863–14868.
4. Ben-Dor A, Chor B, Karp R, Yakhini Z (2003) Discovering local structure in gene expression data: the order-preserving submatrix problem. J Comput Biol 10: 373–384.
5. Cheng Y, Church GM (2000) Biclustering of expression data. Proc Int Conf Intell Syst Mol Biol 8: 93–103.
6. Madeira SC, Oliveira AL (2004) Biclustering algorithms for biological data analysis: a survey. IEEE/ACM Trans Comput Biol Bioinform 1: 24–45.
7. van der Pouw Kraan TC, van Gaalen FA, Huizinga TW, Pieterman E, Breedveld FC, et al. (2003) Discovery of distinctive gene expression profiles in rheumatoid synovium using cDNA microarray technology: evidence for the existence of multiple pathways of tissue destruction and repair. Genes Immun 4: 187–196.
8. van der Pouw Kraan TC, van Gaalen FA, Kasperkovitz PV, Verbeet NL, Smeets TJ, et al. (2003) Rheumatoid arthritis is a heterogeneous disease: evidence for differences in the activation of the STAT-1 pathway between rheumatoid tissues. Arthritis Rheum 48: 2132–2145.
9. van der Pouw Kraan TC, Wijbrandts CA, van Baarsen LG, Voskuyl AE, Rustenburg F, et al. (2007) Rheumatoid arthritis subtypes identified by genomic profiling of peripheral blood cells: assignment of a type I interferon signature in a subpopulation of patients. Ann Rheum Dis 66: 1008–1014.
10. Prieto C, Risueño A, Fontanillo C, De las Rivas J (2008) Human gene coexpression landscape: confident network derived from tissue transcriptomic profiles. PLoS One 3: e3911.
11. Baechler EC, Batliwalla FM, Karypis G, Gaffney PM, Ortmann WA, et al. (2003) Interferon-inducible gene expression signature in peripheral blood cells of patients with severe lupus. Proc Natl Acad Sci U S A 100: 2610–2615.
12. Tan FK, Zhou X, Mayes MD, Gourh P, Guo X, et al. (2006) Signatures of differentially regulated interferon gene expression and vasculotrophism in the peripheral blood cells of systemic sclerosis patients. Rheumatology (Oxford) 45: 694–702.
13. van Baarsen LG, van der Pouw Kraan TC, Kragt JJ, Baggen JM, Rustenburg F, et al. (2006) A subtype of multiple sclerosis defined by an activated immune defense program. Genes Immun 7: 522–531.
14. Bave U, Nordmark G, Lövgren T, Rönnelid J, Cajander S, et al. (2005) Activation of the type I interferon system in primary Sjögren's syndrome: a possible etiopathogenic mechanism. Arthritis Rheum 52: 1185–1195.
15. Reynier F, Pachot A, Paye M, Xu Q, Turrel-Davin F, et al. (2010) Specific gene expression signature associated with development of autoimmune type-I diabetes using whole-blood microarray analysis. Genes Immun 11: 269–278.
16. Huang X, Yuang J, Goddard A, Foulis A, James RF, et al. (1995) Interferon expression in the pancreases of patients with type I diabetes. Diabetes 44: 658–664.
17. Greenberg SA, Pinkus JL, Pinkus GS, Burleson T, Sanoudou D, et al. (2005) Interferon-alpha/beta-mediated innate immune mechanisms in dermatomyositis. Ann Neurol 57: 664–678.

18. Baechler EC, Bauer JW, Slattery CA, Ortmann WA, Espe KJ, et al. (2007) An interferon signature in the peripheral blood of dermatomyositis patients is associated with disease activity. Mol Med 13: 59–68.
19. Kirou KA, Lee C, George S, Louca K, Papagiannis IG, et al. (2004) Coordinate overexpression of interferon-alpha-induced genes in systemic lupus erythematosus. Arthritis Rheum 50: 3958–3967.
20. Bauer JW, Baechler EC, Petri M, Batliwalla FM, Crawford D, et al. (2006) Elevated serum levels of interferon-regulated chemokines are biomarkers for active human systemic lupus erythematosus. PLoS Med 3: e491.
21. Chou JW, Zhou T, Kaufmann WK, Paules RS, Bushel PR (2007) Extracting gene expression patterns and identifying co-expressed genes from microarray data reveals biologically responsive processes. BMC Bioinformatics 8: 427.
22. Ning S, Huye LE, Pagano JS (2005) Regulation of the transcriptional activity of the IRF7 promoter by a pathway independent of interferon signaling. J Biol Chem 280: 12262–12270.
23. Gugliesi F, Mondini M, Ravera R, Robotti A, de Andrea M, et al. (2005) Up-regulation of the interferon-inducible IFI16 gene by oxidative stress triggers p53 transcriptional activity in endothelial cells. J Leukoc Biol 77: 820–829.
24. Mälarstig A, Sigurdsson S, Eriksson P, Paulsson-Berne G, Hedin U, et al. (2008) Variants of the interferon regulatory factor 5 gene regulate expression of IRF5 mRNA in atherosclerotic tissue but are not associated with myocardial infarction. Arterioscler Thromb Vasc Biol 28: 975–982.
25. Akahoshi M, Nakashima H, Sadanaga A, Miyake K, Obara K, et al. (2008) Promoter polymorphisms in the IRF3 gene confer protection against systemic lupus erythematosus. Lupus 17: 568–574.
26. Palucka AK, Blanck JP, Bennett L, Pascual V, Banchereau J (2005) Cross-regulation of TNF and IFN-alpha in autoimmune diseases. Proc Natl Acad Sci U S A 102: 3372–3377.
27. Pisetsky DS (2000) Tumor necrosis factor alpha blockers and the induction of anti-DNA autoantibodies. Arthritis Rheum 43: 2381–2382.
28. Shakoor N, Michalska M, Harris CA, Block JA (2002) Drug-induced systemic lupus erythematosus associated with etanercept therapy. Lancet 359: 579–580.
29. van Baarsen LG, Wijbrandts CA, Rustenburg F, Cantaert T, van der Pouw Kraan TC, et al. (2010) Regulation of IFN response gene activity during infliximab treatment in rheumatoid arthritis is associated with clinical response to treatment. Arthritis Res Ther 12: R11.
30. Arnett FC, Edworthy SM, Bloch DA, McShane DJ, Fries JF, et al. (1988) The American Rheumatism Association 1987 revised criteria for the classification of rheumatoid arthritis. Arthritis Rheum 31: 315–324.
31. Tan E, Cohen A, Fries J, Masi A, McShane D, et al. (1982) The 1982 revised criteria for the classification of systemic lupus erythematosus. Arthritis Rheum 25: 1271–1277.
32. Rainen L, Oelmueller U, Jurgensen S, Wyrich R, Ballas C, et al. (2002) Stabilization of mRNA expression in whole blood samples. Clin Chem 48: 1883–1890.
33. Irizarry RA, Hobbs B, Collin F, Beazer-Barclay YD, Antonellis KJ, et al. (2003) Exploration, normalization, and summaries of high density oligonucleotide array probe level data. Biostatistics 4: 249–264.
34. Bolstad BM, Irizarry RA, Astrand M, Speed TP (2003) A comparison of normalization methods for high density oligonucleotide array data based on variance and bias. Bioinformatics 19: 185–193.
35. Shamir R, Maron-Katz A, Tanay A, Linhart C, Steinfeld I, et al. (2005) EXPANDER: an integrative program suite for microarray data analysis. BMC Bioinformatics 21: 6: 232.
36. Tanay A, Sharan R, Shamir R (2002) Discovering statistically significant biclusters in gene expression data. Bioinformatics 18 Suppl 1: S136–144.
37. Calvano SE, Xiao W, Richards DR, Felciano RM, Baker HV, et al. (2005) A network-based analysis of systemic inflammation in humans. Nature 437: 1032–1037.

8

Autoantibodies to Endothelial Cell Surface ATP Synthase, the Endogenous Receptor for Hsp60, might Play a Pathogenic Role in Vasculatides

Jean-Eric Alard[1], Sophie Hillion[1], Loïc Guillevin[2], Alain Saraux[1,3], Jacques-Olivier Pers[1,3], Pierre Youinou[1,3]*, Christophe Jamin[1,3]

1 EA2216 "Immunology and Pathology" and IFR 148 ScInBioS, Université de Brest and Université Européenne de Bretagne, Brest, France, 2 Department of Internal Medicine, Hôpital Cochin, Paris, France, 3 Centre Hospitalier Universitaire, Brest, France

Abstract

Background: Heat shock protein (hsp) 60 that provides "danger signal" binds to the surface of resting endothelial cells (EC) but its receptor has not yet been characterized. In mitochondria, hsp60 specifically associates with adenosine triphosphate (ATP) synthase. We therefore examined the possible interaction between hsp60 and ATP synthase on EC surface.

Methodology/Principal Findings: Using Far Western blot approach, co-immunoprecipitation studies and surface plasmon resonance analyses, we demonstrated that hsp60 binds to the β-subunit of ATP synthase. As a cell surface-expressed molecule, ATP synthase is potentially targeted by anti-EC-antibodies (AECAs) found in the sera of patients suffering vasculitides. Based on enzyme-linked immunosorbent assay and Western blotting techniques with F1-ATP synthase as substrate, we established the presence of anti-ATP synthase antibodies at higher frequency in patients with primary vasculitides (group I) compared with secondary vasculitides (group II). Anti-ATP synthase reactivity from group I patients was restricted to the β-subunit of ATP synthase, whereas those from group II was directed to the α-, β- and γ-subunits. Cell surface ATP synthase regulates intracellular pH (pHi). In low extracellular pH medium, we detected abnormal decreased of EC pHi in the presence of anti-ATP synthase antibodies, irrespective of their fine reactivities. Interestingly, soluble hsp60 abrogated the anti-ATP synthase-induced pHi down-regulation.

Conclusions/Significance: Our results indicate that ATP synthase is targeted by AECAs on the surface of EC that induce intracellular acidification. Such pathogenic effect in vasculitides can be modulated by hsp60 binding on ATP synthase which preserves ATP synthase activity.

Editor: Graham Pockley, University of Sheffield, United Kingdom

Funding: Jean-Eric Alard was supported by the "Conseil regional de Bretagne". The funders had no role in study design, data collection and analysis, decision to publish, or preparation of the manuscript.

Competing Interests: The authors have declared that no competing interests exist.

* E-mail: youinou@univ-brest.fr

Introduction

Adenosine triphosphate (ATP) synthase, or F0F1-ATPase, produces and hydrolyzes ATP with proton translocation [1]. F0 operates as a proton channel with a rotation driving the F1 to synthesize ATP, depending on the direction of rotation. F1 comprises 3 β-subunits assuming the catalytic activity modulated by 3 α-subunits alternately ordered to form a cylinder, completed by a γ-subunit located at the center of the αβ stalk, that constitutes the key rotary element in the enzyme's catalytic activity [2].

ATP synthase is resident in the inner mitochondrial membrane. However, evidence suggests that it is also localized in cell membranes, and translocate into the lipid rafts (LRs) of normal endothelial cells (EC). Depending on cell type [3], cell surface ATP synthase triggers hydrolysis or synthesis of ATP, modulates angiogenesis, cellular immunity, cholesterol uptake and regulates intracellular pH (pHi).

Cell surface ATP synthase acts also to bind several ligands and to control EC proliferation and differentiation [4]. For example, angiostatin binds to αβ-subunits, blocks ATP synthase activity when EC are in a low extracellular pH (pHe) environment, and is thus responsible for the inhibition of proton flux due to pH stress [5]. The overall consequence is intracellular acidification that induces EC death and inhibits neovascularisation [6]. By contrast, apoliprotein A-I stimulates F1-ATPase activity following binding and generates adenosine diphosphate that inhibits EC apoptosis and promotes proliferation [7].

Alteration in ATP synthase function could therefore cause significant damages to EC homeostasis. Furthermore, in the mitochondria, heat shock protein (hsp)60 specifically associates with ATP synthase [8], and ensures correct assembly of the complex. Hsp60 is also present on EC surface [9]. Though several ligands for different hsps have been listed [10], there is no clear evidence about the one or those which can specifically bind to hsp60 when found on the surface of EC. Thus, hsp60 binds to EC irrespective of TLR2, TLR4, CD91 or CD14 expression [11,12]. Mitochondrial hsp70 has been identified as one ligand for hsp60 on the surface of stressed EC [13], but its receptor remains uncharacterized in non-stressed conditions. Their intra-mitochondrial association suggests that translocation into extra-mitochondrial sites might facilitate ATP synthase and hsp60 interactions. Interestingly, both ATP synthase and hsp60 can cause cytolysis [4,14]. Hsp60 behaves as an antigenic target for antibodies (Abs), such as anti-EC Abs (AECAs) [15] which are frequently associated with vascular inflammation [16], and plays a role in promoting and regulating autoimmunity [17,18]. Therefore, mitochondrial proteins can generate immune responses contributing to damaged EC. Their presence on the EC surface and the subsequent effects of Ab binding might participate in the pathogenesis of vasculitides. Depending on the site and the type of blood vessels affected, clinical and pathological manifestations vary considerably. This awareness has justified nomenclature of vasculitdies [19]. These diseases may be autonomous and referred to as primary vasculitides. They may affect small vessels in Wegener's granulomatosis (WG), Churg-Strauss syndrome (CSS), microscopic polyangiitis (MPA), medium vessels in polyarteritis nodosa (PAN) or large vessels. These primary forms result from vasculitis which is the triggering abnormality. Vasculitides may also be set against a background of autoimmune diseases such as systemic lupus erythematosus (SLE), primary Sjögren's syndrome (pSS), or rheumatoid arthritis (RA) and are then designated as secondary vasculitides [20]. The current work was pursued to first characterize possible interactions between ATP synthase and hsp60 on the EC membrane, and second to evaluate the existence of anti-ATP synthase Abs in vasculitides and their impact on EC.

Results

I – ATP synthase is a receptor for hsp60

A minority of resting human umbilical vein EC (HUVEC) bound to soluble hsp60 [15], suggesting that the "danger" signal provided by hsp60 [21] might be detected by an as yet unidentified receptor. To do so, we opted for a Far Western blot (WB) approach. HUVEC membrane-enriched proteins were resolved on 3 bidimensional gels. The first was stained with Coomassie blue to verify the protein extraction procedure (Figure 1A, left panel). Proteins from the second were blotted onto a PVDF membrane, and probed with anti-hsp60 monoclonal Ab (mAb) to localize the endogenous hsp60 (Figure 1A, middle panel). Proteins from the third were incubated with recombinant hsp60 and probed with anti-hsp60 mAb. This procedure identified 4 additional spots relative to the second gel (Figure 1A, right panel). They were cut out from the Coomassie blue-stained gel, analyzed by mass spectroscopy and their amino acid sequence determined after screening of the Swiss-Prot databank. Actin, ATP synthase β-chain, prolyl-4-hydroxylase β-subunit and gp96 were identified (Figure 1B). We focused on ATP synthase protein, and, to confirm hsp60/ATP synthase β-subunit interaction, performed reverse co-precipitation experiments. Immunoprecipitation with either mAbs co-precipitated the other protein as shown by the 128-kDa molecular weight (MW) complex (Figure 1C). The presence of smears around this MW suggest the persistant interactions between different ATP synthase subunits, and also that other proteins may interact with ATP synthase or with hsp60. Therefore, to demonstrate that ATP synthase could be the receptor for hsp60, recombinant hsp60 was immobilized onto the biosensor chip of a Biacore X system, ATP synthase injected into the cell flow and their interaction followed in real time (Figure 1D). Sensograms indicated that hsp60 interacts with ATP synthase as shown by the curves that did not return to baseline.

Although ATP synthase is abundantly expressed in the cytoplasm of permeabilized EC, a modest level of fluorescence was found on the surface of nonpermeabilized EC by indirect immunofluorescence (Figure 1E). This suggests that ATP synthase could be accessible to hsp60 on the EC surface.

II – Detection of ATP synthase reactivity

We have previously demonstrated that among the EC surface-expressed molecules [16] hsp60 could be a target for AECAs [15]. To assess whether ATP synthase, receptor for hsp60 was recognized by AECAs as well, we screened AECA-positive sera from different patient groups suffering vasculitides with an in-house enzyme-linked immunosorbent assay (ELISA) using bovine F1-ATP synthase as substrate. Sera were considered positive when the optical density (OD) value was over than 0.410 (Figure 2A, left panel). Thus, as shown in right panel of Figure 2A, 20% of controls were reactive and there were more sera from group I patients suffering primary vasculitides (36–73%) positive for ATP synthase binding than from group II patients suffering secondary vasculitides (5–28%, $p < 0.001$).

Because a subgroup of controls displayed positivity, we asked the question as to whether ATP synthase reactivity was similar to that observed in sera from patients and whether those from group I and II were different. To answer this question, reactivities were evaluated by WB. Anti-ATP synthase Abs bound to 3 major bands with a MW of 55, 51 and 30 kDa (Figure 2B), and 3 minor bands of 40, 38 and 32 kDa, that were sequenced. The 3 major bands were the α-, β- and γ-subunits of F1-ATP synthase, and the 3 minor bands were degradation products of the β-subunit. Sera reactivities were considered positive when the OD values after densitometry analysis were over $3.9.10^5$ AU, $4.5.10^5$ AU and $3.8.10^5$ AU for α-, β-, and γ-subunit, respectively (Figure 2C, left panels). Regarding overall reactivities, more than 13% of sera from the controls were positive in the WB. Furthermore, more sera from group I were positive (50–86%) than those from group II (45–78%, $p = 0.005$). In the controls, frequencies of positive sera were 6.7, 10 and 6.7% for α-, β- and γ-subunit, respectively. (Figure 2C, right panels). Reactivity was strikingly homogeneous in sera from group I patients since all were reactive only for the β-subunit. In group II patients, percentages of positivity ranged from 5–15.6% for the α-subunit, 5.6–17.2% for the β-subunit and 18.7–77.8% for the γ-subunit.

We, next, assessed the latent multi-reactivity of positive anti-ATP synthase sera. Positivity for the β-subunit in group I was not associated with other reactivity (Figure 3), and the one positive for the γ-subunit was negative for the others. It is concluded that sera from patients with primary vasculitides exhibited homogeneous reactivity to F1-ATP synthase. By contrast, 1 control serum positive for α-subunit (C24) was also positive for β-, and 1 (C2) was positive for the γ-subunit as well. One control was only positive for the β-subunit (C7), and another 1 (C1) for the γ-subunit. When positive, reactivities of control sera for F1-ATP synthase appeared heterogeneous. In group II patients, 7 SLE sera were only reactive for the α-subunit (SLE1, 8, 36, 50, 51, 52 and 54), 2 (SLE15 and SLE30) were positive for the α-subunit and also for the γ-subunit, and 1 (SLE4) for the α-subunit, the γ-subunit and the β-subunit too. Eleven SLE sera were positive for the β-subunit among which 9 had no other reactivities (SLE2, 28, 42, 56, 57, 58, 59, 61 and 63) and 1 (SLE23) was also positive for the γ-subunit. Finally, 9 of 12 sera positive for the γ-subunit displayed a single reactivity (SLE9, 12, 18, 20, 22, 24, 27, 48 and 64). Reactivities of pSS patients appeared to be less heterogeneous since all positive sera reacted with the γ-subunit, among which only 1 (pSS4) was also positive for the α-subunit and one (pSS6) also positive for the β-

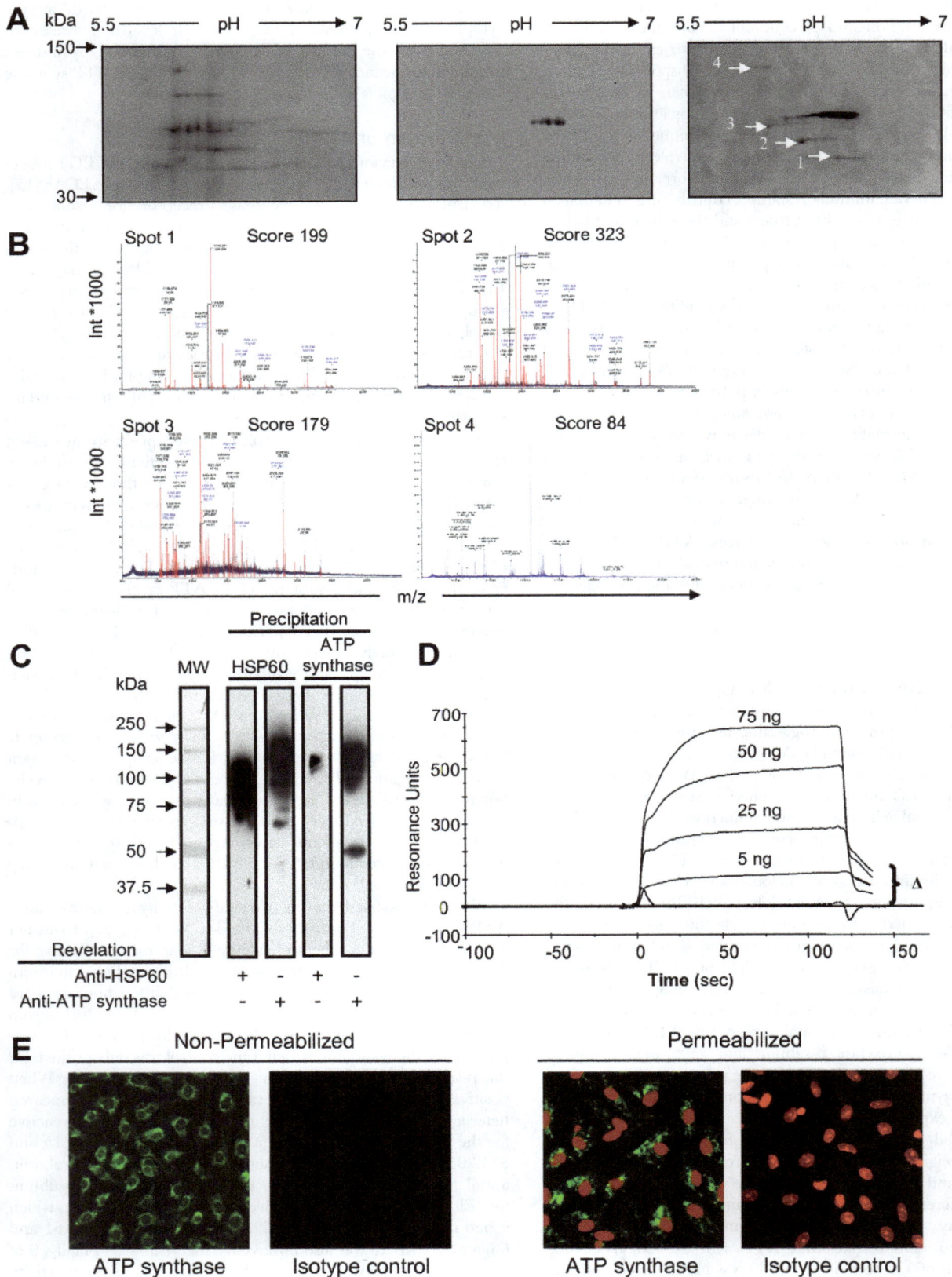

Figure 1. ATP synthase is a receptor for soluble hsp60. A- HUVEC membrane-enriched protein were electrophoresed on bidimensional gels. Left panel: staining with Coomassie blue. Middle panel: WB with anti-hsp60 mAb. Right panel: WB with recombinant hsp60 revealed with anti-hsp60 mAb. **B-** Mass spectrometry data of proteins bound to hsp60. **C-** Hsp60 and ATP synthase were co-immunoprecipitated from membrane-enriched

protein extracts of EAhy926 cells with anti-ATP synthase and anti-hsp60mAbs, respectively. Proteins were analysed by WB using polyclonal anti-hsp60 or anti-ATP synthase Abs. MW markers are on the left. **D-** Increasing amounts of ATP synthase were passed over hsp60 immobilized onto a sensor chip. Sensogram of each amount of analyte with substraction of non-specific binding represent resonance units. Specific binding is shown (Δ). **E-** EAhy926 cells, permeabilized or not, were incubated with a primary anti-ATP synthase Ab revealed by FITC-conjugated anti-Ig Ab, and intracellular as well as cell-surface expression of ATP synthase analyzed by fluorescence microscopy. Propidium iodide was used to visualize nuclei, and isotype control staining performed as negative control.

subunit. Finally, all RA sera were positive for the γ-subunit, but 1 (RA10) reactive with the α-subunit. Two of them (RA9 and RA14) were also positive for the β-subunit. We concluded that among anti-ATP synthase reactive sera, those from patients with secondary vasculitides presented the broadest multi-reactivity pattern ($p = 0.04$) for the F1-ATP synthase subunits (Table 1).

III – Modulation of ATP synthase function

We then asked the question as to whether anti-ATP synthase Abs could alter the ATP synthase-dependent regulation of pHi [3]. EC were stained with $2',7'$-*bis*-carboxyethyl-5,6-carboxyfluorescein (BCECF), and pilot experiments elaborated by flow cytometry to validate the protocol that measures emission intensities of BCECF at 525nm and 640nm. To this end, EAhy926 EC line cells were treated with nigericin and incubated in medium with different pHe from 6.7 to 8. Nigericin is an ionophore that exchanges K^+ and H^+ across cellular membranes [22]. pHi measured in these conditions corresponds to pHe. Intracellular 525/640 ratios increased with pHe (Figure 4A) indicating that flow cytometry analyses were efficient. Moreover, the ratio was left stable without nigericin, demonstrating that nontreated EC retained their ability to maintain constant pHi between pHe 6.7 to 8. Additionally, to evaluate ATP synthase function, EC were pre-treated with piceatannol, an inhibitor of ATP synthase [23], and incubated in an acidic pHe 6.7 medium. pHi decreased to 7.1 ± 0.1 while it was maintained at 7.38 ± 0.11 ($p = 0.004$) in medium free from ATP synthase inhibitor (Figure 4B), demonstrating the importance of ATP synthase activity in pHi regulation. Interestingly, pre-treatment of EC with anti-ATP synthase mAb also reduced pHi to 7.08 ± 0.07 ($p = 0.005$). These results indicate that anti-ATP synthase Abs can inhibit ATP synthase function. By contrast, pHi remained stable at 7.55 ± 0.07 ($p = 0.6$, Figure 4C) and 7.7 ± 0.09 ($p = 0.37$, Figure 4D) when EC were incubated with anti-ATP synthase mAb in neutral (pHe 7.4) or basic (pHe 8) medium, respectively. These experiments demonstrate that anti-ATP synthase mAb alters ATP synthase activity only in acidic environment. This conclusion was confirmed by pre-treatment of EC with oligomycin another inhibitor of ATP synthase [24]. pHi decreased only when EC were incubated in acidic pHe medium. Furthermore, no effects could be observed with anti-hsp Abs, with sodium azide at the concentration found in anti-ATP synthase mAb preparation, nor with DMSO (not shown).

Effect of anti-ATP synthase Abs from sera was therefore evaluated with EC incubated at pHe 6.7 (Figure 5A). Sera from controls, reactive or unreactive for ATP synthase, did not reduce pHi which were maintained at 7.45-7.51. Nearly all sera positive for ATP synthase from group I patients reduced pHi of EC between 6.93 and 7.2. Some had no effect with pHi sustained at 7.46-7.48. ATP synthase positive sera from group II patients displayed diverse effects. A striking down-regulation between 6.85-6.97 was observed with a subgroup of sera from SLE patients, indicating a strong inhibition of ATP synthase function. Another subgroup slightly diminished pHi between 7.23-7.48. Sera from patients with pSS induced intermediate inhibition of ATP synthase activity with pHi decreased between 7.08 and 7.22. Finally, sera from RA patients were variable, from a strong

decrease of pHi to 7.05 to a minor reduction at 7.39. Overall, these data demonstrate varied effects of anti-ATP synthase Abs from sera on ATP synthase function.

To further elucidate this issue, we appraised specific ATP synthase subunit reactivity. Positivity for α-, β- and/or γ-subunits were inspected in sera inducing or not down-regulation of pHi. As shown in Figure 5A, effect on pHi regulation could not be designated with particular ATP synthase reactivities. Thus, while some β-reactive sera decreased pHi others had no effect. Similarly, some α-reactive sera did not affect pHi whilst others reduced it. Moreover, multireactivities did not appear as a decisive factor either. These prompted us to assess Ab titres. The analysis did not show a correlation between OD values for the ELISA and pHi values of EC determined in the presence of sera (Figure 5B), suggesting that effect on pHi was not related to Ab concentration. Nevertheless, down-regulations of pHi were abrogated when sera were depleted of their anti-ATP synthase reactivities by overnight incubation in ATP synthase-coated microplates (Figure 5C). These data confirm that effects of anti-ATP synthase positive sera on pHi modulation are specifically due to ATP synthase recognition.

IV – Regulatory role for hsp60 in ATP synthase activity

Once hsp60 was shown to be a novel ligand for ATP synthase on EC surface, we sought to evaluate its role on the function of ATP synthase. Binding of recombinant hsp60 to EC cultured in acidic pH 6.7 medium had no effect on pHi that was retained at 7.38 ± 0.07, compared with pHi 7.35 ± 0.11 of control EC ($p = 0.76$, Figure 5D). This data indicates that binding of soluble hsp60 does not alter ATP synthase activity. However, reduction of pHi to 7.10 ± 0.07 ($p = 0.03$) following stimulation of EC with anti-ATP synthase β-chain Ab was abrogated when EC were pre-incubated with recombinant hsp60. Thus, pHi was up-regulated to 7.29 ± 0.06 ($p = 0.03$). These results indicate that hsp60 preserved EC from a decrease in pHi subsequent to the binding of anti-ATP synthase Abs at least when they bind to the β chain.

Discussion

This study establishes specific interactions between ATP synthase and hsp60 on the surface of EC, based on Far WB associated with mass spectrometry. Because a single spot may contained several proteins, mass spectrometry will detect the most abundant species. We, therefore, decided to verify the specific interactions using different approaches. Co-immunoprecipitation and surface plasmon resonance analyses confirmed ATP synthase and hsp60 interaction. We determined that soluble hsp60 interacts with the 51 kDa β-subunit of ATP synthase on EC surface. In the mitochondria, hsp60 associates with at least two proteins [8]. One is the 55kDa α-subunit and the second is a 40kDa protein that has not been identified but that could be a product of the β-subunit as suggested herein in Figure 2B. These observations imply that α-subunit and β-subunit of ATP synthase would be able to associate with hsp60 in the mitochondria, whilst cell surface ATP synthase binds hsp60 with its β-subunit only. We did not observe association with the α-subunit. Whether differential conformation of F1-ATP synthase between mitochondrial and cell surface molecules might be responsible for this difference remains to be

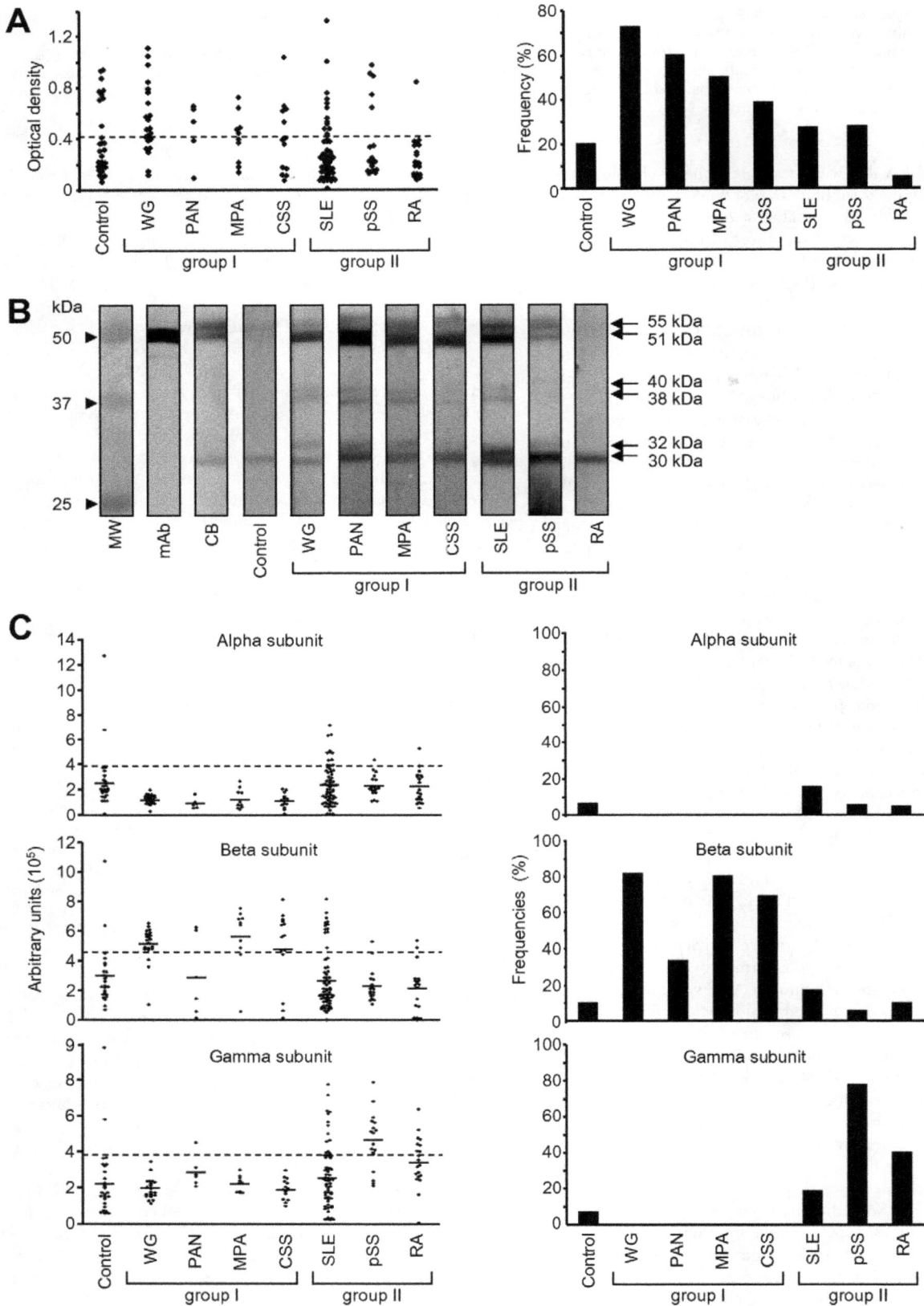

Figure 2. Reactivity of sera with ATP synthase. A- Optical densities (left panel) and percentages of positivity (right panel) of sera from patients in ELISA with purified ATP synthase. Broken line depicts the cut off level for positivity (OD 0.410, representing the mean+2 SD of control values). Group I corresponds to patients with primary vasculitides (WG, PAN, MPA and CSS) and group II to patients with secondary vasculitides associated

with autoimmune diseases (SLE, pSS, RA). **B-** Purified ATP synthase was subjected to electrophoresis and blotted with sera from patients and controls. Representative results from controls, group I and group II patients are shown. MW markers are on the left. Result with anti-β-subunit mAb and Coomassie blue (CB) staining are shown as controls. **C-** Densitometry measurement (left panels) and percentages (right panels) of sera activities against α-, β- and γ-ATP synthase subunits by Western blots. Broken lines show the cut off level for positivity (OD 3.9.10^5, 4.5.10^5 and 3.8.10^5 arbitrary units, representing the mean+2 SD of control values for α-, β-, and γ-subunit, respectively). WG = Wegener's granulomatosis; PAN = polyarteritis nodosa; MPA = microscopic polyangiitis; CSS = Churg-Strauss syndrome; SLE = systemic lupus erythematosus; pSS = primary Sjögren's syndrome; RA = rheumatoid arthritis.

demonstrated. Our findings suggest that hsp60 might serve as a chaperon to protect ATP synthase from degradation on EC membranes. However, chaperon activity requires the presence of ATP which is lacking in our *in vitro* experiments. This aspect is thus unlikely to occur. Moreover, we can not exclude the possibility that other chaperons such as mitochondrial hsp70 may also be able to interact with ATP synthase. Furthermore, the fraction of ATP synthase that co-localized with hsp60 into lipid rafts (not shown) suggest that hsp60/ATP synthase interactions participate also in signaling, and thereby influence ATP synthase-dependent activation and proliferation of EC [25,26]. This is consistent with other observations on extracellular ATP synthase in lipid rafts [27].

The second part of our work focused for the first time on determining the pattern of anti-ATP synthase reactivity in sera from patients containing AECAs known to be potentially pathogenic in vasculitides [28–30]. The frequencies of positivity were higher in patients with primary vasculitides (group I) than in those with secondary vasculitides (group II). The 3 major α-, β- and γ-subunits that constitute the F1 structure [2] were found antigenic. Intriguingly, sera from patients with primary vasculitides had a homogeneous pattern of Ab reactivity to the β-subunit of ATP synthase. By contrast, Abs from secondary vasculitides were multi-reactive. The most heterogeneous pattern was seen in sera from SLE patients with mono-, bi- and tri-reactivities. RA sera had only 2 different mono- and one bi-reactivity patterns, while Abs in the sera of pSS were homogeneous with a striking elevated frequency of mono-reactivity for the γ-subunit and 2 minor bi-reactivities. Overall, there was possiblity that patients with Abs directed to the β-subunit were those with active vasculitic disease at the time they were sampled. However, further analysis could not establish an influence of disease activity nor of medication on the Ab pattern, and reactivity with the β-subunit was not restricted to group I patients. The reasons for mono-

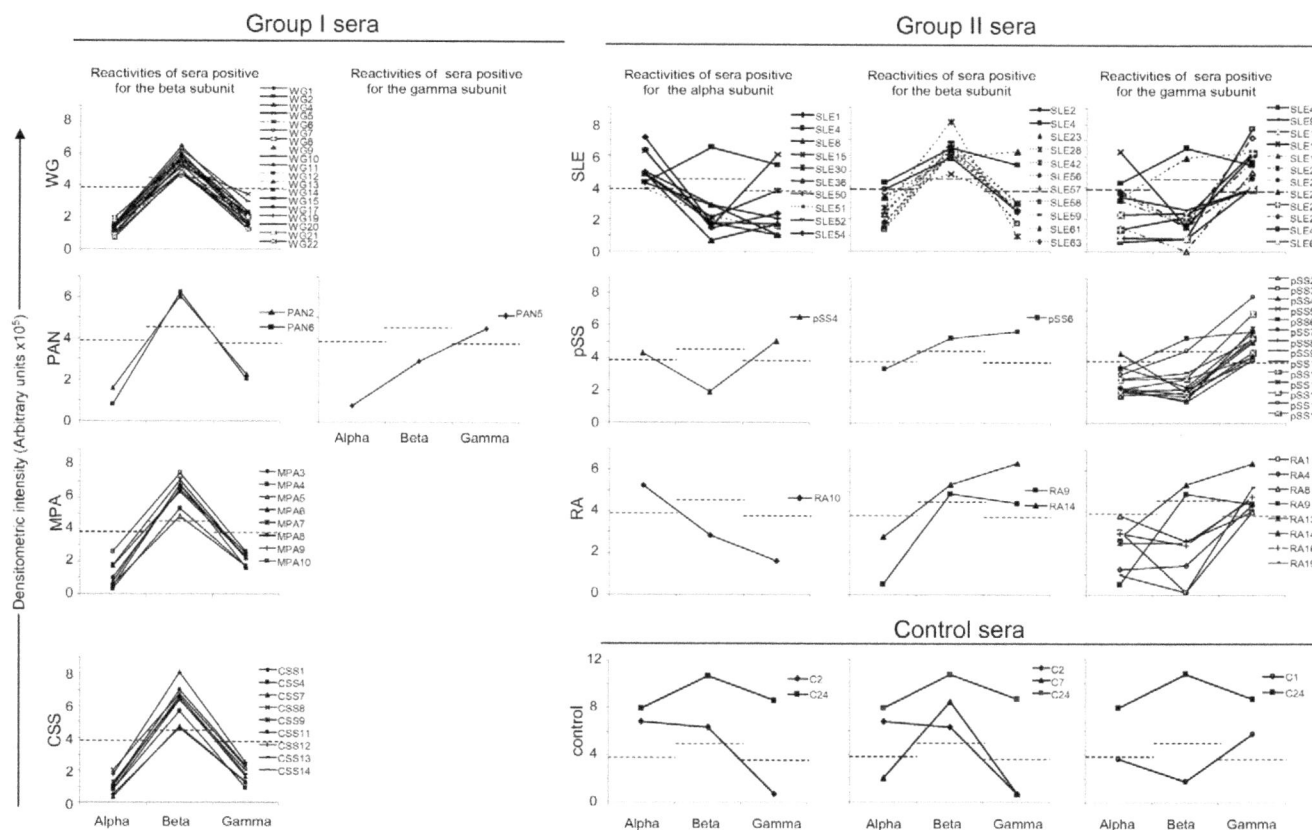

Figure 3. Multireactivity of anti-ATP synthase Ab positive sera. Sera from group I (WG, PAN, MPA, CSS), group II (SLE, pSS, RA) patients and controls positive for the α-, β-, or γ-subunit of ATP synthase were evaluated for their reactivity against all subunits. Densitometry measurements of reactivity by Western blots are shown. Broken lines show the cut off level for positivities against α-subunit (3.9.10^5 AU), β-subunit (4.3.10^5 AU) and γ-subunit (3.9.10^5 AU), corresponding to the mean+2 SD of control values. WG = Wegener's granulomatosis; PAN = polyarteritis nodosa; MPA = microscopic polyangiitis; CSS = Churg-Strauss syndrome; SLE = systemic lupus erythematosus; pSS = primary Sjögren's syndrome; RA = rheumatoid arthritis.

Table 1. ATP synthase multi-reactivities in sera from controls and from patients with primary and secondary vasculitides associated systemic autoimmune diseases found positive by Western blotting*.

	Frequencies (no) of anti-ATP synthase reactivity						
α-subunit	+	−	−	+	−	+	+
β- subunit	−	+	−	+	+	−	+
γ-subunit	−	−	+	−	+	+	+
Control (n = 4)	0	25.0 (1)	25.0 (1)	25.0 (1)	0	0	25.0 (1)
Primary vasculitides							
WG (n = 19)	0	100.0 (19)	0	0	0	0	0
CSS (n = 9)	0	100.0 (9)	0	0	0	0	0
PAN (n = 3)	0	66.6 (2)	33.3 (1)	0	0	0	0
MPA (n = 8)	0	100.0 (8)	0	0	0	0	0
Secondary vasculitides							
SLE (n = 29)	27.6 (8)	31.1 (9)	31.1 (9)	0	3.4 (1)	3.4 (1)	3.4 (1)
pSS (n = 14)	0	0	85.8 (12)	0	7.1 (1)	7.1 (1)	0
RA (n = 9)	11.1 (1)	0	66.7 (6)	0	22.2 (2)	0	0

*ATP synthase reactivities to the 55 kDa α-subunit, the 51 kDa β-subunit and the 30 kDa γ-subunit were determined by Western blotting.

reactivity in group I and multi-reactivity in group II sera remain largely unknown.

Modulation of ATP synthase activity was addressed in the last part of our experiments. The main function of cell surface ATP synthase appears to act as proton transport [3]. Proton flux across the membrane allows rotation of the γ-subunit, which in turn, induces modification of the α- and β-subunit conformation required for ATP synthesis [1]. When incubated in acidic pHe

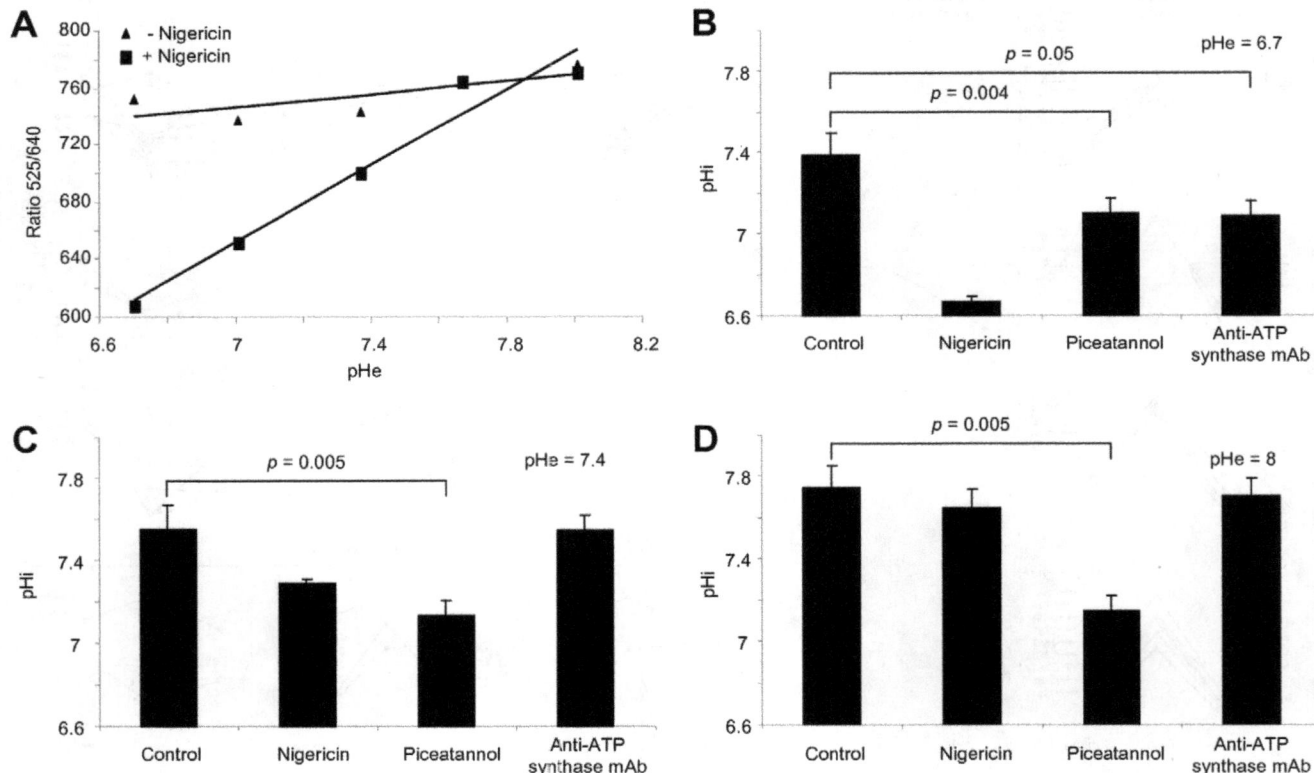

Figure 4. ATP synthase regulates intracellular pH. EAhy926 cells were labelled with BCECF, incubated with or without 40 µM nigericin in medium at different extracellular pH (pHe), and analyzed by flow cytometry. Fluorescence emission ratio 525nm/640nm (green fluorescence/red fluorescence) following BCECF excitation was calculated to determine calibration curves (**A**). BCECF-labelled EAhy926 cells were incubated either alone (control), with 40 µM nigericin, 80 µM piceatannol, or 50 µg/ml anti-ATP synthase mAb in medium at pHe 6.7 (**B**), 7.4 (**C**), or 8 (**D**). Ratio 525/640 was calculated and intracellular pH (pHi) determined with the calibration curves. Mean±SD of 3 experiments.

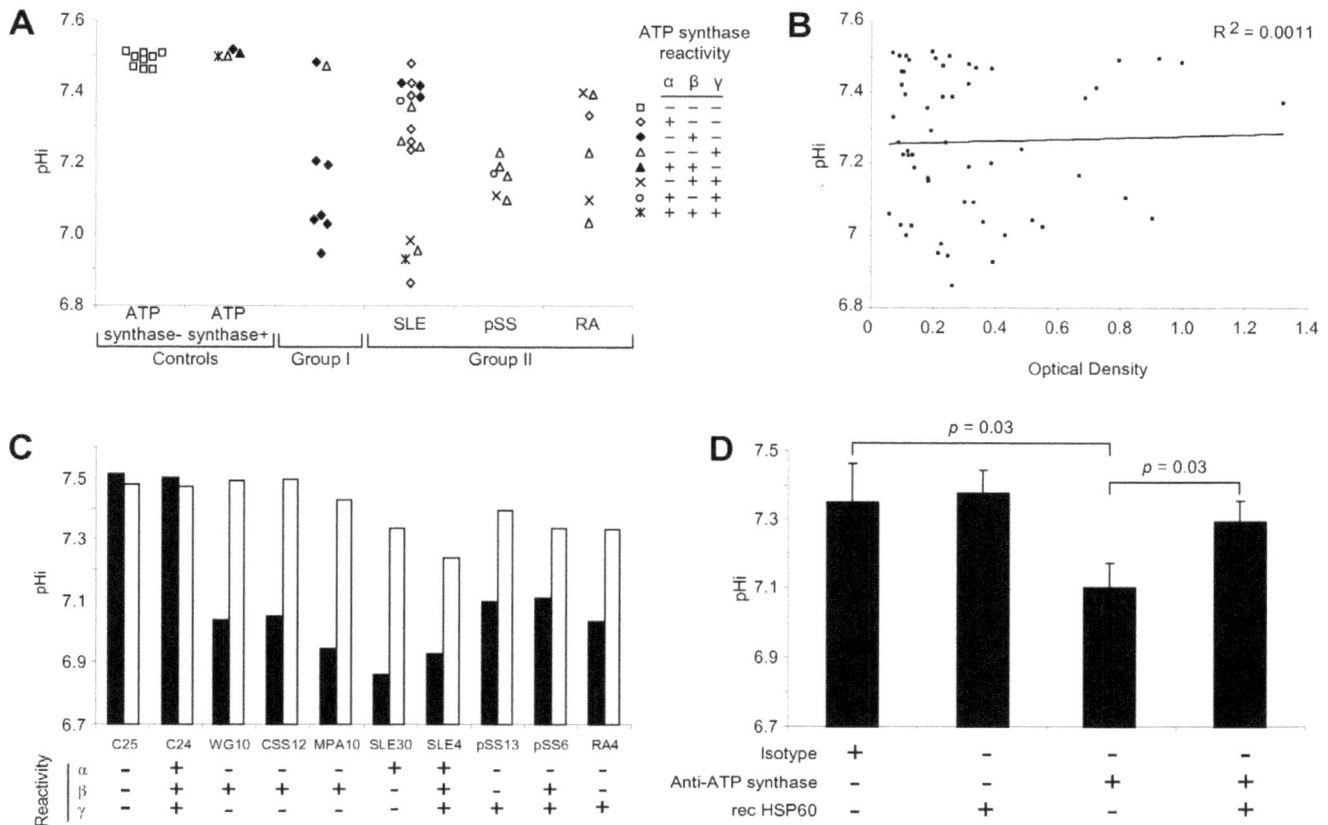

Figure 5. Anti-ATP synthase auto-Abs modulate ATP synthase function. A- EAhy926 cells were labelled with BCECF, incubated in pH 6.7 medium with sera showing different reactivity patterns against α-, β-, and γ-subunit of ATP synthase, and analyzed by flow cytometry. Intracellular pH (pHi) was then calculated from calibration curves. **B-** Correlation between ATP synthase reactivity determined in ELISA and pHi of EAhy926 cells incubated in the presence of sera in pH 6.7 medium. **C-** ATP synthase positive sera were depleted (open bars) or not (solid bars) of their ATP synthase reactivity and incubated with BCECF-loaded EAhy926 cells in pH 6.7 medium. After flow cytometry analyses, pHi were determined using calibration curves. ATP synthase positive (C24) and negative (C25) sera from healthy donors were used as controls. **D-** BCECF-loaded EAhy926 cells were incubated with recombinant hsp60 before suspension in medium pH 6.7 in the presence of 50 µg/ml anti-ATP synthase mAb. After flow cytometry analyses, pHi were determined using calibration curves. Mean±SD of 3 experiments. WG = Wegener's granulomatosis; CSS = Churg-Strauss syndrome; MPA = microscopic polyangiitis; SLE = systemic lupus erythematosus; pSS = primary Sjögren's syndrome; RA = rheumatoid arthritis.

medium, cell surface ATP synthase is activated to preserve pHi and helps EC to survive [4]. Therefore, decreased pHi of EC observed in the presence of anti-ATP synthase Ab from patients may result from different effects. Binding of Abs to the γ-subunit might block its rotation, whilst binding to the α- or β-subunits may alter their conformational changes. Consequently, Abs inhibit ATP synthase activity and decrease pHi of EC. These observations are consistent with others based on the use of polyclonal anti-β-subunit Abs that produce intracellular acidification of EC triggering cell death [5]. However, this interpretation is not in line with other data [5], where any effect was observed with polyclonal anti-γ-subunit Abs. We suggest that inhibition of ATP synthase activity is likely dependent on specific epitope recognition rather than determined by a particular subunit binding. It is noteworthy that anti-ATP synthase mAb 7H10 directed to the α-subunit inhibits ATP synthase activity [5] whereas other anti-α-subunit clones do not [31]. Conceivably, the absence of effects observed with the positive control sera, and the differential responses observed in group I compared with group II sera (Figure 5A) might reflect disparate epitope bindings. Furthermore, piceatannol and oligomycin, inhibitors of ATP synthase [23,24], have different effect on intracellular acidification. When EC were

incubated in neutral or basic pHe, piceatannol still promoted decreases of pHi. This might be due to its ability to inhibit phosphorylation pathway [32]. Consequently, dephosphorylation of NA^+/H^+ transporter would be responsible for pHi diminution [33]. Whether some Abs may affect similarly ATP synthase remains to be determined.

Of interesting note is that the effects of anti-ATP synthase Abs depend on the pHe environment since no variations could be seen in EC incubated in media with neutral or basic pHe. This raises the possibility that anti-ATP synthase Abs, as recently suggested in Alzheimer's disease [34], may contribute to the pathogenicity of renal tubular acidosis that can be observed in patients with primary vasculitides [35] and in pSS patients with secondary vasculitides [36], or in SLE patients developing interstitial nephritis [37]. Furthermore, acidosis, considered as a hallmark of tumor microenvironment [3], is associated with lymphoma in patients with pSS [38]. Thus, among AECAs, anti-ATP synthase Abs should be considered as pathogenic contributors of EC deregulation. It is noteworthy that vasculitides represent hetero-geneous inflammatory diseases that affect different ECs in arteries, arterioles, capillaries, veinules and veins toward major body regions [39]. Therefore, there are possibilities that in *in vivo* situations, effects of anti-ATP synthase Abs may vary from one type of ECs to another.

In addition, binding of hsp60 to ATP synthase might compete with Ab and inhibits the anti-β chain ATP synthase Ab-induced pHi down-regulation (Figure 5D). This indicates that soluble hsp60, whose level is elevated in vasculitides [21], may have protective effects. It remains to determine whether the effectiveness of the protective effect of hsp60 occurs regardless of the specificity of the anti-ATP synthase Ab. Nevertheless, at low pHe environments, this "danger" signal allows EC to maintain normal pHi owing to the preservation of a functional ATP synthase, and promotes cell survival. These effects may depend on the environment. It has thus been suggested that expression of hsp60 increases at sites predisposed to atherosclerotic lesions in response to EC stress [40]. Furthermore, arteriosclerosis can be induced or aggravated by hsp60 immunization [41,42] implying that hsp60 can contribute to the development of cardiovascular diseases [43].

In sum, we provide new insights into the pathogenicity of AECAs in vasculitides. Recognition of cell surface ATP synthase at low pHe microenvironment contributes to intracellular acidification of EC known to induce cell death and the triggering of inflammation. However, the concomitant presence of soluble hsp60 might partly offset this deleterious response due to the specific interaction with ATP synthase. Further investigations are required to design therapeutic strategies derived from these pathogenic mechanisms.

Materials and Methods

Ethics statement

Ethics approval was given by the Institutional Review Board of the Brest University Hospital, of Lyon Hospital and of La Pitié Salpétrière Hospital. Use of samples from WG, CSS, MPA and PAN were approved by the Institutional Review Board of Lyon Hospital and La Pitié Salpétrière Hospital respectively, and those from SLE, RA and pSS by that of the Brest University Hospital. All participants gave their written informed consent to participate in this study.

Cell cultures

HUVEC were prepared by digestion with 0.1% collagenase, grown to confluence [11], and passaged twice in DMEM (Gibco) with 10% fetal calf serum, 2mM glutamine and 100IU/mL polymyxin B prior to use.

The EAhy926 EC were grown in DMEM supplemented with 10% fetal calf serum, 2mM glutamine, 100 μM hypoxanthine, 0.4 μM aminopterin, 16 μM thymidine and 50mg/L gentamycin.

Two-dimensional electrophoresis

HUVEC were detached from culture flasks with trypsin, washed and resuspended in a homogenization buffer (1M sucrose, 100mM Tris-Hcl, 100mM EDTA, 50mM $MgCl_2$, 1 μM leupeptin, 1 μM pepstatin, 1 μM aprotinin). After freezing-thawing cycles, sonication, and centrifugation, membrane-enriched protein fractions were resuspended in solubilization buffer (4% CHAPS, 1% Triton X-100), centrifuged at 10,000g, and protein concentration determined using the Micro BCA protein assay kit (Pierce).

Protein extracts were resuspended in re-hydration buffer (4% CHAPS, 1% Triton X-100, 7M urea, 2M thiourea, 0.48% 3–10 biolyte, 1% tributylphosphine), and loaded onto pH 3–10 or pH 4–8 immobilized pH gradient strips (BioRad) for isoelectric focusing. After passive re-hydration, proteins were focused with a protean immunoelectrofocalisation cell (BioRad). Strips were then incubated in equilibration solutions before subjected to 10% SDS-PAGE. For the spot identifications, proteins of interest were cut out from the Coomassie blue-stained gel, digested with trypsin, desalted and deposited on 600 μm Scout MTP 384 AnchorChip (Brucker Daltonics). Peptidic fingerprints were obtained by mass spectroscopy analysis using the Ultraflex MALDI (Brucker Daltonics). The threshold for positivity was scored at 78. The detected peptide masses were then searched against Swiss-Prot dabatase.

Co-immunoprecipitation

Cell surface proteins were cross-linked with 20 μg/ml bis(sulfo-N-succinimidyl) for 20 min at 4°C. After addition of 1vol of 10mM Tris, membrane-enriched fractions were obtained using a modified solubilization buffer (50mM Tris, 1% Triton X-100, 150mM NaCl). Protein solutions were pre-cleared with protein G-coated beads, and precipitated with polyclonal anti-hsp60 or anti-ATP synthase Ab-coated protein G beads (Abcam). The proteins were washed in modified solubilization buffer, and retained proteins eluted with 0.1% Triton X-100 and 0.1M triethylamin, pH 11.8 and resolved by WB.

Western and Far Western blotting

Proteins were transferred onto PVDF membranes and probed with anti-hsp60 mAb (clone LK-1, Calbiochem) or anti-ATP synthase mAb (clone 3D5, Abcam), amplified with biotinylated anti-Ig Ab (Jackson), and developed with horseradish peroxydase (HRP)-conjugated streptavidin (Amersham). For the Far WB experiments, PVDF membranes were first incubated with 2 μg/ml recombinant hsp60 (Sigma), and then probed with anti-hsp60 mAb before development.

Detection of cellular expression

HUVEC and EAhy926 cells were suspended in PBS, incubated with anti-ATP synthase mAb and FITC-conjugated secondary Abs, washed and analyzed in an Epics XL (Beckman Coulter) flow cytometer. Cells stained with an isotype control Ab and the FITC-conjugated Abs were enabled to set the level of positivity.

For indirect immunofluorescence staining, EC were cultured onto 10-well slides until confluence. They were incubated with anti-ATP synthase or isotype control mAb, and FITC-conjugated secondary Ab and propidium iodide, fixed in paraformaldehyde, and slides mounted in glycerol and examined with a TCS-NT confocal microscope (Leica).

Surface plasmon resonance-based analysis

Surface plasmon resonance analyses were performed using the Biacore X system from GE Healthcare (INSERM U613, Brest). Due to the heterogeneity of the purified bovine ATP synthase complex, recombinant hsp60 was immobilized onto a carboxymethyldextran biosensor chip using amine coupling. Briefly, a continuous flow of 5 μl/min was maintained over the sensor in 10mM HEPES, 150mM NaCl, 2mM EDTA. The matrix of the chip was activated by a 7-min injection of 0.05M N-hydroxy-succinimide with 0.3M N-ethyl-N-(3-diethylaminopropyl) carbodiimide, followed by a 6-min injection of recombinant hsp60 in 10mM sodium acetate, pH4.5. The procedure was completed by a 7-min exposure to ethanolamine hydrochloride to inactivate residual esters. Density of immobilized hsp60 was ~10ng/mm². Purified bovine ATP synthase was injected at a flow rate of 10 μl/min over the immobilized recombinant hsp60 (Flow Cell 2). In control experiments, another part of the same sensor was treated as above but in the absence of recombinant hsp60 (Flow Cell 1).

Sensors were regenerated after each cycle by injection of a 2-μl pulse of 50mM NaOH to dissociate the analyte from the ligand. The final sensograms were calculated by substrating the signal of the control (Flow Cell 1) from that of the test (Flow Cell 2), and results expressed in resonance units.

Patients

Group I sera comprised primary systemic vasculitides: 22 patients with Wegener's granulomatosis (WG), 14 with Churg-Strauss syndrome (CSS), 6 with polyarteritis nodosa (PAN) and 10 with microscopic polyangiitis (MPA). Group II sera comprised secondary systemic vasculitides associated with autoimmune diseases: 64 patients with systemic lupus erythematosus (SLE), 18 with primary Sjögrens' syndrome (pSS) and 20 with rheumatoid arthritis (RA). All patients are Caucasian and fulfilled the criteria for their respective disease and the sera were selected based on their positivity for AECAs [44]. Concurrently, sera from 30 laboratory staff volunteers were studied as controls. They were matched for age and sex to the two groups of patients. Thus, there were 3 women for 1 man, and their ages ranged from 23 to 66 years.

Measurement of ATP synthase reactivity

Anti-ATP synthase autoAbs were detected using an in-house made ELISA [45]. Microtiter plates were sensitized with 0.5 μg of purified bovine ATP synthase at 5 μg/ml, blocked with PBS containing 2% BSA, incubated with 100 μL of serum diluted 1:50 in 1% BSA and developed with alkaline phosphatase-conjugated anti-human IgG (Zymed). Optical density (OD) of control wells without ATP synthase were subtracted from the OD of ATP synthase-coated wells. The mean+2 standard deviations (SDs) of the OD values in negative control sera was taken as the threshold for positivity.

Reactivity was also determined by WB to evaluate the recognition of ATP synthase subunits. The protein complex was subjected to 10% SDS-PAGE, transferred onto PVDF membranes saturated with PBS containing 5% milk proteins, and probed with sera diluted 1:100 in 1% milk proteins. Bound autoAbs were revealed with biotinylated-anti-human IgG Ab (Jackson) and developed with HRP-streptavidin. After densitometry analyses performed with Quantity-One® software (BioRad) for each α-, β- and γ-subunit, the mean+2 SD of the OD values for the control sera were the threshold for positivities.

Assessment of intracellular pH and ATP synthase function

pHi was measured by flow cytometry. Briefly, EAhy926 cells were suspended in HBSS supplemented with 0.32 μM BCECF (Invitrogen). Cells were then incubated at 37°C to allow BCECF to be hydrolyzed by intracellular esterase into pH-dependent fluorescent probe and analyzed in an Epics XL flow cytometer. Excitation at wavelength 488nm led to green and red fluorescences that were selected using a 525nm and a 640nm bandpass filter, respectively. While emission intensity at 525nm is stable that at 640nm decreases with pHi. Therefore, 525/640 nm ratio that increases linearly with pH was considered as an appropriate tool for the evaluation of ATP synthase activity [46]. To ascertain the reproducibility of the method, calibration curves were constructed for each experiment from BCECF-labelled cells suspended in media with different pHe, and in the presence of 40 μM nigericin (Sigma), an ionophore that exchanges K^+ and H^+ across cellular membranes. In these conditions, pHi measured corresponds to pHe [22].

EAhy926 cells labelled with BCECF were incubated 1:20 with 100 μL of serum, or with 50 μg/mL anti-ATP synthase mAb (clone 4.3E8.D10, Sigma-Aldrich) for 1 h at 4°C. The cells were then washed in medium with appropriate pHe and incubated in the same medium for 20 minutes at 37°C before flow cytometry analysis. Modulation of pHi was then evaluated. Positive control was performed using BCECF-loaded cells suspended in medium with different pHe and in the presence of 80 μM piceatannol (Sigma), a tetrahydroxystilbene that inhibits specifically ATP synthase [23].

In some experiments, sera were pre-depleted of their anti-ATP synthase reactivity by overnight incubation at 4°C in ATP synthase-coated microplates. Finally, in some experiments, 5.10^6 BCECF-loaded EC were incubated with 8 μg recombinant hsp60 at 80 μg/ml, before suspension with diluted sera.

Statistical analysis

All data were expressed as the mean±SD. Statistical analysis used chi-square or Fisher's exact test for comparisons of percentages. Mean quantitative values were compared using the Wilcoxon or Mann and Whitney U-test. Significance was assessed at $p = 0.05$.

Acknowledgments

We thank Dr Cora-Jean S. Edgell (University of North Carolina, Chapell Hill, NC) for providing the EAhy926 cells, Prof John E. Walker (Medical Research Council, London, UK) for donating purified bovine F1-ATP synthase. Thanks are also due to Prof Rizgar A. Mageed (William Harvey Research Institute, London, UK) for editorial assistance and to Simone Forest and Genevieve Michel for secretarial assistance.

Author Contributions

Conceived and designed the experiments: JEA PY CJ. Performed the experiments: JEA. Analyzed the data: JEA SH LG AS JOP CJ. Contributed reagents/materials/analysis tools: JEA SH LG AS JOP. Wrote the paper: PY CJ.

References

1. Stock D, Gibbons C, Arechaga I, Leslie AG, Walker JE (2000) The rotary mechanism of ATP synthase. Curr Opin Struct Biol 10: 672–679.
2. Gibbons C, Montgomery MG, Leslie AG, Walker JE (2000) The structure of the central stalk in bovine F(1)-ATPase at 2.4 A resolution. Nat Struct Biol 7: 1055–1061.
3. Chi SL, Pizzo SV (2006) Cell surface F1Fo ATP synthase: a new paradigm? Ann Med 38: 429–438.
4. Moser TL, Kenan DJ, Ashley TA, Roy JA, Goodman MD, et al. (2001) Endothelial cell surface F1-F0 ATP synthase is active in ATP synthesis is inhibited by angiostatin. Proc Natl Acad Sci USA 98: 6656–6661.
5. Champagne E, Martinez LO, Collet X, Barbaras R (2006) Ecto-F1Fo ATP synthase/F1 ATPase: metabolic and immunological functions. Curr Opin Lipido l17: 279–284.
6. Wahl ML, Owen CS, Grant DS (2002) Angiostatin induces intracellular acidosis and anoikis in endothelial cells at a tumor-like low pH. Endothelium 9: 205–216.
7. Radojkovic C, Genoux A, Pons V, Combes G, de Jonge H, et al. (2009) Stimulation of cell surface F1-ATPase activity by apolipoprotein A-I inhibits

endothelial cell apoptosis and promotes proliferation. Arterioscler Thromb Vasc Biol 29: 1125–1130.
8. Prasad TK, Hack E, Hallberg RL (1990) Function of the maize mitochondrial chaperonin hsp60: specific association between hsp60 and newly synthesized F1-ATPase alpha subunits. Mol Cell Biol 10: 3979–3986.
9. Soltys BJ, Gupta RS (1999) Mitochondrial-matrix proteins at unexpected locations: are they exported? Trends Biochem Sci 24: 174–177.
10. Binder RJ, Vatner R, Srivastava P (2004) The heat-shock protein receptors: some answers and more questions. Tissue Antigens 64: 442–451.
11. Habich C, Baumgart K, Kolb H, Burkart V (2002) The receptor for heat shock protein 60 on macrophages is saturable, specific, and distinct from receptors for other heat shock proteins. J Immunol 168: 569–576.
12. Habich C, Burkart V (2007) Heat shock protein 60: regulatory role on innate immune cells. Cell Mol Life Sci 64: 742–751.
13. Alard JE, Dueymes M, Mageed RA, Saraux A, Youinou P, et al. (2009) Mitochondrial heat shock protein (HSP) 70 synergizes with HSP60 in

transducing endothelial cell apoptosis induced by anti-HSP60 autoantibody. FASEB J 23: 2772–2779.

14. Alard JE, Dueymes M, Youinou P, Jamin C (2007) Modulation of endothelial cell damages by anti-hsp60 autoantibodies in systemic autoimmune diseases. Autoimmun Rev 6: 438–443.

15. Jamin C, Dugué C, Alard JE, Jousse S, Saraux A, et al. (2005) Induction of endothelial cell apoptosis by the binding of anti-endothelial cell antibodies to hsp60 in vasculitis-associated systemic autoimmune diseases. Arthritis Rheum 52: 4028–4038.

16. Ronda N (2007) Anti-endothelial cell autoantibodies. In: Shoenfeld Y, Gershwin ME, Meroni PL, eds. Autoantibodies second edition. Amsterdam: Elsevier Science. pp 725–731.

17. Rajaiah R, Moudgil KD (2009) Heat-shock proteins can promote as well as regulate autoimmunity. Autoimmun Rev 8: 388–393.

18. Dubaniewicz A (2010) Mycobacterium tuberculosis heat shock proteins and autoimmunity in sarcoidosis. Autoimmun Rev 9: 419–424.

19. Jennette JC, Falk RJ, Andrassy K, Bacon PA, Churg J, et al. (1994) Nomenclature of systemic vasculitides. Proposal of an international consensus conference. Arthritis Rheum 37: 187–192.

20. Savage CO, Harper L, Cockwell P, Adu D, Howie AJ (2000) ABC of arterial and vascular disease: vasculitis. BMJ 320: 1325–1328.

21. Alard JE, Dueymes M, Youinou P, Jamin C (2008) hsp60 and anti-hsp60 antibodies in vasculitis: they are two of a kind. Clin Rev Allergy Immunol 35: 66–71.

22. Káldi K, Szászi K, Suszták K, Kapus A, Ligeti E (1994) Lymphocytes possess an electrogenic H(+)-transporting pathway in their plasma membrane. Biochem J 301: 329–334.

23. Zheng J, Ramirez VD (1999) Piceatannol, a stilbene phytochemical, inhibits mitochondrial F0F1-ATPase activity by targeting the F1 complex. Biochem Biophys Res Commun 261: 499–503.

24. Stater EC (1967) Application of inhibitors for study of oxidative phosphorylation. Meth Enzymol 10: 48–57.

25. Yegutkin GG, Henttinen T, Jalkanen S (2001) Extracellular ATP formation on vascular endothelial cells is mediated by ecto-nucleotide kinase activities via phosphotransfer reactions. FASEB J 15: 251–60.

26. Arakaki N, Nagao T, Niki R, Toyofuku A, Tanaka H, et al. (2003) Possible role of cell surface H+ -ATP synthase in the extracellular ATP synthesis and proliferation of human umbilical vein endothelial cells. Mol Cancer Res 1: 931–939.

27. Sprenger RR, Speijer D, Back JW, De Koster CG, Pannekoek H (2004) Comparative proteomics of human endothelial cell caveolae and rafts using two-dimensional gel electrophoresis and mass spectrometry. Electrophoresis 25: 156–172.

28. Alessandri C, Bombardieri M, Valesini G (2006) Pathogenic mechanisms of anti-endothelial cell antibodies (AECA): their prevalence and clinical relevance. Adv Clin Chem 42: 297–326.

29. Guilpain P, Mouthon L (2008) Antiendothelial cells autoantibodies in vasculitis-associated systemic diseases. Clin Rev Allergy Immunol 35: 59–65.

30. Domiciano DS, Carvalho JF, Shoenfeld Y (2009) Pathogenic role of anti-endothelial cell antibodies in autoimmune rheumatic diseases Lupus 18: 1233–1238.

31. Chi SL, Wahl ML, Mowery YM, Shan S, Mukhopadhyay S (2007) Angiostatin-like activity of a monoclonal antibody to the catalytic subunit of F1F0 ATP synthase. Cancer Res 67: 4716–4724.

32. Bijli KM, Fazal F, Minhajuddin M, Rahman A (2008) Activation of Syk by protein kinase C-delta regulates thrombin-induced intercellular adhesion molecule-1 expression in endothelial cells via tyrosine phosphorylation of RelA/p65. J Biol Chem 283: 14674–14684.

33. Marches R, Vitetta ES, Uhr JW (2001) A role for intracellular pH in membrane IgM-mediated cell death of human B lymphomas. Proc Natl Acad Sci U S A 98: 3434–3439.

34. Vacirca D, Delunardo F, Matarrese P, Colasanti T, Marhutti P, et al. (2010) Autoantibodies to the adenosine triphosphate synthase play a pathogenic role in Alzheimer's diseases. doi: 10.1016/j.neurobiolaging.2010.05.013.

35. Breedveld FC, Haanen HC, Chang PC (1986) Distal renal tubular acidosis in polyarteritis nodosa. Arch Intern Med 146: 1009–1010.

36. Soy M, Pamuk ON, Gerenli M, Celik Y (2005) A primary Sjögren's syndrome patient with distal renal tubular acidosis, who presented with symptoms of hypokalemic periodic paralysis: Report of a case study and review of the literature. Rheumatol Int 26: 86–89.

37. Gur H, Kopolovic Y, Gross DJ (1987) Chronic predominant interstitial nephritis in a patient with systemic lupus erythematosus: a follow up of three years and review of the literature. Ann Rheum Dis 46: 617–623.

38. Mavragani CP, Moutsopoulos NM, Moutsopoulos HM (2006) The management of Sjögren's syndrome. Nat Clin Pract Rheumatol 2: 252–261.

39. Savage CO, Harper L, Cockwell P, Adu D, Howie AJ (2000) ABC of arterial and vascular disease: vasculitis. BMJ 320: 1325–1328.

40. Wick MC, Mayerl C, Backovic A, van der Zee R, Jaschke W, et al. (2008) In vivo imaging of the effect of LPS on arterial endothelial cells: molecular imaging of heat shock protein 60 expression. Cell Stress Chaperones 13: 275–285.

41. Xu Q, Dietrich H, Steiner HJ, Gown AM, Schoel B, et al. (1992) Induction of arteriosclerosis in normocholesterolemic rabbits by immunization with heat shock protein 65. Arterioscler Thromb 12: 789–799.

42. George J, Shoenfeld Y, Afek A, Gilburd B, Keren P, et al. (1999) Enhanced fatty streak formation in C57BL/6J mice by immunization with heat shock protein-65. Arterioscler Thromb Vasc Biol 19: 505–510.

43. Wick G, Knoflach M, Xu Q (2004) Autoimmune and inflammatory mechanisms in atherosclerosis. Annu Rev Immunol 22: 361–403.

44. Révélen R, D'Arbonneau F, Guillevin L, Bordron A, Youinou P (2002) Comparison of cell-ELISA, flow cytometry and Western blotting for the detection of antiendothelial cell antibodies. Clin Exp Rheumatol 20: 19–26.

45. Révélen R, Bordron A, Dueymes M, Youinou P, Arvieux J (2000) False positivity in a cyto-ELISA for anti-endothelial cell antibodies caused by heterophile antibodies to bovine serum proteins. Clin Chem 46: 273–278.

46. Franck P, Petitipain N, Cherlet M, Dardennes M, Maachi F, et al. (1996) Measurement of intracellular pH in cultured cells by flow cytometry with BCECF-AM. J Biotechnol 46: 187–195.

9

Autoantibodies against the Catalytic Domain of BRAF are not Specific Serum Markers for Rheumatoid Arthritis

Wenli Li[1,2], Wei Wang[1,2], Shipeng Sun[1,2], Yu Sun[1,2], Yang Pan[1,2], Lunan Wang[1], Rui Zhang[1], Kuo Zhang[1], Jinming Li[1]*

1 National Center for Clinical Laboratories, Beijing Hospital, Beijing, People's Republic of China, 2 Graduate School, Peking Union Medical College, Chinese Academy of Medical Sciences, Beijing, People's Republic of China

Abstract

Background: Autoantibodies to the catalytic domain of v-raf murine sarcoma viral oncogene homologue B1 (BRAF) have been recently identified as a new family of autoantibodies involved in rheumatoid arthritis (RA). The objective of this study was to determine antibody responses to the catalytic domain of BRAF in RA and other autoimmune diseases. The association between RA-related clinical indices and these antibodies was also assessed.

Methodology/Principal Findings: The presence of autoantibodies to the catalytic domain of BRAF (anti-BRAF) or to peptide P25 (amino acids 656–675 of the catalytic domain of BRAF; anti-P25) was determined in serum samples from patients with RA, primary Sjögren's syndrome (pSS), systemic lupus erythematosus (SLE), and healthy controls by using indirect enzyme-linked immunosorbent assays (ELISAs) based on the recombinant catalytic domain of BRAF or a synthesized peptide, respectively. Associations of anti-BRAF or anti-P25 with disease variables of RA patients were also evaluated. Our results show that the BRAF-specific antibodies anti-BRAF and anti-P25 are equally present in RA, pSS, and SLE patients. However, the erythrocyte sedimentation rate (ESR) used to detect inflammation was significantly different between patients with and without BRAF-specific antibodies. The anti-BRAF-positive patients were found to have prolonged disease, and active disease occurred more frequently in anti-P25-positive patients than in anti-P25-negative patients. A weak but significant correlation between anti-P25 levels and ESRs was observed ($r = 0.319$, $p = 0.004$).

Conclusions/Significance: The antibody response against the catalytic domain of BRAF is not specific for RA, but the higher titers of BRAF-specific antibodies may be associated with increased inflammation in RA.

Editor: Mehrdad Matloubian, University of California San Francisco, United States of America

Funding: This work was supported by a grant from the National High Technology Reseach and Development Program of China (863 Program) (No. 2011AA02A116). The funders had no role in study design, data collection and analysis, decision to publish, or preparation of the manuscript.

Competing Interests: The authors have declared that no competing interests exist.

* E-mail: ljm63hn@yahoo.com.cn

Introduction

Autoimmune diseases occur when the body's immune system attacks self-antigens. This induces prolonged inflammation and subsequent tissue destruction. Rheumatoid arthritis (RA), a common systemic autoimmune disease of unknown etiology, is characterized by chronically inflamed synovial joints and subsequent destruction of cartilage and bones. Despite decades of research, the pathogenesis of RA is still unresolved. One of the hallmarks of RA is the presence of a broad spectrum of autoantibodies against aberrantly expressed autoantigens. The discovery of autoantibodies to citrullinated proteins such as fibrin and vimentin in patients with RA was one of the most important findings in rheumatology research [1]. Advances in protein array technologies have enabled large-scale analysis of proteins to identify significant biomarkers that contribute to disease pathogenesis. A recently published paper describing 8,268 protein arrays using RA sera indicates that the catalytic domain of v-raf murine sarcoma viral oncogene homologue B1 (BRAF) is a new autoantigen for RA [2].

BRAF is a serine-threonine kinase involved in the mitogen-activated protein kinase (MAPK) pathways that regulate cell survival, proliferation, differentiation, cytokine generation, and metalloproteinase production [3]. BRAF somatic missense mutations are reported in 66% of malignant melanomas and at a lower frequency in a wide range of other human cancers [4]. A mutated BRAF gene with a single amino acid substitution (BRAF V600E) results in higher kinase activity. Thus, the resulting BRAF protein, which has protective activity against Raf kinase inhibitors, has been considered as a potential target for tumor therapy [5]. On the other hand, the MAPK pathways are implicated in the pathogenesis of certain inflammatory autoimmune diseases such as RA via their regulatory effects on the production of cytokines or metalloproteinases [6–9]. Recent data show that serum antibodies to the catalytic domain of BRAF (anti-BRAF) can activate BRAF *in vitro*. This indicates that anti-BRAF may play a role in inflammation in RA through activation of the MAPK pathway [10]. The results of peptide array analysis indicate that the antibody response to P25 (amino acids 656–675 of the catalytic domain of BRAF) is specific to RA. However, antibodies to peptide P25 (anti-P25) were defined as specific markers for RA, based on comparison to small patient cohorts with ankylosing spondylitis (AS) and psoriasis arthritis (PsA), rather than to patients with autoimmune disorders. In the present study, we determined the antibody responses to the catalytic domain of wild-type BRAF and peptide P25 in Chinese patients with RA, primary Sjögren's syndrome (pSS), and systemic lupus erythematosus (SLE) by indirect enzyme-linked immunosorbent assays (ELISAs) and investigated the possible associations between these antibodies and the disease indicators of RA.

Materials and Methods

Ethics statement

Written informed consent was not obtained because of the nature of the study design, which utilized serum samples taken after routine tests. All subjects recruited in this study were informed of the nature of the project and verbal informed consent was obtained from each patient, This was recorded by the physician who explained the study procedure. The study protocol and verbal consent document were approved by the Ethics Committee of the National Center for Clinical Laboratories, where the study was performed.

DNA constructs

The DNA segment corresponding to the catalytic domain of wild-type BRAF (amino acids 416–766) was generated by PCR using specific primers carrying restriction sites. The pEF-myc-BRAF plasmid containing full-length human BRAF cDNA, was kindly provided by Dr. Richard Marais (Institute of Cancer Research, London, United Kingdom). Enzyme-restricted PCR products were ligated into the multiple cloning sites of the pET28b expression vector by T4 DNA ligase. The desired clones were confirmed by sequencing.

Protein expression and purification

The recombinant plasmid carrying the catalytic domain of wild-type BRAF (pET28b-BRAF) was transformed into *Escherichia coli* BL-21(DE3). Further, a $6 \times$ His-tagged protein was expressed with induction by 0.1 mM isopropyl-β-D-thiogalactoside (IPTG) for 4 h at 37°C. Bacterial pellets from a total of 1 L of culture were resuspended in 10 mL lysis buffer (50 mM Tris-Cl, 100 mM NaCl, 5 mM EDTA, 1% NaN_3, 0.5% Triton X-100, 5 mM DTT, pH 8.0). After the suspension was prepared, lysozyme (Sigma-Aldrich, St. Louis, MO, USA) was added to a final concentration of 0.2 mg/mL, followed by incubation at room temperature (RT) for 30 min. The cells were further disrupted by sonication on ice for 10 min (on for 5 s, off for 5 s). The homogenate was then centrifuged at 4°C for 30 min at 6000 *g*. The supernatant was discarded, and the inclusion bodies were collected. The collected precipitates were resuspended in 10 mL washing buffer (100 mM Tris-Cl, 5 mM EDTA, 5 mM DTT, 2 M urea, 2% Triton X-100, pH 8.0) and incubated at RT for 20 min. The inclusion bodies were then recovered by centrifugation at 4°C for 30 min at 8000 *g*. The above washing step was repeated twice, the inclusion bodies were dissolved in binding buffer (20 mM sodium phosphate, 0.5 M NaCl, 40 mM imidazole, 1.5% Triton X-100, 4 mM DTT, 6 M guanidine-HCl, pH 8.0), and the recombinant protein was further purified by affinity chromatography on a Ni-Sepharose Fast flow (FF) column (GE Healthcare, Uppsala, Sweden). The His-tagged protein was eluted with a linear concentration gradient of imidazole from 40 to 400 mM. The fractions containing the target protein were pooled, dialyzed to remove imidazole, and stored in the presence of 6 M guanidine-HCl at −20°C. The protein concentration was determined by a standard bicinchoninic (BCA) protein assay (Pierce, Rockford, USA). To evaluate the size and purity of the recombinant protein,

samples were denatured in SDS loading buffer (25 mM Tris-HCl, pH 6.8, 5% β-mercaptoethanol, 2% SDS, 50% glycerol), separated on a 10% polyacrylamide gel, and stained with Coomassie blue.

Serum samples

Serum samples were obtained from a previously described RA cohort that fulfilled the American College of Rheumatology (ACR) criteria for RA [11,12] and included 101 patients in the final study. For comparison, samples from 250 subjects with other autoimmune diseases were tested, including samples obtained from 132 patients with pSS and samples obtained from 118 patients with SLE. Healthy controls (140) were also included to determine the cutoff value for positivity. Serum samples were stored at −80°C until analysis. The following data were collected from RA patients: gender, age, disease duration, rheumatoid factor (RF), anti-cyclic citrullinated peptide antibodies (anti-CCP), erythrocyte sedimentation rate (ESR), C-reactive protein (CRP), and disease status. Recent-onset RA was defined as RA with disease duration of less than 2 years. RF and CRP levels were determined by an immunonephelometric method. Values >7.9 mg/L for CRP and >20 IU/mL for RF were considered positive. Anti-CCP antibodies were assessed with a commercial ELISA kit (Immunoscan CCPlus, Euro-Diagnostica, Malmo, Sweden) according to the manufacturer's recommendations. The cutoff value for a positive reaction was set at 25 U/mL, as suggested by the manufacturer. The ESR was measured by Westergren's method; values ≤15 mm/h for men and ≤20 mm/h for women were considered normal. Active RA was defined as described previously [12]. The basic characteristics of the RA cohort are described in Table 1.

Table 1. Demographic data and disease indicators of 101 patients with RA.

	Number	Description
Females/Males	101	81/20
Age, years	101	47.3±13.8
Disease duration, years	97	5 (0.1–50)
Recent onset	35	1 (0.1–2)
Prolonged	62	8 (3–50)
RF	97	
RF-positive	83	82.2%
Anti-CCP(U/mL)	101	353 (16–5477)
Anti-CCP-positive	74	811 (25–5477)
ESR, mm/h	81	56±33
Normal	14	12±5
Elevated	67	66±28
CRP	62	
Elevated	25	40.3%
Disease status	101	
Active disease	47	46.5%

RF: rheumatoid factor; anti-CCP: anti-cyclic citrullinated peptide antibodies; ESR: erythrocyte sedimentation rate; CRP: C-reactive protein.
Categorical variables are given as %; normally distributed data are given in mean ± SD; other continuous variables are given in median (range).

Detection of IgG anti-BRAF by ELISA

Specific antibodies to the recombinant catalytic domain of wild-type BRAF were identified in sera by an indirect ELISA. To conduct the assay, 100 μL of the recombinant catalytic domain of BRAF (2.5 μg/mL) was incubated in an ELISA plate (Nunc Maxisorp, Roskilde, Denmark) at 4°C overnight. Microwells were then washed with phosphate-buffered saline (PBS: 0.01 M, pH 7.4) with 0.05% Tween-20 (PBST). Unbound sites were blocked by incubation with 200 μL 20% newborn calf serum (NCS) in PBS at 37°C for 1.5 h. Sera were diluted 1:200 in blocking buffer and aliquots of 100 μL were added to the wells. Wells coated with bovine serum albumin (BSA) were prepared for each sample, to assess non-specific binding. After incubation at 37°C for 1 h, plates were washed 3 times with PBST. Subsequently, the captured antibodies were detected by a horseradish peroxidase (HRP)-conjugated goat anti-human IgG (1:10000) (Sigma), which was diluted with 20% NCS in PBST (100 μL/well). After incubation at 37°C for 30 min, wells were washed 5 times with PBST. Color was developed by application of 100 μL of tetramethylbenzidine (Sigma) at 37°C for 20 min. The reaction was stopped by addition of 0.5 M sulfuric acid, and the optical density at 450 nm (OD450), with 620 nm as the correction wavelength, was obtained using an ELISA plate reader (Labsystems, Finland).

Each sample was assayed in duplicate. A positive serum sample was included in each assay and used to correct for inter-assay variations. Results were expressed as arbitrary units (AU) calculated as ([OD$_{450}$ of sample$-$OD$_{450}$ of the non-specific binding of the sample]/[OD$_{450}$ of the positive control$-$OD$_{450}$ of the non-specific binding of the positive control])$\times$100.

Detection of IgG autoantibodies to P25 by ELISA

To test patient reactivity to peptide P25 (YSNINNRD-QIIFMVGRGYLS, a peptide encompassing amino acids 656–675 of the catalytic domain of BRAF), an indirect ELISA for quantifying IgG autoantibodies to P25 was conducted. Serum samples from RA, pSS, and SLE patients were included in the assay. Eighty-nine of 140 healthy controls were also included to evaluate the cutoff value. To efficiently coat microwells with the peptide, BSA-conjugated P25, synthesized by the Chinese Peptide Company (Hangzhou, Zhejiang, China) via the solid-phase method, was used as an antigen. The purity of the conjugate was greater than 95%. Plates were coated overnight with BSA-P25 at a concentration of 5 μg/mL. After blocking unbound sites, the serum samples were diluted 1:100 and incubated with the plates at RT for 1 h. Wells coated with BSA were prepared for each sample to determine non-specific binding. After washing, HRP-conjugated goat anti-human IgG was added and incubated at RT for 1 h. The plate was read at an OD of 450 nm, with 620 nm as the correction wavelength, using an ELISA plate reader.

Each sample was tested in duplicate. A positive serum sample was included in each assay and used to correct for inter-assay variations. Data was processed as described in the anti-BRAF ELISA procedure.

Statistical analyses

Statistical analyses were performed using SPSS 13.0 for Windows. For normally distributed data, results are expressed as the mean and standard deviation (mean (SD)); differences between groups were assessed by t-tests. For data not distributed normally, results are expressed as the median (range); differences between groups were analyzed using the Mann-Whitney U-test and correlations were determined by computing Spearman rank correlation coefficients. Pearson's 2-tailed χ^2 test or Fisher's exact

test were used to compare proportions. P values<0.05 were considered statistically significant.

Results

Expression and purification of recombinant protein

The recombinant catalytic domain of wild-type BRAF was expressed from pET28b-BRAF-transformed bacteria under IPTG induction. The expressed protein was within insoluble inclusion bodies. To obtain pure antigens, a protocol for inclusion-body extraction followed by affinity chromatography was implemented. Following extraction, recombinant proteins were predominantly identified in collected precipitates, but remained contaminated with a small quantity of host proteins. For further purification, precipitates were solubilized in 6 M guanidine-HCl and purified using nickel affinity chromatography under denaturing conditions. The His-tagged recombinant proteins were eluted with a gradient of increasing imidazole concentration and were detected as a single protein band at a molecular weight of approximately 40 kD on a 10% SDS-PAGE gel (Figure 1). The protein concentration was 1.5 mg/mL as determined by BCA.

Prevalence of antibody responses to BRAF in diseases and controls

The distribution of BRAF-specific antibodies in RA, pSS, SLE and healthy control patients is shown in Figure 2. The cutoff value for positivity was set as 2 SD above the mean AU of the healthy controls. The prevalence of anti-BRAF and anti-P25 is listed in Table 2. There was no significant difference in anti-BRAF or anti-P25 prevalence among RA, pSS, and SLE patients. However, the prevalence of BRAF specific antibodies was significantly higher in disease samples (RA, pSS, and SLE) than in the healthy controls (p = 0.001 for all). 8 serum samples of RA patients were identified

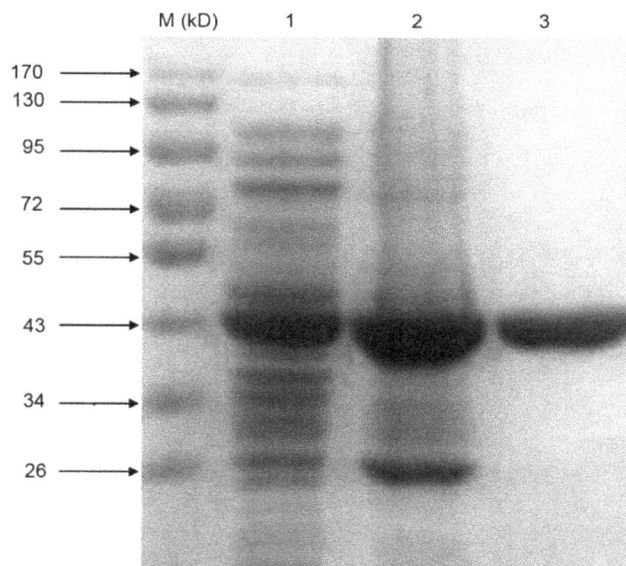

Figure 1. Analysis of the recombinant catalytic domain of BRAF by SDS-PAGE. Samples were separated by electrophoresis on polyacrylamide gels and stained with Coomassie blue. M: molecular mass marker proteins. Lane 1: BL21-(DE3) cells carrying pET28b-BRAF plasmid induced by 0.1 mM IPTG for 4 h at 37°C. Lane 2: inclusion bodies after extraction. Lane 3: 6× His-tagged proteins eluted with imidazole. The weight of the molecular mass markers is indicated on the left side of the figure.

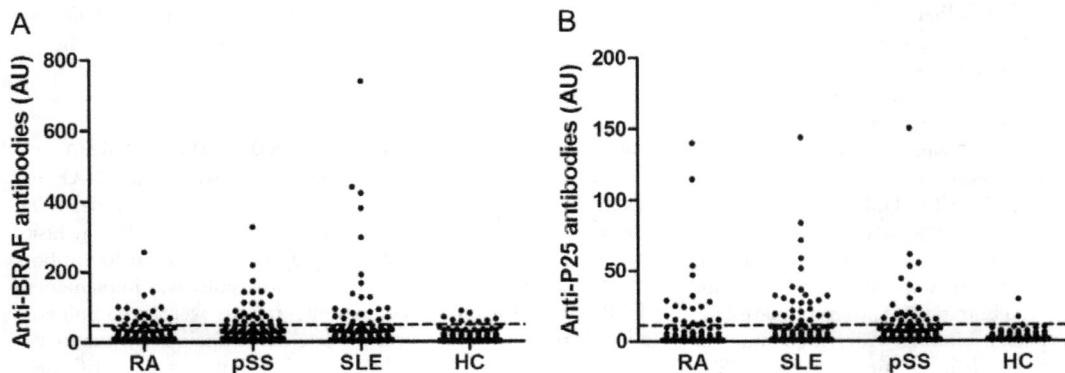

Figure 2. Distribution of BRAF-specific antibodies in diseases and controls. BRAF-specific antibodies were detected in patients with rheumatoid arthritis (RA, n = 101), primary Sjögren's syndrome (pSS, n = 132), systemic lupus erythematosus (SLE, n = 118), and healthy controls (HC, n = 140 for anti-BRAF and n = 89 for anti-P25) using indirect ELISAs based on the recombinant catalytic domain of BRAF (**A**) or a synthesized peptide (**B**). Antibody titers were expressed as arbitrary units (AU). The cutoff value for positivity was set as 2 SD above the mean AU of the healthy controls (dashed line).

as anti-P25 positive and anti-BRAF negative, whereas another 10 RA samples were identified as anti-P25 negative and anti-BRAF positive. A similar tendency was also observed among pSS and SLE patients.

Associations between BRAF-specific antibodies and disease indicators in RA patients

Of the 101 RA patients, 21 (20.8%) and 19 (18.8%) were identified as positive for anti-BRAF and anti-P25, respectively. Patients with BRAF-specific antibodies had significantly higher ESRs than patients without these antibodies (p = 0.040 for anti-BRAF and p = 0.030 for anti-P25). Patients with prolonged disease had a significantly higher prevalence of anti-BRAF (18/62) than patients with recent-onset disease (2/35) (p = 0.006). Furthermore, active disease occurred more frequently in anti-P25-positive patients than in anti-P25-negative patients (p = 0.034). Comparisons of disease indicators between patients with and without BRAF-specific antibodies are shown in Table 3. A weak but significant correlation was found between anti-P25 antibodies and ESRs in the RA patients (r = 0.319, p = 0.004) (Figure 3).

Discussion

Autoantibodies to BRAF, in particular anti-P25 antibodies, have been recently identified as specific markers for RA. However, this suggestion is based on the evidence that anti-P25 is specifically detected in RA patients comparing with AS and PsA. In this report, we developed indirect ELISAs on the basis of the

recombinant catalytic domain of BRAF or the synthesized peptide P25 and determined the prevalence of autoantibodies to BRAF in patients with RA, pSS, or SLE and in healthy controls. Associations between anti-BRAF or anti-P25 and disease variables were investigated in the RA cohort. Our results indicate that neither anti-BRAF nor anti-P25 autoantibodies are specific markers for RA. Nevertheless, the associations between anti-BRAF or anti-P25 and disease variables suggest potential involvement of these antibodies in inflammation in RA patients.

Protein arrays have been used to identify the catalytic domain of BRAF as a new autoantigen involved in RA [2]. Recently, Charpin et al. [10] further identified the peptide targets of anti-BRAF by using 40 overlapping 20-mers encompassing the entire catalytic domain of BRAF. It was shown that 1 peptide, P25 (amino acids 656–675), is specifically recognized by anti-BRAF from serum of RA patients [10]. In the present study, we detected the presence of anti-BRAF and anti-P25 in the serum of RA patients by developing indirect ELISAs on the basis of the recombinant catalytic domain of BRAF in its denatured form and a synthesized peptide P25, respectively. Recombinant proteins dissolved in denaturant have been successfully used to coat antigens in ELISAs. This ensures the validity of our assays for anti-BRAF [13–14]. We unexpectedly observed a considerable prevalence of anti-BRAF and anti-P25 in pSS patients and SLE patients. In the previous 2 studies investigating anti-BRAF in RA patients, the disease controls were AS patients and/or PsA patients, and cohorts used were relatively small [2,10]. Thus, the involvement of autoantibodies to BRAF in other autoimmune

Table 2. Prevalence of BRAF specific antibodies in the test samples.

Disease	anti-BRAF positive (%)	anti-P25 positive (%)	anti-BRAF positive & anti-p25 negative	anti-BRAF negative & anti-p25 positive
RA	21/101 (20.8)	19/101 (18.8)	10	8
SLE	24/118 (20.3)	25/118 (21.2)	9	10
pSS	27/135 (20.5)	24/132 (18.2)	12	9
HC	9/140 (6.4)	2/89 (2.2)	3	0

Since the anti-p25 was not test in all the patients and health controls, the results we list in the last two columns were from the participants that both anti-BRAF and anti-p25 were tested.

Table 3. Comparisons of disease indicators between patients with and without BRAF-specific antibodies.

	Anti-BRAF catalytic domain		p	Anti-P25		p
	Positive	Negative		Positive	Negative	
Female (%)	85.7	78.8	0.685	81.3	86.3	0.604
Age (years)	51.5±12.7	46.2±14.0	0.116	49.6±11.6	46.7±14.3	0.429
Duration (years)	7.5 (0.3–30)	4.8 (0.1–50)	0.073	5.0 (0.2–14)	5.0 (0.1–50)	0.874
Recent onset (%)	10.0	42.9	0.006	22.2	39.2	0.175
RF-positive (%)	80.0	87.0	0.661	94.4	83.5	0.456
Anti-CCP (U/mL)	46 (17–2572)	367 (16–5477)	0.490	357 (17–3799)	338 (16–5477)	0.281
Positive (%)	66.7	75.0	0.443	84.2	70.7	0.232
ESR (mm/h)	69.3±31.6	52.0±32.2	0.040	71.8±26.3	53.0±33.2	0.030
Elevated (%)	90.0	80.3	0.499	92.9	80.6	0.444
CRP elevated	33.3	42.0	0.747	44.4	39.6	1.000
Active disease (%)	42.9	47.5	0.704	68.4	41.5	0.034

RF: rheumatoid factor; anti-CCP: anti-cyclic citrullinated peptide antibodies; ESR: erythrocyte sedimentation rate; CRP: C-reactive protein.
Categorical variables are given as %; normally distributed data are given in mean ± SD; other continuous variables are given in median (range). Recent onset disease is defined as disease duration of less than 2 years.

diseases is still unclear. Here, we detected the presence of BRAF-specific antibodies in larger cohorts of patients with pSS and SLE. The prevalence of anti-BRAF (catalytic domain) or anti-P25 in these 3 diseases (RA, pSS, and SLE) is similar, This suggests that, to some extent, the production of autoantibodies to BRAF might be a common event in systemic autoimmune disorders. There is evidence that different subsets of autoantibodies have different cytokine requirements [15]. Thus, the indistinguishable prevalence of BRAF-specific antibodies among RA, pSS, and SLE patients raises the possibility that the cytokine environment in these diseases is beneficial for anti-BRAF or anti-P25 production. The repertoire of epitopes that elicit antibody responses to the catalytic domain of BRAF might include both linear and conformational forms. For the protein microarray, the catalytic domain of BRAF was adhered to the glass slide under native conditions. In contrast, in the peptide microarray, overlapping linear peptides of the catalytic domain were used as antigens [2,10]. In our study, it is possible that both linear and conformed epitopes of the catalytic

domain of BRAF were involved, as the process by which recombinant BRAF was diluted with coating buffer in denaturant may have caused refolding. Thus, some epitopes probably become inaccessible because of partial refolding or aggregation. This would lead to lower detection sensitivity for a specific peptide. This might account for some samples that were identified as anti-P25 positive but anti-BRAF negative. Furthermore, the difference in the final molar concentration of P25 adsorbed on the microwells between the 2 ELISAs is worthy of consideration.

Multiple signal transduction pathways have been carefully investigated in RA. For instance, NF-κB and MAPK pathways are attractive for intervention in light of their ability to regulate many genes involved in immune responses [16–17]. The enormous diversity of kinases that modulate transduction mechanisms suggests that complex and interrelated events are involved in inflammatory disease. The end results of these pathways may exert influences on the production of proteins such as cytokines and matrix metalloproteinases that are implicated in the pathogenesis of RA [18–20]. BRAF encodes a serine-threonine kinase downstream of RAS in the MAPK pathway and transduces regulatory signals from RAS through MAPK. Autoantibodies to the BRAF protein have been reported in melanoma patients and patients with RA [2,10,21]. Most recently, Charpin, et al. demonstrated that anti-BRAF may activate phosphorylation of MEK1 by using BRAF *in vitro*. This indicates possible involvement of BRAF autoantibodies in the inflammatory responses of RA [10]. Here, we observe a significant difference in ESRs between RA patients with BRAF-specific antibodies and those without these antibodies (p = 0.040 for anti-BRAF and p = 0.030 for anti-P25). Furthermore, a weak but significant correlation was identified between ESRs and anti-P25 antibody levels (r = 0.319, p = 0.004). Patients with BRAF-specific antibodies are likely to have increased ESRs compared to those without these antibodies. Although the ESR is a non-specific marker of inflammation, ESR values are indeed positively correlated with severe inflammation. On the other hand, patients with prolonged disease in our study cohort had significantly higher levels of anti-BRAF antibodies (18/62) than patients with recent onset disease (2/35) (p = 0.006). With respect to disease status, anti-P25-positive patients had a significantly higher risk of incurring active disease than anti-P25-

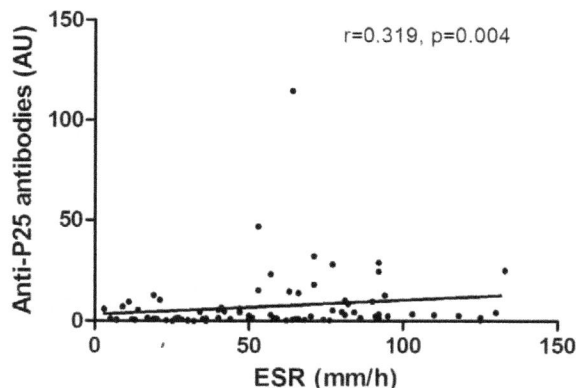

Figure 3. Correlation of anti-P25 antibodies with ESRs in RA patients. The correlation of anti-P25 antibodies and ESRs in 81 RA patients was assessed by Spearman rank correlation coefficients. The coefficient (r = 0.319, p = 0.004) suggests a weak but significant association between anti-P25 antibodies and ESR values.

negative patients (p = 0.034). However, there was no significant difference in the anti-BRAF status among patients with active disease (p = 0.704). This indicates that anti-P25 is more closely correlated with RA than anti-BRAF. The ability of anti-BRAF to activate BRAF, thus activating the MAPK pathway, may be an appropriate explanation for the associations between anti-BRAF and variables of inflammation or disease activity in RA. Charpin, et al. proposed a model to explain how extracellular autoantibodies to BRAF may activate intracellular BRAF [10]. In their model, autoantibodies to BRAF enter the cells as immune complexes via cellular uptake. It is suggested that soluble IgG immune complexes might undergo degradation after uptake [22]. However, it remains unclear how immune complexes formed by BRAF and anti-BRAF antibodies resist degradation from intracellular proteinases.

A limitation of the current study is the inability to collect additional information regarding ESR and other demographic data for SLE and pSS patients who participated in this research as the disease controls, which left us unable to explore the correlation between BRAF-specific antibodies and ESRs for each patient. Further evaluation of BRAF-specific antibodies in autoimmune diseases and other inflammatory diseases would strengthen the conclusions of this study.

In summary, we have observed a similar prevalence of autoantibodies to the intact catalytic domain of wild-type BRAF and a peptide derived from this domain in patients with RA, pSS,

and SLE. The associations of anti-BRAF and anti-P25 with disease variables of RA suggest that BRAF-specific antibodies may participate in the inflammatory responses involved in RA. Our conclusion is that anti-BRAF catalytic domain antibodies and anti-P25 antibodies are not specific markers for RA, but the higher titers of BRAF-specific antibodies may be associated with increased inflammation in RA. This finding is contradictory to that of previous studies. The results presented here contribute to our understanding of the pathogenesis of RA and provide insights into the development of potential intervention targets for repressing inflammation. Extensive studies on antibody responses to BRAF in other autoimmune diseases such as pSS and SLE might contribute to a comprehensive understanding of its role in autoimmune disorders.

Acknowledgments

We thank Dr. Richard Marais of the Institute of Cancer Research, London, United Kingdom, for providing the plasmid pEF-myc-BRAF.

Author Contributions

Conceived and designed the experiments: JL WL WW. Performed the experiments: WL WW SS YS. Analyzed the data: WL WW SS YS. Contributed reagents/materials/analysis tools: YP LW RZ KZ. Wrote the paper: WL WW.

References

1. Raptopoulou A, Sidiropoulos P, Katsouraki M, Boumpas DT (2007) Anti-citrulline antibodies in the diagnosis and prognosis of rheumatoid arthritis: evolving concepts. Crit Rev Clin Lab Sci 44: 339–363.
2. Auger I, Balandraud N, Rak J, Lambert N, Martin M, et al. (2009) New autoantigens in rheumatoid arthritis (RA): screening 8268 protein arrays with sera from patients with RA. Ann Rheum Dis 68: 591–594.
3. Schaeffer HJ, Weber MJ (1999) Mitogen-activated protein kinase: specific messages from ubiquitous messengers. Mol Cell Biol 19: 2435–2444.
4. Davies H, Bignell GR, Cox C, Stephens P, Edkins S, et al. (2002) Mutations of the BRAF gene in human cancer. Nature 417: 949–954.
5. Strumberg D, Voliotis D, Moeller JG, Hilger RA, Richly H, et al. (2002) Results of phase I pharmacokinetic and pharmacodynamic studies of the Raf kinase inhibitor BAY 43-9006 in patients with solid tumors. Int J Clin Pharmacol Ther 40: 580–581.
6. Luo SF, Fang RY, Hsieh HL, Chi PL, Lin CC, et al. (2010) Involvement of MAPKs and NF-kappaB in tumor necrosis factor alpha-induced vascular cell adhesion molecule 1 expression in human rheumatoid arthritis synovial fibroblasts. Arthritis Rheum 62: 105–116.
7. Schett G, Zwerina J, Firestein G (2008) The p38 mitogen-activated protein kinase (MAPK) pathway in rheumatoid arthritis. Ann Rheum Dis 67: 909–916.
8. Thalhamer T, McGrath MA, Harnett MM (2008) MAPKs and their relevance to arthritis and inflammation. Rheumatology (Oxford) 47: 409–414.
9. Sweeney SE, Firestein GS (2004) Signal transduction in rheumatoid arthritis. Curr Opin Rheumatol 16: 231–237.
10. Charpin C, Martin M, Balandraud N, Roudier J, Auger I (2010) Autoantibodies to BRAF, a new family of autoantibodies associated with rheumatoid arthritis. Arthritis Res Ther 12: R194.
11. Arnett FC, Edworthy SM, Bloch DA, McShane DJ, Fries JF, et al. (1988) The American Rheumatism Association 1987 revised criteria for the classification of rheumatoid arthritis. Arthritis Rheum 31: 315–324.
12. Wang W, Li J (2011) Predominance of IgG1 and IgG3 subclasses of autoantibodies to peptidylarginine deiminase 4 in rheumatoid arthritis. Clin Rheumatol 30: 563–567.
13. Yang JC, Blanton RE, King CL, Fujioka H, Aikawa M, et al. (1996) Seroprevalence and specificity of human responses to the *Plasmodium falciparum* rhoptry protein Rhop-3 determined by using a C-terminal recombinant protein. Infect Immun 64: 3584–3591.
14. Di Bonito P, Grasso F, Mochi S, Accardi L, Donà MG, et al. (2006) Serum antibody response to Human papillomavirus (HPV) infections detected by a novel ELISA technique based on denatured recombinant HPV16 L1, L2, E4, E6 and E7 proteins. Infect Agent Cancer 1: 6–14.
15. Richards HB, Satoh M, Shaw M, Libert C, Poli V, et al. (1998) Interleukin 6 dependence of anti-DNA antibody production: evidence for two pathways of autoantibody formation in pristane-induced lupus. J Exp Med 188: 985–990.
16. Chang L, Karin M (2001) Mammalian MAP kinase signalling cascades. Nature 410: 37–40.
17. Tak PP, Firestein GS (2001) NF-kappaB: a key role in inflammatory diseases. J Clin Invest 107: 7–11.
18. Miyazawa K, Mori A, Miyata H, Akahane M, Ajisawa Y, et al. (1998) Regulation of interleukin-1β-induced interleukin-6 gene expression in human fibroblast-like synoviocytes by p38 mitogen-activated protein kinase. J Biol Chem 273: 24832–24838.
19. Lacki JK, Samborski W, Mackiewicz SH (1997) Interleukin-10 and interleukin-6 in lupus erythematosus and rheumatoid arthritis, correlations with acute phase proteins. Clin Rheumatol 16: 275–278.
20. Westermarck J, Li SP, Kallunki T, Han J, Kähäri VM (2001) p38 mitogen-activated protein kinase-dependent activation of protein phosphatases 1 and 2A inhibits MEK1 and MEK2 activity and collagenase 1 (MMP-1) gene expression. Mol Cell Biol 21: 2373–2383.
21. Fensterle J, Becker JC, Potapenko T, Heimbach V, Vetter CS, et al. (2004) B-Raf specific antibody responses in melanoma patients. BMC Cancer 4: 62–70.
22. Johansson AG, Løvdal T, Magnusson KE, Berg T, Skogh T (1996) Liver cell uptake and degradation of soluble immunoglobulin G immune complexes in vivo and in vitro in rats. Hepatology 24: 169–175.

10

Renal Dnase1 Enzyme Activity and Protein Expression is Selectively Shut Down in Murine and Human Membranoproliferative Lupus Nephritis

Svetlana N. Zykova[1][9]**, Anders A. Tveita**[1][9]**, Ole Petter Rekvig**[1,2]*

1 Department of Biochemistry, Institute of Medical Biology, Medical Faculty, University of Tromsø, Tromsø, Norway, **2** Department of Rheumatology, University Hospital of Northern Norway, Tromsø, Norway

Abstract

Background: Deposition of chromatin-IgG complexes within glomerular membranes is a key event in the pathogenesis of lupus nephritis. We recently reported an acquired loss of renal *Dnase1* expression linked to transformation from mild to severe membranoproliferative lupus nephritis in (NZBxNZW)F1 mice. As this may represent a basic mechanism in the progression of lupus nephritis, several aspects of Dnase1 expression in lupus nephritis were analyzed.

Methodology/Principal Findings: Total nuclease activity and Dnase1 expression and activity was evaluated using *in situ* and *in vitro* analyses of kidneys and sera from (NZBxNZW)F1 mice of different ages, and from age-matched healthy controls. Immunofluorescence staining for Dnase1 was performed on kidney biopsies from (NZBxNZW)F1 mice as well as from human SLE patients and controls. Reduced serum Dnase1 activity was observed in both mesangial and end-stage lupus nephritis. A selective reduction in renal Dnase1 activity was seen in mice with massive deposition of chromatin-containing immune complexes in glomerular capillary walls. Mice with mild mesangial nephritis showed normal renal Dnase1 activity. Similar differences were seen when comparing human kidneys with severe and mild lupus nephritis. Dnase1 was diffusely expressed within the kidney in normal and mildly affected kidneys, whereas upon progression towards end-stage renal disease, Dnase1 was down-regulated in all renal compartments. This demonstrates that the changes associated with development of severe nephritis in the murine model are also relevant to human lupus nephritis.

Conclusions/Significance: Reduction in renal Dnase1 expression and activity is limited to mice and SLE patients with signs of membranoproliferative nephritis, and may be a critical event in the development of severe forms of lupus nephritis. Reduced Dnase1 activity reflects loss in the expression of the protein and not inhibition of enzyme activity.

Editor: Pierre Bobé, Institut Jacques Monod, France

Funding: This study was supported by grants from The Health and Rehabilitation organisation Norway, The Northern Norway Regional Health Authority Medical Research Program (Grants SFP-100-04, SFP-101-04), and from University of Tromsoe as a Milieu support given to OPR. The funders had no role in study design, data collection and analysis, decision to publish, or preparation of the manuscript.

Competing Interests: The authors have declared that no competing interests exist.

* E-mail: Ole.Petter.Rekvig@uit.no

[9] These authors contributed equally to this work.

Introduction

Systemic lupus erythematosus (SLE) is a systemic autoimmune disease characterized by the development of autoreactivity against nuclear antigens, including double-stranded DNA (dsDNA) and histones [1,2,3]. The predominance of chromatin-associated antigen targets points at aberrancies in the processing and elimination of chromatin as a potential culprit of such a process [4,5,6,7,8]. It has been postulated that effective degradation of DNA from dying cells is essential to prevent priming of the immune system against chromatin self-antigens, and impaired chromatin degradation has been proposed as a mechanism for the development of antinuclear autoimmunity [9,10].

DNA fragmentation by the activation of various nucleases is considered a key event in apoptotic cell death (reviewed in [11,12]). For elimination of DNA from necrotic cells, secreted nucleases, including Dnase1 are assumed to play a central role in this process (reviewed in [11,13]). Under circumstances of increased cellular stress, such as active infections, malignancies and tissue trauma, increased amounts of DNA can be observed within the circulation, suggesting that the capacity for DNA elimination is exceeded [14,15,16]. Increased levels of circulating DNA and nucleosomes have been reported in SLE [17,18,19], especially in active stages of the disease [20] and in lupus-prone mice [21].

Dnase1 is considered the major serum nuclease, and has been a topic of interest in the context of SLE for several decades. Dnase1 is the founding member of the Dnase1-like (Dnase1l) family of divalent cation-dependent endonucleases, which also include Dnase1l1-3. Reduced serum Dnase1 activity is a common finding in SLE patients [22,23,24] and lupus-prone mice [25]. The basis for increased concentration of DNA in the circulation remains controversial [13], but possible explanations include ineffective elimination of chromatin due to impaired nuclease activity, either by decreased nuclease availability [23] or inhibition by factors such as actin [22,26,27]. Attempts at Dnase1 enzyme replacement therapy in mice and SLE patients have been largely disappointing [28,29], as has experimental over-expression of Dnase1 in T-cells in lupus-prone mice [30]. In contrast, experimental deletion of *Dnase1* in mice resulted in development of lupus-like disease, including anti-chromatin autoantibody production and immune-complex mediated glomerulonephritis [31]. Later studies revealed that these effects were largely eliminated upon backcrossing into one of the parental strains, suggesting that other predisposing genetic aberrancies are required for the development of auto-reactivity in this model. The data, however, suggest that eliminating Dnase1 contributes to the acceleration of renal disease in lupus-prone mice [13].

Taken together, these data suggest that Dnase1 deficiency alone is not sufficient to induce autoimmunity against chromatin, but may play a key role in progression of lupus nephritis. Whereas the activity of Dnase1 in serum has been extensively studied [22,23,25,33], little is known about its expression and activity within different organs. In a recent study, we demonstrated that the appearance of anti-dsDNA antibodies in (NZBxNZW)F1 (B/W) mice coincided with early signs of development of mesangial nephritis, while reduced renal Dnase1 mRNA expression correlated with progression of lupus nephritis into end-stage organ disease [32]. This recent data is indicative of loss of DNase1 serving as a possible factor in the progression of lupus nephritis.

The present study was designed to further characterize these changes in terms of *i.* localization of renal Dnases in different compartments of the kidneys, *ii.* their relative contribution to total renal nuclease activity and *iii.* the relation between renal and serum Dnase1 activity with initiation and progression of lupus nephritis. Furthermore, to evaluate whether changes in Dnase1 expression could also be involved in the progression of the human variant of lupus nephritis, renal Dnase1 expression was also assayed in biopsies from SLE patients and correlated with morphological and immune electron microscopy findings.

Results

Characteristics of the experimental animals

High anti-dsDNA antibody titer was present in all the animals with nephritis irrespective of age (26–38 w.o.) and was elevated for an average of 2 months prior to the development of overt proteinuria [34]. Young B/W mice and BALB/c control mice of all age groups had no clinical or laboratory signs of kidney disease. Pre-proteinuric animals on average had only marginally elevated anti-dsDNA antibody titers. The predominant pattern of glomerular immune complex (IC) deposits was characterized by immune electron microscopy (representative images are presented in Figure S1). Based on these results, the proteinuric mice were divided into two groups, one with mesangial IC deposits (Figure S1A–B), and one with IC deposits in the glomerular capillary walls (Figure S1C–D). The pre-nephritic mice had no glomerular deposits (Figure S1E–F). Data presented below demonstrate the relevance of these groups in identifying pathogenic factors in lupus nephritis.

Gene expression data for major apoptotic nucleases in the kidneys from mice of different ages is presented in Table 1. The results are expressed as fold change relative to 4 weeks old BALB/c control mice and show that of all the renal nucleases studied, only the mRNA level of *Dnase1* was significantly reduced in the group of mice with membranoproliferative nephritis. Lack of down-regulation of other genes, including house-keeping genes or genes encoding other renal nucleases, makes it unlikely that reduced Dnase1 expression was due to renal insufficiency or loss of viable renal cells (see below).

Table 1. Gene expression of apoptotic nucleases in kidneys from (NZBxNZW)F1 and BALB/c mice from different age groups.

Taqman assay	Mouse	Age			
		4 w.o.	8 w.o.	20 w.o.	>26 w.o.
dnase1 Mm01342389_g1	B/W	1.15±0.09[a]	1.82±0.18	1.69±0.42	**0.45±0.59[f]**
	BALB/c	1.07±0.42	1.59±0.27	1.30±0.49	1.49±0.30
dnase2 Mm00438463_m1	B/W	0.82±0.10	0.81±0.18	1.38±0.11	1.43±0.19
	BALB/c	1.01±0.18	1.19±0.23	1.00±0.05	1.16±0.22
endoG[b] Mm00468248_m1	B/W	0.88±0.15	0.78±0.19	1.00±0.11	0.76±0.23
	BALB/c	1.00±0.06	1.18±0.20	1.04±0.17	0.98±0.03
Dffa[c] Mm00438410_m1	B/W	1.09±0.14	0.81±0.12	0.94±0.08	1.24±0.14
	BALB/c	1.00±0.09	1.14±0.24	0.98±0.16	0.86±0.08
Dffb[d] Mm00432822_m1	B/W	0.84±0.10	0.74±0.13	0.89±0.09	0.87±0.13
	BALB/c	1.00±0.09	0.78±0.16	0.81±0.03	0.68±0.20
Cideb[e] Mm00438213_m1[g]	B/W	1.22±0.23	1.04±0.15	1.48±0.33	1.09±0.52
	BALB/c	1.01±0.11	1.28±0.22	1.00±0.17	1.16±0.15

[a]The data are presented as fold change relative to an average level of the 4 w.o. BALB/c mice (mean ± SEM, n = 5), after normalization for the expression level of a house-keeping gene in the same sample (Mouse ACTB (actin, beta) Endogenous Control (4352933E) and TATA-box binding protein (Mm00446973_m1).
[b]endonuclease G.
[c]DNA fragmentation factor, alpha subunit.
[d]DNA fragmentation factor, beta subunit.
[e]cell death-inducing DNA fragmentation factor, alpha subunit-like effector B.
[f]significantly reduced *Dnase1* gene expression only in kidneys from proteinuric B/W mice.
[g]Real time PCR was performed on ABI Prism 7900HT Sequence Detection System with the TaqMan Gene Expression Assay indicated for each gene.

Total renal and serum nuclease activity in progressive murine lupus nephritis

In order to evaluate the Ca^{2+}- and Mg^{2+}-dependent DNase activity in kidneys and sera, kidney homogenates and sera from individual B/W and BALB/c mice of different ages were analyzed by single radial enzyme diffusion (SRED) assay. This allows evaluation of net DNA degrading activity, taking into account the effects of any Dnase1 inhibitory factors present within the samples. There was a significant reduction in total nuclease activity in the proteinuric B/W kidneys compared to those of both younger B/W and age-matched BALB/c mice (Figure 1A). Importantly, the loss of nuclease activity was only observed in mice with glomerular capillary membrane deposits of chromatin fragment-IgG complexes ($p < 0.001$), while nuclease activity was normal in kidneys with deposits confined to the mesangium (Figure 1A). Corresponding assays for total serum nuclease activity revealed a less pronounced but consistent decrease in the proteinuric mice regardless of the pattern of glomerular chromatin-IgG deposits (Figure 1A, $p < 0.001$). No evidence of decreased serum nuclease activity was seen in pre-nephritic mice or in B/W mice prior to anti-dsDNA antibody production. Dnase1 differs from other members of the Dnase1-like family of nucleases by its sensitivity to inhibition by monomeric actin. Pre-incubating the gel in buffer

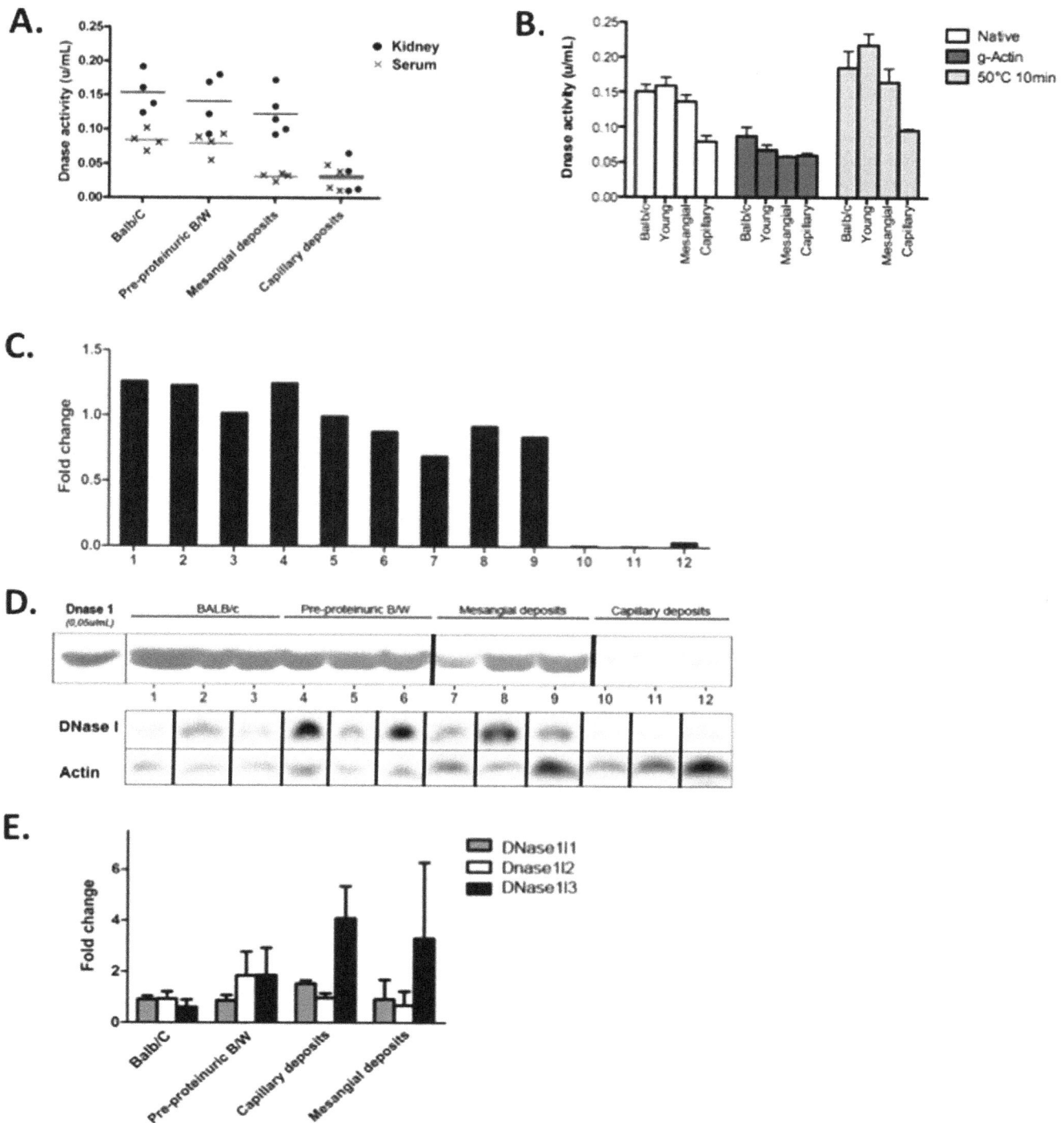

Figure 1. Total nuclease activity, Dnase1 and Dnase1l1-3 expression in kidneys from BALB/c and (NZBxNZW)F1 mice. Pre-proteinuric and proteinuric B/W kidneys were used, the latter divided into 2 groups; one characterized by immune complex deposits in glomerular mesangial matrix only (labeled "Mesangial deposits"), and the other with immune complex deposits in both the mesangial matrix and the capillary membranes (labeled "Capillary deposits"). (*A*) Kidney lysates (black) or sera (grey), in which total protein was measured, and protein content of the samples normalized using BCA assay (Pierce), were applied onto 1% agarose gels containing calf thymus DNA and ethidium bromide in a $CaCl_2$- and $MgCl_2$-containing buffer, pH 7.6, and incubated in a humidified chamber at 37°C for 24 hours. The gel was photographed under UV illumination. The radius of the non-fluorescent area surrounding each well reflected DNase activity in the sample. DNase activity is expressed as Dnase1 equivalent units, by comparison with human recombinant Dnase1. (B) Total nuclease activity in renal homogenates is shown for native samples, after addition of 5µg/mL monomeric actin and after preheating the samples to 50°C for 10 minutes prior to incubation on the gel, reflecting the results of addition and reversal of actin inhibition, respectively. The group labeled "young" represent 10 and 20 week old B/W, whereas the "Mesangial" and "Capillary" groups reflect proteinuric B/W with immune complex deposits in the mesangium and GBM, respectively. DNase activity is expressed as Dnase1 equivalent units, by comparison with human recombinant Dnase1. In panels C and D the order of samples are kidneys from normal age matched BALB/c (lanes 1–3), pre-nephritic B/W kidneys (lanes 4–6), nephritic B/W kidneys with mesangial matrix deposits only (lanes 7–9), and nephritic B/W

kidneys with capillary membrane deposits (lanes 10–12). All kidney samples were analyzed for fold change of renal *Dnase1* mRNA levels relative to 4 weeks old BALB/c mice (C), zymography of Dnase1 activity in 10% SDS-polyacrylamide gel of kidney lysates (D, upper part), and western blot of Dnase1 in the same samples (D, lower part). Western blotting to detect actin in the same samples demonstrated that the low Dnase1 band intensity in lanes 10–12 was not due to unequal loading of the samples on the gel. Renal mRNA expression of Dnase1l1 (TaqMan assay Mm00510102_m1), Dnase1l2 (Mm00481868_g1) and Dnase1l3 (Mm00432865_m1) was not decreased in kidneys from proteinuric mice (E).

containing 5mM actin caused a marked reduced serum and renal SRED activity in mice of all age groups, with similar residual Dnase activity in proteinuric and non-proteinuric mice (Figure 1B). These data suggest that the observed reduction in serum and renal Dnase activity is caused by the loss of one or more actin-inhibitable factors. Preheating the samples to 56°C for 10 minutes, previously reported to reverse Dnase1 inhibition by actin [22,35], caused a proportionally similar increase in SRED activity in both serum and renal homogenates in mice of all ages (Figure 1B), suggesting that inhibition of Dnase1 by actin does not explain the observed differences in nuclease activity in these mice. Inhibition of the actin-resistant Dnase1 homologue Dnase1l3 using the selective inhibitor DR396 showed no differences in Dnase activity by the SRED assay in any mice (data not shown). Gel zymography of sera showed enzyme activity confined to a single band corresponding in size to Dnase1, which was completely inhibited by incubating the gel in the presence of actin (data not shown). While serum nuclease activity was reduced in mesangial and membranoproliferative nephritis, renal Dnase1 activity was reduced only in membranoproliferative nephritis. These results suggest that changes in renal nuclease activity are due to changes intrinsic to the kidney, and not a passive reflection of serum DNase activity. The fact that there is a parallel loss of renal Dnase1 mRNA and the Dnase1 protein (Figure 1C), argue that the loss of Dnase1 in the kidney is a consequence of shut-down of gene expression.

Dnase1 expression and zymography

To evaluate how reduced renal *Dnase1* gene expression affects enzymatic activity in the proteinuric mice, Dnase1 activity in kidney homogenates was assayed after electrophoretic separation of proteins in DNA-containing gels. Renal Dnase1 mRNA expression levels in the individual samples were compared with zymographic renal Dnase1 activity in the same mice (Figure 1C and D for gene expression and zymography, respectively). Zymography revealed DNA-degrading activity predominantly in a band corresponding to the molecular weight of recombinant human Dnase1 (Figure 1D, lanes 1–3 for BALB/c, lanes 4–6 for pre-nephritic B/W mice, and lanes 7–12 for nephritic B/W mice). Activity in this band was completely eliminated in all samples when incubation of the gel was performed in the presence of actin (data not shown), further identifying the responsible enzyme as Dnase1. The samples obtained from nephritic B/W mice clearly separated into two distinct groups: those with mild nephritis and immune complex deposits confined to the mesangial matrix demonstrated normal levels of Dnase1 mRNA and Dnase1 enzyme activity (Figure 1C and D, lanes 7–9), whereas mice with severe nephritis and IC deposits within the capillary membrane showed dramatically reduced Dnase1 mRNA and enzyme activity (Figure 1C and D, lanes 10–12). Thus, there was a consistent correspondence between levels of *Dnase1* mRNA expression and Dnase1 activities within the same kidneys. Several weak bands of high molecular weight (100–150kDa) with DNA-degrading activity were also observed, with similar intensity in all samples from both pre-nephritic and nephritic kidneys (data not shown).

Renal mRNA expression of the Dnase1 homologues Dnase1-like 1, -2, -3 was also assayed in the various groups of mice. The

results demonstrated no evidence of significant nephritic stage reduction or compensatory up-regulation of any of these nucleases (Figure 1E, p = 0.1768 for Dnase1l1, p = 0.1497 for Dnase1l2, p = 0.0780 for Dnase1l3). A tendency for gradual elevation of Dnase1l3 expression with nephritis progression was observed, however, no formal statistical significance was reached when either parametric (ANOVA) or non-parametric (Kruskal-Wallis) tests were applied.

Detection of renal Dnase1 protein by western blotting

In order to clarify whether the low Dnase1 activity in the kidney homogenates from B/W mice with membranoproliferative nephritis was due to inhibition of enzyme activity or to an absolute reduction in renal Dnase1 protein amount, western blotting was performed on the same samples that were used for SDS-PAGE gel zymography (Figure 1D). A single band was seen, corresponding to the MW of recombinant human Dnase1 (rhDnase1, approximately 32 kDa, Figure 1D). Very low band intensities were found in the kidney samples that demonstrated considerably reduced *Dnase1* mRNA levels and Dnase1 enzyme activity (Figure 1D, lanes 10–12), whereas mice with normal mRNA expression and mesangial matrix deposits only, had Dnase1 protein expression comparable to the normal control and pre-proteinuric mice (Figure 1D, lanes 7–9). Immunoblotting to detect actin in the same samples demonstrated that the low Dnase1 band intensity in lanes 10–12 could not be explained by unequal loading of the samples on the gel. (Figure 1D). Immunoblotting against Dnase1l1 showed similar levels of expression in kidneys from B/W mice of all ages (data not shown).

In situ DNA-degradation assay

To visualize areas of renal nuclease activity in situ, non-fixed cryosections of kidneys were incubated in DNase reaction buffer to allow enzymatic cleavage of endogenous nuclear DNA by nucleases present in the tissue. The DNA nicks generated by endogenous nucleases were identified by terminal deoxynucleotidyl transferase-mediated incorporation of dUTPs labeled with a fluorescent marker. The signals generated were present in nuclei of renal cells in BALB/c (Figure 2A and B) and in pre-nephritic B/W (Figure 2C and D) mice, while significantly reduced intensity was observed in proteinuric B/W mice with capillary membrane chromatin-IgG deposits (Figure 2E and F). The reaction was completely blocked by EDTA (Figure 2B, insert labeled B'), confirming that the DNA degradation was divalent cation-dependent, and no signal was seen upon immediate fixation with paraformaldehyde (data not shown). These results corresponded well with data presented in Figure 1.

Detection of the renal Dnase1 protein *in situ* by indirect immunofluorescence in murine and human forms of lupus nephritis

Tissue localization of Dnase1 and its possible contribution to the *in situ* DNA-fragmentation ability as presented in Figure 2, was analyzed by indirect immunofluorescence. For a better overview of morphology of the sections, matched phase contrasts and immunofluorescence micrographs have been included (Figure S2). Staining of normal BALB/c kidneys with an anti-Dnase1 antibody

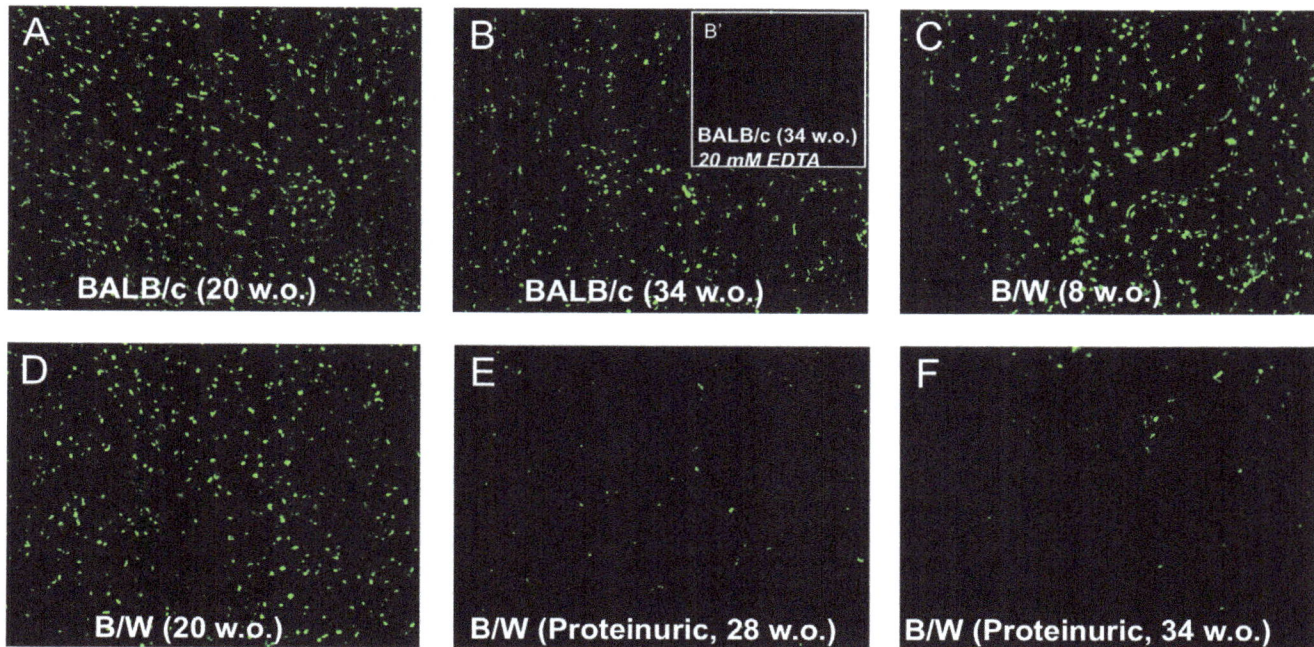

Figure 2. Low rate of nucleolysis in proteinuric (NZBxNZW)F1 kidneys. Non-fixed cryosections of kidneys were incubated in DNase reaction buffer (2mM CaCl$_2$, 2mM MgCl$_2$ in 40mM Tris, pH7.6) to allow enzymatic cleavage of endogenous DNA by nucleases present in the tissue. TUNEL-based detection of DNA fragmentation was performed after 2h incubation at 37°C. Results are given as TUNEL-stained endogenous DNA in kidney sections from 20 w.o. (A) and 32 w.o. (B) BALB/c, 8 w.o. (C), 20 w.o. (D) and proteinuric 28 w.o. (E) and proteinuric 34 w.o. (F) B/W mice. The 2 latter mice suffered from membranoproliferative nephritis with very low renal *Dnase1* mRNA levels and Dnase1 enzyme activity. Control analyses were performed by adding 20 mM EDTA to the reaction buffer. This completely abolished TUNEL staining in 34 w.o. BALB/c kidneys (see inserted panel B' in panel B) as well as in kidneys from young and proteinuric B/W mice (data not shown). Similarly, immediate fixation of the tissue sections with paraformaldehyde also resulted in absence of nicked DNA (data not shown).

(Figure 3A) revealed diffuse intracellular staining throughout the kidney, with weaker staining within glomeruli. Similar staining was observed in B/W mice with mesangial chromatin-IgG deposits (Figure 3B). Proteinuric mice with deposits in capillary membranes had significantly reduced staining of immunoreactive Dnase1 in both tubuli and glomeruli (Figure 3C, see also Figure S2 for details) compared to healthy BALB/c controls and younger pre-diseased B/W mice. Immunofluorescence staining of Dnase1ll showed low levels of staining with comparable intensity in kidneys from mice of all ages (data not shown).

To analyze if the down-regulation of *Dnase1* gene expression and corresponding Dnase1 enzyme activity observed in nephritic BW mice was also relevant in human lupus nephritis, Dnase1 immunostaining was performed on histologically normal human kidney biopsies (Figure 3D) and to biopsies from patients with mild (Patient A, Figure 3E) and membranoproliferative (Patient B, Figure 3F) lupus nephritis. The data revealed a dramatic decrease in Dnase1 immunostaining only in renal sections from the patient with severe nephritis. For a better overview of morphology of the sections, matched phase contrast and immunofluorescence micrographs have been included for biopsies from patients A and B, respectively (Figure S3A–B). This figure demonstrates that the Dnase1 protein is lost both in tubular and glomerular cells in the latter kidney biopsy (Figure S3B). *Crithidia luciliae* immunofluorescence titer (CLIFT) and serum creatinine levels for Patients A and B are shown in Figure 3G. Immune electron microscopy, where in situ bound IgG was detected by rabbit anti-human IgG antibody followed by binding of gold-labeled protein A [36], showed chromatin-IgG deposits predominantly in the mesangial matrix of Patient A (Figures 3H–I), while in the biopsy from Patient B, the

deposits were widely distributed in both glomerular basement membranes (GBM) and the mesangial matrix (Figure 3J). These data parallel the association between reduced renal Dnase1 expression and the occurrence of membranoproliferative lupus nephritis seen in B/W mice. Results from Dnase1 staining of additional biopsies from patients with lupus nephritis revealed a similar relationship between Dnase1 staining intensity and the glomerular loci for chromatin-IgG complex deposits (Figure S4). Moreover, Dnase1 staining in a biopsy of a Wegener's granu-lomatosis patient with severe pauci-immune glomerulonephritis was comparable to that of normal kidneys (Figure S4D), suggesting that the observed reduction in Dnase1 staining is specific for lupus nephritis, and not a general element of particular patterns of nephritis.

Discussion

Dnase1 has been implicated in SLE pathogenesis through a number of studies in both mice and humans [23,25,37]. The kidney is one of the major loci for Dnase1 production and activity. Other organs with Dnase1 expression include salivary glands, liver and gastrointestinal tract cells [38]. In humans but not rodents, the pancreas appears to be an important source of Dnase1 [39]. The relative contribution of each of these organs to the circulating pool of Dnase1 in blood and urine remains uncertain. Dnase1 is the principal renal nuclease, reported to account for more than 80% of the total endonuclease activity within the kidney [40]. Interestingly, decreased levels of urine nuclease activity has been found in lupus-prone B/W mice, preceding the development of renal disease manifestation [25]. Since it has been shown that

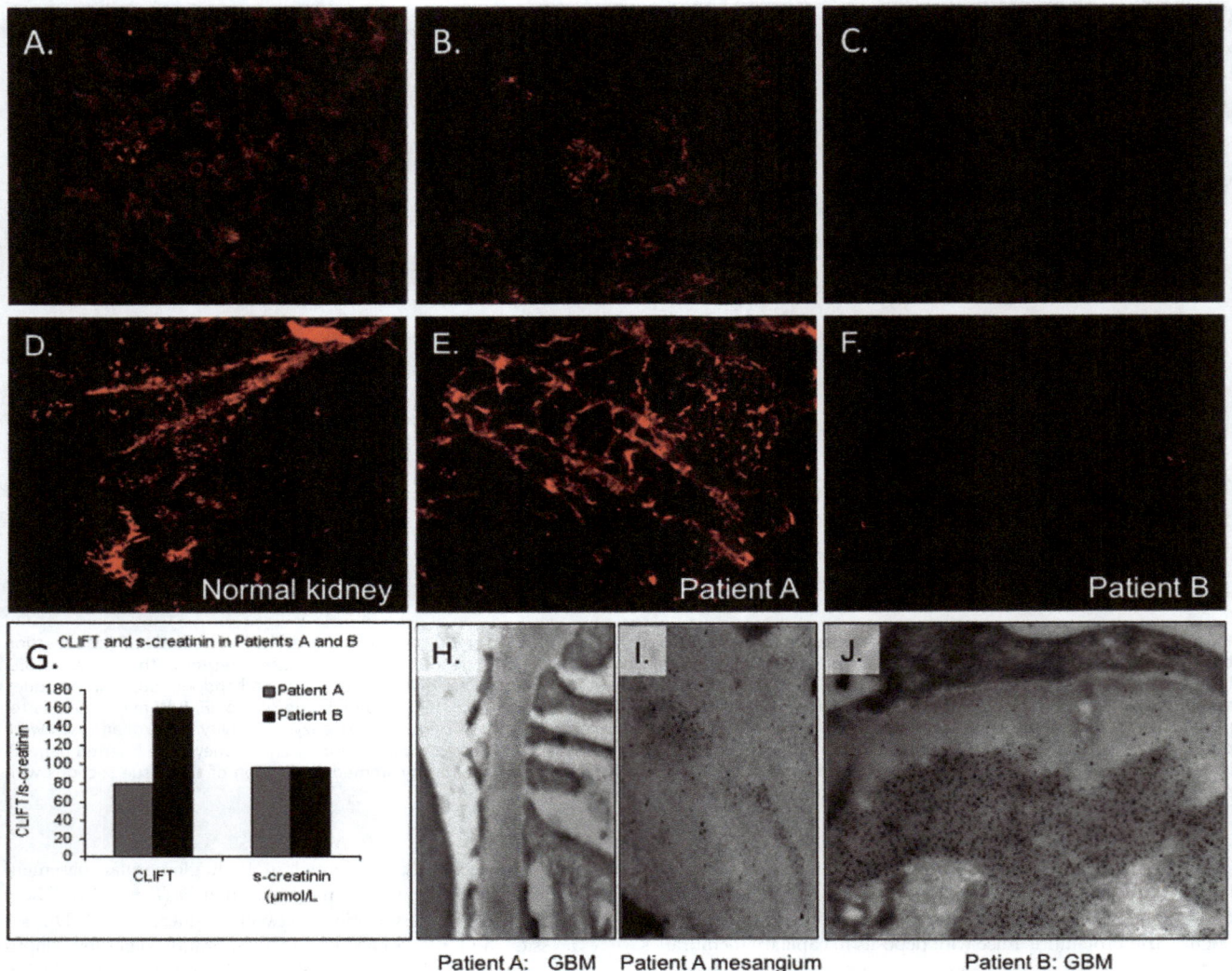

Figure 3. Expression of immunoreactive Dnase1 in kidneys from (NZBxNZW)F1 mice and from patients with lupus nephritis.
Cryosections of B/W and human kidneys were immunostained with rabbit anti-Dnase1 antibody followed by an Alexa488-conjugated F(ab')$_2$ anti-rabbit IgG antibody. The images were taken using identical exposure settings. The images were obtained at 400× magnification on kidney sections from a 32 w.o. BALB/c mouse (A), a 20 w.o. B/W mouse with mesangial nephritis (B) and a 32 w.o. nephritic B/W mouse with membranoproliferative nephritis and low renal Dnase1 activity (C). In the kidneys of the latter mouse, only traces of the Dnase1 enzyme could be detected. Similarly, there was robust Dnase1 staining in a kidney biopsy from a histologically normal kidney (D), a patient with mesangial nephritis (Patient A, panels E, H and I), whereas only traces of Dnase1 staining was detectable in kidneys from a patient with membranoproliferative lupus nephritis (Patient B, panels F and J). Crithidia luciliae immunofluorescence titers (CLIFT) and serum creatinine levels of the two patients are shown (panel G). Immune electron microscopy using protein-A-gold conjugated rabbit anti-human IgG antibodies revealed predominantly mesangial electron-dense structures (EDS) in patient A with mild nephritis (panels H-I), whereas glomerular as well as mesangial EDS were present patient B with severe nephritis (panel J).

urinary nuclease activity correlates with its activity in kidneys [41], renal shut-down of the enzyme could be relevant to explain development of lupus nephritis, including deposition of large chromatin fragments (reviewed in [3,42]).

Using both morphological and zymographic methods, the current work extends previous data demonstrating an acquired, selective down-regulation of renal *Dnase1* gene expression linked to progression towards end-stage lupus nephritis. The existence of several Dnase1-like enzymes with similar biochemical properties makes it important to assay Dnase activity by several methods to verify the identity of the responsible nucleases. Inhibition by actin is only seen for Dnase1 [43] and possibly Dnase1l1 [44]. Quantitative mRNA and immunofluorescence assays demonstrated no

evidence of decreased levels of Dnase1l1 in the kidneys of proteinuric mice. We demonstrate here *i.* that the level of renal Dnase1 mRNA expression is reflected by enzyme activity and Dnase1 protein expression, *ii.* the relative contribution of renal Dnase1 to total renal nuclease activity, *iii.* the renal location of Dnase1 protein expression and loss of Dnase1 protein expression during progression of lupus nephritis, and finally *iv.* the relevance of decreased renal Dnase1 for progression of human lupus nephritis. The discrepancy between serum and renal nuclease activity within the proteinuric group, as well as the consistency of assays of mRNA, protein and enzymatic activity levels, strongly favors reduced renal Dnase1 synthesis as the major contributor to reduced renal Dnase1 activity.

A characteristic feature of lupus nephritis is the appearance of glomerular IC deposits observed as electron dense structures (EDS) by transmission electron microscopy [45,46,47,48]. In a recent report, we correlated patterns of immune complex deposits with renal mRNA expression of *Dnase1* [32]. Whereas mesangial EDS were detectable in all mice that produced anti-dsDNA antibodies, a clear correlation was seen between reduced renal Dnase1 expression and the formation of capillary sub-endothelial and sub-epithelial deposits, and the development of membrano-proliferative nephritis. Our current data confirms that these associations are indeed reflected in a kidney-specific decrease in renal Dnase1 activity. This change may represent an important factor in the progression of mesangial lupus nephritis into end-stage renal disease.

The results of the present immunofluorescence studies on renal biopsies from SLE patients suggest that changes in Dnase1 expression similar to those seen in the B/W mice are relevant to explain disease progression also in humans. Previous data have demonstrated a constitutive defect causing reduced oligonucleosomal DNA fragmentation in kidneys of B/W mice of all ages upon induction of apoptosis in kidneys of B/W mice using the topoisomerase I inhibitor camptothecin [34]. These results therefore led us to investigate whether such a defect could be explained by constitutively reduced expression of one or more of the nucleases responsible for apoptotic DNA fragmentation. In the present report we did not find evidence of decreased total nuclease activity in young B/W mice. This would suggest that the basis of such a camptothecin-related defect lies upstream in the apoptotic signaling cascade. Although not related to the reported reduction in apoptotic DNA fragmentation, there is a striking association between the fall in renal Dnase1 enzyme activity and the accumulation of chromatin fragment-containing IC within the GBM. Because Dnase1 is the major endonuclease within the kidney ([40], present results), an uncompensated reduction in renal Dnase1 activity could contribute to a reduced clearance and secondary exposure of chromatin debris within the kidney. Exposed secondary necrotic chromatin triggers pro-inflammatory signaling in phagocytes, and constitutes an important danger signal [49]. Failure of phagocytic clearance of apoptotic and/or necrotic cells has been postulated as a possible driving force for sustained anti-chromatin autoimmunity [42,46,50,51]. If apoptotic chromatin is exposed, e.g. as a result of diminished renal Dnase1 activity, this could trigger renal inflammation and leukocyte infiltration, and at the same time provide a target for circulating anti-chromatin antibodies. In the face of pre-existing, florid autoreactivity, such changes could conceivably launch a rapidly progressive organ-centered immune attack, causing proteinuria and renal failure.

The fact that down-regulation of Dnase1 in the kidneys appears after initiation of anti-dsDNA antibody production indicates that loss of renal nuclease activity is not responsible for the appearance of anti-chromatin autoimmunity. Moreover, Wilber et al. have identified a mutation in the Dnase1l3 gene in the B/W mice that reduced the ability of this enzyme to fragment DNA [52]. This nuclease has been proposed to play a role during apoptotic chromatin degradation [53,54]. Whether this defect has any impact on development of anti-chromatin antibodies and lupus nephritis has not been determined. Considering such data, and the data presented in this study, several defects in the apoptotic processing and elimination of DNA may together contribute to initiation and progression of e.g. lupus nephritis in these animals. However, inhibition of Dnase1l3 using a specific inhibitor did not significantly alter serum or renal Dnase activity in B/W or BALB/c mice of any ages, suggesting a modest contribution of this endonuclease to total nuclease activity in the circulation and within the kidneys.

Existing data are conflicting on the issue of whether a reduced total serum nuclease activity is present in pre-nephritic B/W mice [25,52]. In the present study, no reduction in activity was found in pre-proteinuric mice. Still, the consistent decrease seen in serum nuclease activity in all proteinuric mice irrespective of the levels of renal total nuclease expression indicate that similar changes could occur in other organs, including the liver. Such changes might therefore be of relevance to the loss of immunological tolerance against DNA and nucleosomes, and is currently being analyzed in our laboratory. Furthermore, the lack of a consistent correlation between serum and renal Dnase1 activity suggests that these reflect separate processes; the latter possibly confined to the kidney and related to the development of particularly unfavorable patterns of progression of the renal disease.

Considering the widespread hypothesis that SLE is related to deficient clearance of apoptotic debris, and in particular to the removal of chromatin-associated antigens, impaired production of a key secreted renal nuclease in a spontaneous model of the disease is a striking observation. An acquired down-regulation of Dnase1 expression during the development of lupus nephritis could be relevant to understand how systemic autoimmunity translates into end-organ disease, and could prove useful as a clinical marker for renal disease in SLE, as discussed by Mortensen et al. [42]. Identifying the processes underlying the observed down-regulation of renal Dnase1 is a complex feat, and is the focus of ongoing investigations.

Materials and Methods

Ethics Statement

The National Animal Research Authority (NARA) approved the study. Treatment and care of animals were conducted in accordance with guidelines of the Norwegian Ethical and Welfare Board for Animal Research. The study was approved by the Regional Ethical Committees in Lund, Sweden, and in Northern Norway.

Collection of samples from B/W and BALB/c mice

Female B/W and BALB/c mice were purchased from Harlan (Blackthorn, UK). Serum samples were collected every second week. Proteinuria was monitored weekly with sticks from Bayer Diagnostics (Bridgend, UK). Staining of $\geq 3+$ (≥ 3 g/L) was regarded as proteinuria indicative of overt nephritis. Kidneys were extirpated from B/W mice of different ages and from gender- and age-matched BALB/c control mice (Table 1), cut and snap-frozen in liquid N_2 with or without OCT (Optimal Cutting Temperature, Tissue-Tek, Terrance, CA), fixed in buffered depolymerised paraformaldehyde for electron microscopy studies, or stored in RNAlater (Ambion Inc, Austin, TX) for studies of gene expression. Treatment and care of animals were conducted in accordance with guidelines of the Norwegian Ethical and Welfare Board for Animal Research, and the institutional review board approved the study.

Human kidney biopsies

Kidney biopsies from female SLE patients with nephritis, and from patients with renal cancer or from a patient with Wegener's granulomatosis, were collected, prepared, and stored as described previously [45]. Baseline data for the SLE patients are presented in Figure 3. The glomeruli from the Wegener kidney were devoid of glomerular chromatin-IgG deposits, and the patient did not produce anti-dsDNA antibodies [55].

Detection of serum anti-dsDNA antibodies by ELISA

Serum anti-DNA autoantibodies were detected by ELISA as previously described [34,36,56].

Renal mRNA levels of nuclease-encoding genes

RNA extraction, cDNA synthesis and real time PCR were performed as previously described [34]. All reagents and assays were from Applied Biosystems. The primers and probes used are presented in Table 1 and in legend to Figure 1 for Dnase1l1/2/3. Expression levels relative to those of 4 w.o. BALB/c mice were calculated for all groups using the ddCT method.

Protein extraction

Nuclear and nucleus-depleted lysates were prepared from 20mg pieces of snap-frozen, lyophilized kidney tissue using Pierce Nuclear and Cytoplasmic Extraction reagent kit (Pierce Biotechnology, Rockford, IL,). Total protein was measured, and protein content of the samples normalized using BCA assay (Pierce).

Radial nuclease diffusion assay

To evaluate nuclease activity within native protein samples, a nuclease radial diffusion assay was performed as described [57], with minor modifications. Briefly, 1μl aliquots of renal lysates or serum samples were loaded in 1mm Ø wells on a 1% agarose gel containing 150 μg/ml calf thymus DNA (Sigma-Aldrich GmbH, Steinheim, Germany) and 1 μg/ml ethidium bromide in DNase reaction buffer (40 mM Tris, pH 7.6, 2 mM $CaCl_2$ and 2 mM $MgCl_2$). The gel was incubated in a humidified chamber at 37°C for 19 hours and photographed under UV illumination.

Heat inactivation of actin was achieved by incubation of samples in a heating block at 56°C for 10 minutes. Dnase1l3 inhibition was performed by addition of 4-(4,6-dichloro-[1,3,5]-triazin-2-ylamino)-2-(6-hydroxy-3-oxo-3H-xanthen-9-yl)-benzoic acid (DR396; Sigma-Aldrich) to a concentration of 5mM. Actin inhibition was achieved by pre-incubating the samples with 5μg/mL bovine g-actin (Sigma-Aldrich) for 10 minutes.

DNase zymography

DNA degrading activity by Dnase1 was determined after protein separation in a 10% SDS-polyacrylamide gel containing 100μg/ml heat-denatured salmon sperm DNA (Invitrogen Corp., Carlsbad, CA) as described [58]. For actin inhibition experiments, the gels were incubated for 4 hours at RT in 40mM Tris pH 7.4 containing g-actin at a concentration of 5μ g/mL, and 5μg/mL actin was also added to the Dnase reaction buffer, adapting a previously published protocol [27].

Western blotting

The renal protein extracts (25μg/lane) were separated using 10% SDS-PAGE gels, transferred onto PVDF membranes, and incubated with goat anti-mouse Dnase1 antibodies or goat anti-human Dnase1l1 antibodies (Santa Cruz Biotechnology, Santa Cruz, CA, USA). Binding was visualized using SuperSignal Chemiluminescent Substrate (Pierce) after incubation with HRP-conjugated anti-goat IgG. Equal loading was confirmed by membrane stripping and reprobing with a rabbit anti-human actin IgG (Sigma-Aldrich).

In situ DNA degradation assay

Four μm thick sections of OCT-embedded kidneys were incubated in DNase reaction buffer (2mM $CaCl_2$, 2mM $MgCl_2$ in 40mM Tris, pH7.6) for 2h at 37°C. The sections were then fixed with 4% paraformaldehyde and assayed using a fluorescent terminal deoxynucleotidyl transferase dUTP nick end labeling (TUNEL) assay kit (Roche Applied Science, Mannheim, Germany).

Direct immunofluorescence microscopy

Four μm thick cryosections from murine and human kidneys were blocked for 1h with 10% goat serum and 1% bovine serum albumin (BSA) in phosphate-buffered saline (PBS) followed by 30 min incubation with Alexa Fluor 488-conjugated F(ab')₂ goat anti-mouse or anti-human IgG (Invitrogen) and overnight washing in 0.05% Tween-20 in PBS at +4°C.

Transmission electron microscopy (TEM) and co-localization immune electron microscopy (IEM)

TEM and co-localization IEM of murine kidney sections were performed exactly as described by Kalaaji et al. [36,46].

Indirect immunofluorescence staining

Four μm sections from mouse kidneys embedded in OCT were blocked for 1 hour with 10% goat serum and 1% BSA in PBS followed by washing with PBS and 30 min incubation with goat anti-mouse Dnase1 or anti-human Dnase1l1 antibody (Santa Cruz Biotechnology) or normal goat IgG (negative control). Slides were washed and incubated for 30 min with Alexa Fluor 488-conjugated F(ab')₂ anti-goat IgG (Invitrogen). Kidney sections from the same mice were incubated with a buffer containing 10% goat serum, 10% fetal calf serum or with 5% BSA in PBS prior to staining with anti-Dnase1 antibody. No difference in Dnase1 staining intensity was seen between these samples. For the human cryopreserved biopsies, rabbit anti-bovine/human Dnase1 antibody (US Biological, Swampscott, Massachusetts) and Alexa Fluor 488-conjugated F(ab')₂ anti-rabbit IgG (Invitrogen) were used as first and second antibody, respectively.

Statistics

Statistics were performed with GraphPad Prism 5 (GraphPad Software, San Diego, CA) using the Mann-Whitney U test for comparison of groups. Differences were considered statistically significant at $p < 0.05$.

Supporting Information

Figure S1 Electron microscopy examination of immune complex deposition in proteinuric (NZBxNZW)F1 mice. Kidney morphology was further studied on ultrathin kidney sections by transmission electron microscopy (A, C, E) to define loci for deposition of electron dense structures, and by co-localization IEM (B, D, F) to detect in vivo-bound IgG (traced by 5nm gold), and chromatin deposits (traced by a monoclonal anti-dsDNA antibody added in vitro to the sections and stained by 10nm gold). In a 28 w.o. B/W mouse with mild proteinuria and sub-normal level of renal Dnase1 activity, the bound anti-dsDNA mAb co-localized with autoantibodies in EDS in the mesangial matrix (Fig. 4A and 4B demonstrate mesangial matrix-associated EDS by TEM, while the anti-dsDNA mAb added to the section in vitro co-localized with in vivo-bound IgG strictly confined to EDS as demonstrated by co-localization IEM, respectively). In a 35 w.o. proteinuric (+3) B/W mouse with low renal Dnase1 activity, the immune complex deposits were observed as EDS in glomerular capillary walls and mesangial matrix by TEM (C). Co-localization IEM demonstrated that these EDS contained IgG molecules and targets for the anti-dsDNA mAb (D). In a 20 w.o. pre-nephritic B/W mouse, TEM (E) revealed normal glomeruli, while co-localization IEM (F) revealed circulating chromatin-containing immune complexes within glomerular capillary lumen (F, enlarged panel), but no immune complexes were associated with membranes or the mesangial matrix. BALB/c mice had normal kidney morphology and no immune complexes were detected by TEM or co-localization IEM (data not shown). In D, it is demonstrated that the anti-dsDNA mAb, added to the sections and traced by 10 nm gold, bound to nuclear DNA.

Figure S2 Phase contrast and indirect immunofluorescence analyses of Dnase1 staining on pre-nephritic and nephritic (NZBxNZW)F1 kidneys. Cryosections of B/W kidneys were analysed by phase-contrast and indirect immunofluorescence using an anti-Dnase1 antibody followed by an Alexa488-conjugated F(ab')2 anti-IgG antibody to stain for Dnase1. The images were taken using identical exposure settings, and were obtained at 200× magnification. Phase-contrast micrographs and corresponding Dnase1 stainings are shown for a pre-nephritic B/W mouse (20 weeks old; panel A), a mouse with mesangial nephritis (panel B) and a mouse with membrano-proliferative nephritis (panel C). Glomeruli have been marked by circles for clarity. As is evident from the figure, Dnase1 is expressed in tubular and glomerular cells, and both compartments loose their Dnase1 expression upon progression of lupus nephritis into end-stage organ disease.

Figure S3 Phase contrast and indirect immunofluorescence analyses of Dnase1 staining of kidney biopsies from patients with lupus nephritis. Cryosections of the kidneys were analysed by phase contrast and indirect immunofluorescence using an anti-Dnase1 antibody followed by an Alexa488-conjugated F(ab')2 anti-IgG antibody to stain for Dnase1. The images were taken

using identical exposure settings at 200× magnification. Corresponding phase-contrast micrographs and Dnase1 immunostainings are shown for a patient with mild mesangial (A) and membrano-proliferative (B) lupus nephritis. Glomeruli have been marked by circles for clarity.

Figure S4 Indirect immunofluorescence analyses of histologically normal kidneys and biopsies from patients with Wegener granulomatosus and lupus nephritis. The renal cryosections were immunostained with rabbit anti-Dnase1 antibody followed by an Alexa488-conjugated F(ab')2 anti-IgG antibody. The images were obtained at 400× magnification using identical exposure settings. Strong staining was visible in histologically normal kidneys (A–C). Comparable levels of staining were present in kidneys from a patient with Wegeners granulomatosis (D) and from mesangial lupus nephritis (E), whereas Dnase1 staining was almost undetectable in kidneys from patients with membrano-proliferative lupus nephritis (F–H).

Acknowledgments

We are thankful to Jørgen Benjaminsen, Randi Olsen and Helga Marie Bye for excellent technical help.

Author Contributions

Conceived and designed the experiments: SNZ AAT OPR. Performed the experiments: SNZ AAT. Analyzed the data: SNZ AAT OPR. Contributed reagents/materials/analysis tools: OPR. Wrote the paper: SNZ AAT OPR.

References

1. Miescher P, Fauconnet M (1954) Absorption of L. E. factor by isolated cell nuclei. Experientia 10: 252–253.
2. Hahn BH (1998) Antibodies to DNA. N Engl J Med 338: 1359–1368.
3. Mortensen ES, Rekvig OP (2009) Nephritogenic potential of anti-DNA antibodies against necrotic nucleosomes. J Am Soc Nephrol 20: 696–704.
4. Gaipl US, Kuhn A, Sheriff A, Munoz LE, Franz S, et al. (2006) Clearance of apoptotic cells in human SLE. Curr Dir Autoimmun 9: 173–187.
5. Gaipl US, Sheriff A, Franz S, Munoz LE, Voll RE, et al. (2006) Inefficient clearance of dying cells and autoreactivity. Curr Top Microbiol Immunol 305: 161–176.
6. Licht R, Dieker JW, Jacobs CW, Tax WJ, Berden JH (2004) Decreased phagocytosis of apoptotic cells in diseased SLE mice. J Autoimmun 22: 139–145.
7. Berden JH, Grootscholten C, Jurgen WC, van der Vlag J (2002) Lupus nephritis: a nucleosome waste disposal defect? J Nephrol 15 Suppl 6: S1–10.
8. Sbarra AJ, Bardawil WA, Shirley W (1963) Relationship between aetiology, LE cell phenomenon and antinuclear antibody in disseminated lupus erythematosus: a hypothesis. Nature 198: 159–161.
9. Su KY, Pisetsky DS (2009) The role of extracellular DNA in autoimmunity in SLE. Scand J Immunol 70: 175–183.
10. Kuenkele S, Beyer TD, Voll RE, Kalden JR, Herrmann M (2003) Impaired clearance of apoptotic cells in systemic lupus erythematosus: challenge of T and B cell tolerance. Curr Rheumatol Rep 5: 175–177.
11. Samejima K, Earnshaw WC (2005) Trashing the genome: the role of nucleases during apoptosis. Nat Rev Mol Cell Biol 6: 677–688.
12. Kawane K, Nagata S (2008) Nucleases in programmed cell death. Methods Enzymol 442: 271–287.
13. Napirei M, Gultekin A, Kloeckl T, Moroy T, Frostegard J, et al. (2006) Systemic lupus-erythematosus: Deoxyribonuclease 1 in necrotic chromatin disposal. Int J Biochem Cell Biol 38: 297–306.
14. Holdenrieder S, Nagel D, Schalhorn A, Heinemann V, Wilkowski R, et al. (2008) Clinical relevance of circulating nucleosomes in cancer. Ann N Y Acad Sci 1137: 180–189.
15. Zeerleder S, Zwart B, Wuillemin WA, Aarden LA, Groeneveld AB, et al. (2003) Elevated nucleosome levels in systemic inflammation and sepsis. Crit Care Med 31: 1947–1951.
16. Lo YM, Rainer TH, Chan LY, Hjelm NM, Cocks RA (2000) Plasma DNA as a prognostic marker in trauma patients. Clin Chem 46: 319–323.
17. Raptis L, Menard HA (1980) Quantitation and characterization of plasma DNA in normals and patients with systemic lupus erythematosus. J Clin Invest 66: 1391–1399.
18. Tan EM, Schur PH, Carr RI, Kunkel HG (1966) Deoxybonucleic acid (DNA) and antibodies to DNA in the serum of patients with systemic lupus erythematosus. J Clin Invest 45: 1732–1740.
19. Amoura Z, Piette JC, Chabre H, Cacoub P, Papo T, et al. (1997) Circulating plasma levels of nucleosomes in patients with systemic lupus erythematosus: correlation with serum antinucleosome antibody titers and absence of clear association with disease activity. Arthritis Rheum 40: 2217–2225.
20. Williams RC, Jr., Malone CC, Meyers C, Decker P, Muller S (2001) Detection of nucleosome particles in serum and plasma from patients with systemic lupus erythematosus using monoclonal antibody 4H7. J Rheumatol 28: 81–94.
21. Licht R, Van Bruggen MC, Oppers-Walgreen B, Rijke TP, Berden JH (2001) Plasma levels of nucleosomes and nucleosome-autoantibody complexes in murine lupus: effects of disease progression and lipopolysaccharide administration. Arthritis Rheum 44: 1320–1330.
22. Frost PG, Lachmann PJ (1968) The relationship of desoxyribonuclease inhibitor levels in human sera to the occurrence of antinuclear antibodies. Clin Exp Immunol 3: 447–455.
23. Chitrabamrung S, Rubin RL, Tan EM (1981) Serum deoxyribonuclease I and clinical activity in systemic lupus erythematosus. Rheumatol Int 1: 55–60.
24. Sallai K, Nagy E, Derfalvy B, Muzes G, Gergely P (2005) Antinucleosome antibodies and decreased deoxyribonuclease activity in sera of patients with systemic lupus erythematosus. Clin Diagn Lab Immunol 12: 56–59.
25. Macanovic M, Lachmann PJ (1997) Measurement of deoxyribonuclease I (DNase) in the serum and urine of systemic lupus erythematosus (SLE)-prone NZB/NZW mice by a new radial enzyme diffusion assay. Clin Exp Immunol 108: 220–226.
26. Lindberg MU (1966) Crystallization from calf spleen of two inhibitors of deoxyribonuclease I. J Biol Chem 241: 1246–1249.
27. Lacks SA (1981) Deoxyribonuclease I in mammalian tissues. Specificity of inhibition by actin. J Biol Chem 256: 2644–2648.
28. Verthelyi D, Dybdal N, Elias KA, Klinman DM (1998) DNAse treatment does not improve the survival of lupus prone (NZB×NZW)F1 mice. Lupus 7: 223–230.
29. Davis JC, Jr., Manzi S, Yarboro C, Rairie J, McInnes I, et al. (1999) Recombinant human Dnase I (rhDNase) in patients with lupus nephritis. Lupus 8: 68–76.

30. Manderson AP, Carlucci F, Lachmann PJ, Lazarus RA, Festenstein RJ, et al. (2006) The in vivo expression of actin/salt-resistant hyperactive DNase I inhibits the development of anti-ssDNA and anti-histone autoantibodies in a murine model of systemic lupus erythematosus. Arthritis Res Ther 8: R68.

31. Napirei M, Karsunky H, Zevnik B, Stephan H, Mannherz HG, et al. (2000) Features of systemic lupus erythematosus in Dnase1-deficient mice. Nat Genet 25: 177–181.

32. Fenton K, Fismen S, Hedberg A, Seredkina N, Fenton C, et al. (2009) Anti-dsDNA antibodies promote initiation, and acquired loss of renal Dnase1 promotes progression of lupus nephritis in autoimmune (NZBxNZW)F1 mice. PLoS One 4: e8474.

33. Tew MB, Johnson RW, Reveille JD, Tan FK (2001) A molecular analysis of the low serum deoxyribonuclease activity in lupus patients. Arthritis Rheum 44: 2446–2447.

34. Zykova SN, Seredkina N, Benjaminsen J, Rekvig OP (2008) Reduced fragmentation of apoptotic chromatin is associated with nephritis in lupus-prone (NZB×NZW)F(1) mice. Arthritis Rheum 58: 813–825.

35. Johnson AJ, Goger PR, Tillett WS (1954) The intravenous injection of bovine crystalline pancreatic desoxyribonuclease into patients. J Clin Invest 33: 1670–1686.

36. Kalaaji M, Sturfelt G, Mjelle JE, Nossent H, Rekvig OP (2006) Critical comparative analyses of anti-alpha-actinin and glomerulus-bound antibodies in human and murine lupus nephritis. Arthritis Rheum 54: 914–926.

37. Yasutomo K, Horiuchi T, Kagami S, Tsukamoto H, Hashimura C, et al. (2001) Mutation of DNASE1 in people with systemic lupus erythematosus. Nat Genet 28: 313–314.

38. Napirei M, Ricken A, Eulitz D, Knoop H, Mannherz HG (2004) Expression pattern of the deoxyribonuclease 1 gene: lessons from the Dnase1 knockout mouse. Biochem J 380: 929–937.

39. Takeshita H, Mogi K, Yasuda T, Nakajima T, Nakashima Y, et al. (2000) Mammalian deoxyribonucleases I are classified into three types: pancreas, parotid, and pancreas-parotid (mixed), based on differences in their tissue concentrations. Biochem Biophys Res Commun 269: 481–484.

40. Basnakian AG, Apostolov EO, Yin X, Napirei M, Mannherz HG, et al. (2005) Cisplatin nephrotoxicity is mediated by deoxyribonuclease I. J Am Soc Nephrol 16: 697–702.

41. Koizumi T (1996) Genetic control of urinary deoxyribonuclease I (DNase I) activity levels in mice. Exp Anim 45: 245–250.

42. Mortensen ES, Fenton KA, Rekvig OP (2008) Lupus nephritis: the central role of nucleosomes revealed. Am J Pathol 172: 275–283.

43. Lazarides E, Lindberg U (1974) Actin is the naturally occurring inhibitor of deoxyribonuclease I. Proc Natl Acad Sci U S A 71: 4742–4746.

44. Shiokawa D, Tanuma S (2001) Characterization of human DNase I family endonucleases and activation of DNase gamma during apoptosis. Biochemistry 40: 143–152.

45. Kalaaji M, Fenton KA, Mortensen ES, Olsen R, Sturfelt G, et al. (2007) Glomerular apoptotic nucleosomes are central target structures for nephritogenic antibodies in human SLE nephritis. Kidney Int 71: 664–672.

46. Kalaaji M, Mortensen E, Jorgensen L, Olsen R, Rekvig OP (2006) Nephritogenic lupus antibodies recognize glomerular basement membrane-associated chromatin fragments released from apoptotic intraglomerular cells. Am J Pathol 168: 1779–1792.

47. Malide D, Londono I, Russo P, Bendayan M (1993) Ultrastructural localization of DNA in immune deposits of human lupus nephritis. Am J Pathol 143: 304–311.

48. Ordonez NG, Gomez LG (1981) The ultrastructure of glomerular haematoxylin bodies. J Pathol 135: 259–265.

49. Scaffidi P, Misteli T, Bianchi ME (2002) Release of chromatin protein HMGB1 by necrotic cells triggers inflammation. Nature 418: 191–195.

50. Napirei M, Wulf S, Mannherz HG (2004) Chromatin breakdown during necrosis by serum Dnase1 and the plasminogen system. Arthritis Rheum 50: 1873–1883.

51. Gaipl US, Beyer TD, Heyder P, Kuenkele S, Bottcher A, et al. (2004) Cooperation between C1q and DNase I in the clearance of necrotic cell-derived chromatin. Arthritis Rheum 50: 640–649.

52. Wilber A, O'Connor TP, Lu ML, Karimi A, Schneider MC (2003) Dnase1l3 deficiency in lupus-prone MRL and NZB/W F1 mice. Clin Exp Immunol 134: 46–52.

53. Shiokawa D, Ohyama H, Yamada T, Tanuma S (1997) Purification and properties of DNase gamma from apoptotic rat thymocytes. Biochem J 326 (Pt 3): 675–681.

54. Mizuta R, Mizuta M, Araki S, Suzuki K, Ebara S, et al. (2009) DNase gamma-dependent and -independent apoptotic DNA fragmentations in Ramos Burkitt's lymphoma cell line. Biomed Res 30: 165–170.

55. Fenton KA, Mjelle JE, Jakobsen S, Olsen R, Rekvig OP (2008) Renal expression of polyomavirus large T antigen is associated with nephritis in human systemic lupus erythematosus. Mol Immunol 45: 3117–3124.

56. Rekvig OP, Moens U, Sundsfjord A, Bredholt G, Osei A, et al. (1997) Experimental expression in mice and spontaneous expression in human SLE of polyomavirus T-antigen. A molecular basis for induction of antibodies to DNA and eukaryotic transcription factors. J Clin Invest 99: 2045–2054.

57. Chitrabamrung S, Bannett JS, Rubin RL, Tan EM (1981) A radial diffusion assay for plasma and serum deoxyribonuclease I. Rheumatol Int 1: 49–53.

58. Rosenthal AL, Lacks SA (1977) Nuclease detection in SDS-polyacrylamide gel electrophoresis. Anal Biochem 80: 76–90.

11

Identification of gp96 as a Novel Target for Treatment of Autoimmune Disease in Mice

Jung Min Han[1,3], Nam Hoon Kwon[1], Jin Young Lee[1], Seung Jae Jeong[1], Hee Jung Jung[4], Hyeong Rae Kim[4], Zihai Li[5], Sunghoon Kim[1,2]*

1 Center for Medicinal Protein Network and Systems Biology, College of Pharmacy, Seoul National University, Seoul, Republic of Korea, **2** Department of Molecular Medicine and Biopharmaceutical Sciences, Graduate School of Convergence Science and Technology, Seoul National University, Suwon, Republic of Korea, **3** Research Institute of Pharmaceutical Sciences, College of Pharmacy, Seoul National University, Seoul, Republic of Korea, **4** Cancer & Infectious Disease Research Center, Bio-Organic Science Division, Korea Research Institute of Chemical Technology, Dae Jeon, Republic of Korea, **5** Center for Immunotherapy of Cancer and Infectious Diseases, University of Connecticut School of Medicine, Farmington, Connecticut, United States of America

Abstract

Heat shock proteins have been implicated as endogenous activators for dendritic cells (DCs). Chronic expression of heat shock protein gp96 on cell surfaces induces significant DC activations and systemic lupus erythematosus (SLE)-like phenotypes in mice. However, its potential as a therapeutic target against SLE remains to be evaluated. In this work, we conducted chemical approach to determine whether SLE-like phenotypes can be compromised by controlling surface translocation of gp96. From screening of chemical library, we identified a compound that binds and suppresses surface presentation of gp96 by facilitating its oligomerization and retrograde transport to endoplasmic reticulum. *In vivo* administration of this compound reduced maturation of DCs, populations of antigen presenting cells, and activated B and T cells. The chemical treatment also alleviated the SLE-associated symptoms such as glomerulonephritis, proteinuria, and accumulation of anti-nuclear and –DNA antibodies in the SLE model mice resulting from chronic surface exposure of gp96. These results suggest that surface translocation of gp96 can be chemically controlled and gp96 as a potential therapeutic target to treat autoimmune disease like SLE.

Editor: Jacques Zimmer, Centre de Recherche Public de la Santé (CRP-Santé), Luxembourg

Funding: This work was supported by the National Research Foundation of Korea Grant funded by the Korean Government (NRF-2008-359-C00024), by FPR08-B1-250 of 21C Frontier Functional Proteomics Project from Korean Ministry of Science and Technology, by R31-2008-000-10103-0 from the WCU project of the Ministry of Education, Science, and Technology and the Korea Science and Engineering Foundation. The funders had no role in study design, data collection and analysis, decision to publish, or presentation of the manuscript.

Competing Interests: The authors have declared that no competing interests exist.

* E-mail: sungkim@snu.ac.kr

Introduction

SLE is a systemic autoimmune disease characterized by abnormalities in dendritic cell (DC), autoreactive T cells and B cells [1],[2]. DCs are important in regulating both immunity and tolerance and have been implicated in the pathogenesis of SLE [1]. DCs induce activation of naïve T cells and stimulate B cell growth and differentiation. Therefore, lupus-associated DCs producing altered signals and amplifying autoreactive specificities in T cells, which, in turn, provide help to autoreactive B cells, inducing an increase in autoantibody production. Glomerulonephritis is induced when DNA specific autoantibodies form complexes in kidney glomerulus [3],[4]. As disease progresses, mesangial proliferation, endocapilliary proliferation, vascular collapse and immune complex accumulation in kidney result in glomerulonephritis and eventual renal failure [3],[4]. SLE is treated by immunosuppressants and cytostatic agents, with extensive use of corticoids when disease is stabilized, but these treatments have numerous side effects [5].

Gp96 is the endoplasmic reticulum (ER)-resident chaperone protein belonging to the HSP90 family [6]. The continuous recycling of escaped ER resident proteins such as gp96, GRP78/Bip, protein disulfide isomerase (PDI), and calreticulin is mediated by retrograde transport form Golgi to ER through COPI-coated vesicles [7]–[10]. ER localization of these proteins is regulated through their C-terminal KDEL sequence. KDEL sequence is recognized by the KDEL receptor ERD2 [11], which is mainly localized to the cis-Golgi [7],[12]. Binding of KDEL proteins to ERD2 leads to its oligomerization [13] and stimulates its rapid transport out of cis-Golgi [14],[15]. Oligomerization seems to be a hallmark of constitutively cycling proteins of the early secretory pathway, as ERGIC-53 is a stable hexamer [16] and the KDEL receptor oligomerizes upon binding to its ligands [13]. gp96 also exists as a homodimer or higher-order oligomer [17]–[19], although it is not known whether dimer or higher-order oligomer is responsible for ERD2 binding. The ERD2-gp96 complex returns to the ER where it dissociates, thus freeing ERD2 for further cycling of transport.

In addition to the intracellular chaperone function, gp96 has been implicated in innate and adaptive immunity [20],[21] and its cell surface exposure is associated with its immunological activities such as the activation or maturation of dendritic cells (DCs) [22]–[24]. Direct interaction between gp96 and DCs via CD91 and TLR2/4 [25]–[27] induces DC maturation, resulting in proinflammatory cytokine secretion and MHC class I and II upregulation [27],[28]. Transgenic mice chronically expressing gp96 on cell surfaces showed significant DC activation and spontaneous systemic lupus erythematosus (SLE)-like autoimmune phenotypes [29]. Gp96 is increased in synovial fluid from the joints of human rheumatoid arthritis patients and the expression of gp96 shows a correlation with inflammation and synovial lining thickness, further supporting the pathological association of gp96 with autoimmune diseases [30].

AIMP1/p43 (ARS-interacting multi-functional protein 1, also known as p43) is a protein involved in diverse physiological processes [31]. Recently, we found that AIMP1 holds gp96 in ER, preventing its extracellular translocation [32]. For this reason, AIMP1-deficient mice contain cells with increased surface levels of gp96, thereby displaying the phenotypes similar to those of gp96tm transgenic mice [32]. Although all of these previous studies demonstrated the importance of the ER retention of gp96 to prevent aberrant autoimmune responses, it is not yet determined whether SLE-like phenotypes resulting from chronic exposure of gp96 can be compromised by suppressing its surface translocation. To address this question, we first screened chemical library to identify a compound that can bind and blocks surface localization of gp96. After determining the mode of action of the selected compound upon binding to gp96, we evaluated its *in vivo* effect on various phenotypes that are associated with SLE symptoms using the transgenic mice displaying SLE-like phenotypes resulting from the chronic surface presentation of gp96.

Results

Screening and Identification of GPM1 as a gp96-Binding Chemical

Since AIMP1 interacts with gp96 and regulates its ER localization, preventing cell surface localization [32], we hypothesize that small molecule, having similar activity like AIMP1, can suppress cell surface localization of gp96 and aberrant autoimmune responses although small molecule may compete with AIMP1 for gp96 binding. For this, we set up modified ELISA assay method using recombinant AIMP1 and gp96 proteins. The screening assay was designed to select the compounds that block the interaction of gp96 with AIMP1 as described in Methods. In the chemical screening, we chose 6,482 representative chemicals with different pharmacophore representing 150,000 chemicals deposited in Korea Chemical Bank (http://www.chembank.org/).

Each of the tested compounds gave different inhibitory effect on the interaction of the two proteins (Fig. 1A), and we have selected 12 compounds that inhibited the interaction more than 95% of the control at 0.1µM (Table S1). These 12 compounds had no effect on the interaction between lysyl-tRNA synthetase (KRS) and superoxide dismutase 1 (SOD1) [33] indicating the specificity of compounds. We obtained 1251 additional derivative compounds from the 12 initial hits and tested them again for the activities against the gp96-AIMP1 interaction. Among them, 77 compounds showed negative effect while 1174 compounds gave no effect (Table S1). The chemicals that would block the interaction of gp96 and AIMP1 are expected to either enhance or suppress the surface localization of gp96 depending on their binding sites. If chemicals bind to AIMP1 side, they are expected to enhance the surface localization of gp96 since it would release gp96 from its intracellular anchor, AIMP1. But if chemicals bind to gp96 side, they may suppress the surface translocation of gp96 by interfering with the subsequent processes for the molecular trafficking of gp96 to the plasma membrane. We thus examined the effects of the 77 compounds on the surface expression of gp96 by flow cytometry as described. Out of 77 compounds, 8 reduced gp96 positive cells to below 10% whereas 12 compounds increased gp96 positive cells to

more than 20% and the rest 57 compounds gave the effects within the range between them (Fig. 1B and Table S1). Among the 8 selected compounds, four were discarded for the following experiments due to their cellular toxicity (data not shown). In the next step, we subjected the remaining 4 compounds to the single dose toxicity test (single i.p. injection, 500mg/kg, 1 week) using mice. Among them, [(S)-methyl 2-(4,6-dimethoxypyrimidine-2-yloxy)-3-methylbutanoate] (designated as GPM1, Fig. 1C upper), showed no toxicity (data not shown) and gave high score in leadlikeness rule [34]. Among other 3 compounds, one gave severe toxicity to mice and the other two showed low lead-likeness score (data not shown). Based on these results, we finally chose GPM1 for further experiments. Among the total screened compounds, 2-(4,6-dimethoxypyrimidin-2-yloxy)-3-phenylpropanoic acid showed only 4% inhibition on the interaction of gp96 and AIMP1 despite it shares dimethoxypyrimidine ring with GPM1. We thus selected it as a control (NC1) (Fig. 1C lower).

We compared the dose-dependent effect of GPM1 and NC1 on the interaction of gp96 and AIMP1. GPM1 showed 50% inhibition at around 30nM whereas NC1 gave no effect on the binding of the two proteins (Fig. 1D). We monitored the binding kinetics of GPM1 to gp96 or AIMP1 by surface plasmon resonance (SPR) using BIAcore 3000. GPM1 showed the binding to gp96 with K_D of 87.9nM (Fig. 1E and F), but no apparent binding to AIMP1 (data not shown). We also determined whether GPM1 can bind to protein disulfide isomerase (PDI) and GRP78/Bip that are also an ER-resident KDEL protein like gp96. GPM1 showed extremely weak binding to PDI and GRP78/Bip compared to gp96 ($K_D = 249$ µM and 11.9 mM, respectively) (Fig. S1A and S1B). To further define the GPM1-binding region of gp96, we introduced point mutations at L707, V706, V712, L713, F714, Y731 and M738 that are located within AIMP1-binding region of gp96 [32] and monitored how the mutations at these sites would affect the binding of GPM1 to gp96 using SPR method. All the mutants retained the normal ATPase activity of gp96 (Fig. S2), suggesting that the mutations did not affect their native conformation. However, GPM1 showed significantly decreased affinity to the mutants except for V706A/L707A mutant, suggesting the importance of the C-terminal dimerization domain of gp96 for the binding to GPM1.

Suppression of Cell Surface gp96 by GPM1 through Increased ER Retention

First, we tested the effect of GPM1 on the surface localization of gp96. We isolated splenocytes from C57BL/6 mice, treated with vehicle, GPM1, or NC1 (10µM, 24h), and monitored the surface levels of gp96 by flow cytometry. The surface gp96 levels in GPM1-treated splenocytes were lower compared to those of the vehicle- or NC1-treated cells (Fig. 2A). We also determined whether GPM1 can affect the cell surface level of GRP78/Bip, PDI, and calreticulin that are also an ER-resident KDEL protein like gp96. GPM1 had no effect on the populations of the surface GRP78/Bip, PDI, and calreticulin positive cells while it reduced gp96-positive cell population, suggesting the specificity of GPM1 for gp96 (Fig. 2B). Next, we examined the action mechanism of GPM1 for suppression of cell surface gp96. Since GPM1 has no effect on the cellular protein level of gp96, GPM1 is expected to have two action points. The first possibility is that GPM1 directly enhances the endocytosis of cell surface gp96 and the second possibility is that GPM1 enhances the retrograde transport from Golgi to ER, resulting in the decreased movement of gp96 to the cell surface. Since surface expression of gp96 was abrogated in the presence of brefeldin A (BFA), which leads to Golgi disturbance and protein accumulation inside the ER [35], we monitored the

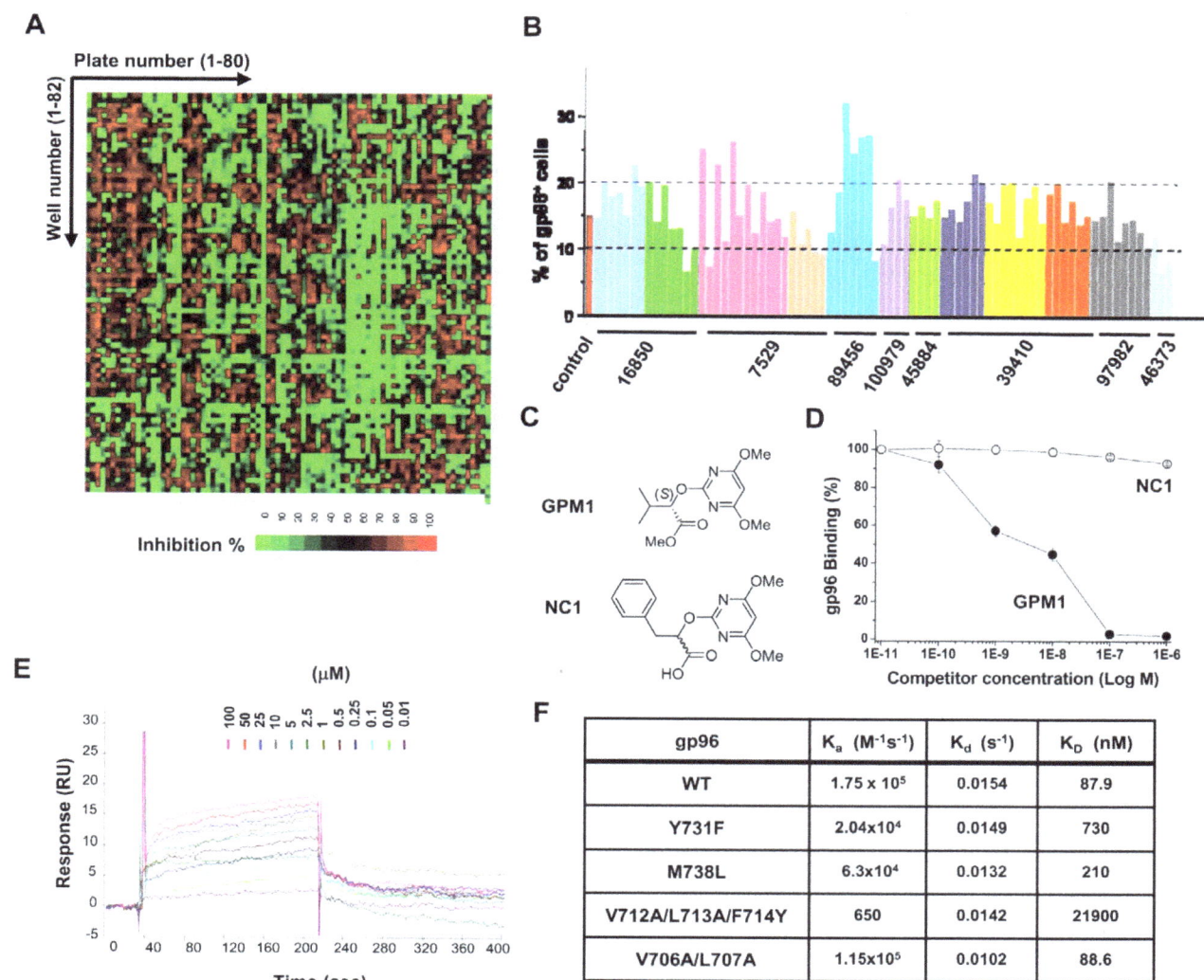

Figure 1. Identification of gp96-binding compound that suppresses plasma membrane levels of gp96. (A) Heat map of primary screening data. Inhibitory effects of 6,482 chemicals on the interaction of gp96 and AIMP1 were monitored by modified ELISA method as described. Taking the value of DMSO as 0%, the inhibition of each chemical was indicated as relative percentage and the degree of the inhibition was represented by a heat map in a 10% scale from 0 (green) to 100% (red). (B) Effect of the derivatives of the primary hits on surface expression of gp96. RAW264.7 cells were treated with 77 compounds (10μM, 24h) and the effects on surface expression of gp96 were analyzed by flow cytometry. We took 5% changes compared to the control group (15% of the gp96⁺ cells) as cut-off values. Out of 77 compounds, 8 compounds showed suppressive effect on surface expression of gp96 below 10% whereas 12 compounds showed increased gp96⁺ cells more than 20%. The numbers indicate the primary hits (see table S1) and the effects of their derivatives are shown as bar graphs. The compounds in the same plate are displayed as one color. (C) Chemical structure of GPM1 and negative control (NC1) used in this study. (D) The dose-dependent effect of GPM1 or NC1 on the AIMP1-gp96 interaction using ELISA method as described. The indicated concentrations of the two compounds and biotin-conjugated murine gp96 were added to AIMP1 coated on the surface of microtiter wells, and gp96 bound to AIMP1 was detected with strepavidin-conjugated peroxidase. (E) The binding of GPM1 to gp96 was examined by surface plasmon resonance (SPR). GPM1 at the indicated concentrations was injected to immobilized gp96 and the binding was measured using Biacore 3000. The response data were processed using data from a reference surface and buffer injections. Each concentration was tested in triplicate. (F) Association rate constant (K_a), dissociation rate constant (K_d), and equilibrium dissociation constant (K_D) were determined for the interactions of GPM1 with various mutants of gp96 by the SPR experiments as described in Methods.

effect of GPM1 on the cell surface gp96 in the absence of the translocation of gp96 from the Golgi to the cell surface by BFA treatment. If GPM1 has an effect on endocytosis of cell surface gp96, it should additionally suppress cell surface gp96 in the presence of BFA. But, GPM1-induced suppression of surface gp96 was abrogated in the presence of BFA (Fig. 2C), suggesting that the target point of GPM1 is the translocation of gp96 from the ER to the cell surface. To determine the functional importance of KDELR1 for the suppressive effect of GPM1 on the surface

localization of gp96, we introduced siRNA to knockdown KDELR1 transcript and examined how GPM1 would affect the surface levels of gp96. In the control cells, GPM1 reduced gp96 positive cell population (Fig. 2D). When the cells were transfected with KDELR1 siRNA, GPM1 effect was ablated while gp96 positive cells were increased due to the depletion of KDELR1 (Fig. 2D). These results demonstrate that the suppressive effect of GPM1 on the surface translocation of gp96 requires KDEL receptor. We tested whether GPM1 would affect the binding of

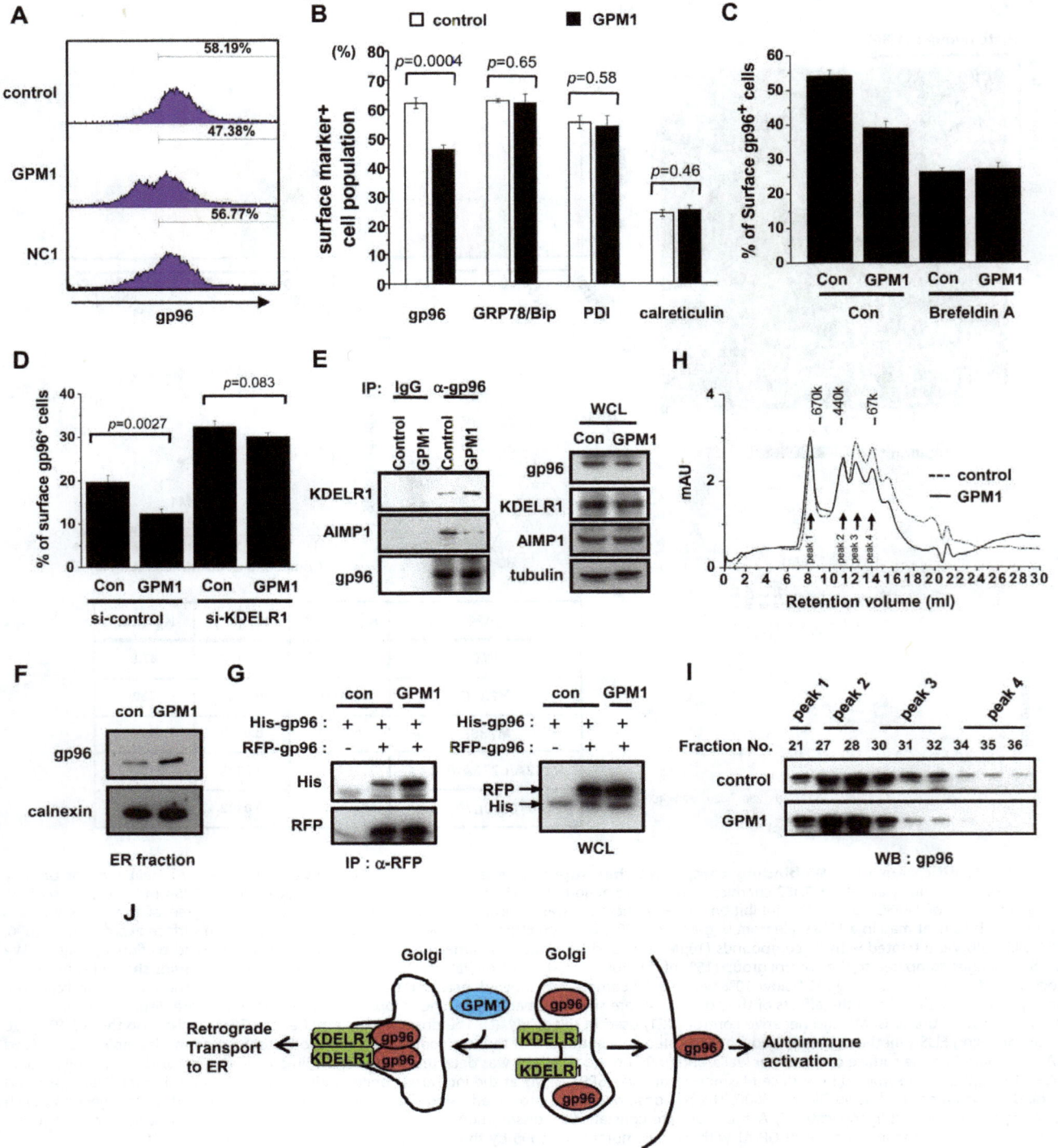

Figure 2. The effect of the selected chemical on gp96 oligomerization and surface levels of gp96. (A) Splenocytes isolated from C57BL/6 mice were treated with vehicle (5% DMSO in PBS), GPM1, or NC1 (10μM, 24h), stained for cell surface gp96, and followed by flow cytometry. The numbers indicate the percentage of gp96+ splenocytes. (B) The effect of GPM1 on cell surface gp96, GRP78/Bip, PDI, and calreticulin. RAW264.7 cells were treated with DMSO or GPM1 (10μM) for 24h. Cells were stained for cell surface gp96, GRP78/Bip, PDI, and calreticulin, followed by flow cytometry. (C) RAW264.7 cells were treated with DMSO, GPM1 (10μM), or brefeldin A (1μg/ml) for 4h. Cells were stained for cell surface gp96, followed by flow cytometry. (D) RAW264.7 cells were transfected with si-control or si-KDELR1 for 48h and then further treated with DMSO or GPM1 (10μM) for 24h. Cells were stained for cell surface gp96, and followed by flow cytometry. (E) RAW24.7 cells were treated with 10μM GPM1 for 24h. Cell lysates were immunoprecipitated with control IgG or anti-gp96 antibody and the immunoprecipitated proteins were immunoblotted with anti-KDELR1, anti-AIMP1 and gp96 antibodies. WCL means whole cell lysate. (F) RAW264.7 cells were treated with 10μM GPM1 for 24h. Cell lysates were fractionated using sucrose density gradient. Proteins from ER fraction were immunoblotted with anti-gp96 antibody. Calnexin was used as an ER marker. (G) The effect of GPM1 on gp96 oligomerization. 293 cells were transfected with RFP-tagged gp96 and His-tagged gp96. Cells were then treated with DMSO or GPM1 (10μM) for 4h. Cell lysates were immunoprecipitated with anti-RFP antibody, and the precipitated proteins were immunoblotted using anti-

His antibody. WCL, whole cell lysates. (H) FPLC gel filtration chromatography of gp96 protein. The purified gp96 (5µM) was incubated with DMSO or GPM1 (50µM) for 1h on ice and then injected into a Superdex 200 10/300 GL size exclusion column. The positions of mass standards used for calibration are indicated at the top of the chromatogram. Molecular weight: thyroglobin (670 kDa), ferritin (440kDa) and BAS (67kDa). Peak 1, 2, 3, and 4 indicate the position of oligomer, tetramer, dimer, and monomer of gp96 protein, respectively. (I) Peak fractions from gel filtration of DMSO or GPM1-treated gp96 proteins were immunoblotted with anti-gp96 antibody. (J) Model for GPM1 action. In the absence of KDEL proteins such as gp96, KDEL receptor exists mainly in monomeric form. GPM1 treatment leads to gp96 oligomerization and binding to KDEL receptor, which induces retrograde transport of gp96 to ER. The data represent the means ± S.D. Student t-test P values are shown.

gp96 to KDEL receptor 1 (KDELR1) by co-immunoprecipitation between the two proteins. GPM1 increased the amount of gp96 bound to KDELR1 while blocking the binding of gp96 to AIMP1 (Fig. 2E left). However, GPM1 did not decrease the cellular levels of three proteins (Fig. 2E right) and the ATPase activity of gp96 (Fig. S3A). The ER retention of gp96 is enhanced via its interaction with AIMP1 that facilitates the oligomerization of gp96 [32]. We thus examined whether GPM1 would functionally mimic AIMP1 for the ER residency of gp96. When we isolated ER fraction from control-treated or GPM1-treated cells, the ER residency of gp96 was increased by GPM1 treatment (Fig. 2F). The retrograde transport of gp96 from Golgi to ER is mediated through the recognition of the C-terminal KDEL motif of gp96 by the KDEL receptor [11]. Binding of gp96 to KDEL receptor leads to its oligomerization [13] and retrieval to ER [14]. Thus, oligomerization status of gp96 can be a signature for its ER residency. Indeed, GPM1 treatment increased the amount of His-tagged gp96 coimmunoprecipitated with RFP-tagged gp96 (Fig. 2G), suggesting that GPM1 can regulate gp96 oligomer formation. When we monitored the conformational change of gp96 induced by GPM1, the α-helicity of gp96 was slightly increased as shown by circular dichroism spectroscopy (Fig. S3B). Here we examined whether GPM1 would directly affect oligomerization of gp96 using size exclusion chromatography. When the purified gp96 was mixed with GPM1, the monomer fraction of gp96 was shifted to the oligomers (Fig. 2H and I), suggesting that the oligomerization of gp96 can be facilitated by the binding to GPM1.

Based on these results, we propose the working mechanism of GPM1 as schematically shown in Fig. 2J. Namely, gp96 can be exposed to extracellular space upon various cellular stresses to trigger autoimmune responses. GPM1 binds to the C-terminal dimerization domain of gp96 and enhances oligomerization, leading to the KDEL receptor-mediated retrograde transport to ER.

Suppression of Cell Surface gp96 by GPM1 Reduces DC Maturation

In vivo effects of GPM1 were determined on cell surface presentation of gp96 and DC maturation associated with SLE. GPM1 was systemically delivered to gp96tm transgenic mice in which the surface levels of gp96 are chronically enhanced [29]. We used phosphate-buffered saline containing 5% DMSO and dexamethasone (Dex), an immunosuppressant of glucocorticoid family as negative and positive control, respectively. Each group consisted of age-matched nine female mice. During intraperitoneal administration for 2 months at the dose of 30mg/kg, GPM1-treated mice did not give apparent adverse effects whereas two of the nine Dex-treated mice died during the treatment (Fig. 3A). After 2 month, we isolated splenocytes from vehicle-, Dex-, and GPM1-treated mice and determined the viability of splenocytes. GPM1 did not affect the viability of splenocytes whereas Dex significantly damaged cell viability (Fig. 3B). We then confirmed the effect of GPM1 on the surface localization of gp96 of splenocytes from vehicle-, dexamethasone-, or GPM1-treated mice. We isolated MHC class II⁺ splenocytes and lymph nodes from vehicle-, Dex-, and GPM1-

treated mice and determined the portion of gp96⁺ cells by flow cytometry. The percentages of gp96⁺ MHC class II⁺ cells in the control, Dex- and GPM1-treated groups were about 57, 25 and 41%, respectively, suggesting the suppressive effect of GPM1 on the surface translocation of gp96 (Fig. 3C).

Gp96 has been implicated in the activation and maturation of DCs via CD91 and Toll-like receptor (TLR) 2/4 [25]–[27]. Also, DCs from gp96tm transgenic mice and AIMP1-deficient mice were shown to be hyperfunctional [29],[32]. We tested whether suppression of cell surface gp96 through the increase of retrograde transport to ER affected DC maturation in GPM1-treated mice. GPM1-treated mice showed little difference in CD11b⁺CD11c⁺ myeloid DC and CD11b⁻CD11c⁺ lymphoid DC populations (Fig. 3D upper). We monitored the maturity of DCs by measuring the surface levels of inducible costimulator ligand (ICOSL), one of the known DC maturation markers using flow cytometry and found that GPM1 significantly reduced ICOSL levels in splenic CD11b⁺CD11c⁺ myeloid DC and splenic CD11b⁺CD11c⁻ macrophages (Fig. 3D lower), and also reduced lymph node ICOSL⁺CD11b⁺CD11c⁺ myeloid DCs (Fig. 3E). However, GMP1 gave little effect on the ICOSL levels in CD11b⁻CD11c⁺ lymphoid DCs (Fig. 3E right graph). The decreased expression of cell surface ICOSL correlates with the decreased ability of GPM1-treated splenic DCs to activate allogeneic naïve CD4⁺ T cells, as measured by TNFa secretion (Fig. 3F) and IFNγ secretion (Fig. 3G). Based on these results, we conclude that suppression of cell surface gp96 affected DC maturation in GPM1-treated mice.

Suppression of Cell Surface gp96 by GPM1 Reduces B Cells, Memory T cells in gp96tm Transgenic Mice

We then examined whether GPM1 could influence the cellular phenotypes that can influence SLE-like phenotypes. The GPM1-treated mice showed reduced populations of B220⁺ and MHC class II⁺ cells in the spleen and in the lymph nodes (Fig. 4A and B left two graphs, respectively). GPM1 gave little effect on the T cell populations in both organs (Fig. 4A and B right three graphs). SLE involves abnormal activation of CD4⁺ T cells that accumulate as activated memory cells and contributes to B cell activation and expansion, and hypergammaglobulinemia [3],[4]. We found a reduction in the population of CD4⁺ memory cells and activated CD4⁺ T cells in the spleen and lymph nodes of GPM1-treated mice (CD4⁺CD44ʰⁱᵍʰ, CD4⁺CD62Lˡᵒʷ, and CD4⁺CD69⁺ cells; Fig. 4C and D). GPM1 treatment also decreased mature B cell population (B220⁺IgM⁺IgD⁺; data not shown).

Suppression of Cell Surface gp96 by GPM1 Reduces Renal Disease in gp96tm Transgenic Mice

We checked whether the typical SLE-like phenotypes are also compromised by systemic administration of GPM1. Although vehicle-treated mice displayed severe glomerulonephritis phenotypes such as thickening of basement membrane and capillary walls, vascular obliteration, increased mesangial cells, and renal tubules packed with pink proteinaceous materials (Fig. 5A left column and Table S2) and glomerular immunoglobulin deposition (Fig. 5B top), GPM1 as well as Dex treatment alleviated the

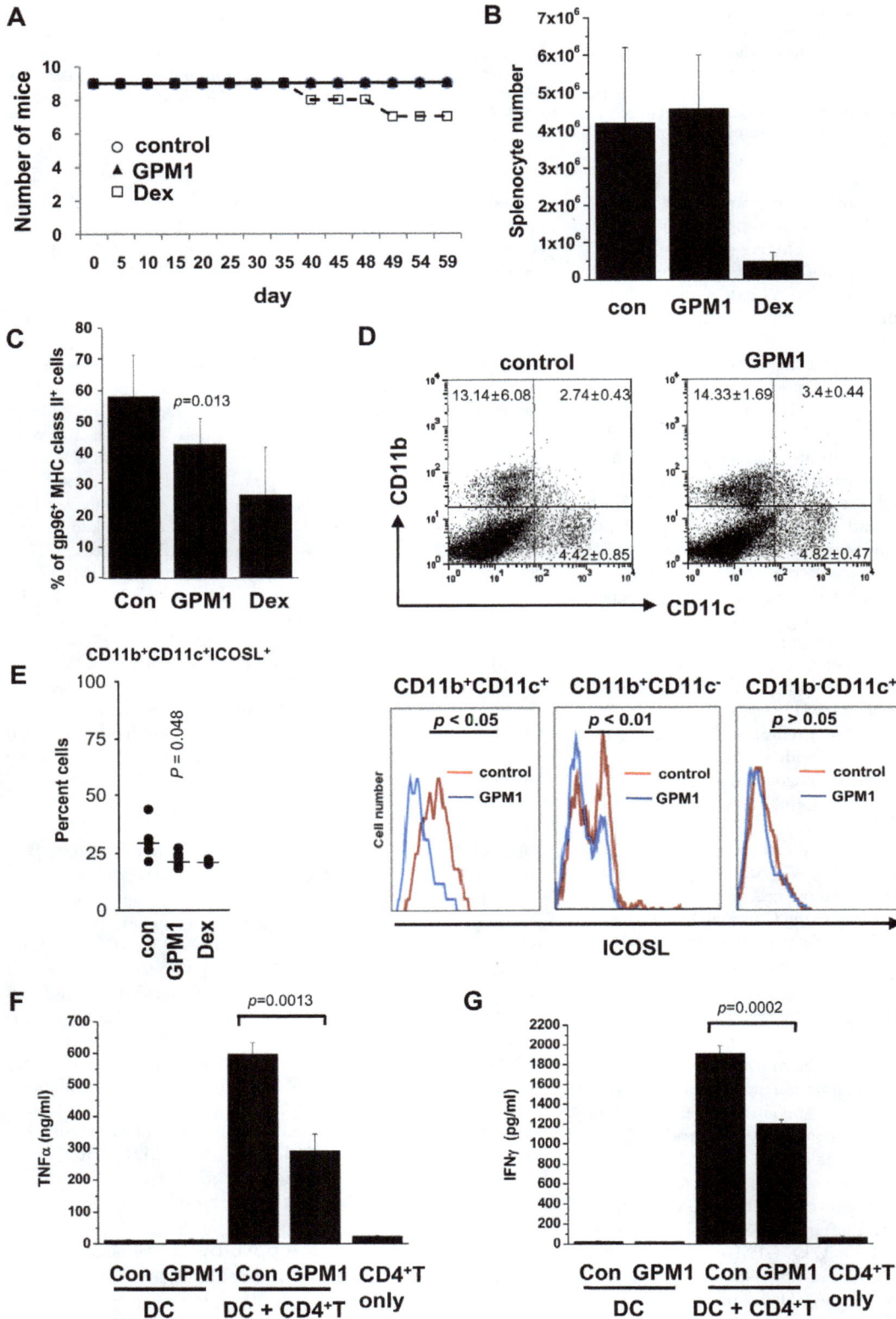

Figure 3. *In vivo* **effect of the selected compound on DC maturation.** (A) Survival rate of gp96tm transgenic female mice treated with vehicle (n = 9), GPM1 (n = 9), and dexamethasone (n = 9) at 30mg/kg/day. (B) The numbers of total splenocytes isolated from vehicle- (n = 9), GPM1- (n = 9), and Dex (dexamethasone)- (n = 7) treated mice. (C) Percentage of gp96[+] MHC class II[+] cell population in splenocytes from gp96tm transgenic female mice treated with vehicle (control) (n = 9), GPM1 (n = 9), and dexamethasone (n = 7) at 30mg/kg. (D) Cell surface ICOSL of CD11b[+]CD11c[+] (myeloid DCs), CD11b[−]CD11c[+] (lymphoid DCs), and CD11b[+]CD11c[−] (macrophages) cell populations in splenocytes from gp96tm transgenic female mice treated with vehicle (n = 9) and GPM1 (n = 9) at 30mg/kg. (E) Cell surface ICOSL[+]CD11b[+]CD11c[−] cell populations in lymph nodes from gp96tm

transgenic female mice treated with vehicle (n = 9) and GPM1 (n = 9) at 30mg/kg. Freshly isolated CD11c$^+$ splenic DCs from vehicle- or GPM1-treated mice were tested for their abilities to stimulate allogeneic naïve WT CD4$^+$ T cells to produce TNFα (F) and IFNγ (G). Student t-test P values are indicated.

symptoms (Fig. 5A and 5B, middle columns). Proteinuria, the sign of kidney dysfunction, the serum levels of nuclear antigen-specific and double stranded DNA-specific autoantibodies were also reduced in GPM1-treated mice (Fig. 5C, D and E, respectively). GPM1 treatment improved hypergammaglobulinemia symptom shown in these mice [29] as determined by total serum levels of IgG1, IgG2b, IgG3, IgM, and IgA (Fig. 5F).

These results show that the selective suppression of cell surface gp96 in gp96tm transgenic mice reduced SLE disease severity. We document possible one mechanism for this recovery, the reduction of DC maturation. These results suggest that the surface gp96 is critical cause of SLE-like disease and may be a useful target in the treatment of SLE.

Discussion

SLE is a clinically heterogeneous autoimmune disorder with diverse genetic causes [36], and the genes encoding HLA class II, mannose binding protein (MBP), TNFα, the T cell receptor,

interleukin 6 (IL-6), CR1, immunoglobulin Gm and Km allotypes, FcgRIIA and FcgRIIIA (both IgG Fc receptors), and heat shock protein 70 are thought to be associated with SLE [37]. Despite the complex molecular etiology of SLE, corticosteroids are commonly used to treat most of the SLE patients but long term usage of these drugs may induce numerous side effects, urging a need to develop more target- or mechanism-based therapy with less adverse effect. In this study, Dex showed several side effects on mouse and splenocyte survival (Fig. 3A and B), and abdominal obesity (data not shown) although Dex reduced phenotypes associated with SLE. However, GPM1 did not show any effect on survival or organ problems (data not shown) according to the long-term treatment. At this moment, we do not yet know how much portion of human SLE results from aberrant localization of gp96, and how the effect of GPM1 is in other spontaneous lupus animal models. These issues are currently under investigation.

The clinical need for novel targets and therapies for human autoimmune disease is high. Previous reports have demonstrated that several novel targets and drug-like compounds for autoim-

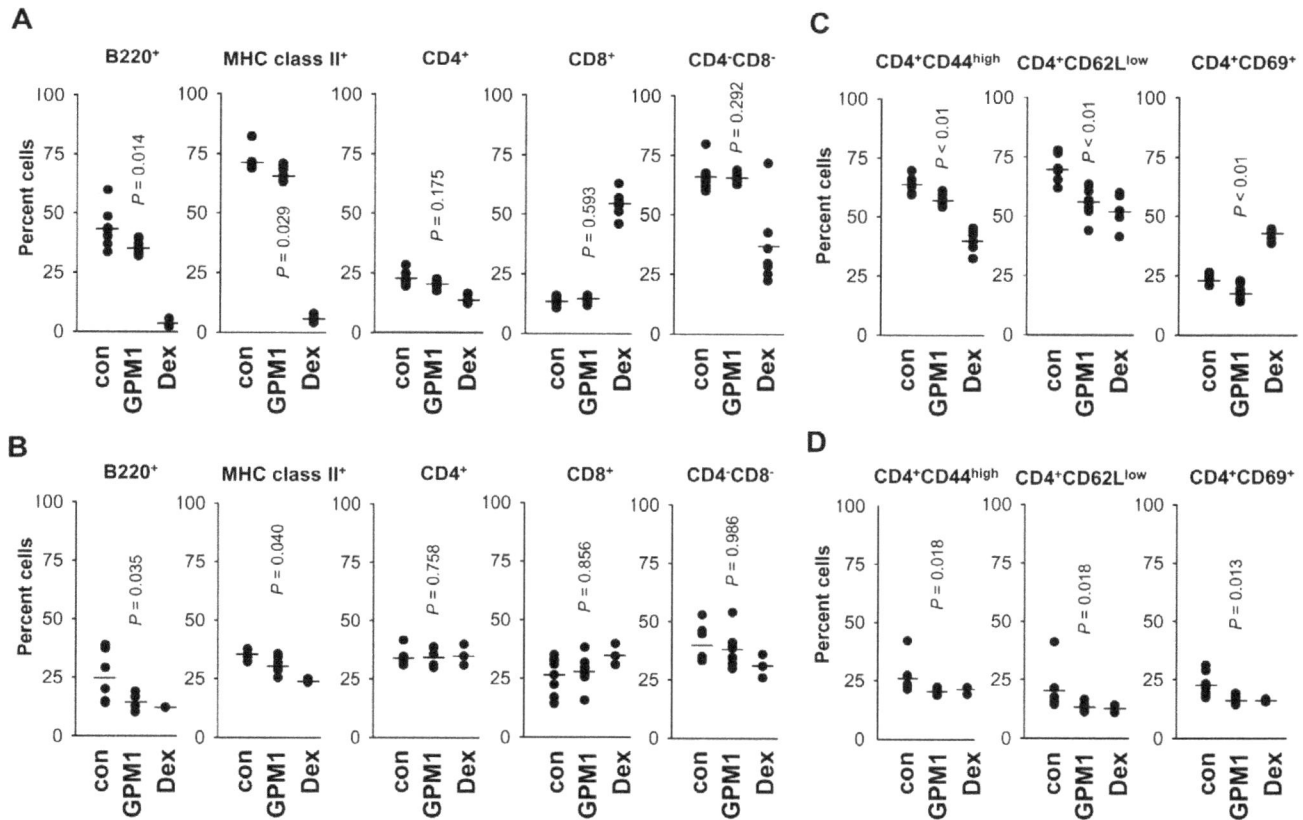

Figure 4. *In vivo* effect of the selected compound on various immune cells. (A) Percentage of B220$^+$, MHC class II$^+$, CD4$^+$, CD8$^+$, CD4 and CD8 double negative cell populations in splenocytes from gp96tm transgenic female mice treated with vehicle (n = 9), GPM1 (n = 9), and dexamethasone (n = 7) at 30mg/kg. (B) Percentages of B220$^+$, MHC class II$^+$, CD4$^+$, CD8$^+$, CD4 and CD8 double negative cell populations in lymph nodes from gp96tm transgenic female mice treated with vehicle (n = 9), GPM1 (n = 9), and dexamethasone (n = 7) at 30mg/kg. (C) Percentage of CD4$^+$CD44^{high} (memory T cells), CD4$^+$CD62L^{low} (effector T cells), and CD4$^+$CD69$^+$ (activated T cells) in splenocytes from gp96tm transgenic female mice treated with vehicle (n = 9), GPM1 (n = 9), and dexamethasone (n = 7) at 30mg/kg. (D) Percentages of CD4$^+$CD44^{high}, CD4$^+$CD62L^{low}, and CD4$^+$CD69$^+$ lymph node cells in vehicle- (n = 9), GPM1- (n = 9), and dexamethasone- (n = 7) treated mice. Student t-test P values comparing GPM1-treated mice with control are indicated.

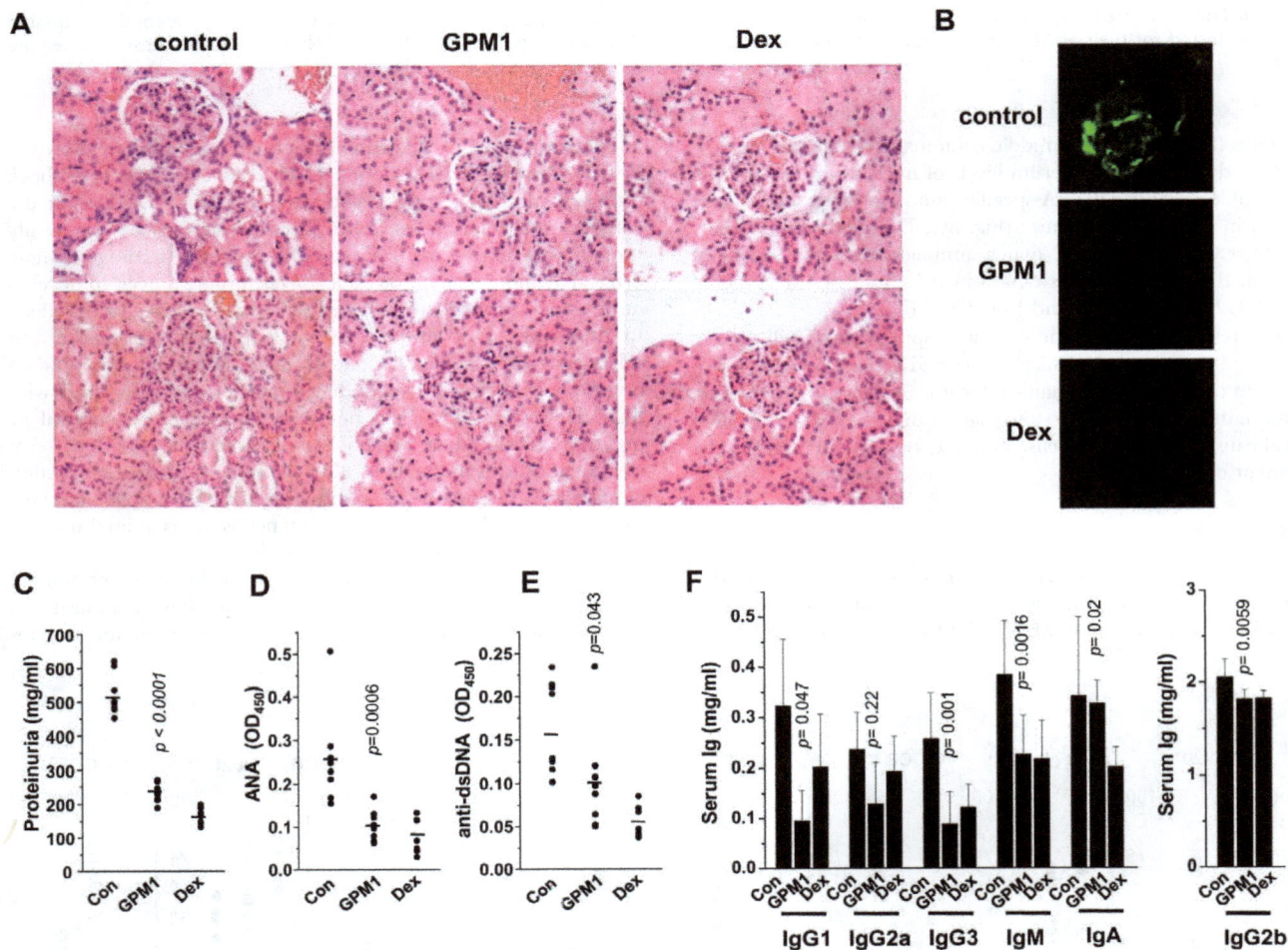

Figure 5. *In vivo* **effect of the selected compound on SLE-associated phenotypes in gp96tm transgenic mice.** (A) Representative kidney sections stained with hematoxylin and eosin from control (n = 9), GPM1- (n = 9) and dexamethasone (Dex)-treated (n = 7) groups. (B) Glomerular immunoglobulin deposition is shown by green fluorescence with FITC-conjugated goat anti-mouse Ig antibody in vehicle and GPM1-treated kidney. (C) Protein concentrations (mg/ml) in the urines, serum levels of nuclear antigen-specific (D) and double strand DNA-specific antibody (E) were compared between control (n = 9), GPM1- (n = 9) and dexamethasone (Dex)-treated (n = 7) groups. Arbitrary units represent autoantibody absorbance at OD_{450nm} at 1: 101 serum dilution. (F) Serum Ig levels from control (n = 9), GPM1- (n = 9), and Dex-treated (n = 7) groups by ELISA. Total IgG1, IgG2a, IgG2b, IgG3, IgM, and IgA levels were determined using sandwich ELISA kits from Southern Biotechnology Associates (Birmingham, AL). Data represent the mean±S.D. Student t-test *P* values comparing GPM1-treated mice with control are shown.

mune diseases are identified. Björk *et al.* identified human S100A9 as a novel target for autoimmune disease via binding to Quinoline-3-carboxamides [38]. Neubert *et al.* reported that proteosome inhibitor bortezomib successfully depletes plasma cells and protects mice from lupus [39]. Barber *et al.* reported that PI3Kγ inhibitor blocks SLE symptoms [40]. Johnson *et al.* reported that mitochondrial F_1F_0-ATPase, which is a target of benzodiazepine Bz-423, is a useful target for lupus [41]. In this study, we are suggesting that cell surface gp96 is also candidate target for lupus.

GPM1 directly interacts with gp96 and hydrophobic residues of gp96 within dimerization domain are important to GPM1 binding (Fig. 1E and F). Crystal structure of mammalian gp96 shows that along with the dimerization interface, helix C4 and helix C5 of the C domain of gp96 contains GPM1 binding motifs [18]. In the vicinity of helix C4 and C5, Helix C6 of the C-terminal domain of gp96 forms disordered straps to give stability to the gp96 dimer. In our result, since GPM1 confers slight helical change of gp96 (Fig. S2C) and dimer/oligomer formation

of gp96 (Fig. 2G–I), we speculate that GPM1 stabilizes disordered helix C6 straps of the C-terminal domain of gp96 to lead gp96 dimer formation.

SLE is characterized by abnormalities in dendritic cell (DCs), autoreactive T cells and B cells [1],[2]. DCs are important in regulating both immunity and tolerance and have been implicated in the pathogenesis of SLE [1]. DCs induce naïve T cell activation and stimulate B cell growth and differentiation. The lupus-associated DCs producing altered signals amplify autoreactive specificities in T cells, which, in turn, stimulate autoreactive B cells, leading to the increase of autoantibodies. Since cell surface gp96 induced significant DC activations [29],[32], we employed a chemical method to intervene over-maturation of DCs via gp96. The results of this work consistently show that aberrant surface exposure of gp96 can be chemically controlled. The selective suppression of cell surface gp96 reduced the incidence and severity of SLE-associated phenotypes, suggesting gp96 as a potential target to control autoimmune disease like SLE.

Materials and Methods

Drug Administration

Female gp96tm transgenic mice were bred and maintained at the animal center for pharmaceutical research, Seoul National University. We used age-matched, 12~26 weeks old mice in each experimental group. To suppress cell surface gp96 we used GPM1 compound. Dexamethasone and GPM1 were dissolved in 5% DMSO in phosphate-buffered saline (PBS) and control vehicle was 5% DMSO in PBS. Compounds were administered i.p. every 24h for 2 months (30mg/kg/day). Three groups of each 9 mice were examined. All procedures were conducted in accordance with the *Guide for the Care and Use of Laboratory Animals*, published by the Korean National Institute of Health. This study was approved by Review Board of Institute of Laboratory Animal Resources of Seoul National University.

Flow Cytometry

Spleen and lymph node cell suspensions were prepared by grinding tissue through sterile mesh and erythrocytes were lysed with RBC lysis buffer (eBioscience, CA). For surface staining, antibodies were fluoresceinisothiocyanate (FITC)-, phycoerythrin (PE)-, PerCP-, or APC-conjugated. Antibodies used were CD4 (RM4-5, H129.12), CD8 (53-6,7), B220 (RA3-6B2), CD11b (M1/70), CD11c (HL3), CD44 (IM7), CD62L (MEL-14), CD69 (H1.2F3), CD25 (PC61.5), IgM (11/41), IgD (11-26C.2a), calreticulin (BD Pharmingen, CA), MHC class II (M5/114.15.2), Foxp3 (FJK-16s) (eBioscience, CA), gp96(Santacruz, CA), and PDI (Assay Designs, MI). After staining, cells were washed and analyzed on a FACScan flow cytometer using CellQuest software (BD Bioscience, Mountain View, CA).

Mixed Lymphocyte Reaction

Splenic DCs (8×10^3) from vehicle- or GPM1-treated mice were purified using CD11c magnetic beads (Miltenyi Biotec, Auburn, CA), fixed with 1% paraformaldehyde, and co-cultured with 1.5×10^5 purified allogeneic CD4$^+$ T cells. Culture supernatants were collected for TNFα assay using ELISA kit from Pierce Biotechnology Inc. (Rockford, IL).

ELISA Assay for Chemical Screening

96-well plates (Maxisorp., F96; Nunc) were coated with 500ng/well AIMP1in PBS (pH 7.4). After washing, the remaining sites were blocked with PBS containing 1% BSA for 1h. Binding of 10ng/well biotin-conjugated gp96 was performed in Tris buffer (25 mM Tris, 10 mM NaCl and 0.4% Triton X-100). Each of the 6,580 compounds was added to the well at 100nM and the plates were washed and incubated with HRP-conjugated streptavidin in PBS containing 0.1% BSA and 0.1% Tween 20 for 30 min. The plates were washed, and then substrate was added to each well. The absorbance was monitored at 450 nm.

Histology

Kidney tissue sections of gp96tm transgenic mice were fixed in 10% formaldehyde in PBS and dehydrated using an alcohol gradient. After paraffin infiltration, the tissues were sectioned using a microtome, stained with hematoxylin and eosin (H&E) and analyzed by light microscopy. For immunofluorescent staining, kidneys were sectioned with a cryostat. These cryosections were blocked with normal goat serum, stained with FITC-conjugated goat anti-mouse Ig (BD pharmingen, CA), and then observed by fluorescent microscopy. Glomerulonephitis was quantitated according to Berden scores [42].

Surface Plasmon Resonance (SPR)

Human gp96 was expressed as His tag fusion protein in *Escherichia coli* BL21 (DE3) and purified by nickel affinity chromatography. His-tagged human gp96 was immobilized onto CM5 sensor chips using standard amine coupling[2]. PBS was used as a running buffer. The carboxymethyl dextran surface within one side of the flow cell was activated with a 7-min injection of a 1:1 ratio of 0.4M EDC and 0.1M NHS. The protein was coupled to the surface with a 7-min injection of gp96 diluted in 10mM sodium acetate, pH 3.7. Remaining activated groups were blocked with a 7-min injection of 1.0M ethanolamine, pH 8.5. GPM1 compound was dissolved directly in the PBS running buffer containing 1% DMSO and injected at a flow rate of 20μl/min at 25°C and the binding was determined by the change in resonance units (RU). The compound concentration varied from 10nM to 25μM and each concentration was tested at least three times. All of the bound complexes dissociated back to baseline within a reasonable time frame; therefore, no regeneration was required. Sensorgram was processed by subtracting the binding response recorded from the control surface, followed by subtracting an average of the buffer blank injections from the reaction spot[3]. To determine kinetic rate constants, all data sets were fit to a simple 1:1 binding with drifting baseline model using BIAevaluation program.

Purification of gp96

His-tagged gp96 protein was expressed in *E. coli* BL21 (DE3) and purified by nickel affinity chromatography and by gel filtration chromatography, and dialyzed against buffer (25mM Tris-HCl, pH7.5, 50 mM NaCl).

Circular dichroism (CD)

The gp96-GPM1 complex was prepared at a molar ratio 1:10 (5μM:50μM) in 250μl of buffer (25mM Tris-HCl, pH7.5, 50mM NaCl). The final concentration of DMSO was 0.1%. The complex was incubated at 20°C for 1h before CD measurements were taken. Samples were loaded in a 0.2 cm CD cell, and the spectra were acquired at 20°C using Jasco J-810. Wavelength scans were performed between 195 and 260 nm. The signal was digitized at 1nm intervals and each final scan was an average of 3 repeats and is presented after baseline buffer correction.

FPLC of gp96

FPLC gel filtration was used to separate gp96 monomer, dimer, and oligomer. gp96 or gp96-GPM1 complex containing a 1:10 molar ratio of gp96 to GPM1 were injected into a Superdex 200 10/300 GL (GE healthcare, 10 mm i.d. ×30 cm length) size exclusion column. The elution (0.5 ml/min) was carried out with buffer (20mM KH$_2$PO$_4$, 500mM NaCl, pH7.8, 2mM β-mercaptoethanol, 300mM imidazole). Fractions of a volumn of 0.5 ml were collected during 60 min.

Statistical analysis

The student's *t*-test was used for statistical analysis. *P* values of <0.05 were considered to represent statistically significant differences.

Supporting Information

Figure S1 The binding of GPM1 to protein disulfide isomerase (PDI) (A) and GRP78/Bip (B) were examined by surface plasmon resonance (SPR). GPM1 at the indicated concentrations was injected to immobilized PDI and GRP78/Bip, and the binding was measured using Biacore 3000. The response data were processed using data from a reference surface and buffer injections. Equilibrium dissociation constant (KD) was determined for the interaction of GPM1 with PDI and GRP78/Bip.

Figure S2 The effect of point mutations on the ATPase activity of gp96. The effect of gp96 point mutations on its ATPase activity was examined using ATPase assay kit (Innova Biosciences, Cambridge, UK). One unit is the amount of enzyme that catalyzes the reaction of 1µmol substrate per minute. The enzymatic activity was calculated according to manufacturer's instruction.

Figure S3 The effect of GPM1 on gp96 ATPase activity and conformational change. (A) The dose-dependent effect of GPM1 on the ATPase activity of gp96. The gp96 activity in the absence of GPM1 was 0.02066 ± 0.00334 unit/ml and GPM1 showed little effect on the ATPase activity within the range of the tested concentration (0 vs. 100µM, p = 0.071). (B) Circular dichroism spectrum of free and GPM1-bound gp96 protein. GPM1 (50µM, >95% purity) was mixed with gp96 (5µM). The CD spectra were normalized by buffer containing 0.1% DMSO.

Table S1 Summary of the screening of the chemicals derived from the primary hits that inhibit the interaction between gp96 and AIMP1 more than 95% of the control at 0.1µM.

Table S2 Comparison of glomerulonephritis in gp96tm transgenic mice treated with vehicle (n = 9), GPM1 (n = 9), or dexamethasone (n = 7). Glomerulonephitis was quantitated according to Berden scores [26].

Acknowledgments

We thank Dr. Bairagi C. Mallick and Dr. Sa-Ouk Kang, Seoul National University, for CD analysis.

Author Contributions

Conceived and designed the experiments: JMH. Performed the experiments: JMH NHK JYL SJJ. Analyzed the data: JMH NHK JYL. Contributed reagents/materials/analysis tools: HJJ HRK ZL SK. Wrote the paper: JMH ZL SK.

References

1. Monrad S, Kaplan MJ (2007) Dendritic cells and the immunopathogenesis of systemic lupus erythematosus. Immunol Res 37: 135–145.
2. Nagy G, Koncz A, Perl A (2005) T- and B-cell abnormalities in systemic lupus erythematosus. Crit Rev Immunol 25: 123–140.
3. Singer GG, Carrera AC, Marshak-Rothstein A, Martinez C, Abbas AK (1994) Apoptosis, Fas and systemic autoimmunity: the MRL-lpr/lpr model. Curr Opin Immunol 6: 913–920.
4. Wakeland EK, Wandstrat AE, Liu K, Morel L (1999) Genetic dissection of systemic lupus erythematosus. Curr Opin Immunol 11: 701–707.
5. Chatham WW, Kimberly RP (2001) Treatment of lupus with corticosteroids. Lupus 10: 140–147.
6. Li Z, Dai J, Zheng H, Liu B, Caudill M (2002) An integrated view of the roles and mechanisms of heat shock protein gp96-peptide complex in eliciting immune response. Front Biosci 7: d731–751.
7. Pelham HR (1991) Recycling of proteins between the endoplasmic reticulum and Golgi complex. Curr Opin Cell Biol 3: 585–591.
8. Letourneur F, Gaynor EC, Hennecke S, Demolliere C, Duden R, et al. (1994) Coatomer is essential for retrieval of dilysine-tagged proteins to the endoplasmic reticulum. Cell 79: 1199–1207.
9. Wieland F, Harter C (1999) Mechanisms of vesicle formation: insights from the COP system. Curr Opin Cell Biol 11: 440–446.
10. Barlowe C (2000) Traffic COPs of the early secretory pathway. Traffic 1: 371–377.
11. Semenza JC, Hardwick KG, Dean N, Pelham HR (1990) ERD2, a yeast gene required for the receptor-mediated retrieval of luminal ER proteins from the secretory pathway. Cell 61: 1349–1357.
12. Griffiths G, Ericsson M, Krijnse-Locker J, Nilsson T, Goud B, et al. (1994) Localization of the Lys, Asp, Glu, Leu tetrapeptide receptor to the Golgi complex and the intermediate compartment in mammalian cells. J Cell Biol 127: 1557–1574.
13. Majoul I, Straub M, Hell SW, Duden R, Soling HD (2001) KDEL-cargo regulates interactions between proteins involved in COPI vesicle traffic: measurements in living cells using FRET. Dev Cell 1: 139–153.
14. Lewis MJ, Pelham HR (1992) Ligand-induced redistribution of a human KDEL receptor from the Golgi complex to the endoplasmic reticulum. Cell 68: 353–364.
15. Majoul I, Sohn K, Wieland FT, Pepperkok R, Pizza M, et al. (1998) KDEL receptor (Erd2p)-mediated retrograde transport of the cholera toxin A subunit from the Golgi involves COPI, p23, and the COOH terminus of Erd2p. J Cell Biol 143: 601–612.
16. Neve EP, Lahtinen U, Pettersson RF (2005) Oligomerization and intracellular localization of the glycoprotein receptor ERGIC-53 is independent of disulfide bonds. J Mol Biol 354: 556–568.
17. Nemoto T, Sato N (1998) Oligomeric forms of the 90-kDa heat shock protein. Biochem J 330(Pt 2): 989–995.
18. Dollins DE, Warren JJ, Immormino RM, Gewirth DT (2007) Structures of GRP94-nucleotide complexes reveal mechanistic differences between the hsp90 chaperones. Mol Cell 28: 41–56.
19. Chadli A, Ladjimi MM, Baulieu EE, Catelli MG (1999) Heat-induced oligomerization of the molecular chaperone Hsp90. Inhibition by ATP and geldanamycin and activation by transition metal oxyanions. J Biol Chem 274: 4133–4139.
20. Srivastava P (2002) Interaction of heat shock proteins with peptides and antigen presenting cells: chaperoning of the innate and adaptive immune responses. Annu Rev Immunol 20: 395–425.
21. Srivastava P (2002) Roles of heat-shock proteins in innate and adaptive immunity. Nat Rev Immunol 2: 185–194.
22. Hilf N, Singh-Jasuja H, Schwarzmaier P, Gouttefangeas C, Rammensee HG, et al. (2002) Human platelets express heat shock protein receptors and regulate dendritic cell maturation. Blood 99: 3676–3682.
23. Basu S, Binder RJ, Suto R, Anderson KM, Srivastava PK (2000) Necrotic but not apoptotic cell death releases heat shock proteins, which deliver a partial maturation signal to dendritic cells and activate the NF-kappa B pathway. Int Immunol 12: 1539–1546.
24. Banerjee PP, Vinay DS, Mathew A, Raje M, Parekh V, et al. (2002) Evidence that glycoprotein 96 (B2), a stress protein, functions as a Th2-specific costimulatory molecule. J Immunol 169: 3507–3518.
25. Binder RJ, Han DK, Srivastava PK (2000) CD91: a receptor for heat shock protein gp96. Nat Immunol 1: 151–155.
26. Basu S, Binder RJ, Ramalingam T, Srivastava PK (2001) CD91 is a common receptor for heat shock proteins gp96, hsp90, hsp70, and calreticulin. Immunity 14: 303–313.
27. Vabulas RM, Braedel S, Hilf N, Singh-Jasuja H, Herter S, et al. (2002) The ER-resident heat shock protein Gp96 activates dendritic cells via the TLR2/4 pathway. J Biol Chem.
28. Singh-Jasuja H, Scherer HU, Hilf N, Arnold-Schild D, Rammensee HG, et al. (2000) The heat shock protein gp96 induces maturation of dendritic cells and down-regulation of its receptor. Eur J Immunol 30: 2211–2215.
29. Liu B, Dai J, Zheng H, Stoilova D, Sun S, et al. (2003) Cell surface expression of an endoplasmic reticulum resident heat shock protein gp96 triggers MyD88-dependent systemic autoimmune diseases. Proc Natl Acad Sci U S A 100: 15824–15829.
30. Huang QQ, Sobkoviak R, Jockheck-Clark AR, Shi B, Mandelin AM, 2nd, et al. (2009) Heat shock protein 96 is elevated in rheumatoid arthritis and activates macrophages primarily via TLR2 signaling. J Immunol 182: 4965–4973.
31. Lee SWKG, Kim S (2008) Aminoacyl-tRNA synthetase-interacting multi-functional protein 1/p43: an emerging therapeutic protein working at systems level. Exp Opinion Drug Discovery 3: 945–957.
32. Han JM, Park SG, Liu B, Park BJ, Kim JY, et al. (2007) Aminoacyl-tRNA Synthetase-Interacting Multifunctional Protein 1/p43 Controls Endoplasmic Reticulum Retention of Heat Shock Protein gp96: Its Pathological Implications in Lupus-Like Autoimmune Diseases. Am J Pathol 170: 2042–2054.
33. Kunst CB, Mezey E, Brownstein MJ, Patterson D (1997) Mutations in SOD1 associated with amyotrophic lateral sclerosis cause novel protein interactions. Nat Genet 15: 91–94.
34. Teague SJ, Davis AM, Leeson PD, Oprea T (1999) The Design of Leadlike Combinatorial Libraries. Angew Chem Int Ed Engl 38: 3743–3748.
35. Robert J, Menoret A, Cohen N (1999) Cell surface expression of the endoplasmic reticular heat shock protein gp96 is phylogenetically conserved. J Immunol 163: 4133–4139.
36. Schur PH (1995) Genetics of systemic lupus erythematosus. Lupus 4: 425–437.
37. Mok CC, Lau CS (2003) Pathogenesis of systemic lupus erythematosus. J Clin Pathol 56: 481–490.

38. Bjork P, Bjork A, Vogl T, Stenstrom M, Liberg D, et al. (2009) Identification of human S100A9 as a novel target for treatment of autoimmune disease via binding to quinoline-3-carboxamides. PLoS Biol 7: e97.
39. Neubert K, Meister S, Moser K, Weisel F, Maseda D, et al. (2008) The proteasome inhibitor bortezomib depletes plasma cells and protects mice with lupus-like disease from nephritis. Nat Med 14: 748–755.
40. Barber DF, Bartolome A, Hernandez C, Flores JM, Redondo C, et al. (2005) PI3Kgamma inhibition blocks glomerulonephritis and extends lifespan in a mouse model of systemic lupus. Nat Med 11: 933–935.
41. Johnson KM, Chen X, Boitano A, Swenson L, Opipari AW, Jr., et al. (2005) Identification and validation of the mitochondrial F1F0-ATPase as the molecular target of the immunomodulatory benzodiazepine Bz-423. Chem Biol 12: 485–496.
42. Berden JH, Hang L, McConahey PJ, Dixon FJ (1983) Analysis of vascular lesions in murine SLE. I. Association with serologic abnormalities. J Immunol 130: 1699–1705.

12

Risk of Subsequent Coronary Heart Disease in Patients Hospitalized for Immune-Mediated Diseases

Bengt Zöller[1]*, **Xinjun Li**[1], **Jan Sundquist**[1,2], **Kristina Sundquist**[1]

1 Center for Primary Health Care Research, Lund University/Region Skåne, Clinical Research Centre, Skåne University Hospital, Malmö, Sweden, 2 Stanford Prevention Research Center, Stanford University School of Medicine, Stanford, California, United States of America

Abstract

Background: Certain immune-mediated diseases (IMDs), such as rheumatoid arthritis and systemic lupus erythematosus, have been linked to cardiovascular disorders. We examined whether there is an association between 32 different IMDs and risk of subsequent hospitalization for coronary heart disease (CHD) related to coronary atherosclerosis in a nationwide follow up study in Sweden.

Methods and Findings: All individuals in Sweden hospitalized with a main diagnosis of an IMD (n = 336,479) without previous or coexisting CHD, between January 1, 1964 and December 31 2008, were followed for first hospitalization for CHD. The reference population was the total population of Sweden. Standardized incidence ratios (SIRs) for CHD were calculated. Overall risk of CHD during the first year after hospitalization for an IMD was 2.92 (95% CI 2.84–2.99). Twenty-seven of the 32 IMDs studied were associated with an increased risk of CHD during the first year after hospitalization. The overall risk of CHD decreased over time, from 1.75 after 1–5 years (95% CI 1.73–1.78), to 1.43 after 5–10 years (95% CI 1.41–1.46) and 1.28 after 10+ years (95% CI 1.26–1.30). Females generally had higher SIRs than males. The IMDs for which the SIRs of CDH were highest during the first year after hospitalization included chorea minor 6.98 (95% CI 1.32–20.65), systemic lupus erythematosus 4.94 (95% CI 4.15–5.83), rheumatic fever 4.65 (95% CI 3.53–6.01), Hashimoto's thyroiditis 4.30 (95% CI 3.87–4.75), polymyositis/dermatomyositis 3.81 (95% CI 2.62–5.35), polyarteritis nodosa 3.81 (95% CI 2.72–5.19), rheumatoid arthritis 3.72 (95% CI 3.56–3.88), systemic sclerosis 3.44 (95% CI 2.86–4.09), primary biliary cirrhosis 3.32 (95% CI 2.34–4.58), and autoimmune hemolytic anemia 3.17 (95% CI 2.16–4.47).

Conclusions: Most IMDs are associated with increased risk of CHD in the first year after hospital admission. Our findings suggest that many hospitalized IMDs are tightly linked to coronary atherosclerosis.

Editor: Thomas Forsthuber, University of Texas at San Antonio, United States of America

Funding: This work was supported by grants from the Swedish Research Council (2008-3110 and 2008-2638), the Swedish Council for Working Life and Social Research (2006-0386, 2007-1754 and 2007-1962), and Formas (2006-4255-6596-99 and 2007-1352), and from Region Skåne (REGSKANE-124611). The funders had no role in study design, data collection and analysis, decision to publish, or preparation of the manuscript.

Competing Interests: The authors have declared that no competing interests exist.

* E-mail: bengt.zoller@med.lu.se

Introduction

Coronary heart disease (CHD) and myocardial infarction are major causes of morbidity and mortality worldwide [1]. During recent years it has become clear that systemic inflammation can enhance atherogenesis [2],[3],[4]. Immune-mediated diseases (IMDs) are a heterogeneous group of disorders that are characterized by acute or chronic inflammation. Certain IMDs have been linked to an increased risk for cardiovascular disease (CVD) [5]. IMDs may increase the CVD risk through several mechanisms such as autoantibodies, autoantigens, autoreactive lymphocytes, epigenetic mechanisms, and inflammatory components driving the formation, progression and rupture of atherosclerotic plaques [2],[3],[4],[5],[6],[7]. Inflammation may also modulate the thrombotic responses by upregulating procoagulants, downregulating anticoagulants and suppressing fibrinolysis [7]. It

is therefore not surprising that inflammatory IMDs such as rheumatoid arthritis (RA) [3],[5],[6],[8],[9],[10],[11],[12] and systemic lupus erythematosus (SLE) [3],[5],[6],[8],[13],[14],[15] have been linked to an increased risk of CVD. An enhanced atherogenesis has also been suggested in several other IMDs such as Sjögren's disease [3],[5],[6],[16], systemic vasculitis [3],[5], inflammatory bowel disease [3],[5],[8][17], and psoriasis [8], [18].

We postulated that not only immune-mediated diseases such as RA and SLE, but also a number of other less well studied IMDs or related diseases have an increased risk of CVD. More specifically we aimed at determining whether IMDs increase the risk for hospitalized CHD related to coronary atheroslerosis. In a nationwide follow-up study from 1964–2008 we have estimated the risk of hospitalization with CHD in patients hospitalized with 32 different immune-mediated diseases whithout previous or coexisting CHD.

Methods

MigMed 2 Database

The study was approved by the Ethics Committee at Lund University and recommendations of the Declaration of Helsinki were complied with. Informed consent was waived as a requirement by the ethics committee. Data used in this study represented information on all individuals registered as residents of Sweden. It included individual-level information on age, sex, occupation, geographic region of residence, hospital diagnoses, and dates of hospital admissions in Sweden (1964–2008), as well as date of emigration, and date and cause of death. The datasources were several national Swedish data registers (reviewed by Rosen and Hakulinen) [19], including the Swedish National Population and Housing Census (1960–1990), the Total Population Register, the Multi-Generation register, and the Swedish Hospital Discharge register (1964–2008) [20], provided to us by Statistics Sweden and the National Board of Health and Welfare.

Information retrieved from the various registers was linked, at the individual level, via the national 10-digit personal identification number assigned to each resident of Sweden for his or her lifetime. Registration numbers were replaced by serial numbers to preserve anonymity. As well as being used to track all records in the dataset at the individual level, these serial numbers were used to check that individuals with hospital diagnoses of CHD appeared only once in the data set (for the first hospital diagnosis of CHD during the study period).

The follow-up period for analysis of these data in the present study started on January 1, 1964 and continued until hospitalisation for CHD, death, emigration, or the end of the study period (December 31, 2008). Data for first hospitalisation for CHD (main or secondary diagnosis) during the study period were retrieved from the Hospital Discharge Register (1964–2008), provided to us by the National Board of Health and Welfare. This register does not include data for hospital outpatients or patients treated at primary health care centres.

Predictor variable

The predictor variable was first hospitalization for a main diagnosis of an IMD, diagnosed according to ICD-7, ICD-8, ICD-9 and ICD-10 (Table S1). IMD patients with CHD (main or secondary diagnosis) before or at the same time as first hospitalization for IMD (n = 32,352) were excluded.

Outcome variable

Diagnosis of CHD was based on the 7th, 8th, 9th and 10th revisions of the International Classification of Diseases (ICD-7, ICD-8, ICD-9 and ICD-10). Cases with a main or secondary diagnosis of CHD were identified using the following ICD codes: 420 (ICD-7); 410-410 (ICD-8); 410-414 (ICD-9); and I20–I25 (ICD-10).

ICD 7
420.0: CHD
420.1: acute cardiac infarction
420.2: angina pectoris
420.9: old cardiac infarction
ICD 8
410: acute cardiac infarction
411: other acute and subacute forms of CHD
412: old cardiac infarction or chronic CHD
413: angina pectoris
414: asymptomatic CHD
ICD 9
410: acute cardiac infarction

411: other acute and subacute forms of CHD
412: old cardiac infarction
413: angina pectoris
414: other forms of chronic CHD
ICD 10
I20: angina pectoris
I21: acute cardiac infarction
I22: reinfarction (within 4 weeks)
I23: complications due to acute cardiac infarction
I24: other acute forms of CHD
I25: chronic CHD

Individual-level variables adjusted for in the model

The individual-level variables included in the analysis were sex, age, time period, geographic region of residence, socioeconomic status (SES) and comorbidity.

Sex: male or female.

Time period: time was divided into five periods in order to allow for adjustment for any change in incidence over time: 1964–1973, 1974–1983, 1984–1993, 1994–2003, and 2003–2008.

Age was divided into 5-year categories. Subjects of all ages were included in the study. Geographic region of residence was included as an individual-level variable to adjust for possible differences in hospital admissions for CHD between different geographic regions in Sweden. It was categorized as 1) large city (city with a population of >200,000 (i.e., Stockholm, Gothenburg or Malmo), 2) Southern Sweden (both rural and urban), and 3) Northern Sweden (both rural and urban).

Occupation was used as a proxy for SES. Occupational data were retrieved from national census records. We classified each individual's occupation into one of six categories: 1) manual worker, 2) lower-level employee, 3) middle-level employee/professional, 4) self-employed, 5) farmer, and 6) other. Homemakers and students without an occupation were categorized on the basis of their father's or mother's occupation. If that was not possible, they were included in the "other" category. Individuals without paid employment were also included in the "other" category. For individuals aged <20 years, parental occupation was used.

Comorbidity was defined as the first hospitalization with a main or secondary diagnosis at follow up from 1964–2008) of the following: 1) chronic lower respiratory diseases (500, 501 and 502 (ICD-7), 490–493 (ICD-8), 490–496 (ICD-9) and J40–J49 (ICD-10)); 2) obesity (287.00 and 287.99 (ICD-7), 277.99 (ICD-8), 278A (ICD-9) and E65–E68 (ICD-10)); 3) alcoholism (307, 322 and 581 (ICD-7), 291, 303 and 571 (ICD-8), 291 and 303 (ICD-9) and F10 and K70 (ICD-10)); 4) type 2 diabetes mellitus (260 (age>29 yr) (ICD-7), 250 (age>29 yr) (ICD-8), 250 (age>29 yr) (ICD-9) and E11–E14 (ICD-10); 5) hypertension (440–447 (ICD-7), 400 and 402–404 (ICD-8), 401–405 (ICD-9) and I10–I15 (ICD-10)); 6) atrial fibrillation (433.12 and 433.13 (ICD-7), 427.92 (ICD-8), 427D (ICD-9) and I48 (ICD-10)); 7) heart failure (434.10, 434.20 and 782.40 (ICD-7), 427.00, 427.10, 428.99 and 782.40 (ICD-8), 428 (ICD-9) and I50 (ICD-10)); 8) renal disease (590–601 and 757.10 (ICD-7), 580–591 and 753.1 (ICD-8), 580–591 and 753B (ICD-9) and N00–N19, Q61 (ICD-10)).

Statistical analysis

Person-years of risk (i.e., number of persons at risk multiplied by time at risk) were calculated from the time at which subjects were included in the study (in 1964 or later) until first hospitalization for a main or secondary diagnosis of CHD, death, emigration, or the end of the study period (December 31, 2008). Person-years for IMD patients (without main or secondary diagnosis of CHD before or at the same time as first hospitalization) were counted from discharge of the first hospitalization for IMD. The expected number of cases was based on the number of cases in the reference group. SIRs were calculated as the ratio of observed (O) and expected (E) number of CHD cases using the indirect standardization method [21]:

$$SIR = \frac{\sum_{j=1}^{J} o_j}{\sum_{j=1}^{J} n_j \lambda_j^*} = \frac{O}{E^*},$$

where $O = \sum o_j$ denotes the total observed number of cases in the study group; E^* (expected number of cases) is calculated by applying stratum-specific standard incidence rates (λ_j^*) obtained from the reference group to the stratum-specific person-years (n_j) of risk for the study group; o_j represents the observed number of cases that the cohort subjects contribute to the jth stratum; and J represents the strata defined by cross-classification of the different adjustment variables: age, sex, time period, SES, geographic region of residence, and comorbidity [21]. Ninety-five percent confidence intervals (95% CIs) were calculated assuming a Poisson distribution [21]. All analyses were performed using SAS version 9.2 (SAS Institute, Cary, NC, USA).

Results

Table S2 shows the number of people in the study who were admitted to hospital with any of the selected IMDs during the study period. Totally 32,352 IMD patients, with a CHD diagnosis before or at the same time as the first hospitalization for IMD, were excluded from the study. After this exclusion, a total of 336,479 patients hospitalized with an IMD (128,536 males and 207,943 females) remained in the study (Table S2). The three most common IMDs were rheumatoid arthritis (62,064 cases), Graves' disease (40,557) and ulcerative colitis (29,698).

Table 1 shows the total number of CHD cases in the entire population (1,934,822 individuals). Of these, 56,135 had had a previous hospitalization for IMDs. The comorbidities (defined as main or second hospital diagnosis) adjusted for are presented in Table 1. The risk of CHD was increased during the first year after hospitalization for 27 of the 32 IMDs studied (Table 2). The overall risk of CHD during the first year after hospitalization for an IMD was 2.92 (95% confidence interval (CI) 2.84–2.99). The overall risk of CHD decreased over time, from 1.75 after 1–5 years (95% CI 1.73–1.78), to 1.43 after 5–10 years (95% CI 1.41–1.46) and 1.28 after 10+ years (95% CI 1.26–1.30).

The risk of CHD was ≥3 during the first year after hospitalization for 13 IMDs (Table 2). For 18 IMDs, the risk of CHD was increased 10+ years after hospitalization, i.e., ankylosing spondylitis, Behçet's disease, type 1 diabetes mellitus, discoid lupus erythematosus, Graves'disease, Hashimoto's thyroiditis, immune thrombocytopenic purpura, pernicious anemia, polymyalgia rheumatica, polymyositis/dermatomyositis, psoriasis, rheumatic fever, rheumatoid arthritis, Sjögren's syndrome, systemic lupus erythematosus, systemic sclerosis, ulcerative colitis and Wegener's granulomatosis (Table 2).

The SIR for CHD was highest among individuals younger than 50 years but was increased also among older IMD patients (Table 3). The overall risk of CHD was increased in both males and females at different times after hospitalization with an IMD (Tables S3 and S4) and in all studied age groups (<50, 50–59, 60–69,70–79 and >80 years) (Tables S5 and S6). The SIR for CHD tended to be slightly higher for females with IMDs than males with IMDs (Tables S3, S4, S5, and S6). The overall risk of CHD for

females during the first year after hospitalization for an IMD was 3.06 (95% CI 2.96–3.17) versus 2.72 (95% CI 2.61–2.83) for males.

The overall risk of CHD was somewhat lower between 1994 and 2008 (SIR 1.42, 95% CI 1.40–1.44) than between 1964 and 1993 (SIR 1.58, 95% CI 1.56–1.60) (Table S7). This was observed both for females and males (Tables S8 and S9).

Overall risks of CHD were slightly higher for IMD patients who stayed in hospital for less than 7 days (overall SIR 1.63, 95% CI 1.61–1.64), compared to those who stayed 7 days or more (SIR 1.41, 95% CI 1.40–1.44) (Table S10).

Discussion

The present study is the first nationwide study of immune-mediated diseases and CHD. The results indicate that hospitalized immune-mediated diseases affect the risk of hospitalization for CHD in both males and females in all studied ages. The relative risk of hospitalized CHD during the first year after hospitalization with an IMD was even higher than for many traditional risk factors for CHD [22]. Although the CHD risk declined over time, the overall risk of CHD remained increased for 10 or more years. The results of our study are in line with previous studies linking rheumatoid arthritis [3][5][6][8][9][10][11][12], systemic lupus erythematosus [3],[5],[6],[8],[13],[14],[15], Sjögren's disease [3],[5],[6],[16], systemic vasculitis [3],[5], inflammatory bowel disease [3][5][8][17], and psoriasis [8],[18] to an increased risk of CVD. However, our study is unique because it includes a comparison of patients with a wide spectrum of IMDs with the general population in a nationwide setting, as well as a long-term follow-up of patients for CHD. Moreover, we also found a number of novel associations between IMDs and CHD. The results of the present study suggest that CHD due to coronary atherosclerosis is a common feature of several hospitalized IMDs. This risk is not limited to the period immediately following hospital admission: in the case of IMD for which there were sufficient numbers of cases for analysis it was sustained over time.

The increased risk of CHD may have different underlying causes in different IMDs although a general link between systemic inflammation and atherothrombosis is well established [2],[3],[4],[5],[6],[7]. It may be a reflection of more extreme cases of IMDs with severe inflammation, since the patients in our study had been admitted to hospital. The risk was also slightly higher among IMD patients who stayed in hospital for less than 7 days (SIR 1.63), compared to those who stayed 7 days or more (SIR 1.41). Although we cannot explain these findings, it is possible that those patients who stayed for more than a week also received some treatment for CHD risk factors, which could have decreased their CHD risk.

The effects of treatment (corticosteroids promote hemostasis) may contribute to the identified associations [23]. The fact that the risk of CHD decreased over time may suggest that the CHD risk is linked to the inflammatory activity of the IMD, which is likely to decrease over time due to treatment. In line with this hypothesis, several studies have suggested that disease activity is linked with atherosclerosis progression [24],[25]. Moreover, the risk of CHD for IMD patients was somewhat lower between 1994 and 2008 (SIR 1.42) than between 1964 and 1993 (SIR 1.58), which may reflect a general decrease in CHD rates over time or progressively more intensive antiinflammatoric treatment regimes in the recent decades. However, as we lack treatment data, we cannot test this hypothesis.

The present study has certain limitations. For example, we had no data on general cardiovascular risk factors such as body mass

Table 1. Number of cases of coronary heart disease (CHD), 1964–2008.

Characteristics	All CHD events		Subsequent CHD events of IMD patients	
	No.	%	No.	%
Gender				
Men	1109456	57.3	22270	39.7
Women	825366	42.7	33865	60.3
Age at diagnosis (yrs)				
<50	66777	3.5	1670	3.0
50–59	184444	9.5	3963	7.1
60–69	382388	19.8	9207	16.4
70–79	612816	31.7	18306	32.6
>=80	688397	35.6	22989	41.0
Period of diagnosis (yrs)				
1964–73	355086	18.4	1908	3.4
1974–83	497005	25.7	10221	18.2
1984–93	472520	24.4	17089	30.4
1994–03	424548	21.9	18546	33.0
2004–08	185663	9.6	8371	14.9
Socioeconomic status				
Farmers	186832	9.7	5225	9.3
Self-employed	130747	6.8	3700	6.6
Professionals	79564	4.1	2099	3.7
White collar workers	383918	19.8	13735	24.5
Workers	754431	39.0	25003	44.5
Others	399330	20.6	6373	11.4
Hospitalization for obesity				
Yes	4566	0.2	226	0.4
No	1930256	99.8	55909	99.6
Hospitalization for alcoholism				
Yes	41752	2.2	1509	2.7
No	1893070	97.8	54626	97.3
Hospitalization for chronic lower respiratory diseases				
Yes	82665	4.3	3912	7.0
No	1852157	95.7	52223	93.0
Hospitalization for hypertension				
Yes	43046	2.2	1783	3.2
No	1891776	97.8	54352	96.8
Hospitalization for diabetes type II				
Yes	115547	6.0	4963	8.8
No	1819275	94.0	51172	91.2
Hospitalization for artrial flutter				
Yes	122027	6.3	5171	9.2
No	1812795	93.7	50964	90.8
Hospitalization for heart failure				
Yes	289675	15.0	11796	21.0
No	1645147	85.0	44339	79.0
Hospitalization for renal disease				
Yes	62748	3.2	3606	6.4
No	1872074	96.8	52529	93.6
All	1934822	100.0	56135	100.0

Table 2. SIR for subsequent CHD of patients with IMD.

Immune-mediated diseases	Follow-up interval (years)																			
	<1				1–5				5–10				>=10				All			
	O	SIR	95% CI		O	SIR	95% CI		O	SIR	95% CI		O	SIR	95% CI		O	SIR	95% CI	
Addison's disease	36	3.06	2.14	4.24	90	1.78	1.43	2.18	51	1.38	1.03	1.81	35	1.03	0.71	1.43	212	1.59	1.38	1.82
Amyotrophic lateral sclerosis	153	2.47	2.10	2.90	183	2.21	1.90	2.56	65	1.43	1.11	1.83	81	1.23	0.97	1.52	482	1.88	1.72	2.06
Ankylosing spondylitis	53	2.61	1.95	3.41	215	1.82	1.58	2.08	170	1.38	1.18	1.61	415	1.12	1.02	1.24	853	1.35	1.26	1.45
Autoimmune hemolytic anemia	32	3.17	2.16	4.47	61	1.50	1.15	1.93	43	1.61	1.17	2.17	42	1.31	0.95	1.78	178	1.63	1.40	1.88
Behcet's disease	55	3.13	2.36	4.08	172	1.82	1.56	2.11	146	1.69	1.43	1.99	293	1.12	1.00	1.26	666	1.45	1.34	1.56
Celiac disease	37	2.57	1.81	3.54	116	1.43	1.18	1.71	95	1.25	1.01	1.52	138	0.86	0.72	1.01	386	1.16	1.05	1.28
Chorea minor	3	6.98	1.32	20.65	11	5.50	2.73	9.88	3	2.10	0.40	6.21	4	2.58	0.67	6.67	21	3.88	2.40	5.94
Crohn's disease	135	2.22	1.86	2.63	376	1.15	1.03	1.27	291	0.99	0.88	1.11	502	0.92	0.84	1.01	1304	1.06	1.01	1.12
Diabetes mellitus type I	0				8	5.56	2.37	11.00	16	4.97	2.83	8.09	488	3.02	2.76	3.30	512	3.08	2.82	3.36
Discoid lupus erythematosus	5	1.85	0.58	4.34	36	2.38	1.67	3.30	25	1.73	1.12	2.56	60	1.68	1.29	2.17	126	1.86	1.55	2.21
Grave's disease	474	2.43	2.21	2.66	1737	1.34	1.27	1.40	1621	1.23	1.18	1.30	3391	1.10	1.06	1.14	7223	1.23	1.20	1.25
Hashimoto's thyroiditis	375	4.30	3.87	4.75	903	2.03	1.90	2.16	533	1.58	1.45	1.72	774	1.39	1.30	1.49	2585	1.81	1.74	1.88
Immune thrombocytopenic purpura	46	2.69	1.97	3.60	127	1.60	1.34	1.91	82	1.40	1.11	1.73	86	1.28	1.03	1.58	341	1.53	1.38	1.71
Localized scleroderma	11	1.82	0.90	3.26	50	1.19	0.89	1.57	50	1.19	0.88	1.57	81	1.25	0.99	1.55	192	1.24	1.07	1.43
Lupoid hepatitis	4	2.34	0.61	6.05	8	1.29	0.55	2.55	7	1.54	0.61	3.19	14	0.81	0.44	1.37	33	1.11	0.77	1.56
Multiple sclerosis	150	2.96	2.50	3.47	382	1.54	1.39	1.70	257	1.30	1.14	1.47	330	0.97	0.87	1.08	1119	1.34	1.26	1.42
Myasthenia gravis	47	2.46	1.81	3.28	143	1.56	1.31	1.84	80	1.23	0.97	1.53	93	1.12	0.90	1.37	363	1.40	1.26	1.55
Pernicious anemia	294	1.90	1.69	2.13	1163	1.25	1.18	1.32	1001	1.33	1.25	1.42	1058	1.43	1.35	1.52	3516	1.36	1.32	1.41
Polyarteritis nodosa	40	3.81	2.72	5.19	97	2.12	1.72	2.58	43	1.13	0.82	1.53	68	1.19	0.93	1.51	248	1.64	1.44	1.86
Polymyalgia rheumatica	468	2.18	1.98	2.38	2031	1.65	1.58	1.72	1429	1.54	1.46	1.62	1741	1.42	1.35	1.49	5669	1.57	1.53	1.62
Polymyositis/ dermatomyositis	33	3.81	2.62	5.35	76	2.17	1.71	2.72	40	1.55	1.11	2.12	68	1.55	1.20	1.96	217	1.92	1.67	2.19
Primary biliary cirrhosis	37	3.32	2.34	4.58	51	1.71	1.28	2.26	30	1.40	0.95	2.01	43	1.36	0.98	1.83	161	1.72	1.46	2.00
Psoriasis	305	2.99	2.67	3.35	1197	2.02	1.91	2.14	799	1.52	1.42	1.63	1424	1.35	1.28	1.42	3725	1.64	1.59	1.69
Reiter's disease	2	2.02	0.19	7.43	10	1.43	0.68	2.64	9	1.31	0.59	2.50	13	1.69	0.90	2.91	34	1.51	1.04	2.11
Rheumatic fever	58	4.65	3.53	6.01	156	2.03	1.72	2.37	149	1.62	1.37	1.90	434	1.25	1.14	1.37	797	1.51	1.41	1.62
Rheumatoid arthritis	2088	3.72	3.56	3.88	6125	2.35	2.29	2.40	2970	1.73	1.67	1.80	2806	1.52	1.46	1.57	13989	2.08	2.04	2.11
Sarcoidosis	124	3.11	2.59	3.71	322	1.41	1.26	1.57	283	1.09	0.97	1.22	876	1.00	0.94	1.07	1605	1.15	1.09	1.20
Sjögren's syndrome	18	2.22	1.31	3.51	94	2.04	1.65	2.50	45	1.18	0.86	1.59	60	1.48	1.13	1.91	217	1.63	1.42	1.87
Systemic lupus erythematosus	138	4.94	4.15	5.83	357	2.78	2.50	3.09	225	2.11	1.84	2.41	288	1.60	1.42	1.79	1008	2.27	2.14	2.42
Systemic sclerosis	125	3.44	2.86	4.09	317	1.66	1.48	1.85	229	1.32	1.16	1.51	397	1.20	1.08	1.32	1068	1.46	1.37	1.55
Ulcerative colitis	205	2.07	1.80	2.38	756	1.33	1.24	1.43	609	1.17	1.07	1.26	998	1.08	1.01	1.15	2568	1.21	1.17	1.26
Wegener's granulomatosis	333	2.21	1.98	2.46	1417	1.47	1.39	1.55	1220	1.37	1.30	1.45	1747	1.54	1.47	1.62	4717	1.50	1.46	1.55
All	5884	2.92	2.84	2.99	18787	1.75	1.73	1.78	12616	1.43	1.41	1.46	18848	1.28	1.26	1.30	56135	1.55	1.53	1.56

O = observed number of cases; SIR = standardized incidence ratio; CI = confidence interval.
Bold type: 95% CI does not include 1.00.
Adjusted for age, period, socioeconomic status, hospitalization of chronic lower respiratory diseases, obesity, alcohol, hypertension, diabetes, arterial flutter, heart failure, and renal disease.

index (BMI), smoking, and diet, because it would be unrealistic to gather such data for an entire national population. However, we did adjust for socioeconomic status, which is associated with factors such as smoking. Adjustment was also made for eight different comorbidities (COPD, obesity, alcoholism and alcohol-related liver disease, hypertension, type 2 diabetes mellitus, atrial fibrillation, heart failure, and renal disease). We had no access to outpatient data, which means that only the most severe cases of immune-mediated diseases (i.e. those requiring hospitalization) were included in the analyses. Thus, although we adjusted for

Table 3. SIR for subsequent CHD of patients with IMD after one year of follow-up.

| Immune-mediated diseases | Age at diagnosis of CHD (years) | | | | | | | | | | | |
| | <50 | | | 50–59 | | | 60–69 | | | >=70 | | |
	O	SIR	95% CI	O	SIR	95% CI	O	SIR	95% CI	O	SIR	95% CI
Addison's disease	8	1.83	0.78 3.62	19	1.43	0.86 2.23	27	1.33	0.88 1.94	122	**1.46**	**1.21 1.74**
Amyotrophic lateral sclerosis	3	1.02	0.19 3.02	29	**2.90**	**1.94 4.17**	68	**2.04**	**1.58 2.58**	229	**1.55**	**1.36 1.76**
Ankylosing spondylitis	59	**1.58**	**1.21 2.04**	173	**1.33**	**1.14 1.55**	228	**1.19**	**1.04 1.36**	340	**1.35**	**1.21 1.50**
Autoimmune hemolytic anemia	1	0.63	0.00 3.58	3	0.68	0.13 2.02	18	1.45	0.86 2.29	124	**1.53**	**1.27 1.83**
Behcet's disease	48	**1.82**	**1.34 2.42**	81	**1.30**	**1.03 1.61**	114	**1.29**	**1.06 1.55**	368	**1.39**	**1.25 1.54**
Celiac disease	12	1.07	0.55 1.88	36	1.19	0.83 1.64	75	1.12	0.88 1.40	226	1.08	0.94 1.23
Chorea minor	1	9.09	0.00 52.11	3	**21.43**	**4.04 63.43**	2	3.57	0.34 13.13	12	**2.88**	**1.48 5.05**
Crohn's disease	70	0.95	0.74 1.21	173	0.85	0.73 0.99	265	0.93	0.82 1.05	661	**1.09**	**1.01 1.18**
Diabetes mellitus type I	453	**3.49**	**3.18 3.83**	58	**1.64**	**1.24 2.12**	1	0.93	0.00 5.31	0		
Discoid lupus erythematosus	3	1.71	0.32 5.07	16	**2.11**	**1.20 3.44**	41	**2.63**	**1.88 3.57**	61	**1.52**	**1.16 1.95**
Grave's disease	115	**1.27**	**1.05 1.52**	425	**1.23**	**1.12 1.35**	1084	**1.18**	**1.11 1.26**	5125	**1.18**	**1.15 1.21**
Hashimoto's thyroiditis	21	1.55	0.96 2.38	133	**2.33**	**1.95 2.76**	335	**1.90**	**1.70 2.11**	1721	**1.58**	**1.50 1.65**
Immune thrombocytopenic purpura	9	1.52	0.69 2.90	19	1.40	0.84 2.20	57	**1.85**	**1.40 2.39**	210	**1.36**	**1.18 1.55**
Localized scleroderma	1	0.98	0.00 5.62	4	1.12	0.29 2.91	10	0.70	0.33 1.28	166	**1.28**	**1.09 1.49**
Lupoid hepatitis	1	0.88	0.00 5.07	6	1.91	0.69 4.19	8	1.39	0.59 2.75	14	0.78	0.43 1.32
Multiple sclerosis	47	**1.94**	**1.43 2.59**	151	**1.46**	**1.24 1.72**	276	**1.40**	**1.24 1.57**	495	1.07	0.98 1.17
Myasthenia gravis	10	**2.19**	**1.04 4.04**	17	1.24	0.72 1.99	52	**1.40**	**1.04 1.83**	237	**1.28**	**1.13 1.46**
Pernicious anemia	3	0.75	0.14 2.21	39	1.37	0.98 1.88	176	1.15	0.99 1.34	3004	**1.34**	**1.29 1.39**
Polyarteritis nodosa	9	**3.24**	**1.47 6.17**	18	**1.88**	**1.11 2.98**	43	**1.59**	**1.15 2.14**	138	**1.36**	**1.14 1.61**
Polymyalgia rheumatica	78	**2.17**	**1.72 2.71**	308	**2.01**	**1.79 2.25**	582	**1.45**	**1.34 1.58**	4233	**1.51**	**1.47 1.56**
Polymyositis/dermatomyositis	4	1.85	0.48 4.79	20	**2.50**	**1.52 3.86**	36	**1.62**	**1.13 2.24**	124	**1.72**	**1.43 2.05**
Primary biliary cirrhosis	5	2.44	0.77 5.74	9	1.15	0.52 2.19	27	1.17	0.77 1.71	83	**1.67**	**1.33 2.07**
Psoriasis	121	**1.65**	**1.37 1.97**	457	**1.93**	**1.75 2.11**	783	**1.65**	**1.54 1.77**	2059	**1.49**	**1.42 1.55**
Reiter's disease	4	2.21	0.57 5.71	9	1.94	0.88 3.71	12	**2.42**	**1.24 4.24**	7	0.69	0.27 1.43
Rheumatic fever	69	**2.04**	**1.59 2.58**	139	**1.69**	**1.42 2.00**	184	**1.39**	**1.19 1.60**	347	**1.30**	**1.16 1.44**
Rheumatoid arthritis	110	**2.64**	**2.17 3.18**	505	**2.32**	**2.12 2.53**	2043	**2.47**	**2.37 2.58**	9243	**1.82**	**1.78 1.85**
Sarcoidosis	67	1.11	0.86 1.41	187	1.04	0.90 1.20	366	**1.17**	**1.05 1.29**	861	**1.07**	**1.00 1.14**
Sjögren's syndrome	3	2.33	0.44 6.88	9	1.26	0.57 2.40	51	**2.30**	**1.71 3.03**	136	**1.45**	**1.21 1.71**
Systemic lupus erythematosus	66	**5.90**	**4.56 7.51**	114	**3.04**	**2.51 3.65**	200	**2.40**	**2.08 2.75**	490	**1.73**	**1.58 1.89**
Systemic sclerosis	28	1.35	0.89 1.95	76	**1.41**	**1.11 1.76**	187	**1.58**	**1.36 1.82**	652	**1.30**	**1.20 1.40**
Ulcerative colitis	122	1.11	0.93 1.33	319	1.07	0.95 1.19	474	1.06	0.97 1.16	1448	**1.25**	**1.18 1.31**
Wegener's granulomatosis	5	1.38	0.44 3.25	48	**2.08**	**1.54 2.77**	279	**1.48**	**1.31 1.66**	4052	**1.46**	**1.42 1.51**
All	1556	**1.87**	**1.77 1.96**	3603	**1.51**	**1.46 1.56**	8104	**1.52**	**1.49 1.55**	36988	**1.44**	**1.42 1.45**

O = observed number of cases; SIR = standardized incidence ratio; CI = confidence interval.
Bold type: 95% CI does not include 1.00.
Adjusted for age, period, socioeconomic status, region of residence, hospitalization of chronic lower respiratory diseases, obesity, alcohol, hypertension, diabetes, arterial flutter, heart failure, and renal disease.

comorbidites residual confounding may still be present. However, we excluded all IMD cases with previous or coexisting CHD (n = 32,352) in order to minimize the risk for selection bias, which instead may have lead to an underestimation of the actual CHD risk in IMD patients. In fact, the relative risks for CHD among patients with RA or SLE in the present study are within the range previously reported for CVD for these two immune-mediated diseases [3],[5],[6],[8],[9],[10],[11],[12],[13],[14],[15]. It is therefore likely that risk estimates in the present study are fairly valid. Moreover, the present findings reflect the "real world" and the risk for subsequent CHD among hospitalized IMD patients without previous or coexisting CHD. Another problem might be that not all CHD are hospitalized. However, most cases of acute coronary syndrome should have been treated at hospitals in Sweden during the study period [26]. Moreover, incidence rates were calculated for the whole follow-up period, divided into time periods, and adjustments were made for possible changes in hospitalization rates over time due to different admission criteria.

This study also had a number of strengths. For instance, the study population included all patients hospitalized with IMD (without previous or coexisting CHD) and subsequently with CHD in Sweden during the study period, which eliminated recall bias.

Because of the personal identification number assigned to each resident in Sweden, it was possible to trace the records for every subject for the whole follow-up period. Data on occupation were 99.2% complete (1980 and 1990 census), which enabled us to adjust our models for socioeconomic status. A further strength of the present study was the use of validated hospital discharge data. The Hospital Discharge Register has high validity [19],[27],[28],[29], especially for cardiovascular disorders such as stroke, and myocardial infarction, for which approximately 95% of diagnoses have been shown to be correct [27],[28],[29]. Although, the positive predictive value (PPV) may differ between diagnoses in the Swedish Hospital Dicharge Register, the PPV is generally around 85–95% [29].

In summary, the risk of hospitalization for CHD was, for most immune-mediated diseases, found to be significantly increased during the first year after hospitalization. The risk for CHD decreased with time, but for many IMDs persisted for more than 10 years. The findings of the present study suggest that many hospitalized IMDs are tightly linked to coronary atherosclerosis. Further studies need to clarify the mechanisms behind our findings.

Supporting Information

Table S1 ICD codes of IMD and related conditions.

Table S2 Number of hospitalizations with a main diagnosis of IMD, 1964–2008.

Table S3 SIR for subsequent CHD of male patients with IMD.

Table S4 SIR for subsequent CHD of female patients with IMD.

Table S5 SIR for subsequent CHD of male patients with IMD after one year of follow-up.

Table S6 SIR for subsequent CHD of female patients with IMD after one year of follow-up.

Table S7 SIR for subsequent CHD of patients with IMD after one year of follow-up for time periods 1964–1993 and 1994–2008.

Table S8 SIR for subsequent CHD of male patients with IMD after one year of follow-up for time periods 1964–1993 and 1994–2008.

Table S9 SIR for subsequent CHD of female patients with IMD after one year of follow-up for time periods 1964–1993 and 1994–2008.

Table S10 SIR for all subsequent CHD of patients with IMD hospitalization length <7 days or 7 or more days.

Acknowledgments

The authors wish to thank the CPF's Science Editor Stephen Gilliver for his useful comments on the text. The registers used in the present study are maintained by Statistics Sweden and the National Board of Health and Welfare.

Author Contributions

Conceived and designed the experiments: BZ XL JS KS. Performed the experiments: BZ XL JS KS. Analyzed the data: BZ XL JS KS. Contributed reagents/materials/analysis tools: JS KS. Wrote the paper: BZ XL JS KS.

References

1. White HD, Chew DP (2008) Acute myocardial infarction. Lancet 372: 570–584.
2. Libby P (2002) Inflammation in atherosclerosis. Nature 420: 868–374.
3. van Leuven SI, Franssen R, Kastelein JJ, Levi M, Stroes ES, et al. (2008) Systemic inflammation as a risk factor for atherothrombosis. Rheumatology 47: 3–7.
4. Hansson GK, Hermansson A (2011) The immune system in atherosclerosis. Nature Immunology 12: 204–212.
5. Shoenfeld Y, Gerli R, Doria A, Matsuura E, Cerinic MM, Ronda N, et al. (2005) Accelerated atherosclerosis in autoimmune rheumatic diseases. Circulation 112: 3337–3347.
6. López-Pedrera C, Pérez-Sánchez C, Ramos-Casals M, Santos-Gonzalez M, Rodriguez-Ariza A, et al. (2012) Cardiovascular risk in systemic autoimmune diseases: epigenetic mechanisms of immune regulatory functions Clin Dev Immunoldoi:10.1155/2012/974648.
7. Xu J, Lupu F, Esmon CT (2010) Inflammation, innate immunity and blood coagulation. Hamostaseologie 30: 5–6, 8–9.
8. El-Gabalawy H, Guenther LC, Bernstein CN (2010) Epidemiology of immune-mediated inflammatory diseases: incidence, prevalence, natural history, and comorbidities. J Rheumatol Suppl 85: 2–10.
9. Lévy L, Fautrel B, Barnetche T, Schaeverbeke T (2008) Incidence and risk of fatal myocardial infarction and stroke events in rheumatoid arthritis patients. A systematic review of the literature. Clin Exp Rheumatol 26: 673–679.
10. Solomon DH, Karlson EW, Rimm EB, Cannuscio CC, Mandl LA, et al. (2003) Cardiovascular morbidity and mortality in women diagnosed with rheumatoid arthritis. Circulation 107: 1303–1307.
11. Gabriel SE (2008) Cardiovascular morbidity and mortality in rheumatoid arthritis. Am J Med 121: S9–S14.
12. Libby P (2008) Role of inflammation in atherosclerosis associated with rheumatoid arthritis. Am J Med 121: S21–S31.
13. Manzi S, Meilahn EN, Rairie JE, Conte CG, Medsger TA, Jr., et al. (1997) Age-specific incidence rates of myocardial infarction and angina in women with systemic lupus erythematosus: comparison with the Framingham Study. Am J Epidemiol 145: 408–415.
14. Asanuma Y, Oeser A, Shintani AK, Turner E, Olsen N, et al. (2003) Premature coronary-artery atherosclerosis in systemic lupus erythematosus. N Engl J Med 349: 2407–2415.
15. Roman MJ, Shanker BA, Davis A, Lockshin MD, Sammaritano L, et al. (2003) Prevalence and correlates of accelerated atherosclerosis in systemic lupus erythematosus. N Engl J Med 349: 2399–2406.
16. Vaudo G, Bocci EB, Shoenfeld Y, Schillaci G, Wu R, et al. (2005) Precocious intima-media thickening in patients with primary Sjogren's syndrome. Arthritis Rheum 52: 3890–3897.
17. van Leuven SI, Hezemans R, Levels JH, Snoek S, Stokkers PC, et al. (2007) Enhanced atherogenesis and altered high density lipoprotein in patients with Crohn's disease. J Lipid Res 48: 2640–2646.
18. Vizzardi E, Raddino R, Teli M, Gorga E, Brambilla G, et al. (2010) Psoriasis and cardiovascular diseases. Acta Cardiol 65: 337–340.
19. Rosen M, Hakulinen T (2005) Use of disease registers. In: Ahrens W, Pigeot I, eds. Handbook of epidemiology Springer-Verlag, Berlin. pp 231–52.
20. The Swedish Hospital Discharge Register 1987–1996: quality and contents. (1998) National Board of Health and Welfare, Stockholm.
21. Rothman KJ, Greenland S (1998) Modern Epidemiology, Second Edition Lippincott-Raven, Philadelphia.
22. O'Keefe JH, Carter MD, Lavie CJ (2009) Primary and secondary prevention of cardiovascular diseases: a practical evidence-based approach. Mayo Clin Proc 84: 741–757.
23. Jilma B, Cvitko T, Winter-Fabry A, Petroczi K, Quehenberger P, et al. (2005) High dose dexamethasone increases circulating P-selectin and von Willebrand factor levels in healthy men. Thromb Haemost 94: 797–801.
24. Westlake SL, Colebatch AN, Baird J, Kiely P, Quinn M, et al. (2010) The effect of methotrexate on cardiovascular disease in patients with rheumatoid arthritis: a systematic literature review. Rheumatology 49: 295–307.
25. Westlake SL, Colebatch AN, Baird J, Curzen N, Kiely P, et al. (2011) Tumour necrosis factor antagonists and the risk of cardiovascular disease in patients with rheumatoid arthritis: a systematic literature review. Rheumatology 50: 518–531.
26. Nationella riktlinjer för hjärtsjukvård 2008. Beslutsstöd för prioriteringar. (2008) In Swedish. National Board of Health and Welfare, Stockholm.
27. Validity of the diagnoses from the Swedish In-Care Register 1987 and 1995. (2000) In Swedish. National Board of Health and Welfare, Stockholm.

13

Deficiency of Activating Fcγ-Receptors Reduces Hepatic Clearance and Deposition of IC and Increases CIC Levels in Mercury-Induced Autoimmunity

Klara Martinsson[1]*[¤], Thomas Skogh[2], Seyed Ali Mousavi[4], Trond Berg[5], Jan-Ingvar Jönsson[3], Per Hultman[1]

1 Division of Molecular and Immunological Pathology (AIR), Department of Clinical and Experimental Medicine, Linköping University, Linköping, Sweden, 2 Rheumatology Unit (AIR), Department of Clinical and Experimental Medicine, Linköping University, Linköping, Sweden, 3 Experimental Hematology Unit, Department of Clinical and Experimental Medicine, Linköping University, Linköping, Sweden, 4 Medical Genetics Laboratory, Department of Medical Genetics, Rikshospitalet University Hospital, Oslo, Norway, 5 Department of Molecular Biosciences, University of Oslo, Oslo, Norway

Abstract

Background: Inorganic mercury (Hg) induces a T-cell dependent, systemic autoimmune condition (HgIA) where activating Fcγ-receptors (FcγRs) are important for the induction. In this study we examined the influence of activating FcγRs on circulating levels and organ localization of immune complexes (IC) in HgIA.

Methods and Principal Findings: Mercury treated BALB/c wt mice showed a significant but modest increase of circulating IC (CIC) from day 12 until day 18 and day 35 for IgG2a- and IgG1- CIC, respectively. Mercury-treated mice lacking the trans-membrane γ-chain of activating FcγRs (FcRγ$^{-/-}$) had significantly higher CIC levels of both IgG1-CIC and IgG2a-CIC than wt mice during the treatment course. The hepatic uptake of preformed CIC was significantly more efficient in wt mice compared to FcγR$^{-/-}$ mice, but also development of extrahepatic tissue IC deposits was delayed in FcRγ$^{-/-}$ mice. After 35 days of Hg treatment the proportion of immune deposits, as well as the amounts was significantly reduced in vessel FcRγ$^{-/-}$ mice compared to wt mice.

Conclusions: We conclude that mice lacking functional activating FcγRs respond to Hg with increased levels and altered quality of CIC compared with wt mice. Lack of functional activating FcγRs delayed the elimination of CIC, but also significantly reduced extrahepatic tissue localization of CIC.

Editor: Pierre Bobé, Institut Jacques Monod, France

Funding: The project was supported by the Swedish Research Council Branch of Medicine (project no. 9453), funds from the County Council of Ostergotland and Ingrid Asp foundation. The funders had no role in study design, data collection and analysis, decision to publish, or preparation of the manuscript.

Competing Interests: The authors have declared that no competing interests exist.

* E-mail: klara.martinsson@liu.se

¤ Current address: Department of Pharmacology and Therapeutics, MRC Centre for Drug Safety Science, University of Liverpool, Liverpool, United Kingdom

Introduction

The deposits of glomerular immune complexes (IC) is a hallmark of certain systemic autoimmune diseases with glomerulonephritis (GN) [1]. However, the formation of ICs is also a physiological function of the immune system in order to eliminate antigens and to regulate immune responses [2,3] . IgG-containing circulating ICs (CIC) are cleared via Fc-gamma receptor (FcγR) dependent uptake by Kupffer cells as well as liver sinusoidal endothelial cells [4–8]. In addition, hepatic elimination and extrahepatic deposition of CIC are affected by complement and complement receptors [9,10]. If the physiological mechanisms of hepatic IC-elimination fails, extrahepatic tissue deposition of IC may occur and lead to tissue inflammation and organ damage [1]. The damage following tissue IC deposits depends on the mechanism and site of formation, but especially on the amount of deposits and their composition [1]. Thus, tissue ICs in systemic inflammatory disease may be derived from the circulation, as indicated by murine autoimmune models [11,12], and in human diffuse proliferative lupus nephritis [13], or membranous GN [14]. The amount of CIC correlates with disease severity in systemic lupus erythematosus (SLE), where patients with overt nephritis show higher levels of CIC than patients with silent nephritis [15,16]. Tissue IC deposits may, however, also form *in situ*, either by the interaction of antibodies (abs) with antigens planted in the glomerulus, or by binding of abs to intrinsic glomerular antigens [17,18]. Formation of tissue IC deposits in SLE may be due to abnormal handling by FcγRs since hepatic FcγR-mediated IC clearance is less efficient in SLE patients than in healthy individuals [19].

All murine FcγRs ligate exposed Fcγ parts of ICs via the surface-exposed γ-chain: FcγRI, FcγRIII and FcγRVI, but not the inhibitory FcγRIIb, then promote cell activation via a signal-transducing trans-membrane dimeric γ-chain (FcRγ) residing the immune receptor tyrosine-based activation motif (ITAM) [20]. Furthermore, the trans-membrane FcRγ is essential for endocytosis of surface-bound soluble IgG-ICs and phagocytosis of IgG-opsonized particles via the stimulating FcγRs, although Fc-ligation remains intact [20,21]. FcγRIII is the predominant receptor in triggering immune effector functions following murine IgG1-IC binding [22]. The response is also influenced by the inhibitory FcγRIIb, where the immune receptor tyrosine-based inhibitory motif (ITIM) becomes phosphorylated upon Fc-ligation, thereby inhibiting ITAM- signalling [20]. In rats, the FcγRIIb2 of liver sinusoidal endothelial cells (LSEC) is used not only as a receptor for efficient CIC clearance, but also as a recycling receptor with or without ligated ICs [8].

Lack of FcγRIIB increases the incidence of nephritis in murine pristane-induced lupus [23], and may even cause spontaneous GN in some mouse strains [24]. A delicate balance between activating and inhibitory signals emanating from the FcγRs characterizes a normal immune response. This balance may be disturbed in autoimmune diseases [2,3,25].

The importance of the activating FcγRs (FcγRI, FcγRIII and FcγRIV in mice) and the inhibiting FcγRIIb in autoimmune diseases has been elucidated in mouse strains with targeted knockout mutations for these FcγRs [25,26]. We have previously used FcγR-deficient mice to explore the role of these receptors in HgIA [27,28], a model characterized by Hg-induced lymphopro-liferation, hypergammaglobulinaemia, antinucleolar autoantibod-ies (ANoA) and IC deposits in the renal glomerular mesangium and systemically in vessel walls in susceptible mouse strains [29]. In HgIA, activating FcγRs affect development of ANoA [28] as well as IC deposits [27], while the inhibiting FcγRIIb down-regulates the hyper-gammaglobulinaemic response [27,28].

In this study we aimed at elucidating the effect of the signal-transducing trans-membrane dimeric γ-chain of activating FcγRs in HgIA on levels of CIC, hepatic IC uptake, and the development and composition of IC deposits in typical target organs in systemic autoimmune disease.

Results

Firstly, we compare the levels of CIC in wildtype (wt) and FcRγ$^{-/-}$ BALB/c mice in relation to the development of tissue IC deposits during five weeks of Hg treatment. Secondly, we report differences regarding blood clearance and hepatic uptake of preformed model immune complexes in the two BALB/c strains. Thirdly, we analyse the composition of tissue IC deposits in the two mouse strains after five weeks of Hg treatment.

Increased levels of IgG1- and IgG2a-containing CIC are associated with development of high-titred tissue IC deposits in wt BALB/c mice but not in FcRγ$^{-/-}$ mice

Wt mice. BALB/c wt mice treated with Hg had significantly higher concentrations of CIC containing IgG1 (Figure 1A) and IgG2a (Figure 2) after 12 ($p<0.001$) and 18 ($p<0.001$) days of treatment, and regarding IgG1-CIC after 26 ($p<0.001$) and 35 ($p<0.001$) days as compared to untreated mice. Renal mesangial (Figure 1B) and splenic vessel wall (Figure 1C) IgG1 deposits were first seen after 16 days of Hg treatment, and the fraction of mice with IC deposits and/or the titre of the deposits increased until end of treatment after 35 days. Despite the increase of IgG2a-CIC in Hg-treated wt mice (Figure 2) neither renal mesangial nor splenic vessel wall deposits contained IgG2a (data not shown). While C3c deposits were seen already after 12 days treatment in the renal mesangium, C3c deposits were not seen in splenic vessel walls until the end of treatment after 35 days of Hg treatment (data not shown). None of the untreated wt mice showed IgG1, IgG2a

or C3c deposits in glomeruli or vessel walls at any time during the 35 days of Hg treatment (data not shown).

FcRγ$^{-/-}$ mice. In FcRγ$^{-/-}$ mice the levels of IgG1-containing CIC were highest after 12 days of Hg treatment (Figure 1A), but remained significantly increased compared to untreated FcRγ$^{-/-}$ mice during an additional 14 days of treatment (for 12 days $p<0.01$, 18 days $p<0.001$ and 26 days $p<0.01$). The IgG1-CIC level was significantly higher in Hg-treated FcRγ$^{-/-}$ mice as compared to wt mice during all of the 35 days (12 days $p<0.001$, 18 days $p<0.001$, 26 days $p<0.01$ and 35 days $p<0.05$). In the FcRγ$^{-/-}$ mice, traces of renal mesangial (Figure 1B) and splenic vessel wall (Figure 1C) IgG1 deposits were seen after 12–18 days of Hg treatment, but higher titres of IgG1 deposits were not seen until 26 days of treatment (Figure 1B–C). After 18 days of Hg treatment the titre of IgG1 deposits in the renal mesangium of FcRγ$^{-/-}$ mice was significantly lower than in wt mice ($p<0.05$).

The level of IgG2a-containing CIC was significantly increased in FcRγ$^{-/-}$ mice after 26 and 35 days of Hg treatment compared to both untreated FcRγ$^{-/-}$ mice ($p<0.001$) and Hg-treated wt mice (26 days $p<0.01$ and 35 days $p<0.05$, respectively) (Figure 2). However, IgG2a deposits were not detected in renal mesangium or splenic vessel walls at any time (data not shown). C3c deposits first appeared in the renal mesangium of Hg-treated FcRγ$^{-/-}$ mice after 12 days but with significantly lower titres than in wt mice ($p<0.05$) (data not shown). C3c deposits were seen in splenic vessel wall of Hg-treated FcRγ$^{-/-}$ mice after 26 days, and the fraction of positive mice was significantly higher ($p<0.05$) than in Hg-treated wt mice. However, the amount of deposits was low with a score of 0.5 ± 0.7 (mean $\pm$ SD). None of the untreated FcRγ$^{-/-}$ mice developed IgG1, IgG2a or C3c deposits (data not shown).

The levels of C1q-binding CIC were measured in the above sera but there was no difference, neither between Hg-treated and untreated mice nor between wt and FcRγ$^{-/-}$ mice (data not shown).

In conclusion, increased levels of IgG1- and IgG2a-containing CIC were associated with development of tissue IC deposits in Hg-treated wt BALB/c mice. While significantly higher levels of CIC were seen in FcRγ$^{-/-}$ mice, the development of high-titred tissue IC deposits was delayed as compared to wt mice.

Intact functional activating FcγRs are important for the elimination of CIC by the liver

BALB/c wt and FcRγ$^{-/-}$ mice treated with Hg for 15–17 days showed a similar clearance rate of preformed dinitrophenyl (DNP)- conjugated human serum albumin (HSA)/IgG IC. No difference was seen in clearance rate comparing Hg-treated and untreated mice (data not shown). In contrast, Hg-treated wt mice showed a significantly higher hepatic uptake of DNP-HSA/IgG IC compared to Hg-treated FcRγ$^{-/-}$ mice ($p<0.05$) demonstrating the importance of intact functional activating FcγRs for the elimination of CIC by the liver (Figure 3).

Lack of intact functional activating FcγRs reduces tissue IC deposits

Splenic vessel wall IC deposits in wt mice. All nine wt mice showed IgG1-IC deposits in splenic vessel walls (Figure 4A) after 5 weeks of Hg treatment, while none of the untreated mice ($p<0.001$) showed such deposits (Table 1). Hg treatment caused slight deposits of IgG2b and IgG3 in one and two mice, respectively. The proportion of mice with C3c deposits in the splenic vessel walls was significantly higher ($p<0.001$) in Hg-

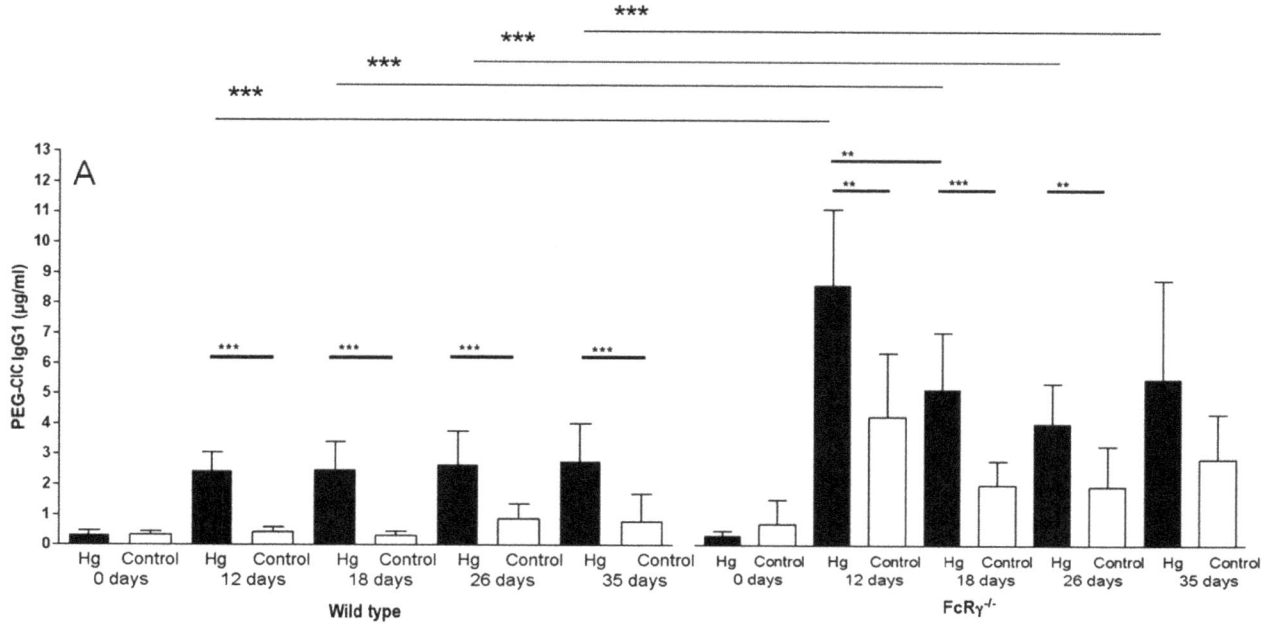

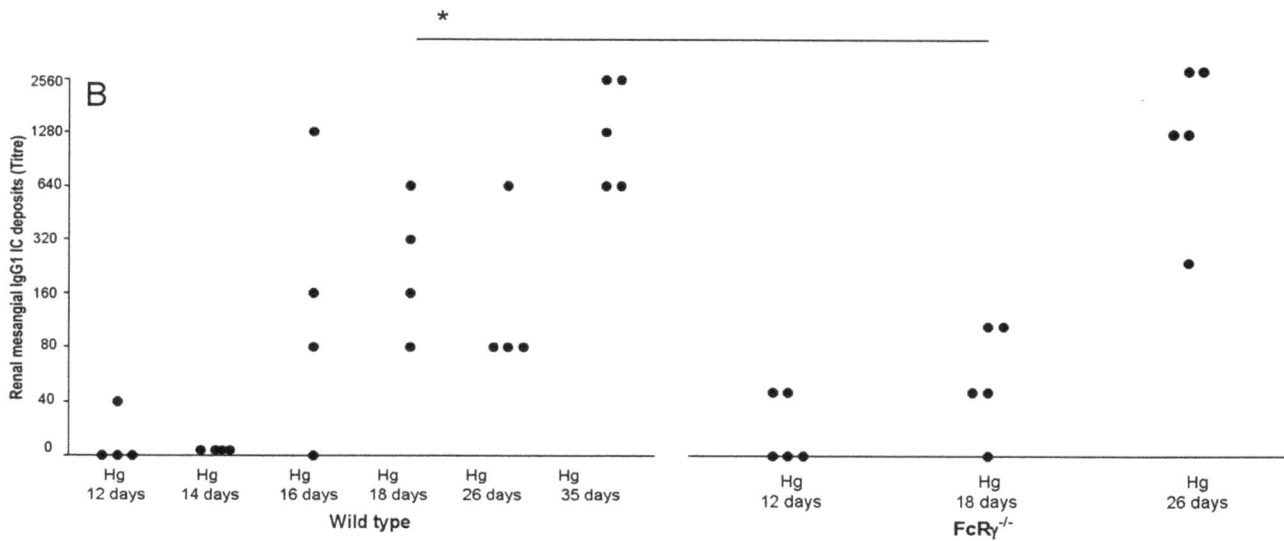

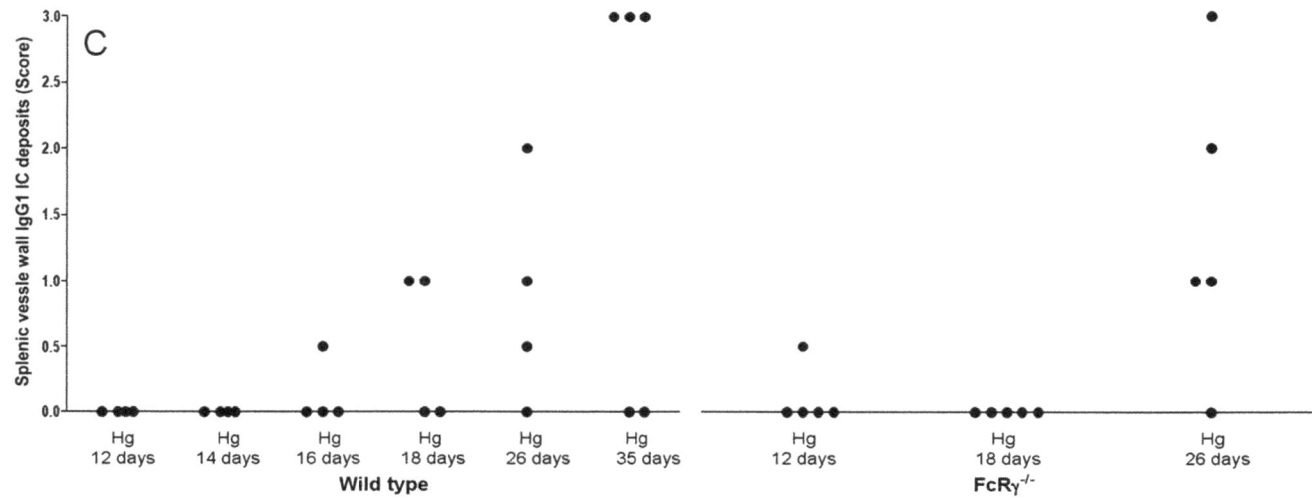

Figure 1. Development of circulating IgG1 immune complexes and tissue IgG1 immune complex deposits. Development of circulating IgG1-containing immune complexes and tissue IgG1 immune complex deposits during 26–35 days of treatment of female BALB/c wild type and FcR$\gamma^{-/-}$ mice with 15 mg/L HgCl$_2$ in the drinking water or drinking water without any addition of Hg (controls). (A) PEG-precipitated circulating immune complexes containing IgG1 antibodies. The bars denote mean ± SD. ** $p<0.01$ and *** $p<0.001$ (Mann-Whitney's test). (B) Renal mesangial IgG1 and (C) splenic vessel wall IgG1 deposits. Each symbol represents a single mouse. * $p<0.05$ (Mann-Whitney's test).

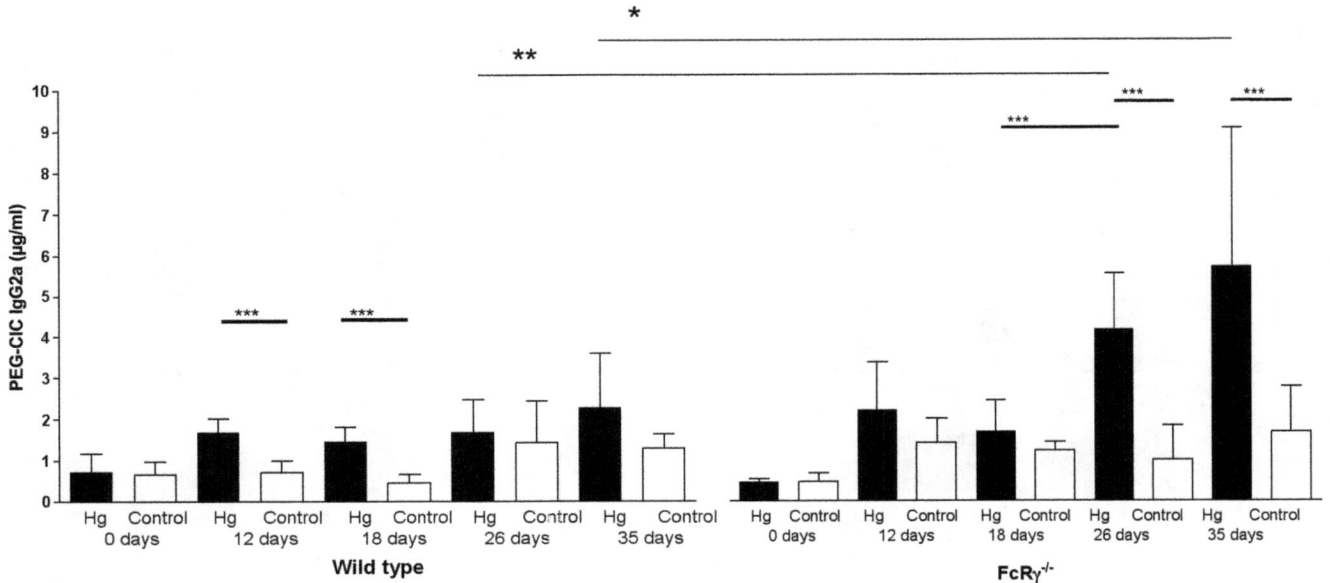

Figure 2. Development of circulating IgG2a immune complexes. Development of PEG-precipitated circulating IgG2a-containing immune complexes during 26–35 days of treatment of female BALB/c wild type and FcR$\gamma^{-/-}$ mice with 15 mg/L HgCl$_2$ in the drinking water or drinking water without any addition of Hg (controls). The bars denote mean ± SD. * $p<0.05$, ** $p<0.01$ and *** $p<0.001$ (Mann-Whitney's test).

treated mice than in untreated mice (Table 1). None of the wt mice showed C1q deposits (Table 1).

Splenic vessel wall IC deposits in FcR$\gamma^{-/-}$ mice. Eight out of 9 (89%) Hg-treated FcR$\gamma^{-/-}$ mice had developed IgG1 deposits in the splenic vessel walls after 5 weeks (Figure 4B), which was significantly higher than in the untreated FcR$\gamma^{-/-}$ mice

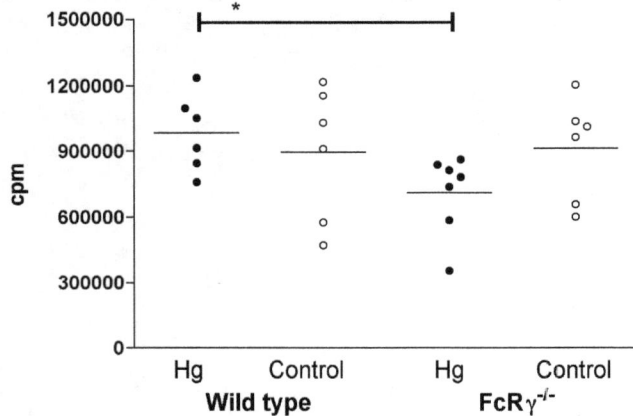

Figure 3. Uptake of circulating immune complexes in the liver. Uptake of preformed circulating HSA/DNP-IgG immune complexes in the liver of female BALB/c wild type and FcR$\gamma^{-/-}$ mice following 15–17 days of treatment with 15 mg/L HgCl$_2$ in the drinking water or drinking water without any addition of Hg (controls). The bars denote mean ± SD. * $p<0.05$ (Mann-Whitney's test).

($p<0.001$) (Table 1). The amount of IgG1 deposits was significantly ($p<0.05$) lower in Hg-treated FcR$\gamma^{-/-}$ compared to Hg-treated wt mice (Table 1). Fifty-six percent of the Hg-treated FcR$\gamma^{-/-}$ mice showed C3c deposits in the splenic vessel walls, which was significantly higher than in untreated mice ($p<0.05$). However, the percentage of mice with C3c deposits as well as the amount of deposits ($p<0.05$, $p<0.001$, respectively) were significantly lower in Hg-treated FcR$\gamma^{-/-}$ mice than in wt mice (Table 1). None of the untreated FcR$\gamma^{-/-}$ mice developed C3c deposits. Neither Hg-treated nor untreated FcR$\gamma^{-/-}$ mice showed C1q deposits in the splenic vessel walls (Table 1).

Renal glomerular and vessel wall IC deposits in wt mice. After 5 weeks of Hg treatment renal mesangial IC deposits were dominated by IgG1 (Figure 4C), although most mice also showed a relatively low titre of IgG2b. IgG2a and IgG3 deposits were less frequent and of a low titre (Table 2). IgG1 and IgG2a deposits were not observed in untreated mice. The Hg-treated wt mice developed mesangial C3c deposits, which were present also in untreated mice but with only a low titre. None of the wt mice developed C1q deposits (Table 2).

A single wt mouse treated with Hg but none of the untreated wt mice showed IC deposits of the IgG1 isotype in the renal vessel walls (Table 2). Neither Hg-treated nor untreated wt mice developed C1q or C3c renal vessel wall IC deposits.

Renal glomerular and vessel wall IC in FcR$\gamma^{-/-}$ mice. The Hg-treated FcR$\gamma^{-/-}$ mice also developed renal mesangial IC deposits mainly containing IgG1 and IgG2b (Table 2). The IgG1 titre was significantly lower in Hg-treated FcR$\gamma^{-/-}$ mice than in Hg-treated wt mice (Figure 4D) ($p<0.05$) (Table 2). There was no significant difference in the titre of C3c

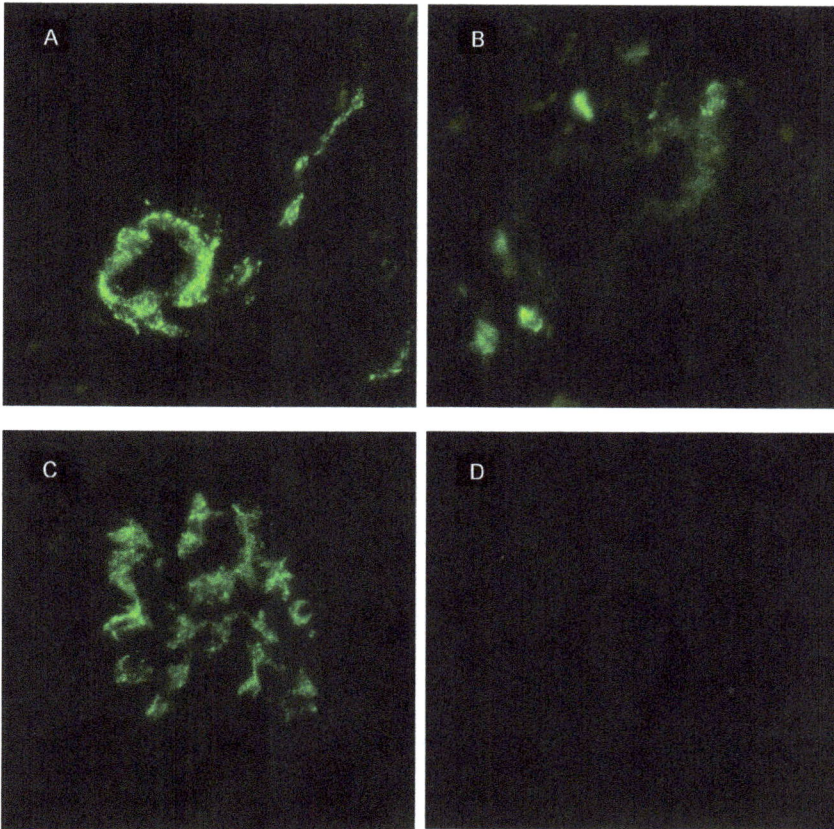

Figure 4. Tissue IgG1 immune complex deposits. Direct immunofluorescence using FITC-conjugated anti-IgG1 antibodies on cryostate sections from female BALB/c wild type (A, C) and FcRγ$^{-/-}$ (B, D) mice treated with 15 mg/l HgCl$_2$ in the drinking water for 5 weeks. Heavy granular staining in splenic vessel walls (A) and renal mesangium (C) in wild type mice, but only slight deposits in the corresponding tissues of FcRγ$^{-/-}$ mice (B, D).

Table 1. Composition of immune complex deposits in splenic vessel walls from HgCl$_2$-treated and untreated BALB/c mice after 5 weeks.

Strain	No	Treatment	Splenic vessel walls						
			IgG1	IgG2a	IgG2b	IgG3	Total IgG	C1q	C3c
Wt	9	Hg[a]	100[b, c]	0	11	22	100	0	100[c]
			(3.1±0.8)[d]		(0.1±0.3)	(0.2±0.4)			(2.1±0.6)
Wt	10	Untreated	0	0	ND	ND	0	0	0
FcRγ$^{-/-}$	9	Hg[a]	89[e]	0	0	11	89	0	56[f,g]
			(1.7±1.1)[h]			(0.1±0.2)			(0.3±0.4)[i]
FcRγ$^{-/-}$	10	Untreated	0	0	ND	ND	0	0	0

[a]15 mg/L HgCl$_2$ in the drinking water,
[b]Fraction of mice with immune complex deposits,
[c]significantly different from untreated wt mice (Fisher's exact test $p<0.001$),
[d]Grading, 0–4: figures denote mean ± SD,
[e]significantly different from untreated FcRγ$^{-/-}$ mice (Fisher's exact test $p<0.001$),
[f]significantly different from untreated FcRγ$^{-/-}$ mice (Fisher's exact test $p<0.05$),
[g]significantly different from Hg-treated wt mice (Fisher's exact test $p<0.05$),
[h]significantly different from Hg-treated wt mice (Mann-Whitney's test $p<0.05$),
[i]significantly different from Hg-treated wt mice (Mann-Whitney's test $p<0.001$)
Wt, wild type mice; ND, not determined.

Table 2. Composition of immune complex deposits in renal mesangial and vessel walls from $HgCl_2$-treated and untreated BALB/c mice after 5 weeks.

Strain	No	Treatment	Renal mesangial IC deposits							Renal vessel wall IC deposits					
			IgG1	IgG2a	IgG2b	IgG3	Total IgG	C1q	C3c	IgG1	IgG2a	IgG2b	IgG3	C3c	C1q
Wt	9	Hg[a]	100[b]	22	89	67	100	0	100	11	0	0	0	0	0
			(1351±747)[c]	(13±28)	(169±123)	(44±37)			(391±198)	(0.1±0.3)[d]					
	10	Untreated	0	0	ND	ND	0	0	100	0	0	ND	ND	0	0
									(80±0)						
FcRγ[−/−]	9	Hg[a]	100[e]	25[e]	88[e]	13[e]	100	0	100[f]	25	0	0	0	0	0
			(620±470)[g]	(20±37)	(200±113)	(10±28)			(389±242)	(0.4±1)					
	10	Untreated	0	0	ND	ND	0	0	100	0	0	ND	ND	0	0
									(176±51)						

[a]15 mg/L $HgCl_2$ in the drinking water,
[b]Fraction of mice with immune complex deposits,
[c]Reciprocal titre, figures denote mean ± SD,
[d]Grading, 0–4, figures denote mean ± SD,
[e]results from 8 mice,
[f]results from 7 mice,
[g]significantly different from Hg-treated wt mice (Mann-Whitney's test $p < 0.05$).
Wt, wild type mice; ND, not determined.

deposits between Hg-treated and untreated FcRγ[−/−] mice and none of the mice developed C1q deposits (Table 2). Two FcRγ[−/−] mice treated with Hg developed IgG1 renal vessel wall deposits without C1q or C3c deposits (Table 2), whereas none of the untreated FcRγ[−/−] mice showed IgG1, IgG2a, C1q or C3c deposits.

Taken together these results show that FcRγ[−/−] mice develop less IgG1 and C3c deposits in the splenic vessel walls and lower IgG1 titre in the renal mesangium compared to Hg-treated wt mice.

Discussion

The present study demonstrates that BALB/c mice with Hg-induced systemic autoimmunity respond with significantly increased concentrations of CIC containing IgG1 and IgG2a compared to untreated mice. Confirming previous results [12] we conclude that Hg treatment *per se* does not affect the elimination rate of CIC, suggesting that Hg-induced IC formation accounts for the raised levels of CIC. We also demonstrated that the concentration of IgG-CIC was significantly higher in FcRγ[−/−] mice than in wt animals, and that this functional deficiency in trans-membrane signalling of activating FcγRs is associated with deficient hepatic clearance of circulating IgG-IC. This accords with the findings of Ahmed *et al*, who reported that reduced FcγR expression on hepatic non-parenchymal cells was associated with spontaneous development of IC-mediated-GN in NZB/WF1 mice [30]. In SLE reduced expression of FcγRIII and FcγRII is association with high levels of CIC, prolonged FcγR-mediated clearance and high disease activity [31]. Willocks *et al* reported that a low copy number of the human FCGR3B gene correlates with reduced neutrophil expression of FcγRIIIB as well as with reduced neutrophil adherence to and uptake of IC in SLE patients [32].

The levels of circulating IgG and IgG-containing IC depend on several factors *e.g.* (i) the rate of antibody production, which in turn depend on the balance between exposure of activating/inhibiting FcγRs [2,3], (ii) elimination from the circulation via non-specific escape/tissue deposits [10], and (iii) FcγR-mediated binding and

endocytosis or recirculation [3–5,8]. It is likely that the increased CIC concentration in the Hg-treated FcRγ[−/−] mice as compared to wt mice is caused by a disturbance of the normal hepatic IC clearance. The uptake of CIC was not completely lost in mice deficient for trans-membrane signalling by activating FcγRs. This may to some extent be explained by IC-adherence to the stimulating FcγRs although endocytosis was deficient, and to some extend by binding to and endocytosis via FcγRIIB2 exposed on liver sinuoisdal endothelial cells as shown in rats [8].

The profile of CIC increase in Hg-treated mice was quite different between wt and FcRγ[−/−] mice, the former showing a modest but steady increase from day 12, while the latter showed an initially 4-fold higher concentrations of IgG1-CIC on day 12 which subsequently declined but with a vigorous increase of IgG2a-CIC on day 26–35. FcRγ[−/−] mice did not respond with a rise of serum IgG1 following Hg treatment as seen in wt mice [27,28] indicating another mechanism for the elevation of CIC levels. The higher and also more variable CIC levels in the Hg-treated FcRγ[−/−] mice might be due both to the reduced ability by these mice to handle normal levels of CIC and to the extensive Hg-induced IC-production. The higher concentration of CIC of first IgG1 and then IgG2a in Hg-treated FcRγ[−/−] mice was associated with a delayed and reduced deposition of IgG1 IC in the renal mesangium as well as IgG1 and C3c systemically in vessel walls.

IC deposits can be generated from preformed CIC or by *in situ* formation due to adsorption of circulating abs to antigen exposed in the tissue [11,12,18]. The immune deposits seen in Hg-treated wt BALB/c mice may thus originated from serum IgG binding either to antigen planted in the tissue or to endogenouse tissue antigen, or from tissue deposition/binding of IgG-containing CIC. There are observations indicating that formation of IC, containing nucleosomes as antigens, take place within the kidney or in the circulation prior to deposition [33–35]. The only identified autoantigen in HgIA is fibrillarin (AFA) [36], which has also been indicated to be present in murine IC deposits [37]. However, the presence of AFA is not necessarily followed by IC formation

[38,39]. On the other hand, IC deposits may develop without formation of AFA as seen in Hg-treated BALB/c mice [27,40]. Anti-nuclear abs (ANA), especially anti-nuclesomal have been implicated to be important in lupus nephritis [33–35]. Although anti-nucleosomal abs are seldom induced by Hg treatment of BALB/c mice, we have previously reported that ANA of IgG1 and IgG2a subclass is common, indicating antigen-specific induction [27]. Although the antigen has not yet been identified the typical ANA pattern in sera from Hg-treated BALB/c mice is fine-speckled with a distinct staining of nuclear membrane and of condensed chromosomes in dividing cells [27].

Mesangial cells express FcγRs and may mediate binding of IC by recognition of exposed Fc-part [41]. The loss of functionally activating FcγRs will hinder this particular mechanism of deposition as shown in the present study as well as in experimental autoimmune myasthenia gravis. FcγRIII deficient mice show reduction of immune deposits in neuromuscular junctions [42]. An additional consequence of lost FcγRs function is retarded CIC clearance [31,32] leading to further accumulation of CIC in the circulation as seen in the present study.

In glomerular diseases IgG-IC may cause tissue damage due to FcγR activation as well as complement activation [43]. In an experimental model of IC-mediated disease induced by intravenous injection of soluble IgG-IC, Stokol et al showed that the damaging effect of IC deposits was primarily dependent on C1q, followed by neutrophil recruitment [44]. The effect of renal mesangial and systemic vascular IC deposits in Hg-treated BALB/c mice is a mild glomerular endocapillary cell proliferation and slight widening of the mesangium, neither of which is affected by the loss of activating FcγRs, or by vasculitis [27]. How might this mild histological reaction be explained? The frequencies and/or the amounts of the strongly complement-activating IgG2b, IgG3, and especially IgG2a antibodies [45] are low in the IC deposits of HgIA. Instead the IgG1 isotype, which does not activate complement via the classical pathway, dominates [27] as shown also by the lack of C1q in the deposits (present study). Another explanation for the mild renal reaction in HgIA might be that the glomerular IC deposits in HgIA are strictly localised to the mesangium [46], which leads to less histological damage [47]. In fact, when the spontaneously developing glomerular IC-deposits of NZB/WF1 mice, preferentially situated in the capillary loops, are relocalised to the mesangium, the histological damage is greatly reduced [48]. IgG-Fc modulation by in vivo administration of endoglycosidase-S is a novel and fascinating possibility to treat autoantibody-/IC-mediated diseases [49]. In the future, other strategies to specifically interfere with FcγR-mediated IC handling may also become options to treat IC-mediated disease.

In conclusion, mice deficient regarding the function of activating FcγRs respond to an Hg-induced autoimmune stimulus with increased levels and altered quality of CIC compared with mice expressing the intact receptors. The lack of increased IC deposits in target organs for tissue IC deposits and the reduced uptake of CIC in the liver speak in favour of a reduced elimination of CIC but at the same time protection from a more pronounced histological kidney damage.

Methods

Animals and housing

Female BALB/c mice with a targeted knockout mutation for the signal-transducing (ITAM-containing) intracellular γ-chain dimer (FcRγ$^{-/-}$), causing a functional loss of the activating FcγRs, were obtained from Taconic M&B (Georgetown, NY, USA). Corresponding BALB/c mice without a mutation (wild type - wt mice)

were obtained from Taconic M&B (Ry, Denmark). All mice were 11–14 weeks old at onset of the experiments except for the animals in the studies of blood clearance and tissue uptake of CIC, where the mice were 39–44 weeks old. The mice were kept under specific pathogen-free conditions and housed under 12-hour dark-/12-hour light cycles in steel-wire cages. They were fed with pellets (Transbreed E, Special Diets services, Witham, UK) and tap water ad libitum. The animal ethics committee in Linköping approved the study protocol (ID 14-06).

Treatment

Groups of wt and FcRγ$^{-/-}$ mouse strains were exposed to 15 mg/L HgCl$_2$ (Fluka Chemie, Buchs, Germany) in the sterilised drinking water given ad libitum for 26–35 days. Control mice received sterilised tap water only.

Blood and tissue sampling

Blood samples were obtained from the retro-orbital vein plexus.

The first groups of wt and FcRγ$^{-/-}$ mice were bled before onset of treatment and then after 12, 18, 26, and 35 days. At sacrifice after 35 days treatment samples of the kidney and spleen were obtained for examination of tissue IC deposits. The blood was allowed to clot at 4°C for 2 hours, and CIC measured using these fresh sera.

The second groups of wt and FcRγ$^{-/-}$ mice were treated with Hg for 12–35 days in order to assess the specific time needed for formation of tissue IC deposit. Pieces of the kidney and spleen were collected at sacrifice after 12, 14, 16, 18, 26, and 35 days of treatment in wt mice, and after 12, 18, and 26 days of treatment in FcRγ$^{-/-}$ mice.

The third group of wt and FcRγ$^{-/-}$ mice were treated with Hg for 15–17 days and then given a single tail vein injection of 0.2 ml preformed isotope-labelled soluble ICs (see below) at concentration of 0.7 mg/ml to analyse blood clearance and liver uptake of CIC. Blood samples (50 μl) were taken after 0, 2, 4, 6, 8, 12, 22 and 32 minutes following the injection and the liver was collected at sacrifice.

Assessment of circulating immune complexes

Circulating immune complexes assessed by PEG precipitation followed by analyses of IgG1, IgG2a and IgG2b ELISA. CIC in serum was measured by polyethylene glycol (PEG)-induced precipitation of immune complexes [12,50]. Equal volumes of serum and 8% PEG (Fluka) were incubated at 4°C for 1 h and then centrifuged at 1000 g for 1 h. The pellet was washed, resuspended in phosphate-buffered saline (PBS pH 7.4) and stored at −20°C. The method used for detection of IgG1 has been described before [27]. A standard curve using mouse myeloma protein of the IgG1 (LO-IMEX) isotype was used to obtain the actual concentration. The IgG2a and IgG2b content were measured by a commercially available enzyme-linked immunosorbent (ELISA) kit (Bethyl Laboratories Inc, Montgomery, Texas, USA). To obtain the actual IgG2a or IgG2b concentration the standard supplied with the kit was used.

Circulating immune complexes assessed by a C1q-binding assay. CIC containing C1q were measured using a mouse specific ELISA kit from Alpha Diagnostic International (San Antonio, TX, USA). Briefly, serum was added to wells pre-coated with C1q. A horseradish-peroxidise- (HRP-) conjugated anti-mouse IgG detection antibody (ab) was added followed by substrate buffer. After adding stop solution the absorbance was measured at 450 nm and background values were subtracted. Positive and negative controls included in the kit gave the expected results.

Assessment of tissue immune complex deposits

Pieces of the left kidney and the spleen were examined for IC deposits with direct immunofluorescence microscopy as described before [27]. Briefly, snap frozen tissue pieces were sectioned and incubated with either a fluorescein-isothiocyanate- (FITC-) conjugated goat anti-mouse ab against the IgG1, IgG2a, IgG2b or IgG3 isotype (Southern Biotechnology, Birmingham, AL, USA), C1q (Cedarlane, Burlington, Canada), or C3c (Organon-Technica, West Chester, PA, USA). Kidneys from aged NZB/WF1 mice were used as a positive control. The presence of deposits in glomeruli, renal and splenic vessel walls was examined with a fluorescence microscope (Nikon, Tokyo, Japan). The endpoint titre for the IgG isotypes, C1q and C3c was defined as the highest dilution of detection ab giving a specific staining of the tissue. No staining at an ab dilution of 1:40 was considered as negative and given the value 0. The amount of the IgG isotypes, C1q and C3c in renal and splenic vessel walls was scored from 0–4 (0, no specific staining; 1, slight staining; 2, moderate staining; 3, strong staining and 4, very strong staining). All examinations were done without knowledge of treatment given or other results.

Immune complex formation and isotope labeling

DNP-conjugated HSA was prepared essentially as described previously [51]. Briefly, 1 g of HSA (Sigma, St Louis, Missouri, USA) and 1 g potassium carbonate was dissolved in distilled water and allowed to react with 1 g 2,4-dinitrobenzene sulfonate in the dark, at 37°C under continuous agitation, for approximately 5 h to achieve DNP-HSA with a conjugation degree of 4–6 DNP per HSA. The DNP-HSA protein was then passed through a Sephadex G-10 column and dialysed against distilled water at 4°C for 24 h, lyophilized and stored at 4°C.

^{125}I-TC labelling and CIC formation

The radioactive tyramine cellbiose (TC) label has the advantage of remaining intracellularly over a long time after endocytosis and degradation, allowing analysis of accumulated intracellular uptake of labelled IC. Radiolabelling of HSA was accomplished by the TC method as previously described [52] with some modifications. In brief, iodinated TC (^{125}I-TC) was prepared by reacting TC (6 μl of 10 mM solution in PBS) with Na^{125}I (1.2 mCi, Perkin-Elmer) in Iodo-Gen tubes (Pierce) for 30 min at room temperature and was then activated by transferring the solution to a tube containing cyanuric chloride (6 μl of 1.8 mg solution in acetone) and potassium iodide (6 μl of 0.1 M solution) for 3 min. The activated ^{125}I-TC adduct was then covalently coupled to DNP-HSA (0.5 mg in 200 μl 10 mM borate buffer, pH 8.8). To remove unincorporated ^{125}I-TC, the labelled protein (^{125}I-TC-DNP-HSA) was passed through a Sephadex G-10 column (GE Healthcare) eluated with PBS. Radiolabelled preparations were>95% trichloroaetic acid-precipitable. Specific activities obtained were in the range of $7-8\times10^5$ cpm/μg. The ^{125}I-TC moiety formed after degradation of ^{125}I-TC-labeled proteins is not released to the medium but remains trapped in degradative compartments [52], thus enabling assessment of the accumulated uptake of radioactive protein over time. ^{125}I-TC-labelled DNP-HSA was diluted with PBS and allowed to react with polyclonal rabbit IgG anti-DNP ab (AbD Serotec, Oxford, England) at 4-fold ab excess for 45 min at 37°C.

Statistical methods

Differences between the groups were analysed by the non-parametric Mann-Whitney test or Fisher's exact test. *P<0.05* was considered statistically significant.

Acknowledgments

We thank our colleagues Marie-Louise Eskilsson and Christer Bergman for technical assistance.

Author Contributions

Conceived and designed the experiments: KM TS TB PH. Performed the experiments: KM SAM JIJ. Analyzed the data: KM. Contributed reagents/materials/analysis tools: SAM. Wrote the paper: KM TS TB JIJ PH.

References

1. Nangaku M, Couser WG (2005) Mechanisms of immune-deposit formation and the mediation of immune renal injury. Clinical and experimental nephrology 9: 183–191.
2. Heyman B (2003) Feedback regulation by IgG antibodies. Immunology letters 88: 157–161.
3. Ravetch J. In vivo veritas: the surprising roles of Fc receptors in immunity. Nature immunology 11: 183–185.
4. Bogers WM, Stad RK, Janssen DJ, van Rooijen N, van Es LA, et al. (1991) Kupffer cell depletion in vivo results in preferential elimination of IgG aggregates and immune complexes via specific Fc receptors on rat liver endothelial cells. Clinical and experimental immunology 86: 328–333.
5. Johansson AG, Lovdal T, Magnusson KE, Berg T, Skogh T (1996) Liver cell uptake and degradation of soluble immunoglobulin G immune complexes in vivo and in vitro in rats. Hepatology (Baltimore, Md 24: 169–175.
6. Kosugi I, Muro H, Shirasawa H, Ito I (1992) Endocytosis of soluble IgG immune complex and its transport to lysosomes in hepatic sinusoidal endothelial cells. Journal of hepatology 16: 106–114.
7. Lovdal T, Andersen E, Brech A, Berg T (2000) Fc receptor mediated endocytosis of small soluble immunoglobulin G immune complexes in Kupffer and endothelial cells from rat liver. Journal of cell science 113(Pt 18): 3255–3266.
8. Mousavi SA, Sporstol M, Fladeby C, Kjeken R, Barois N, et al. (2007) Receptor-mediated endocytosis of immune complexes in rat liver sinusoidal endothelial cells is mediated by FcgammaRIIb2. Hepatology (Baltimore, Md 46: 871–884.
9. Skogh T, Blomhoff R, Eskild W, Berg T (1985) Hepatic uptake of circulating IgG immune complexes. Immunology 55: 585–594.
10. Skogh T, Stendahl O (1983) Complement-mediated delay in immune complex clearance from the blood owing to reduced deposition outside the reticuloendothelial system. Immunology 49: 53–59.
11. Izui S, McConahey PJ, Theofilopoulos AN, Dixon FJ (1979) Association of circulating retroviral gp70-anti-gp70 immune complexes with murine systemic lupus erythematosus. The Journal of experimental medicine 149: 1099–1116.

12. Hultman P, Skogh T, Enestrom S (1989) Circulating and tissue immune complexes in mercury-treated mice. Journal of clinical & laboratory immunology 29: 175–183.
13. Sasaki T, Muryoi T, Hatakeyama A, Suzuki M, Sato H, et al. (1991) Circulating anti-DNA immune complexes in active lupus nephritis. The American journal of medicine 91: 355–362.
14. Kotnik V, Premzl A, Skoberne M, Malovrh T, Kveder R, et al. (2003) Demonstration of apoptosis-associated cleavage products of DNA, complement activation products SC5b-9 and C3d/dg, and immune complexes CIC-C3d, CIC-IgA, and CIC-IgG in the urine of patients with membranous glomerulonephritis. Croatian medical journal 44: 707–711.
15. Zabaleta-Lanz M, Vargas-Arenas RE, Tapanes F, Daboin I, Atahualpa Pinto J, et al. (2003) Silent nephritis in systemic lupus erythematosus. Lupus 12: 26–30.
16. Zabaleta-Lanz ME, Munoz LE, Tapanes FJ, Vargas-Arenas RE, Daboin I, et al. (2006) Further description of early clinically silent lupus nephritis. Lupus 15: 845–851.
17. Kain R, Exner M, Brandes R, Ziebermayr R, Cunningham D, et al. (2008) Molecular mimicry in pauci-immune focal necrotizing glomerulonephritis. Nature medicine 14: 1088–1096.
18. Oates JC, Gilkeson GS (2002) Mediators of injury in lupus nephritis. Current opinion in rheumatology 14: 498–503.
19. Davies KA, Robson MG, Peters AM, Norsworthy P, Nash JT, et al. (2002) Defective Fc-dependent processing of immune complexes in patients with systemic lupus erythematosus. Arthritis and rheumatism 46: 1028–1038.
20. Nimmerjahn F, Ravetch JV (2008) Fcgamma receptors as regulators of immune responses. Nature reviews 8: 34–47.
21. Takai T, Li M, Sylvestre D, Clynes R, Ravetch JV (1994) FcR gamma chain deletion results in pleiotrophic effector cell defects. Cell 76: 519–529.
22. Hazenbos WL, Heijnen IA, Meyer D, Hofhuis FM, Renardel de Lavalette CR, et al. (1998) Murine IgG1 complexes trigger immune effector functions predominantly via Fc gamma RIII (CD16). J Immunol 161: 3026–3032.

23. Clynes R, Calvani N, Croker BP, Richards HB (2005) Modulation of the immune response in pristane-induced lupus by expression of activation and inhibitory Fc receptors. Clinical and experimental immunology 141: 230–237.
24. Bolland S, Ravetch JV (2000) Spontaneous autoimmune disease in Fc(gamma)RIIB-deficient mice results from strain-specific epistasis. Immunity 13: 277–285.
25. Kleinau S (2003) The impact of Fc receptors on the development of autoimmune diseases. Current pharmaceutical design 9: 1861–1870.
26. Kleinau S, Martinsson P, Heyman B (2000) Induction and suppression of collagen-induced arthritis is dependent on distinct fcgamma receptors. The Journal of experimental medicine 191: 1611–1616.
27. Martinsson K, Hultman P (2006) The role of Fc-receptors in murine mercury-induced systemic autoimmunity. Clinical and experimental immunology 144: 309–318.
28. Martinsson K, Carlsson L, Kleinau S, Hultman P (2008) The effect of activating and inhibiting Fc-receptors on murine mercury-induced autoimmunity. Journal of autoimmunity 31: 22–29.
29. Havarinasab S, Hultman P (2005) Organic mercury compounds and autoimmunity. Autoimmunity reviews 4: 270–275.
30. Ahmed SS, Muro H, Nishimura M, Kosugi I, Tsutsi Y, et al. (1995) Fc receptors in liver sinusoidal endothelial cells in NZB/W F1 lupus mice: a histological analysis using soluble immunoglobulin G-immune complexes and a monoclonal antibody (2.4G2). Hepatology (Baltimore, Md 22: 316–324.
31. Kavai M, Szegedi G (2007) Immune complex clearance by monocytes and macrophages in systemic lupus erythematosus. Autoimmunity reviews 6: 497–502.
32. Willcocks LC, Lyons PA, Clatworthy MR, Robinson JI, Yang W, et al. (2008) Copy number of FCGR3B, which is associated with systemic lupus erythematosus, correlates with protein expression and immune complex uptake. The Journal of experimental medicine 205: 1573–1582.
33. Fenton KA, Tommeras B, Marion TN, Rekvig OP. Pure anti-dsDNA mAbs need chromatin structures to promote glomerular mesangial deposits in BALB/c mice. Autoimmunity 43: 179–188.
34. Fismen S, Hedberg A, Fenton KA, Jacobsen S, Krarup E, et al. (2009) Circulating chromatin-anti-chromatin antibody complexes bind with high affinity to dermo-epidermal structures in murine and human lupus nephritis. Lupus 18: 597–607.
35. Mjelle JE, Rekvig OP, Fenton KA (2007) Nucleosomes possess a high affinity for glomerular laminin and collagen IV and bind nephritogenic antibodies in murine lupus-like nephritis. Annals of the rheumatic diseases 66: 1661–1668.
36. Hultman P, Enestrom S, Pollard KM, Tan EM (1989) Anti-fibrillarin autoantibodies in mercury-treated mice. Clinical and experimental immunology 78: 470–477.
37. Hultman P, Enestrom S (1988) Mercury induced antinuclear antibodies in mice: characterization and correlation with renal immune complex deposits. Clinical and experimental immunology 71: 269–274.
38. Hultman P, Ganowiak K, Turley SJ, Pollard KM (1995) Genetic susceptibility to silver-induced anti-fibrillarin autoantibodies in mice. Clinical immunology and immunopathology 77: 291–297.
39. Hultman P, Johansson U, Turley SJ, Lindh U, Enestrom S, et al. (1994) Adverse immunological effects and autoimmunity induced by dental amalgam and alloy in mice. Faseb J 8: 1183–1190.
40. Hultman P, Bell LJ, Enestrom S, Pollard KM (1992) Murine susceptibility to mercury. I. Autoantibody profiles and systemic immune deposits in inbred, congenic, and intra-H-2 recombinant strains. Clinical immunology and immunopathology 65: 98–109.
41. Bergtold A, Gavhane A, D'Agati V, Madaio M, Clynes R (2006) FcR-bearing myeloid cells are responsible for triggering murine lupus nephritis. J Immunol 177: 7287–7295.
42. Tuzun E, Saini SS, Yang H, Alagappan D, Higgs S, et al. (2006) Genetic evidence for the involvement of Fcgamma receptor III in experimental autoimmune myasthenia gravis pathogenesis. Journal of neuroimmunology 174: 157–167.
43. Berger SP, Daha MR (2007) Complement in glomerular injury. Seminars in immunopathology 29: 375–384.
44. Stokol T, O'Donnell P, Xiao L, Knight S, Stavrakis G, et al. (2004) C1q governs deposition of circulating immune complexes and leukocyte Fcgamma receptors mediate subsequent neutrophil recruitment. The Journal of experimental medicine 200: 835–846.
45. Baudino L, Azeredo da Silveira S, Nakata M, Izui S (2006) Molecular and cellular basis for pathogenicity of autoantibodies: lessons from murine monoclonal autoantibodies. Springer seminars in immunopathology 28: 175–184.
46. Enestrom S, Hultman P (1984) Immune-mediated glomerulonephritis induced by mercuric chloride in mice. Experientia 40: 1234–1240.
47. Weening JJ, D'Agati VD, Schwartz MM, Seshan SV, Alpers CE, et al. (2004) The classification of glomerulonephritis in systemic lupus erythematosus revisited. Kidney international 65: 521–530.
48. Havarinasab S, Hultman P (2006) Alteration of the spontaneous systemic autoimmune disease in (NZB x NZW)F1 mice by treatment with thimerosal (ethyl mercury). Toxicology and applied pharmacology 214: 43–54.
49. Allhorn M, Collin M (2009) Sugar-free antibodies—the bacterial solution to autoimmunity? Annals of the New York Academy of Sciences 1173: 664–669.
50. Chia D, Barnett EV, Yamagata J, Knutson D, Restivo C, et al. (1979) Quantitation and characterization of soluble immune complexes precipitated from sera by polyethylene glycol (PEG). Clinical and experimental immunology 37: 399–407.
51. Skogh T, Stendahl O, Sundqvist T, Edebo L (1983) Physicochemical properties and blood clearance of human serum albumin conjugated to different extents with dinitrophenyl groups. International archives of allergy and applied immunology 70: 238–244.
52. Pittman RC, Carew TE, Glass CK, Green SR, Taylor CA, Jr., et al. (1983) A radioiodinated, intracellularly trapped ligand for determining the sites of plasma protein degradation in vivo. The Biochemical journal 212: 791–800.

14

Patterns of Antibody Binding to Aquaporin-4 Isoforms in Neuromyelitis Optica

Simone Mader[1], Andreas Lutterotti[1], Franziska Di Pauli[1], Bettina Kuenz[1], Kathrin Schanda[1], Fahmy Aboul-Enein[2], Michael Khalil[3], Maria K. Storch[3], Sven Jarius[4], Wolfgang Kristoferitsch[2], Thomas Berger[1], Markus Reindl[1]*

1 Clinical Department of Neurology, Innsbruck Medical University, Innsbruck, Austria, 2 Department of Neurology, SMZ-Ost Donauspital, Vienna, Austria, 3 Department of Neurology, Medical University of Graz, Graz, Austria, 4 Division of Molecular Neuroimmunology, Department of Neurology, University of Heidelberg, Heidelberg, Germany

Abstract

Background: Neuromyelitis optica (NMO), a severe demyelinating disease, represents itself with optic neuritis and longitudinally extensive transverse myelitis. Serum NMO-IgG autoantibodies (Abs), a specific finding in NMO patients, target the water channel protein aquaporin-4 (AQP4), which is expressed as a long (M-1) or a short (M-23) isoform.

Methodology/Principal Findings: The aim of this study was to analyze serum samples from patients with NMO and controls for the presence and epitope specificity of IgG and IgM anti-AQP4 Abs using an immunofluorescence assay with HEK293 cells expressing M-1 or M-23 human AQP4. We included 56 patients with definite NMO (n = 30) and high risk NMO (n = 26), 101 patients with multiple sclerosis, 27 patients with clinically isolated syndromes (CIS), 30 patients with systemic lupus erythematosus (SLE) or Sjögren's syndrome, 29 patients with other neurological diseases and 47 healthy controls. Serum anti-AQP4 M-23 IgG Abs were specifically detected in 29 NMO patients, 17 patients with high risk NMO and two patients with myelitis due to demyelination (CIS) and SLE. In contrast, IgM anti-AQP4 Abs were not only found in some NMO and high risk patients, but also in controls. The sensitivity of the M-23 AQP4 IgG assay was 97% for NMO and 65% for high risk NMO, with a specificity of 100% compared to the controls. Sensitivity with M-1 AQP4 transfected cells was lower for NMO (70%) and high risk NMO (39%). The conformational epitopes of M-23 AQP4 are the primary targets of NMO-IgG Abs, whereas M-1 AQP4 Abs are developed with increasing disease duration and number of relapses.

Conclusions: Our results confirm M-23 AQP4-IgG Abs as reliable biomarkers in patients with NMO and high risk syndromes. M-1 and M-23 AQP4-IgG Abs are significantly associated with a higher number of relapses and longer disease duration.

Editor: Christoph Kleinschnitz, Julius-Maximilians-Universität Würzburg, Germany

Funding: Research grant (no. 2007104) of the interdisciplinary center for research and treatment (IFTZ), Innsbruck Medical University, Research Fellowship from the European Committee for Treatment and Research in Multiple Sclerosis (ECTRIMS) to S.J. The funders had no role in study design, data collection and analysis, decision to publish, or preparation of the manuscript.

Competing Interests: The authors have declared that no competing interests exist.

* E-mail: markus.reindl@i-med.ac.at

Introduction

Neuromyelitis optica (NMO) is a demyelinating neurological disease defined by optic neuritis (ON) and longitudinally extensive transverse myelitis (LETM) [1,2]. NMO often leads to severe disability and even death within several years of disease onset [1,3]. Since the discovery and validation of NMO-IgG serum antibodies (Abs) in NMO patients [4,5], NMO is considered to be a separate disease entity to multiple sclerosis (MS) [6,7,8,9]. Compared to MS, NMO patients have a worse prognosis and require different treatment strategies according to the dominant humoral immunopathogenesis in NMO. Thus, early discrimination from MS enables specific attention for and treatment of NMO patients [10,11,12,13]. The specificity of NMO-IgG Abs for the disease led to addition of NMO-IgG Abs to the diagnostic criteria of NMO [14]. NMO-IgG are especially useful in the early phase of disease after a first episode of LETM or recurrent ON. More than half of NMO-IgG seropositive patients with first LETM relapse within half a year [15]. NMO-IgG Abs have also been detected in patients with non organ specific autoimmunity such as in systemic lupus erythematosus (SLE) or Sjögren syndrome (SS) patients [16]. NMO-IgG Abs target AQP4 [17], the predominant water-channel protein within the central nervous system (CNS) [18]. AQP4 exists as two different heterotetramers [19], M-1 and M-23 AQP4, which result from usage of different start codons [20,21] and vary in the 23 amino acids in the N terminus of the protein [19]. Contrary to full length AQP4, M-23 AQP4 forms orthogonally arranged particles (OAPs) [20], which were shown to be potential targets for antibody binding [20,22].

Although AQP4 antibodies have now been analyzed in several cohorts of NMO patients worldwide and the importance of AQP4 OAPs has been demonstrated in all of these studies, it is not clear whether the specificity and sensitivity of the antibody response to AQP4 differs between these two isoforms. To the best of our knowledge no systematic study has so far analyzed the immune response to both AQP4 M-1 and M-23 isoforms in NMO and high risk NMO and their follow-up samples. We therefore screened serum probes of patients with NMO, MS, clinically isolated syndromes (CIS), other neurological diseases (OND), SLE and healthy controls (HC) for M-1 and M-23 AQP4-IgG and- IgM. We were also interested to compare clinical characteristics of patients showing the antibody response and, in addition, to assess the value of anti-AQP4 IgM antibodies in our cohort.

Materials and Methods

Patients and serum samples

Serum samples from 30 patients with NMO and 26 patients with high risk NMO were recruited prospectively from 2007 to 2009 by the Austrian NMO Study-Group from several Austrian Neurological Departments, or were sent in for AQP4 antibody testing by the Department of Neurology, University of Heidelberg, Germany (n = 10). The Austrian NMO Study-Group was established to obtain clinical, neuroradiological and immunological data of Austrian patients with definite and high risk NMO, to enable an early and appropriate treatment, and to determine the so far unknown prevalence of NMO in Austria. The present study was approved by the ethical committee of Innsbruck Medical University (study no. UN3041 257/4.8) and all Austrian patients gave written informed consent to the study protocol. All German samples were tested in an anonymized fashion as requested by the institutional review board of the University of Heidelberg. All NMO patients met the revised diagnostic criteria of 1999 [1] and 97% of patients showed longitudinally extensive transverse myelitis extending over more than three vertebral segments. Ninety-seven percent of definite NMO cases were females (Table 1). The high risk group of NMO patients comprised two patients with recurrent ON (8%) and 24 patients with a single episode or recurrent LETM (92%), including three neuropsychiatric SLE patients and two patients with neurosarcoidosis. Additionally, we included 101 patients with MS according to the revised "McDonald Criteria" [23]: 64 patients with relapsing remitting MS (RRMS), 13 patients with primary progressive MS (PPMS) and 24 patients with secondary progressive MS (SPMS). Moreover, 27 patients with CIS, 29 patients with various OND (ischemic infarct, parkinson disease, epileptic seizure, radiculopathy, insomnia, sleep apnoea

syndrome, CNS lymphoma, traumatic brain injury, myasthenia gravis, chronic inflammatory demyelinating polyneuropathy, vestibular neuritis, orthostatic syncope, psychogenic neurological symptoms, CNS vasculitis, hereditary neuropathy, analgesic-induced headache, neuroborreliosis, viral encephalitis, chronic tension-type headache, glioblastoma multiforme), 30 patients with SLE or SS and 47 HC were screened for AQP4-Ig.

Serial blood samples were available from two patients with recurrent ON who converted to NMO after 2.6 and 8.7 years.

None of the patients was under high-dose methylprednisolone treatment (HDMP) at the time of blood sampling.

All samples were stored at $-20°C$ until use.

Expression of AQP4 in HEK-293A cells

Human M-1 and M-23 AQP4 isoforms were amplified from a human adult spinal cord Quick Clone^{Tm} cDNA library (Clontech-Takara Bio Europe, Saint-Germain-en-Laye, France) and cloned into the mammalian expression vector Vivid Colours^{TM} pcDNA^{TM} 6.2C-EmGFP-GW/TOPO (Invitrogen, Carlsbad, CA, USA). The correct M-1 and M-23 AQP4 insert sequences were verified by DNA sequencing (Microsynth, Balgach, Switzerland). HEK-293A cells (ATCC, LGC Standards GmbH, Wesel, Germany) were transiently transfected (Fugene 6 transfection reagent, Roche Applied Sciences, Mannheim, Germany) achieving over-expression of AQP4 isoforms fused C-terminally to emerald green fluorescence protein (EmGFP), respectively. The empty vector served as control. Furthermore, both AQP4 isoforms were cloned into the pcDNA3.1 Directional TOPO Expression vector (Invitrogen, Carlsbad, CA, USA), to express M-1 and M-23 AQP4 without the EmGFP fusion protein.

Efficiency of transfection was determined by flow cytometry (FACScan and Cell Quest pro software, BD Biosciences, San Jose, CA, USA). The topology of AQP4 was determined via intracellular staining using a rabbit anti-AQP4 Ab detecting amino acids 249–323 (Sigma-Aldrich). Cells were fixed with 4% paraformaldehyde, blocked with goat IgG (Sigma-Aldrich), incubated with the antibody, washed with phosphate buffered saline (PBS)/10% FCS and incubated with Cy^{Tm}3-conjugated AffiniPure Goat anti-rabbit IgG (Jackson ImmunoResearch Laboratory, West Grove, PA).

Table 1. Serum antibody binding AQP4 M-1 and M-23 isoforms in different disease groups.

AQP4	NMO	High risk NMO	MS	CIS	SLE/SS	OND	HC	p-value
Number	30	26	101	27	30	29	47	
Females	29 (97%)	16 (62%)	65 (64%)	21 (78%)	27 (90%)	20 (69%)	39 (83%)	0.001 [2]
Age (y) [1]	49 (18–80)	49 (26–75)	40 (16–68)	35 (19–63)	41 (22–92)	44 (18–84)	43 (21–68)	0.001 [3]
M-23 IgG	29 (97%) *#	17 (65%) *	0 (0%)	1 (4%)	1 (3%)	0 (0%)	0 (0%)	<0.001 [2]
M-23 IgG Titer (1:) [1]	2,560 (160–20,480)	1,280 (40–10,240)	-	640	320	-	-	
M-1 IgG	21 (70%) *	10 (39%) *	0 (0%)	1 (4%)	0 (0%)	0 (0%)	0 (0%)	<0.001 [2]
M-1 IgG Titer (1:) [1]	160 (40–5,120)	80 (20–2,560)	-	40	-	-	-	
M-23 IgM	8 (27%) *	3 (12%)	4 (4%)	1 (4%)	0 (0%)	1 (4%)	0 (0%)	<0.001 [2]
M-23 IgM Titer (1:) [1]	40 (20–80)	80 (20–80)	50 (20–80)	20	-	20	-	
M-1 IgM	3 (10%)	2 (8%)	0 (0%)	0 (0%)	0 (0%)	0 (0%)	0 (0%)	0.001 [2]
M-1 IgM Titer (1:) [1]	40 (20–40)	30 (20–40)	-	-	-	-	-	

[1]data are shown as median (range), p-value: groups were compared using [2] Chi-Square test and [3] Kruskal-Wallis test and Dunn's multiple comparison post-hoc test,
*statistically different from HC group at p<0.01,
statistically different from high risk NMO group at p<0.01.
Abbreviations: n = number of patients, y = years.

AQP4-Ig Immunofluorescence (IF) assay

All serum samples were analyzed for the presence of AQP4-IgG and- IgM by an extracellular live cell staining IF technique as previously described [24,25,26].

HEK-293A cells were transfected using the expression plasmids mentioned above and cultured for 72 h. Then, cells were blocked with goat IgG (Sigma-Aldrich) in PBS/10%FCS, incubated with pre-absorbed (rabbit liver powder, Sigma-Aldrich) serum samples (screening dilution 1:20 and 1:40, positive sera were further diluted until loss of signal), washed and detected with Cy^{Tm}3-conjugated goat anti-human IgG or IgM antibody (Jackson ImmunoResearch Laboratory, West Grove, PA). Dead cells were visualized with DAPI staining (Sigma-Aldrich) and live cells were analyzed for AQP4-Ig binding. All samples were assessed by two independent investigators blinded for any clinical information. Anti-AQP4 antibodies purified from a NMO patient's plasma by affinity chromatography served as positive control [25].

Statistical analysis

Statistical analysis (means, medians, range, standard deviations), significance of group differences and linear regression were evaluated using SPSS software (release 16.0, SPSS Inc., USA) or GraphPad Prism 5 (GraphPad, San Diego, USA). Between-group comparisons were performed with Kruskal-Wallis test, Dunn's multiple comparison post-hoc test, Mann-Whitney U test, Fisher's exact test and Chi-square test. Correlation of parameters was analyzed with Spearman's non-parametric correlation. Statistical significance was defined as two-sided p-value <0.05 and Bonferroni corrections were applied for multiple comparisons when appropriate.

Results

M-1 and M-23 AQP4-IgG binding results in different staining patterns

With the advent of AQP4 Abs as biomarkers in NMO [4,17], various NMO-IgG antibody assays have been developed so far. In our study we screened serum samples by a live cell staining IF assay, based on the publication of Takahashi et al [24].

In a first step we verified the AQP4 topology of transfected cells with the rabbit anti-water channel AQP4 antibody, followed by the determination of the transfection efficiency via flow cytometry staining (EmGFP 68±5%; M-23 AQP4 64±2%; M-1 AQP4 58±5%; statistically non-significant). We then analyzed the presence of anti-AQP4 Abs in patients' sera by our immunofluorescence assay. As shown in Figure 1 we found co-localization of NMO Abs (red) with the AQP4 protein (green), whereas NMO Abs did not bind to EmGFP transfected cells. All serum samples were screened for the presence of AQP4 M-23 (Figure 1A) and M-1 IgG (Figure 1B), which resulted in different staining patterns. Antibody binding to M-23 AQP4 showed a laminar staining pattern, which could resemble the formation of OAPs. In contrast, M-1 AQP4 did not form visible OAPs and therefore had a more point shaped staining pattern (Figure 1).

In order to exclude that EmGFP might influence the formation of large arrays compared to the non-fused AQP4 proteins we have also over-expressed M-1 and M-23 proteins without EmGFP. We observed the same NMO-IgG binding patterns using M-1 and M-23 AQP4 transfected cells without the EmGFP fusion protein, as illustrated in Figure 2. Consequently we can exclude that EmGFP has an influence on the formation of OAPs. Furthermore, EmGFP fused versus unfused AQP4 M-1 and M-23 transfected cells gave identical results in a subset of 15 M-1 and M-23 seropositive and 15 M-1 and M-23 seronegative patients.

NMO-IgG mainly targets M-23 AQP4

Anti-AQP4 M-23 specific IgG was detected in 29 of 30 definite NMO patients and in 17 of 26 patients with high risk NMO (Table 1). Thus the sensitivity of our assay using M-23 AQP4 transfected cells was 97% for NMO patients and 65% for patients with suspected NMO. In the high risk NMO group, three patients with SLE associated LETM and one patient with recurrent ON were seropositive for anti-AQP4 M-23 IgG. Additionally, M-23 AQP4-IgG was detected in two patients with myelitis due to demyelination (CIS) and SLE, respectively. Furthermore, all HCs, patients with MS, OND and non-neuropsychiatric SLE patients were seronegative for anti-AQP4 M-1 and M-23 IgG. In contrast, sensitivity with M-1 AQP4 transfected cells was remarkably lower for clinically definite NMO (70%) and high risk NMO (39%). Additionally, serum Abs to full length AQP4 were also detected in the patient with isolated myelitis, but not in the patient with SLE-myelitis, who were both positive for M-23 AQP4-IgG.

To summarize, weaker binding was observed to full length AQP4, which is also evident from the lower titer values of M-1 AQP4-IgG (Table 1).

NMO and high risk patients can be classified into three groups

According to their NMO-IgG serostatus, we classified definite and high risk NMO patients into three different groups (Table 2): 1) seronegative patients (n = 10); 2) patients with Abs against M-23 AQP4 but not against full length AQP4 (n = 15); and 3) patients with Abs against both AQP4 isoforms (n = 31). As described before, AQP4-IgG were predominantly detected in the sera of female patients: 93% of patients with M-23 AQP4-IgG, 94% of cases with M-1 and M-23 AQP4-IgG, but only 20% of seronegative patients.

Whereas only one NMO patient was seronegative for AQP4-IgG, the majority of patients with Abs against both AQP4 isoforms (68%) and with Abs against M-23 AQP4 (53%) were diagnosed as NMO. We found no significant differences in the percentage of patients with myelits, LETM, ON, cerebral MRI lesions and oligoclonal bands in the three groups.

M-1 AQP4-IgG seropositivity is significantly associated with a longer median disease duration (70 months), compared to patients who were only positive for M-23 AQP4-IgG (45 months) and the subjects without AQP4 Abs (8 months). Additionally, the median number of relapses was higher in the M-1 and M-23 AQP4-IgG double positive group (6) and in the M-1 negative but M-23 AQP4-IgG positive group (4) than in the seronegative patients (1).

Furthermore, median antibody titers to M-23 AQP4 were significantly higher in the M-1+M-23 AQP4-IgG double positive group (1:2,560) than those cases only positive for M-23 AQP4-IgG (1:640).

Additionally, our results show an increase of NMO-IgG titers in the serum of two patients with recurrent ON after converting into definite NMO (Figure 3). With increasing M-23 AQP4-IgG titers, the patient with the longer disease duration developed Abs against full length AQP4, whereas the second patient remained M-1 AQP4-IgG negative.

NMO-IgM is elevated in definite and high risk NMO patients

A higher percentage of M-23 IgM Abs was detected in NMO patients (n = 8; 27%) and in the high risk group (n = 3; 12%) compared to the other groups (Table 1). M-23 IgM Abs were also present in the NMO-IgG seropositive patient with isolated

A M23 AQP4

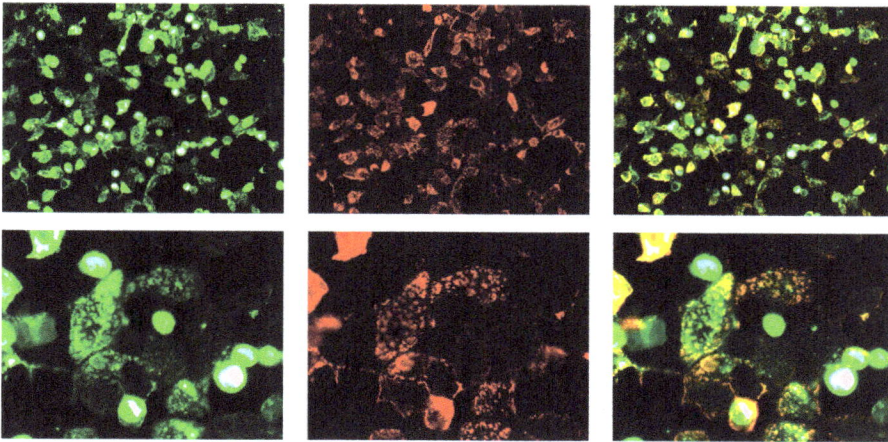

B M1 AQP4

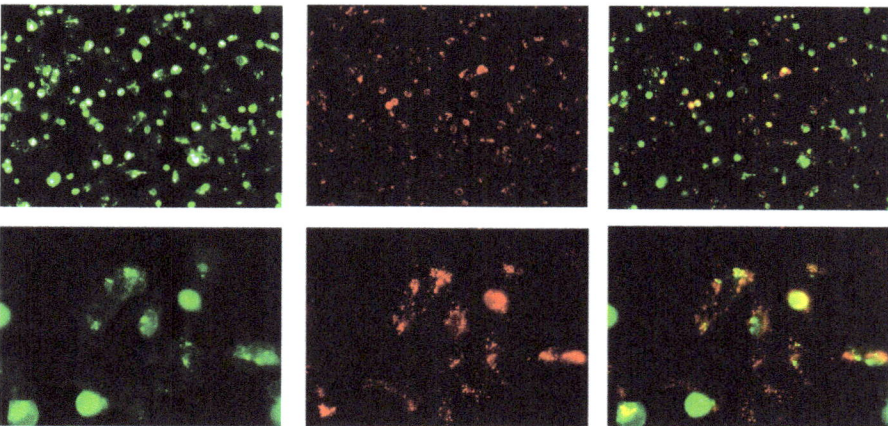

Figure 1. Different staining patterns of NMO-IgG in M-1 and M-23 AQP4 transfected cells. Anti-AQP4 IgG (red) in NMO patient's serum targets AQP4 (green), which is expressed by transiently transfected HEK cells. Performing the assay for M-23 AQP4 (**A**, green) versus M-1 AQP4 (**B**, green), results in different staining patterns of NMO-IgG (red). Weaker binding was observed to M-1 AQP4, which contrary to M-23 AQP4 forms only few orthogonal arrays of particles.

myelitis, in four patients with MS (4%) and in one OND patient (4%).

Furthermore, anti-AQP4-IgM Abs to M-1 AQP4 were only detectable in a small subgroup of patients with definite NMO (n = 3) and high risk NMO (n = 2). In contrast to NMO-IgG, AQP4-IgM positive samples yield much lower titer values (Table 1).

Discussion

Our assay with living AQP4 M-23 transfected cells is highly sensitive for detecting anti-AQP4-IgG Abs in definite (97%) and high risk (65%) NMO patients. Furthermore, we detected M-23 AQP4-IgG in two patients with myelitis (CIS and SLE), who harbour the risk of later developing NMO and could benefit from an appropriate early treatment. In contrast, AQP4-IgG Abs were not present in patients with MS, OND, and non-neuropsychiatric SLE and in HC, which supports their high relevance as biological markers. Our results are in concordance with studies showing highest sensitivity for NMO-IgG detection in cell based assays [27].

Recent papers suggest stronger NMO-IgG Ab binding directed to the shorter M-23 AQP4 isoform [22], which in contrast to M-1 AQP4 can form orthogonal arrays (OAPs) [20,28]. Our study confirms weaker binding of NMO-IgG to full length AQP4, resulting in a lower sensitivity for clinically definite NMO (70%) and high risk NMO (39%) patients, besides also the M-23 IgG seropositive patient with SLE associated myelitis was negative for full length AQP4-IgG. Consequently the assay with M-23 AQP4 transfected cells is much more reliable for an early identification of NMO-IgG Abs in serum samples, whereas numerous patients turned out to be "false negative" when performing the assay with M-1 AQP4 transfected cells.

NMO-Ig Abs resulted in different staining patterns when binding to full length AQP4 in contrast to the M-23 AQP4 isoform. We speculate that the laminar staining pattern of M-23 AQP4-IgG is due to the capability of M-23 AQP4 to form OAPs, which are suggested to be potential targets for Ab binding. On the contrary, IgG binding to full length AQP4, resulted in a more point shaped staining pattern. In order to exclude the possibility that EmGFP has an influence on the formation of OAPs, we performed the immunofluorescence assay with both AQP4

A
M23 AQP4-EmGFP   M23 AQP4

B
M1 AQP4-EmGFP   M1 AQP4

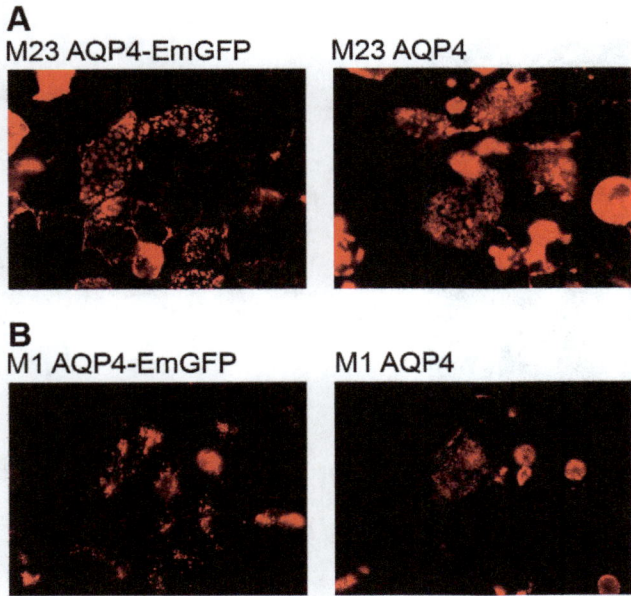

Figure 2. NMO-IgG staining patterns in AQP4-EmGFP versus AQP4 expressing cells. Fusion of EmGFP to AQP4 molecules has no effect on the formation of the different staining patterns of NMO-IgG in M-1 and M-23 AQP4 transfected cells. NMO-IgG has the same laminar staining pattern when binding M-23 AQP4 with and without EmGFP fusion (A). In contrast, cells transfected with M-1 AQP4-EmGFP and M-1 AQP4 have a more point shaped staining pattern (B).

isoforms without EmGFP fusion protein, and obtained same staining patterns and identical results for serum M-1 and M-23 AQP4-IgG and- IgM seropositive and seronegative samples.

As recent studies suggest a strong correlation of NMO-IgG titres with the clinical status of disease [24,29] we performed serial dilutions of NMO Ig positive samples, resulting in higher titer levels of M-23 AQP4-IgG. Moreover, none of the patients were only positive for M-1 AQP4-IgG and negative for M-23 AQP4-IgG, or had higher titer levels for full length AQP4. Possibly, the differences in sensitivity and specificity of the various published NMO-IgG Ab assays could be due to the AQP4 isoform [30], in particular earlier papers do not differentiate between M-1 versus M-23 AQP4-IgG. According to their AQP4-IgG serostatus, we could classify definite and high risk NMO patients into three different groups: AQP4-IgG seronegative patients, patients with Abs against M-23 AQP4 but not against full length AQP4 and patients with Abs against both AQP4 isoforms.

Our results indicate a primary NMO-IgG response directed to an epitope present in the shorter M-23 AQP4 isoform, which could be an epitope present in OAPs. It seems, however, that with increasing disease duration and severity, patients develop higher titers for M-23 AQP4-IgG and additionally target epitopes present in full length AQP4, thus also M-1 AQP4-IgG titer values increase with time. This hypothesis is supported by the significant higher number of relapses and the longer disease duration in patients with M-1 and M-23 IgG compared to patients who target only M-23 AQP4. Moreover, AQP4-IgG negative patients (definite and high risk) had the shortest disease duration and lowest number of relapses. Alternatively, this finding could also be explained by an affinity maturation of these antibodies like it has been shown for other high-affinity IgG autoantibodies that have undergone somatic hypermutation and class switching thus reflecting a pathologic process [31].

The difference in titer levels was also seen in two patients who were initially diagnosed with recurrent ON. The M-23 AQP4-IgG titer was much higher after they had developed definite NMO, and the patient with longer disease duration developed Abs against M-1 AQP4.

In comparison to AQP4-IgG, AQP4-IgM Abs are not a reliable biomarker, although they were elevated in definite and high risk NMO patients. However, AQP4-IgM were also detected in a low percentage of patients with MS and OND.

In this study we confirm that AQP4-IgG are useful biomarkers for early diagnosis of NMO and high risk patients. Our results suggest M-23 AQP4 as initial and major target antigen for

Table 2. Different features of NMO and High risk patients according to their AQP4 Ab status.

	M1-M23-	M1-M23+	M1+M23+	p-value
Number	10	15	31	
Females	2 (20%)	14 (93%) *	29 (94%) *	<0.001 [2]
Age (y) [1]	40 (26–65)	54 (18–77)	49 (19–80)	0.095 [3]
Duration (m) [1]	8 (0.8–60)	45 (0.1–114)	70 (0.4–540) *#	0.009 [3]
NMO	1 (10%)	8 (53%)	21 (68%) *	0.006 [2]
Myelitis	9 (90%)	15 (100%)	30 (97%)	0.413 [2]
LETM	9 (90%)	15 (100%)	29 (94%)	0.179 [2]
ON	2 (20%)	8 (53%)	22 (71%) *	0.026 [2]
Cerebral MRI	0 (0%)	5 (33%)	8 (26%)	0.131 [2]
OCBs	2 (20%) [5]	2 (13%) [6]	2 (7%) [7]	0.675 [2]
Relapses [1]	1 (0–4)	4 (1–13) *	6 (1–15) *	<0.001 [3]
M-23 IgG Titer [1]	-	640 (40–10,240)	2,560 (160–20,480) #	<0.001 [4]
M-1 IgG Titer [1]	-	-	160 (20–5,120)	

[1] data are shown as median (range), p-value: groups were compared using [2] Chi-Square test and [3] Kruskal-Wallis test and Dunn's multiple comparison post-hoc test, [4] Mann-Whitney U test * statistically different from M1-M23- group at p<0.01, # statistically different from M1-M23+ group at p<0.01. data available of [5] 8, [6] 13 and [7] 23 patients.
Abbreviations: n = number of patients, y = years, m = months.

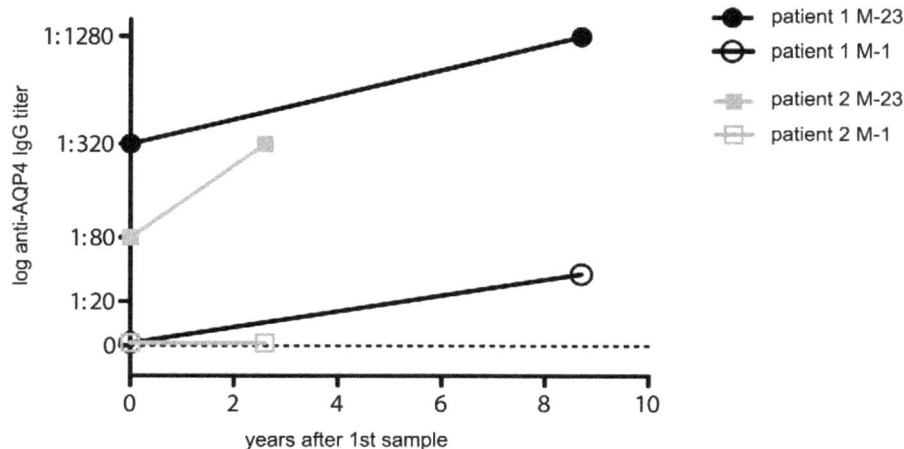

Figure 3. M-1 and M-23 AQP4-IgG titer values in follow-up samples. Higher titer values of NMO-IgG in two patients with recurrent ON (1st sample) after conversion into NMO (2nd sample) after 2.6 and 8.7 years. With increasing M-23 AQP4-IgG titers, patient one developed Abs against full length AQP4, whereas patient two remained M-1 AQP4-IgG negative.

antibody binding in definite and high risk NMO patients, whereas Abs to M-1 AQP4 are predominantly developed with increasing disease duration and severity. Thus we suggest that only M-23 AQP4 should be used as target antigen for the early detection of AQP4-IgG. AQP4-IgM was elevated in AQP4-IgG positive patients, however because of lower sensitivity and specificity its role as biomarker in NMO remains unclear.

Acknowledgments

The authors wish to thank Carolyn Rainer for excellent technical assistance and Benjamin Obholzer for image processing.
Special thank to the following people for providing serum samples for the Austrian NMO-study group: Florian Deisenhammer, Christian Eggers, Franz Fazekas, Elisabeth Fertl, Stefan Guggenberger, Julia Jecel, Mario Jeschow, Josef Kaar, Peter Kapeller, Reinhard Kalchmayr, Herbert Kollross-Reisenbauer, Barbara Kornek, Christian Lampl, Wilfried Lang, Astrid Ursula Leinweber-Thiel, Fritz Leutmezer, Kurt Mihalkovits, Alexander Moser, Armin Muigg, Barbara Niessner, Agnes Pirker, Werner Poewe, Bettina Raber, Gerhard Ransmayr, Helmut Rauschka, Martin Reisz, Paulus Rommer, Kevin Rostasy, Georg Safoschnik, Franz Schautzer, Mascha Schmied, Alena Skrobal, Viktor Stellamor, Karl Vass.

Author Contributions

Conceived and designed the experiments: SM FDP KS MR. Performed the experiments: SM KS. Analyzed the data: SM FDP WK MR. Contributed reagents/materials/analysis tools: AL FDP BK FAE MK MKS SJ WK TB. Wrote the paper: SM AL FDP SJ WK TB MR.

References

1. Wingerchuk DM, Hogancamp WF, O'Brien PC, Weinshenker BG (1999) The clinical course of neuromyelitis optica (Devic's syndrome). Neurology 53: 1107–1114.
2. Cree B (2008) Neuromyelitis optica: diagnosis, pathogenesis, and treatment. Curr Neurol Neurosci Rep 8: 427–433.
3. Wingerchuk DM, Weinshenker BG (2003) Neuromyelitis optica: clinical predictors of a relapsing course and survival. Neurology 60: 848–853.
4. Lennon VA, Wingerchuk DM, Kryzer TJ, Pittock SJ, Lucchinetti CF, et al. (2004) A serum autoantibody marker of neuromyelitis optica: distinction from multiple sclerosis. Lancet 364: 2106–2112.
5. Jarius S, Franciotta D, Bergamaschi R, Wright H, Littleton E, et al. (2007) NMO-IgG in the diagnosis of neuromyelitis optica. Neurology 68: 1076–1077.
6. Weinshenker BG (2007) Neuromyelitis optica is distinct from multiple sclerosis. Arch Neurol 64: 899–901.
7. Roemer SF, Parisi JE, Lennon VA, Benarroch EE, Lassmann H, et al. (2007) Pattern-specific loss of aquaporin-4 immunoreactivity distinguishes neuromyelitis optica from multiple sclerosis. Brain 130: 1194–1205.
8. Misu T, Fujihara K, Kakita A, Konno H, Nakamura M, et al. (2007) Loss of aquaporin 4 in lesions of neuromyelitis optica: distinction from multiple sclerosis. Brain 130: 1224–1234.
9. Jarius S, Paul F, Franciotta D, Waters P, Zipp F, et al. (2008) Mechanisms of disease: aquaporin-4 antibodies in neuromyelitis optica. Nat Clin Pract Neurol 4: 202–214.
10. Wingerchuk DM (2007) Diagnosis and treatment of neuromyelitis optica. Neurologist 13: 2–11.
11. Cree BA, Lamb S, Morgan K, Chen A, Waubant E, et al. (2005) An open label study of the effects of rituximab in neuromyelitis optica. Neurology 64: 1270–1272.
12. Keegan M, Pineda AA, McClelland RL, Darby CH, Rodriguez M, et al. (2002) Plasma exchange for severe attacks of CNS demyelination: predictors of response. Neurology 58: 143–146.
13. Jacob A, Weinshenker BG, Violich I, McLinskey N, Krupp L, et al. (2008) Treatment of neuromyelitis optica with rituximab: retrospective analysis of 25 patients. Arch Neurol 65: 1443–1448.
14. Wingerchuk DM, Lennon VA, Pittock SJ, Lucchinetti CF, Weinshenker BG (2006) Revised diagnostic criteria for neuromyelitis optica. Neurology 66: 1485–1489.
15. Weinshenker BG, Wingerchuk DM, Vukusic S, Linbo L, Pittock SJ, et al. (2006) Neuromyelitis optica IgG predicts relapse after longitudinally extensive transverse myelitis. Ann Neurol 59: 566–569.
16. Pittock SJ, Lennon VA, de Seze J, Vermersch P, Homburger HA, et al. (2008) Neuromyelitis optica and non organ-specific autoimmunity. Arch Neurol 65: 78–83.
17. Lennon VA, Kryzer TJ, Pittock SJ, Verkman AS, Hinson SR (2005) IgG marker of optic-spinal multiple sclerosis binds to the aquaporin-4 water channel. J Exp Med 202: 473–477.
18. Satoh J, Tabunoki H, Yamamura T, Arima K, Konno H (2007) Human astrocytes express aquaporin-1 and aquaporin-4 in vitro and in vivo. Neuropathology 27: 245–256.
19. Neely JD, Christensen BM, Nielsen S, Agre P (1999) Heterotetrameric composition of aquaporin-4 water channels. Biochemistry 38: 11156–11163.
20. Furman CS, Gorelick-Feldman DA, Davidson KG, Yasumura T, Neely JD, et al. (2003) Aquaporin-4 square array assembly: opposing actions of M1 and M23 isoforms. Proc Natl Acad Sci U S A 100: 13609–13614.
21. Jung JS, Bhat RV, Preston GM, Guggino WB, Baraban JM, et al. (1994) Molecular characterization of an aquaporin cDNA from brain: candidate osmoreceptor and regulator of water balance. Proc Natl Acad Sci U S A 91: 13052–13056.
22. Nicchia GP, Mastrototaro M, Rossi A, Pisani F, Tortorella C, et al. (2009) Aquaporin-4 orthogonal arrays of particles are the target for neuromyelitis optica autoantibodies. Glia 57: 1363–1373.
23. Polman CH, Reingold SC, Edan G, Filippi M, Hartung HP, et al. (2005) Diagnostic criteria for multiple sclerosis: 2005 revisions to the "McDonald Criteria". Ann Neurol 58: 840–846.
24. Takahashi T, Fujihara K, Nakashima I, Misu T, Miyazawa I, et al. (2007) Anti-aquaporin-4 antibody is involved in the pathogenesis of NMO: a study on antibody titre. Brain 130: 1235–1243.

25. Bradl M, Misu T, Takahashi T, Watanabe M, Mader S, et al. (2009) Neuromyelitis optica: pathogenicity of patient immunoglobulin in vivo. Ann Neurol 66: 630–643.

26. Takahashi T, Fujihara K, Nakashima I, Misu T, Miyazawa I, et al. (2006) Establishment of a new sensitive assay for anti-human aquaporin-4 antibody in neuromyelitis optica. Tohoku J Exp Med 210: 307–313.

27. Waters P, Vincent A (2008) Detection of anti-aquaporin-4 antibodies in neuromyelitis optica: current status of the assays. Int MS J 15: 99–105.

28. Crane JM, Tajima M, Verkman AS (2009) Live-cell imaging of aquaporin-4 diffusion and interactions in orthogonal arrays of particles. Neuroscience.

29. Jarius S, Aboul-Enein F, Waters P, Kuenz B, Hauser A, et al. (2008) Antibody to aquaporin-4 in the long-term course of neuromyelitis optica. Brain 131: 3072–3080.

30. Graber DJ, Levy M, Kerr D, Wade WF (2008) Neuromyelitis optica pathogenesis and aquaporin 4. J Neuroinflammation 5: 22.

31. Elkon K, Casali P (2008) Nature and functions of autoantibodies. Nat Clin Pract Rheumatol 4: 491–498.

Amelioration of Lupus Nephritis by Serum Amyloid P Component Gene Therapy with Distinct Mechanisms Varied from Different Stage of the Disease

Weijuan Zhang[1]◟, Jin Wu[1]◟, Bin Qiao[1], Wei Xu[1], Sidong Xiong[1,2]*

1 Institute for Immunobiology and Department of Immunology, Shanghai Medical College, Fudan University, Shanghai, People's Republic of China, **2** Institutes of Biology and Medical Sciences, Soochow University, Suzhou, People's Republic of China

Abstract

Background: Our previous study revealed that administration of syngeneic female BALB/c mice with excessive self activated lymphocyte-derived DNA (ALD-DNA) could induce systemic lupus erythematosus (SLE) disease, indicating that overload of self-DNA might exceed normal clearance ability and comprise the major source of autoantigens in lupus mice. Serum amyloid P component (SAP), an acute-phase serum protein with binding reactivity to DNA in mice, was proved to promote the clearance of free DNA and prevent mice against self-antigen induced autoimmune response. It is reasonable to hypothesize that SAP treatment might contribute to alleviation of SLE disease, whereas its role in ALD-DNA-induced lupus nephritis is not fully understood.

Methodology/Principal Findings: The ratios of SAP to DNA significantly decreased and were negatively correlated with the titers of anti-dsDNA antibodies in ALD-DNA-induced lupus mice, indicating SAP was relatively insufficient in lupus mice. Herein a pcDNA3-SAP plasmid (pSAP) was genetically constructed and intramuscularly injected into BALB/c mice. It was found that SAP protein purified from the serum of pSAP-treated mice bound efficiently to ALD-DNA and inhibited ALD-DNA-mediated innate immune response *in vitro*. Treatment of ALD-DNA-induced lupus mice with pSAP in the early stage of SLE disease with the onset of proteinuria reversed lupus nephritis via decreasing anti-dsDNA autoantibody production and immune complex (IC) deposition. Further administration of pSAP in the late stage of SLE disease that had established lupus nephritis alleviated proteinuria and ameliorated lupus nephritis. This therapeutic effect of SAP was not only attributable to the decreased levels of anti-dsDNA autoantibodies, but also associated with the decreased infiltration of lymphocytes and the reduced production of inflammatory markers.

Conclusion/Significance: These results suggest that SAP administration could effectively alleviated lupus nephritis via modulating anti-dsDNA antibody production and the inflammation followed IC deposition, and SAP-based intervening strategy may provide new approaches for treating SLE disease.

Editor: Pierre Bobe, Institut Jacques Monod, France

Funding: This work was supported by grants of National Natural Science Foundation of China (30890141, 30671952), Major State Basic Research Development Program of China (2007CB512401), Shanghai STC grant (10JC1401400, 07JC14004), Program for Outstanding Medical Academic Leader of Shanghai (LJ06011), Research Fellow Fund and Startup Fund for Young Backbone Scholars of Shanghai Medical College, Fudan University. The funders had no role in study design, data collection and analysis, decision to publish, or preparation of the manuscript.

Competing Interests: The authors have declared that no competing interests exist.

* E-mail: sdxiongfd@126.com

◟ These authors contributed equally to this work.

Introduction

Defect in clearance of self nuclear antigen is the hallmark of systemic lupus erythematosus (SLE), an autoantibody-mediated chronic autoimmune disease characterized by the deposition of immune complexes and its followed inflammation that contribute to sever organ damage [1–3]. However, the precise means by which clearance of self antigen is inefficient in SLE remain obscure. Studies of both mice and humans suggest that SLE could arise from excessive production of self antigen released from unremoved apoptotic cells and impairment in the ability of macrophages to clear self antigen [4,5].

Our previous study revealed that the syngeneic female BALB/c mice immunized with activated lymphocyte-derived DNA (ALD-DNA) develop high titers of anti-dsDNA antibodies, immune complex (IC) deposition, proteinuria, and glomerular nephritis which closely resemble human SLE [6–8], thus being used as a model to investigate pathogenesis and potential new therapies for human disease. These findings indicate that ALD-DNA, which mimics large amount of self-DNA released from unremoved apoptotic lymphocytes in SLE patients, might serve as an important self-immunogen to trigger the autoimmune responses which eventually lead to the pathogenesis of SLE in the murine model.

In addition to DNA overload in SLE, insufficiency of DNA clearance represents the other side of the coin [4]. Emerging studies reveal that serum amyloid P component (SAP) would be one of the candidates responsible for DNA clearance [2,4]. SAP is a member of the pentraxin family of proteins and an acute phase reactant, which is produced primarily in the liver in response to infection, inflammation, and trauma [9]. SAP could recognize DNA and other ligands, activate complement, and facilitate pathogen and nuclear antigen phagocytosis, hence playing a nonredundant role in protection against autoimmune disease and in resistance against selected pathogens [10]. Furthermore, SAP shares many properties in common with IgG, including the capacity to interact with FcγR and the ability to bind to ligands [11,12]. The interaction of SAP with FcγR mediates several functions that are analogous or opposite to those of IgG, including modulation the response to inflammatory stimuli and opsonization of bacteria and altered or exposed self-molecules on damages cells [4,11], thus could compete with antibody and be used to treat antibody-mediated disease such as SLE.

As the major DNA- and chromatin-binding protein in plasma of mice, SAP could bind to nuclear antigens that are the target of the autoantibodies of patients with SLE, as well as to damaged membranes and microbial antigens [13,14]. Furthermore, SAP−/− mice spontaneously developed antinuclear autoimmunity and sever glomerulonephritis, a phenotype resembling human SLE [15], which strongly supported a role for SAP in the protection against self-DNA and chromatin-induced autoimmunity.

Although the pathological relevance of SAP to autoimmune disease and the significance of self-DNA in the pathogenesis of SLE attracted much attention in recent years, whether SAP takes responsibility for self-DNA clearance and plays a protective role in self-DNA-induced SLE in a mouse model with clear genetic background remain poorly understood. In the present study, we tested the ratios of SAP to DNA and found that they decreased in ALD-DNA-induced lupus mice as compared to controls, and were negatively correlated with SLE disease. Further SAP gene administration in the early stage of SLE disease could reversed lupus nephritis via reduced pathogenic anti-dsDNA antibody production, while in the late stage of disease, SAP gene treatment alleviated proteuria and lupus nephritis via reducing the infiltration of leukocytes and the production of inflammatory markers besides decreasing the levels of anti-dsDNA antibodies. These results indicated that SAP administration would ameliorate self-DNA-induced lupus nephritis via regulating pathogenic anti-dsDNA antibody production and inflammation in lupus mice, which might provide SAP as a potential therapeutic strategy for self-antigen induced SLE and other autoimmune disease.

Results

ALD-DNA immunization induces SLE syndrome in non-autoimmune-prone mice

Levels of serum anti-dsDNA antibodies, which represent a serological hallmark of SLE, tend to reflect disease severity for SLE patients [1]. According to our previously reported procedure, SLE murine model was generated by immunizing female BALB/c mice with ALD-DNA (Fig. 1A) [6,7]. Compared with PBS or unactivated lymphocyte-derived DNA (UnALD-DNA) injection, ALD-DNA immunization generated higher levels of anti-dsDNA IgG antibody (Fig. 1B), which was evident from week 4 and reached the maximum at week 8 after initial injection (Fig. 1B). Glomerulonephritis was also confirmed by urine protein quantification, H&E staining of renal tissues, and immune complex deposition assay (Fig. 1C–G). Remarkably up-regulated urine protein (Fig. 1C), notable glomerulonephritis (Fig. 1D and E), and increased IgG deposition (Fig. 1F and G) were found in ALD-DNA-immunized lupus mice as compared to PBS- or UnALD-

DNA-treated controls (Fig. 1C–G). These results demonstrate that SLE murine model could be established through ALD-DNA immunization.

The ratios of SAP to DNA decrease in lupus mice and are negatively correlated with SLE disease

To study whether SAP has a correlation to SLE disease, the levels of SAP and circulating DNA in the serum of lupus mice generated by ALD-DNA immunization were assayed. Slightly increased serum SAP levels accompanied with remarkably enhanced circulating DNA levels were found in lupus mice as compared with those in controls (Fig. 2A–D). Pearson correlation analysis showed that the serum SAP levels were closely correlated to the circulating DNA levels (Fig. 2E). However, the ratios of SAP to DNA were lower in lupus mice than in controls, which suggested that SAP protein were relatively insufficient in lupus mice (Fig. 2F). Notably, the ratios of SAP to DNA were negatively correlated with the levels of anti-dsDNA antibodies in SLE mice (Fig. 2G). Taken together, these results indicate that SAP was relatively insufficient in lupus mice.

Efficiently expressed SAP protein could inhibit ALD-DNA-mediated innate immune responses *in vitro*

Our results described above provided the basis for the hypothesis that SAP administration *in vivo* may modulate the immune response in SLE disease. Consequently, pcDNA3-SAP recombinant (pSAP) was constructed for expression of SAP. As shown in Fig. 3A, ELISA analysis for the expression of SAP in culture supernatants of NIH3T3 cell line transfected with pSAP shown that SAP cDNA cloned into pcDNA3 could be correctly transcribed, translated and the protein could be efficiently secreted. To detect the expression of SAP *in vivo*, BALB/c mice were injected intramuscularly with pSAP (100 μg/mice). Immunohistochemistry examination showed an obvious expression of SAP in the muscle received pSAP compared with that receiving pcDNA3 (Fig. 3B). Consistently, quantitative analysis of SAP levels in serum of mice revealed that SAP reached maximal levels at day 10 after injection and then declined (Fig. 3C). 21 days after plasmid injection, the concentration of serum SAP protein went back to the baseline level (Fig. 3C). In contrast, the levels of serum SAP protein in the mice treated with parental plasmid pcDNA3 or physiological saline were not significantly increased over the course of the experiments (Fig. 3C). To further confirm the expression of SAP *in vivo*, serum was collected on day 10 after pSAP injection and subjected to western blot analysis using specific anti-SAP antibody. Marked immune-reactive bands were observed in the serum from mice receiving pSAP injection (Fig. 3D), indicating that SAP could be efficiently expressed *in vivo*. Accumulating data indicate that SAP has the capacity of binding to DNA under physiological conditions [9]. To explore the biological function of SAP purified from the serum of mice receiving pSAP injection, the binding ability of the purified SAP protein to ALD-DNA was evaluated. It was found that the purified SAP protein had the capacity to bind to ALD-DNA (Fig. 3E). Previous studies have shown that SAP can bind macrophage and opsonize the ligands for phagocytosis [11,16]. In order to investigate whether the binding of SAP to ALD-DNA had any effects on the uptake of ALD-DNA by macrophages, we performed flow cytometry to determine the uptake of ALD-DNA or the complexes of purified SAP protein and ALD-DNA (SAP plus ALD-DNA). However, the intracellular DNA did not increase in macrophages in the presence of SAP (Fig. 3F). As endocytic naked DNA was always degraded rapidly by endosomal nucleases, we used chloroquine to prevent

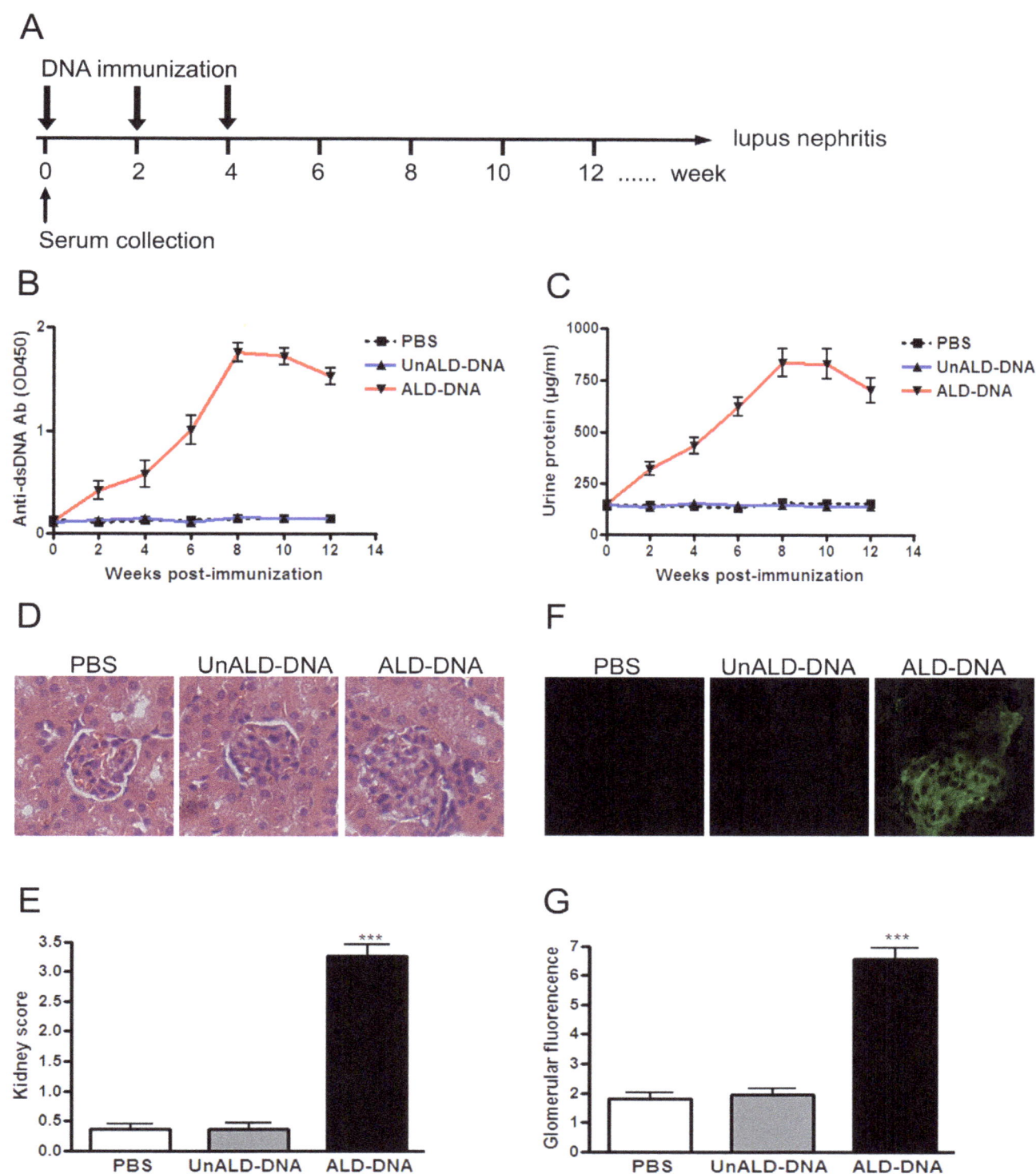

Figure 1. ALD-DNA immunization induces high levels of anti-dsDNA antibody and lupus nephritis. (A) Schematic diagram of animal immunization. 6- to 8-week old female BALB/c mice were immunized subcutaneously with ALD-DNA (50 µg/mice) plus CFA at week 0, followed by two booster immunizations of ALD-DNA (50 µg/mice) emulsified with IFA at week 2 and week 4 after initial immunization. (B) Serum anti-dsDNA IgG levels were measured by ELISA every 2 weeks after initial immunization. Data are means ± SD from 10 mice in each group. (C) Urine protein levels of the mice were assessed by BCA Protein Assay Kit every 2 weeks. Data are means ± SD from 10 mice in each group. (D) 8 weeks after initial immunization, nephritic pathology was evaluated by H&E staining of renal tissues. Imagines (magnification×200) are representative of at least 10 mice in each group. (E) The kidney score was assessed using paraffin sections stained with H&E in (D). ***, $p < 0.001$. (F) Glomerular immune deposition were detected by direct immunofluorescence for IgG in frozen kidney section from ALD-DNA-immunized lupus mice or control mice. Representative images (magnification×200) of 10 mice are shown for each group. (G) Mean glomerular fluorescence intensity (arbitrary units) was determined for IgG in ALD-DNA-immunized lupus mice (n = 10) and control mice (n = 10). ***, $p < 0.001$.

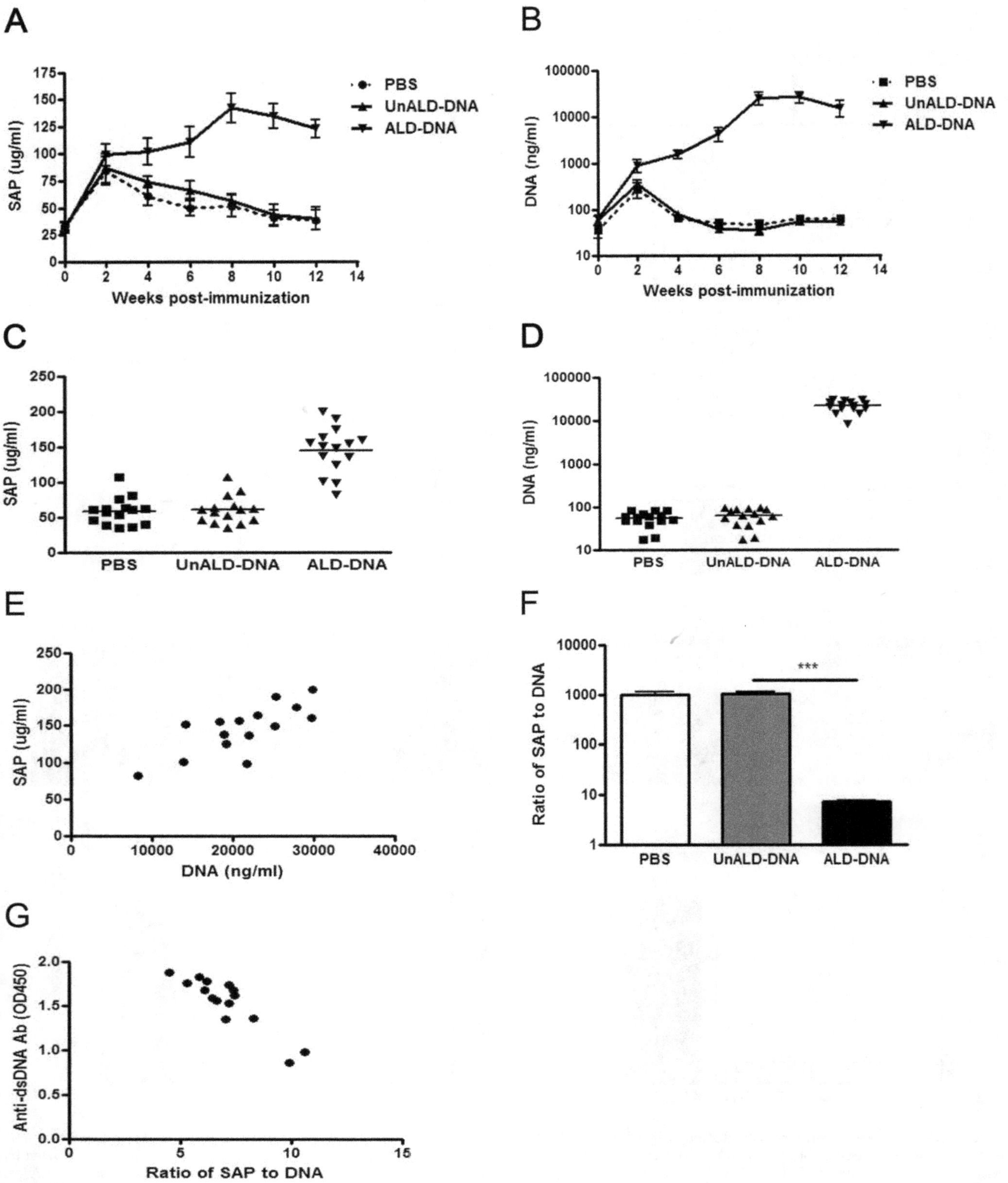

Figure 2. The ratios of SAP to DNA decrease in SLE murine model. 6-week-old female BALB/c mice were immunized subcutaneously with ALD-DNA, UnALD-DNA, or PBS (n = 15) for 3 times in 4 weeks. (A) The dynamics of SAP level in serum of mice immunized with ALD-DNA, UnALD-DNA, or PBS were determined by ELISA assay every 2 weeks. (B) The dynamics of circulating DNA level in serum of mice immunized with ALD-DNA, UnALD-DNA, or PBS were determined using a PicoGreen DNA detection kit (Invitrogen) every 2 weeks. (C) SAP levels in the serum of SLE murine model and controls were tested by ELISA at week 8 after initial immunization. n = 15. (D) Circulating DNA levels in the serum of SLE murine model and controls were determined using a PicoGreen DNA detection kit at week 8 after initial immunization. n = 15. (E) The correlation between SAP and DNA levels in

ALD-DNA-immunized lupus mice. n = 15. Pearson correlation analysis was used to carry out the correlation study. r = 0.76; P<0.05. (F) The ratios of SAP to DNA in SLE murine model and controls. Data are means ± SD from 15 mice in each group. ***, P<0.001. (G) The correlation between the ratio of SAP to DNA and anti-dsDNA IgG level in SLE murine model. Pearson correlation analysis was used to carry out the correlation study. r = 0.90; P<0.001.

endosome acidification. It was found that SAP increased the intracellular fluorescence rates of treated macrophages, indicating that SAP binding to ALD-DNA promoted the uptake of ALD-DNA by macrophages (Fig. 3F). Furthermore, we performed real-time PCR to detect cytokine expression in the macrophages cultured with ALD-DNA or the complexes of purified SAP protein and ALD-DNA (SAP plus ALD-DNA), and found that mRNA levels of inflammatory cytokines including TNF-α, IL-1β, IL-6, IL-12, and MCP-1 were notably decreased in the macrophages cultured with SAP plus ALD-DNA; however, mRNA level of IL-10 was significantly increased in the macrophages cultured with SAP plus ALD-DNA as compared with those of macrophages cultured with ALD-DNA alone (Fig. 3G). These data suggest that pSAP plasmid could be correctly transcribed, translated and the expressed SAP protein could inhibit ALD-DNA-mediated innate immune responses *in vitro*.

pSAP treatment in the early stage of SLE disease reverses lupus nephritis via reducing anti-dsDNA antibody production and IC deposition

To evaluate the effect of pSAP treatment in mice, ALD-DNA-induced lupus mice with the onset of proteinuria (at week 4 after the initial ALD-DNA immunization) were treated with pSAP (ALD-DNA plus pSAP group). Significantly increased serum SAP levels accompanied with remarkably decreased circulating DNA levels were found in pSAP-treated lupus mice as compared with those in pcDNA3-treated lupus mice (Fig. 4A and B). The ratios of SAP to DNA were simultaneously increased in pSAP-treated lupus mice as compared with those in pcDNA3-treated lupus mice, which suggested that pSAP injection could reverse the insufficiency of SAP in lupus mice (Fig. 4C). 12 weeks after the initial ALD-DNA immunization, the levels of anti-dsDNA autoantibodies, IC deposition, proteinuria, renal pathology, and kidney score were analyzed. Notably reduced the levels of anti-dsDNA autoantibodies (Fig. 4D and E), urine protein (Fig. 4F), IC deposition (Fig. 4G and H), renal pathology (Fig. 4I), and kidney score (Fig. 4J) were found in the pSAP-treated lupus mice as compared with those of pcDNA3-treated lupus mice. These results show that pSAP treatment in the early stage of SLE disease could reverse lupus nephritis via decreasing anti-dsDNA antibody production and IC deposition in lupus mice.

pSAP administration in the late stage of SLE disease alleviates lupus nephritis via reducing leukocyte infiltration and inflammatory marker production

To further evaluate the protective effect of pSAP treatment in mice in the late stage of SLE disease, ALD-DNA-induced lupus mice with the established lupus nephritis (at week 8 after the initial ALD-DNA immunization) were treated with pSAP (ALD-DNA plus pSAP group). Significantly increased serum SAP levels accompanied with remarkably decreased circulating DNA levels were found in pSAP-treated lupus mice as compared with those in pcDNA3-treated lupus mice (Fig. 5A and B). The ratios of SAP to DNA were simultaneously increased in pSAP-treated lupus mice as compared with those in pcDNA3-treated lupus mice, which suggested that pSAP injection could partly improve the insufficiency of SAP in lupus mice (Fig. 5C). 12 weeks after the initial

ALD-DNA immunization, the levels of anti-dsDNA autoantibodies, IC deposition, proteinuria, renal pathology, and kidney score were analyzed in the lupus murine model receiving pSAP injection at week 8 after the initial ALD-DNA immunization when lupus mice already had the highest levels of anti-dsDNA autoantibodies and established lupus nephritis (ALD-DNA plus pSAP group). Twelve weeks after the initial immunization, notably decreased levels of urine protein (Fig. 5F) and ameliorated glomerulonephritis (Fig. 5I and J) but slowly reduced levels of autoantibody titers (Fig. 5D and E) and IC deposition (Fig. 5G and H) were found in pSAP-treated lupus mice as compared with pcDNA3-treated lupus mice, indicating the improved lupus nephritis was not exclusively ascribed to the decreased anti-dsDNA antibody levels and IC deposition.

Other than the pathogenic anti-dsDNA autoantibody production and IC deposition, severe renal injury can be mediated by infiltrating proinflammatory leukocyte populations [17]. Flow cytometry analysis of cells extracted from kidneys of lupus mice showed a marked decrease in the number of CD45+ leukocytes in kidneys isolated from pSAP-treated lupus mice as compared with pcDNA3-treated lupus mice (Fig. 6A). Further flow cytometry analysis of infiltrating leukocyte populations revealed that pSAP-treated lupus mice displayed a decrease in renal T cells (CD4+) and B cells (CD19+) as compared to pcDNA3 treated lupus mice (Fig. 6A), but T and B cells only account for a portion of the decreased infiltrating cells in the kidneys of pSAP-treated lupus mice. Flow cytometry analysis of the presence of myeloid cells showed that pSAP-treated lupus mice exhibited a notable decrease in the number of F4/80+ macrophages (Fig. 6A), but there was no significant decrease in the number of CD11c+ dendritic cells (data not shown), suggesting that macrophages were the key cells that was influenced by pSAP treatment. As a set of inflammatory markers mainly secreted by macrophages were expressed in kidneys following glomerular immune complex deposition [8,18,19], further studies using ELISA analysis allowed us to determine several key markers in kidneys of mice. It was found that TNF-α, IL-1β, IL-6, IL-12 and MCP-1, which were upregulated in kidneys of ALD-DNA-induced lupus mice, were decreased in the pSAP-treated lupus mice (Fig. 6B). However, levels of IL-10 were notably increased in the pSAP-treated lupus mice (Fig. 6B). Analysis of the cytokine profile in serum of mice further confirmed that the inflammatory markers (including TNF-α, IL-1β, IL-6, IL-12, and MCP-1) were extensively and dramatically decreased in pSAP-treated lupus mice as compared with other control groups (Fig. 6C). These data suggest that pSAP treatment in the late stage of SLE disease could ameliorate the lupus nephritis via reducing the number of infiltrating inflammatory cells and decreasing the levels of inflammatory markers.

Discussion

We have provided here evidence that relative insufficiency of SAP played a critical role in the pathological process of the ALD-DNA-induced lupus nephritis, and verified that administration of SAP *in vivo* by a plasmid encoding the SAP, could significantly ameliorated the severity of SLE disease, as demonstrated by decreased levels of anti-dsDNA antibodies, reduced immune complex deposition, less proteinuria, less lupus nephritis, and decreased kidney score of

A

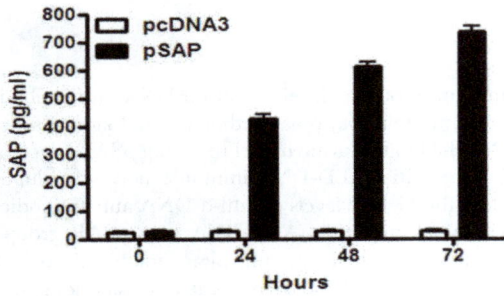

B

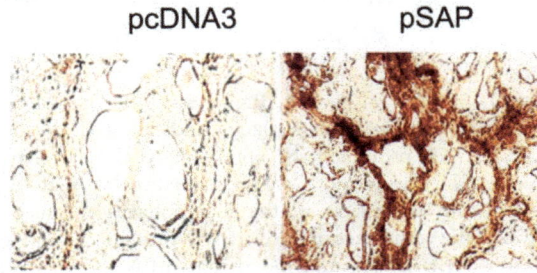

C

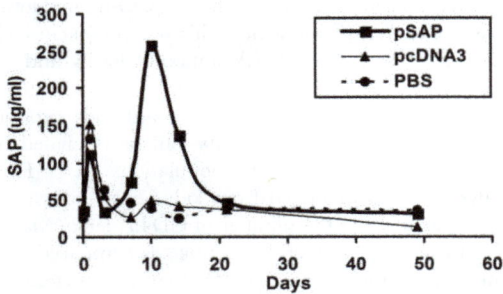

D

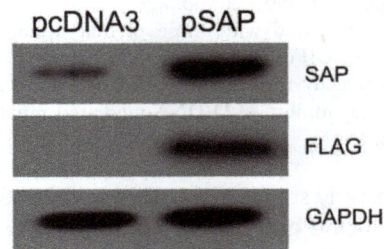

E

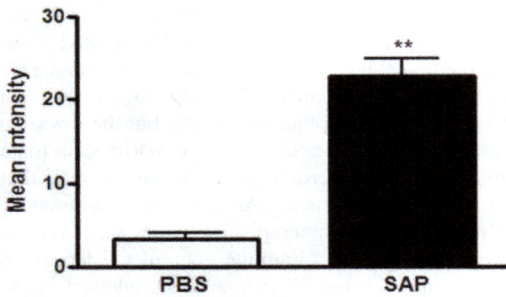

F

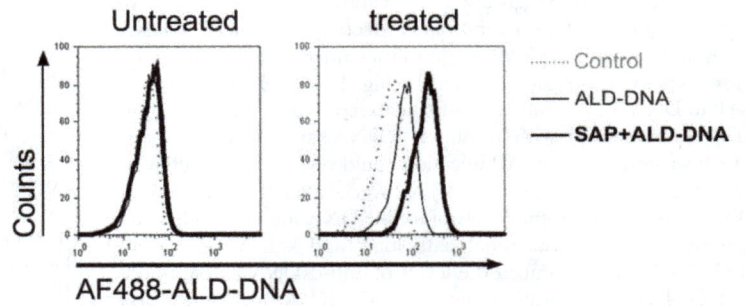

G

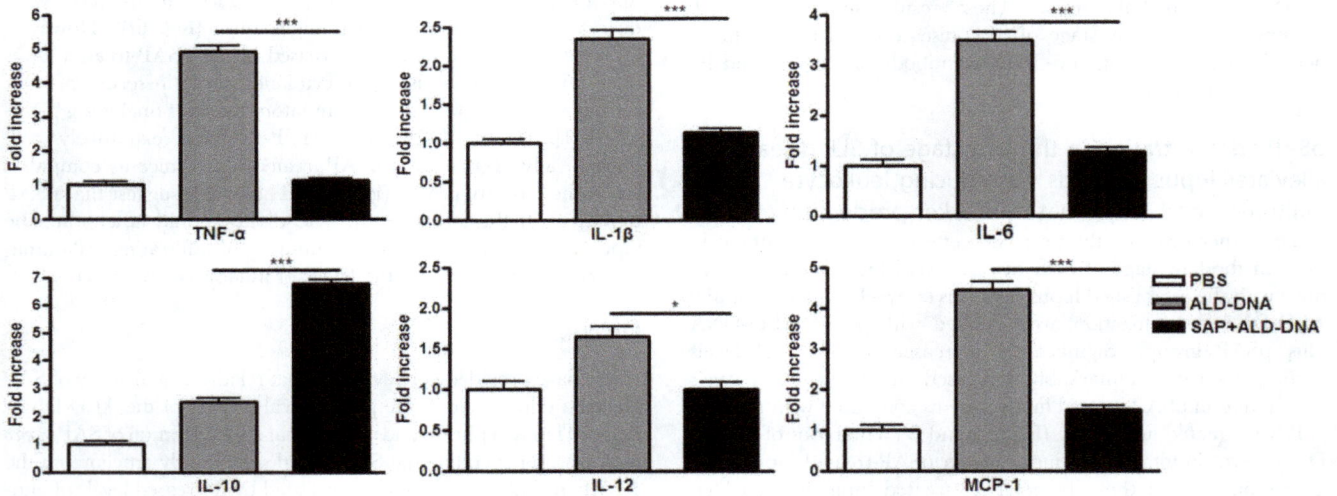

Figure 3. Efficiently expressed SAP could inhibit ALD-DNA-induced innate immune response. (A) NIH 3T3 cells were transfected with pcDNA3 or pcDNA3-SAP plasmid (pSAP) using Lipofectamine 2000 transfection reagent, and cell supernatants were collected and subjected to ELISA assay for the expression of SAP protein at 24 h, 48 h, and 72 h post transfection. Data are means ± SD of three independent experiments. (B–D) 6-week-old female BALB/c mice were injected intramuscularly with pSAP (100 µg/mice). (B) Immunohistochemistry examination was performed to determine the expression of SAP protein with anti-mouse SAP Ab in the muscle received pSAP injection. Imagines (×400) are representative of at least 10 mice in each group. (C) ELISA assay was performed to determine the levels of SAP protein in the serum of mice received pSAP injection. Data are means ± SD of three independent experiments. n = 10. (D) The serum was collected on day 10 after pSAP injection. Western blot analysis was performed to detect the expression of SAP in serum of mice received pSAP injection. Data are representative of at least 10 mice in each group. (E–G) SAP protein was purified from the serum of mice received pSAP injection. (E) The binding ability of the purified mouse SAP protein to DNA was detected by dot blot analysis. Quantitative analysis of blots was reflected as mean intensity. Data are means ± SD of three independent experiments. **, $P<0.01$. (F) Alexa Fluor 488 labeled ALD-DNA (AF488-ALD-DNA) was incubated with or without the purified SAP protein for 2 h (SAP plus ALD-DNA). BMDMs were treated with or without chloroquine (100 µg/ml) before DNA incubation. The intracellular Alexa Fluor 488 labeled ALD-DNA (AF488-ALD-DNA) in chloroquine-treated or untreated macrophages was determined by flow cytometry. Data are representative of results obtained in three independent experiments. (G) The purified SAP protein was incubated with ALD-DNA (SAP plus ALD-DNA) for 2 h. RAW264.7 cells were treated with PBS, ALD-DNA, or SAP plus ALD-DNA. 12 h later, levels of TNF-α, IL-1β, IL-6, IL-10, IL-12, and MCP-1 in the RAW264.7 cells were measured by real-time PCR. Data are means ± SD of three independent experiments. * $P<0.05$; ***, $P<0.001$.

glomerulonephritis. This therapeutic effect was closely associated with reduced production of anti-dsDNA antibodies in the early stage of the disease and significantly decreased infiltrating lymphocytes and reduced levels of inflammatory markers in kidneys of pSAP-treated mice in the late stage of the disease.

In previous study, the crucial and versatile functions of SAP in autoimmune disease have been well established [9,10]. SAP$^{-/-}$ mice spontaneously develop antinuclear autoimmunity and severe glomerulonephritis, a phenotype resembling human SLE [15]. However, people doubt if SAP deficiency or strain combination

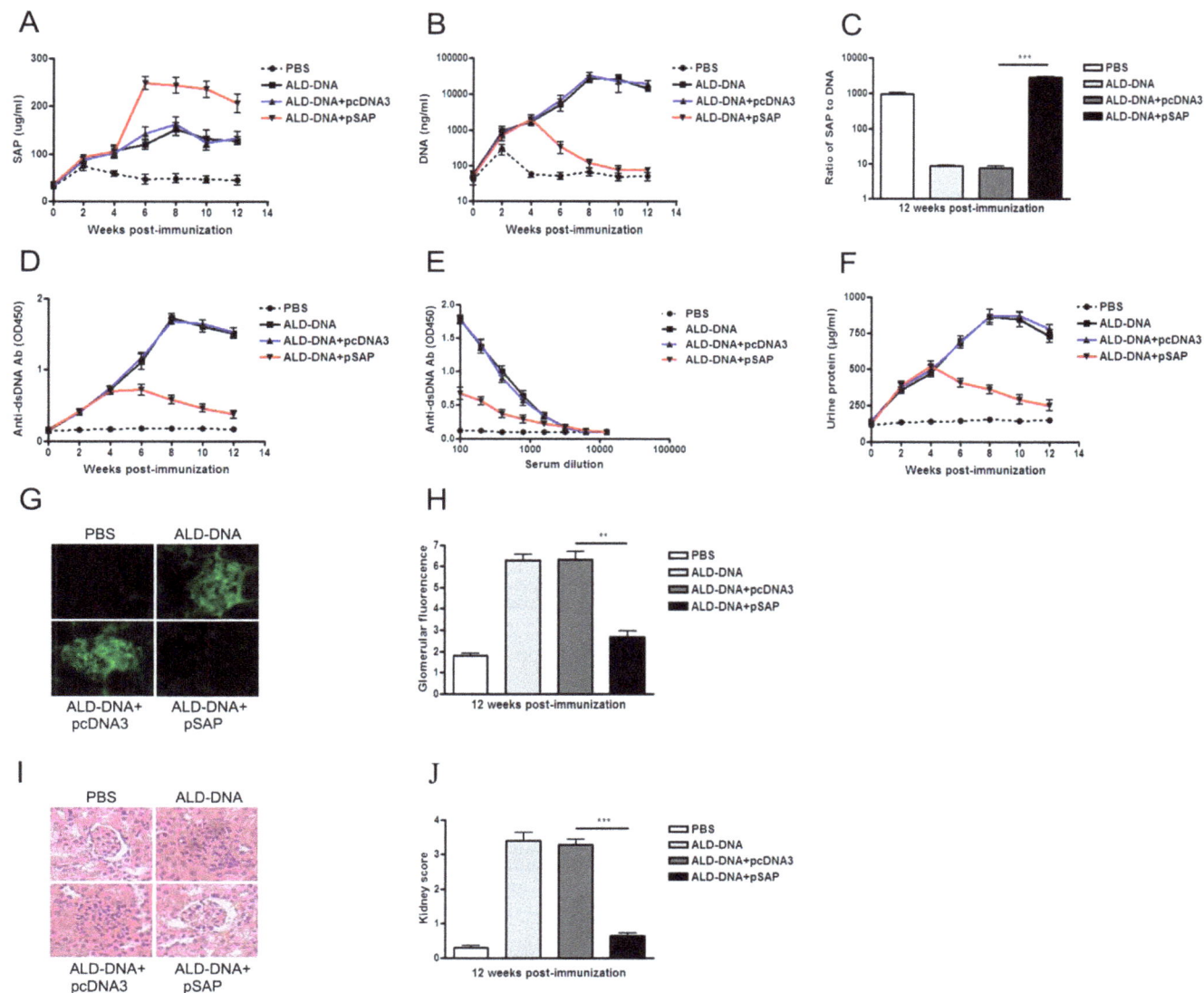

Figure 4. pSAP administration in the early stage of SLE disease reverses ALD-DNA-induced lupus nephritis. BALB/c mice were immunized subcutaneously with ALD-DNA (50 µg/mouse) or PBS for total 3 times in 4 weeks. Mice immunized with ALD-DNA were administrated intramuscularly with pSAP (100 µg/mice) from week 4 after initial immunization (with the onset of proteinuria) and injected every 2 weeks for total 5 times. (A) The dynamics of SAP level in serum of lupus mice injected with pSAP (ALD-DNA plus pSAP) or pcDNA3 (ALD-DNA plus pcDNA3) were determined by ELISA assay every 2 weeks. (B) The dynamics of circulating DNA level in serum of lupus mice injected with pSAP (ALD-DNA plus pSAP) or pcDNA3 (ALD-DNA plus pcDNA3) were determined by ELISA assay every 2 weeks. (C) The ratios of SAP to DNA in SLE murine model injected with pSAP (ALD-DNA plus pSAP) or pcDNA3 (ALD-DNA plus pcDNA3) at week 12 after initial immunization. Data are means ± SD from 10 mice in each group. ***, $P<0.001$. (D) Serum anti-dsDNA IgG levels of the mice were measured by ELISA assay every 2 weeks. (E) Anti-dsDNA IgG antibody titers in serum of pSAP-treated lupus mice (ALD-DNA plus pSAP) or pcDNA3-treated lupus mice (ALD-DNA plus pcDNA3) were detected by ELISA assay at week 8 after the initial ALD-DNA immunization. n = 10. (F) Urine protein levels of the mice were assessed by BCA Protein Assay Kit (Thermo Fisher Scientific) every 2 weeks. n = 10. (G) The deposition of IgG-containing IC in glomeruli at week 12 after initial immunization. Imagines (×200) are representative of at least 10 mice in each group. (H) Mean glomerular fluorescence intensity (arbitrary units) was determined for IgG in ALD-DNA-immunized lupus mice and control mice at week 12 after initial immunization. n = 10. **, $P<0.01$. (I) 12 weeks after initial immunization, nephritic pathological changes were shown by H&E staining of renal tissues surgical resected from the mice. Imagines (×200) are representative of at least 10 mice in each group. (J) The kidney score was assessed using paraffin sections stained with H&E. n = 10. ***, $P<0.001$.

contributes to the pathogenesis of SLE [20,21]. And the SAP-linked genes co-deficiency may confuse the elucidation of the role of SAP in autoimmunity [22]. Therefore, study of SLE pathogenesis in regarding to SAP in a mouse model with clear genetic background is very critical and should be a prerequisite. Herein, we use ALD-DNA-induced SLE murine model to

extensively study the role of SAP in SLE pathogenesis. In this study, it was found that the ratios of SAP to DNA significantly decreased in ALD-DNA-induced lupus mice as compared to controls. SAP plasmid (pSAP) treatment *in vivo* could significantly increase the levels of serum SAP and notably decreased the levels of circulating DNA, thus simultaneously increasing the ratios of

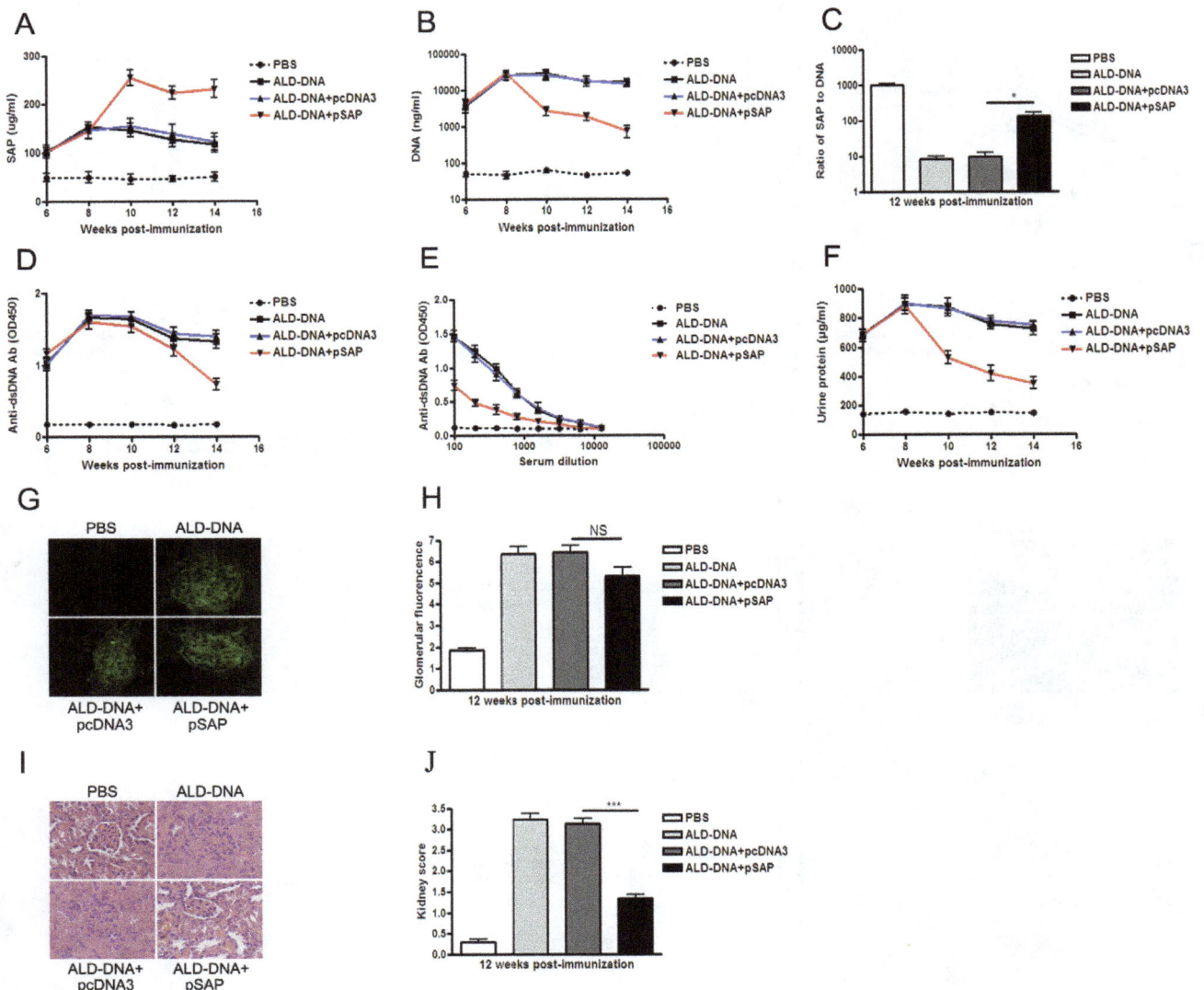

Figure 5. pSAP administration in the late stage of SLE disease ameliorates ALD-DNA-induced lupus nephritis. BALB/c mice were immunized subcutaneously with ALD-DNA (50 µg/mouse) or PBS for total 3 times in 4 weeks. Mice were administrated intramuscularly with pSAP (100 µg/mice) from week 8 after initial immunization (when sever lupus nephritis has been established) and injected every 2 weeks for total 4 times. (A) The dynamics of SAP level in serum of lupus mice injected with pSAP (ALD-DNA plus pSAP) or pcDNA3 (ALD-DNA plus pcDNA3) were determined by ELISA assay every 2 weeks. (B) The dynamics of circulating DNA level in serum of lupus mice injected with pSAP (ALD-DNA plus pSAP) or pcDNA3 (ALD-DNA plus pcDNA3) were determined by ELISA assay every 2 weeks. (C) The ratios of SAP to DNA in SLE murine model injected with pSAP (ALD-DNA plus pSAP) or pcDNA3 (ALD-DNA plus pcDNA3) at week 12 after initial immunization. Data are means ± SD from 10 mice in each group. ***, $P<0.001$. (D) Serum anti-dsDNA IgG levels were measured by ELISA assay every 2 weeks. (E) Anti-dsDNA IgG antibody titers in serum of pSAP-treated lupus mice (ALD-DNA plus pSAP) or pcDNA3-treated lupus mice (ALD-DNA plus pcDNA3) were detected by ELISA assay at week 14 after the initial ALD-DNA immunization. n = 10. (F) Urine protein levels of the mice were assessed by BCA Protein Assay Kit (Thermo Fisher Scientific) every 2 weeks. n = 10. (G) The deposition of IgG-containing IC in glomeruli at week 12 after initial immunization. Imagines (×200) are representative of at least 10 mice in each group. (H) Mean glomerular fluorescence intensity (arbitrary units) was determined for IgG in ALD-DNA-immunized lupus mice and control mice at week 12 after initial immunization. n = 10. NS, not significant. (I) 12 weeks after initial immunization, nephritic pathological changes were shown by H&E staining of renal tissues surgical resected from the mice. Imagines (×200) are representative of at least 10 mice in each group. (J) The kidney score was assessed using paraffin sections stained with H&E. n = 10. ***, $P<0.001$.

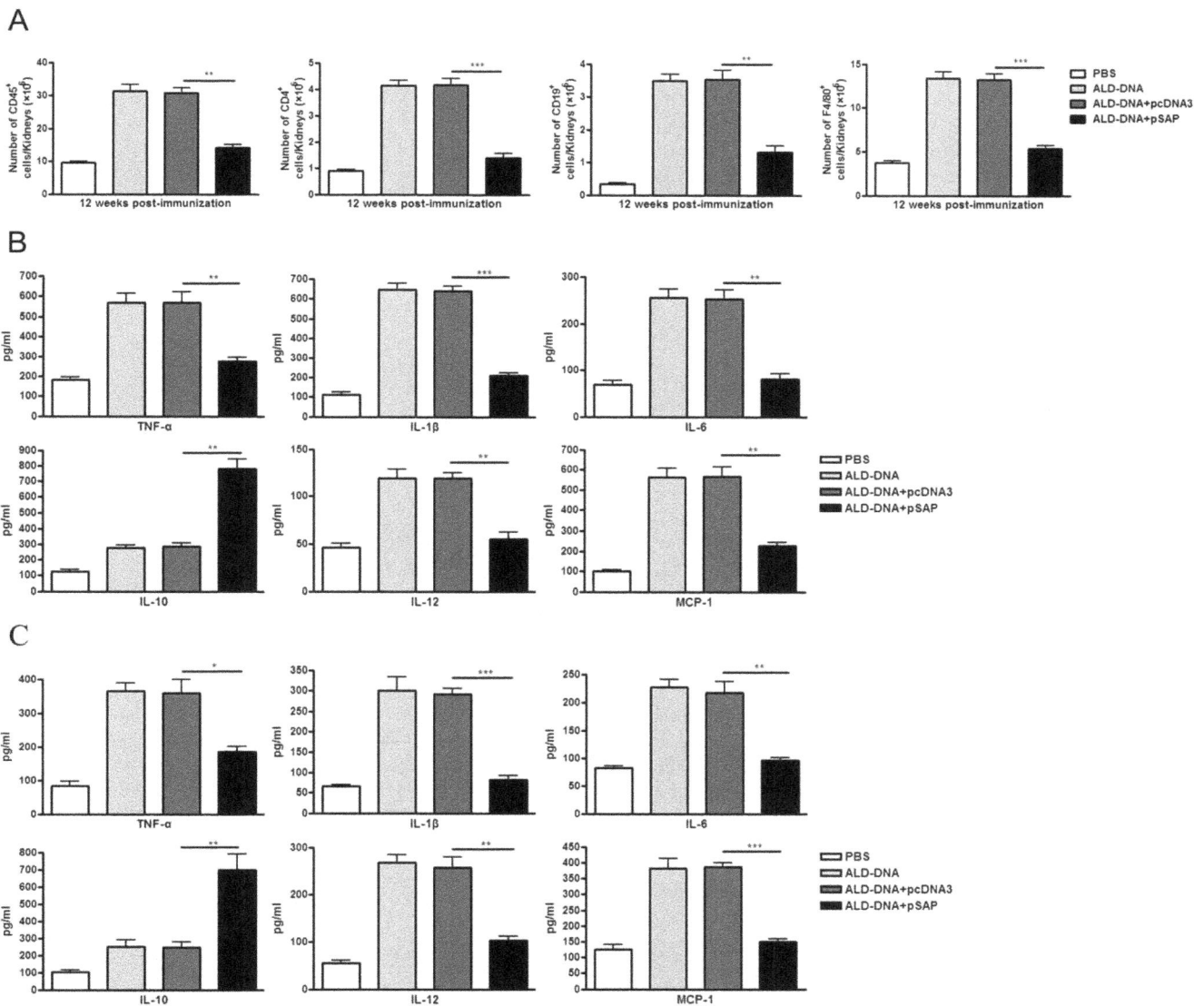

Figure 6. pSAP administration in the late stage of SLE disease reduces inflammation in kidneys of mice. BALB/c mice were immunized subcutaneously with ALD-DNA (50 µg/mouse) for total 3 times in 4 weeks. Mice were administrated intramuscularly with pSAP (100 µg/mice) from week 8 after initial immunization and injected every 2 weeks for total 4 times. (A) 12 weeks after initial immunization, the infiltration of leukocyte populations in kidneys of treated mice were assessed by flow cytometry. Decreased CD45+ cells, CD19+ cells, CD4+ cells, and F4/80+ cells were found in kidneys of pSAP-treated lupus mice. Data are representative of results obtained in three independent experiments. n = 10. (B) At week 12, the kidney tissues were collected and homogenized, the expression of TNF-α, IL-1β, IL-6, IL-10, IL-12, and MCP-1 were determined by ELISA assay. Data are means ± SD of three independent experiments. n = 8. ** $P<0.01$, *** $P<0.001$. (C) At week 12 after initial immunization, expression of TNF-α, IL-1β, IL-6, IL-10, IL-12, and MCP-1 in serum of the mice were determined by ELISA assay. Data are means ± SD of three independent experiments. n = 8. * $P<0.05$, ** $P<0.01$, *** $P<0.001$.

SAP to DNA. These results indicated that SAP was relative insufficient in ALD-DNA-induced SLE mice, which further provide the evidence that SAP defect rather than the deficiency of SAP linked genes might contribute to the pathogenesis of antinuclear autoimmunity in $SAP^{-/-}$ mice [15,20–22]. Notably, the ratios of SAP to DNA were negatively correlated with the titers of anti-dsDNA antibodies in lupus mice, which verified the critical role of SAP insufficiency in ALD-DNA-induced autoimmunity, although we did not exclude other factors contributing to the pathogenesis of the SLE disease [23,24]. As SAP and IgG shared the same binding site on FcγR and competed for FcγR binding, SAP could be used to inhibit antibody or immune complex-mediated immune response [11]. All these results strongly support a role for SAP in the protection against self-DNA-induced autoimmunity.

We thus adopted a gene therapy method using the pcDNA3-SAP plasmid (pSAP) to treat lupus nephritis. The SAP protein could be efficiently expressed and secreted into the culture supernatants when pSAP was transfected into NIH3T3 cell line, indicating that SAP cDNA cloned into pcDNA3 could be correctly transcribed, translated and the protein was efficiently secreted *in vitro*. Further study confirmed that the SAP protein could be efficiently expressed and secreted into the systemic circulation via intramuscular injection of pSAP, and SAP protein purified from pSAP-treated mice could promote self-DNA clearance via binding to self-DNA, indicating that efficiently expressed SAP protein could perform the biological functions. Analysis of cytokine levels of macrophages cultured with the complexes of SAP and DNA revealed that levels of inflammatory cytokines including TNF-α, IL-1β, IL-6, IL-12, and MCP-1 were notably decreased in the macrophages cultured with SAP plus ALD-DNA; however, level of IL-10 was significantly increased in the macrophages cultured with SAP plus ALD-DNA as compared with those of macrophages cultured with ALD-DNA alone, indicating that SAP inhibited ALD-DNA-mediated innate immune response *in vitro*. However, the mechanism of how SAP promotes the clearance of ALD-DNA needs to be further revealed. The protective effect of SAP had also been noticed by other groups and testified that the interaction of SAP with FcγR is able to mediate phagocytosis of apoptotic cells, as well as mediate protective immune response [12,25]. In our study, injection of pSAP in the early stage of SLE disease with the onset of proteinuria notably reversed lupus nephritis. The beneficial effect of pSAP treatment was associated with its inhibitory effect on ALD-DNA-induced anti-dsDNA antibody production and immune complex deposition, which was consistent with the findings from other groups that anti-dsDNA antibodies promoted initiation of lupus nephritis [26]. Furthermore, injection of pSAP at the late stage of SLE disease with the established lupus nephritis remarkably reduced proteinuria and lupus nephritis, while slowly decreased levels of anti-dsDNA antibodies and immune complex deposition were noticed in these pSAP-treated mice, indicating that the protective effect of SAP treatment in the late stage of SLE disease was not exclusively attributable to the decreased levels of anti-dsDNA autoantibodies.

SAP is the main acute-phase reactants in mice and its capacity to bind with DNA has been identified for more than 20 years [13,14,27,28]. However, recent emerging evidences indicate that SAP also plays a critical role in modulating cytokine production in inflammatory reactions [10,11]. The inflamed kidneys of patients with SLE, NZB/W F_1 mice, and ALD-DNA-induced lupus mice contain many lymphocytes around glomeruli, blood vessels, and in the interstitium [8,29–31]. Our study verified again that $CD45^+$ leucocytes were infiltrated into kidneys of ALD-DNA-induced lupus mice. SAP treatment in the late stage of SLE disease significantly decreased the numbers of $CD45^+$ leucocytes including T cells, B cells, and macrophages but not dendritic cells in kidney tissue of ALD-DNA-induced lupus mice and the underlying mechanisms need to be elucidated in the future. Further analysis of inflammatory markers revealed that SAP treatment notably decreased systemic and local inflammatory cytokine levels of TNF-α, IL-1β, IL-6, IL-12, and MCP-1, which were closely associated with the severity of lupus nephritis [18]. However, inhibitory cytokine IL-10 was notably increased in pSAP-treated lupus mice, which might also partly contribute to the alleviation of lupus nephritis. Our results were in good agreement with previous studies, and further confirmed the immunomodulatory function and potential protective and therapeutic effect of SAP in ALD-DNA-induced lupus nephritis.

In conclusion, we showed that SAP gene administration at the onset of proteinuria could reverse lupus nephritis. The main mechanism seems to be associated with the effective inhibiting the production of anti-dsDNA antibodies and immune complex deposition. While SAP gene treatment in the stage of established lupus nephritis could reduce the disease severity, which was possibly attributable to the decreased infiltration of lymphocytes and reduced levels of inflammatory markers beyond decreased anti-dsDNA autoantibody production. Our findings may provide an insight into better understanding of the underlying mechanism of ALD-DNA-induced lupus nephritis, and provide the preclinical data indicating that SAP administration can alleviate lupus nephritis. This strategy may be a clinically relevant and feasible therapeutic method for patients suffering from self-DNA-induced nephritis or other autoimmune diseases which accompany with decreased clearance of apoptotic cells.

Materials and Methods

Ethics statement

All experiments carried out in this study were strictly performed in a manner to minimize suffering of laboratory mice. All animal procedures were performed according to the Guide for the Care and Use of Medical Laboratory Animals (Ministry of Health, P.R. China, 1998) and with the ethical approval of the Shanghai Medical Laboratory Animal Care and Use Committee (Permit number: SYXK 2007-0036) as well as the Ethical Committee of Fudan University (Permit number: 2007016).

Mice and plasmid

Six-week-old female BALB/c mice were purchased from the Experimental Animal Center of Chinese Academy of Sciences (Shanghai, P. R. China). Mice were housed in a specific pathogen-free room under controlled temperature and humidity. The full length of SAP cDNA was amplified from total RNA of murine liver using the primers 5′-CGA AGC TTG CCA CCA TGG ACA AGC TGC TGC-3′ and 5′-CGG AAT TCC CTC TTA CAC ATC GGC AAT C-3′. 24 nucleotides encoding FLAG epitope (DYKDDDDK) were added directly at the carboxyl-terminal of SAP gene sequence by primer design. SAP cDNA with a FLAG tag was inserted into the pcDNA3 vector (Invitrogen) to generate pcDNA3-SAP plasmid (pSAP). The plasmid construct was confirmed by DNA sequencing.

Generation of bone marrow-derived macrophages (BMDMs)

Bone marrow (BM) cells were harvested from uninfected, normal BALB/c mice and filtered through nylon mesh. BM cells were cultured in L929 cell-conditioned medium at a density of 3×10^5 cells/ml of medium and maintained in a 5% CO_2

incubator at 37°C as described previously [32,33]. Six days after initial BM cells culture, the medium was changed and the purity of F4/80+ cells was more than 90%, as determined by flow cytometry (FACSCalibur; BD Biosciences).

DNA preparation

ALD-DNA and UnALD-DNA were prepared with murine splenocytes which were generated from surgical resected spleens of six- to eight-week-old female BALB/c mice and cultured with or without Con A (Sigma-Aldrich) in vitro as previously described [7]. Briefly, for generation of ALD-DNA, splenocytes were seeded at 2×10^6 cells/ml in 75 cm^2 cell culture flask and cultured in the presence of Con A (5 μg/ml) for 6 days to induce apoptosis. The apoptotic cells were stained with FITC-labeled Annexin V (BD Biosciences) and propidium iodide (PI; Sigma-Aldrich), and sorted using a FACSAria (BD Biosciences). Genomic DNAs from syngeneic apoptotic splenocytes were treated with S1 nuclease (TaKaRa) and proteinase K (Sigma-Aldrich), and then purified using the DNeasy Blood & Tissue Kits (Qiagen) according to the manufacturer's instructions. UnALD-DNA was prepared with unactivated (resting) splenocytes and extracted using the same methods. To exclude contaminations with LPS, sterile endotoxin-free plastic ware and reagents were used for DNA preparation. DNA samples were also monitored for low level of endotoxin by the Limulus amoebocyte lysate assay (BioWhittaker) according to the manufacturer's instructions. The concentration of DNA was determined by detection of the absorbance (A) at 260 nm. The apoptotic DNA ladder of ALD-DNA was confirmed by agarose gel electrophoresis (AGE).

Generation of SLE murine model

To generate SLE murine model, 6- to 8-wk-old syngeneic female BALB/c mice were divided into several groups of 8–10 mice and actively immunized by subcutaneous injection on the back with 0.2 ml of an emulsion containing ALD-DNA (50 μg/ mouse) in phosphate-buffered saline (PBS) plus equal volume of complete Freund's adjuvant (CFA; Sigma-Aldrich) at week 0, and followed by two booster immunizations of ALD-DNA (50 μg/ mouse) emulsified with IFA (Sigma-Aldrich) at week 2 and week 4 for total 3 times as previously described [6,7]. Eight to 10 mice in each group received an equal volume of PBS plus CFA or IFA, or UnALD-DNA (50 μg/mouse) plus CFA or IFA were used as contols. Mice were bled from retro-orbital sinus prior to immunization and at 2-week internals until 3 months after the initial immunization. 8 or 12 weeks later, mice were sacrificed and surgical resected spleens and kidneys were collected for further cellular function and tissue histology analysis.

Autoantibody and proteinuria examination

Anti-dsDNA antibodies in the mice serum were determined by ELISA assay as described previously [6]. In briefly, ELISA plates (Costar) were pretreated with protamine sulphate (Sigma-Aldrich) and then coated with calf thymus dsDNA (Sigma-Aldrich). After incubation with mouse serum, the levels of anti-dsDNA Abs were detected with the horseradish peroxidase (HRP)-conjugated goat anti-mouse IgG (Southern Biotech). Tetramethylbenzidine (TMB) substrate was used to develop colors and absorbance at 450 nm was measured on a microplate reader (BIO-TEK ELX800). Proteinuria of the mice was measured with the BCA Protein Assay Kit (Thermo Scientific) according to the manufacturer's instructions.

Measurement of anti-dsDNA antibody titers

Anti-dsDNA antibody titers in the mice serum were determined by ELISA assay as described previously [34]. In briefly, protamine

sulphate pre-treated 96-well microtitre plates (Costar) were coated with calf thymus dsDNA (Sigma-Aldrich; 50 μg/ml) for 2 h at 37°C and then placed overnight at 4°C. After washing three times with PBS containing 0.05% Tween-20 (PBST), the plates were blocked with 1% BSA for 1 h, and serial dilutions of serum in PBS–1% BSA were added for 1 h at 37°C. After washing, the plates were incubated with 1:1000 dilution of horseradish peroxidase (HRP)-conjugated goat anti-mouse IgG (Southern Biotech) for 1 h at 37°C. Tetramethylbenzidine (TMB) substrate was used to develop colors and absorbance at 450 nm was measured on a microplate reader (BIO-TEK ELX800).

Measurement of SAP level

To assess protein levels of SAP in serum of mice or in the culture supernatants, ELISA assays were performed with the following anti-SAP Abs and SAP standards: sheep anti-mouse SAP (Calbiochem), rabbit anti-mouse SAP (Calbiochem), and mouse SAP (Calbiochem) as previously described [35].

Measurement of circulating DNA level

DNA was extracted from serum samples and then quantified using a PicoGreen DNA detection kit (Invitrogen) according to the manufacturer's instructions [36]. In briefly, DNA was extracted from 200 μl of serum samples using a QIAamp Blood Kit (Qiagene) using the blood and body fluid protocol as recommended by the manufacturer. After the removal of most proteins by digestion with proteinase K, the sample was applied to the QIAamp 96 plate. DNA was adsorbed onto the silica membrane during a brief centrifugation step, while any remaining protein, salt and other contaminants were completely removed by three consecutive washes. Membrane-bound DNA was then eluted in double deionized H$_2$O or Tris–EDTA buffer. A final elution volume of 200 μl was used. Quantification of DNA was carried out using a PicoGreen DNA detection kit (Invitrogen). Calf thymus DNA (100 mg/ml; Sigma-Aldrich) was used as the standard. The concentration of DNA in the standard curve ranged from 0 to 100 ng/ml. Briefly, 20 ml of final DNA eluated was mixed with 1 ml of Tris–EDTA (10 mmol/l Tris–HCl, 1 mmol/l EDTA, pH 7.5) diluted with PicoGreen reagent. Fluorescence intensity was measured on an F-2000 spectrofluorometer (Molecular Devices) at excitation wavelength of 480 nm and an emission of 520 nm. Standard curve used to determine the levels of circulating DNA in the samples was established by the linear relationship between the known concentrations of calf thymus DNA (Sigma-Aldrich) and the corresponding fluorescence intensities.

Immunohistochemistry examination

The expression of SAP protein in the muscle tissue received pcDNA3-SAP (pSAP) injection was analyzed by immunohistochemistry. In briefly, mice were injected with pSAP (100 μg/mice) at the site of femoral muscle. 3 days later, the muscle tissue harvested from pSAP treated mice were fixed in 4% paraformaldehyde, processed on a standard histology processor, embedded in paraffin, and cut into 5 micron sections. Paraffin sections were dewaxed in xylene and rehydrated in decreasing concentrations of alcohol. Sections were exposed to citrate buffer and heat antigen retrieval and then blocked and incubated with rabbit anti-mouse SAP antibody (Calbiochem). Sections were subsequently assayed with the Super Sensitive Polymer-HRP IHC Detection System (Vector Laboratories) according to the manufacturer's instructions. 3, 3′-Diaminobenzidine (DAB) substrate (Dako) was used to develop slides. Slides were counterstained with hematoxylin (Dako) and coverslipped using Permount mounting media (Fisher Scientific). Pictures were acquired with a 20×/0.45 Plan Fluor object on a Nikon SCLIPSS TE2000-S microscope (Nikon) equipped with ACT-1 software (Nikon). Original magnification was 400×.

Western blot analysis

Six-week-old female BALB/c mice were injected intramuscularly with pSAP (100 μg/mice). 10 days later, the serum was collected and western blot analysis was performed as described previously [37]. In briefly, serum was electrophoresed on SDS-PAGE gels and then transferred to the PVDF membrane. The membrane was probed with rabbit anti-SAP (Calbiochem), mouse anti-FLAG (Santa Cruz), or rabbit anti-GAPDH antibody (Santa Cruz), followed by HRP-conjugated goat anti-rabbit antibody (Santa Cruz) or goat anti-mouse antibody (Southern Biotech). The signals were developed by chemiluminescence (Pierce).

Binding ability of SAP to DNA

The binding ability of SAP to DNA was detected by dot blot analysis with mouse SAP protein purified from pSAP treated mice and rabbit anti-mouse SAP (Calbiochem) as previously described [38]. In briefly, DNA (1 μg) was spotted on the nitrocellulose membranes. After the incubation of SAP protein (1 μg/ml), anti-SAP Abs, and peroxidase-labeled IgG Abs (Southern Biotech), the blots were developed with 3, 3′-Diaminobenzidine (DAB) to measure the binding ability of SAP to DNA. Quantitative analysis of blots was done using Mini-Transilluminator (Bio-Rad) equipped with molecular analysis software. The binding ability of SAP to DNA was reflected as mean intensity.

DNA uptake in vitro

ALD-DNA was labeled with Alexa Fluor 488 (Invitrogen) according to the manufacturer's instructions. The labeled ALD-DNA (referred as AF488-ALD-DNA) was purified using Bio-Rad Micro Bio-Spin P-30 column (Bio-Rad, Hercules, CA) according to the manufacturer's protocol. AF488-ALD-DNA was incubated with purified mouse SAP protein (SAP plus ALD-DNA) at 37°C for 2 h. BMDMs were treated with chloroquine (100 μg/ml) before DNA incubation. The intracellular Alexa Fluor 488 labeled ALD-DNA (AF488-ALD-DNA) was determined by flow cytometry (FACSCalibur) as previously described [39]. All flow cytometry data were acquired on a BD FACSCalibur (BD Biosciences) in CellQuest (BD Biosciences) and analyzed by FlowJo software (Tree Star).

Real-time PCR analysis

Total RNA was isolated from cultured cells with TRIzol reagent (Invitrogen) and was reverse-transcribed (RT) using a cDNA synthesis kit (MBI Ferments) according to the manufacturer's instructions. Subsequently, cDNA was subjected to quantitative real-time PCR using a Lightcycler480 and SYBR Green system (Roche Diagnostics) following the manufacturer's protocol [40].

Flow cytometry analysis

Murine renal tissues were surgical resected and dispersed in RPMI 1640 contained 5% FBS and 0.1% collagenase (Sigma-Aldrich) at 37°C for 30 min, followed by progressive sieving to obtain single-cell suspensions. To assess the infiltration of leucocyte populations in kidneys of mice, flow cytometry analysis were performed with PE-labeled anti-CD45, PerCP-labeled anti-CD4, FITC-labeled anti-CD19, and FITC-labeled anti-F4/80 (BD Biosciences). All flow cytometry data were acquired on a BD FACSCalibur (BD Biosciences) in CellQuest (BD Biosciences) and analyzed by FlowJo software (Tree Star).

ELISA Assay

To assess protein levels of TNF-α, IL-1β, IL-6, IL-10, IL-12, and MCP-1 in the homogenized kidney tissue and in serum of mice, ELISA assays were performed with relative ELISA Kits (eBioscience) according to the manufacturer's instructions.

Pathological analysis

For histology analysis, murine renal tissues were surgical resected and fixed in 4% paraformaldehyde (Sigma-Aldrich), processed, and embedded in paraffin. H&E staining of renal tissue sections were performed according to the manufacturer's instructions and assessed by a pathologist blinded to treatment group. The kidney score of glomerulonephritis was determined by using the ISN/RPS2003 classification. Fluorescent staining of cryosections was used for autoantibody deposition analysis in the glomeruli. Sections were fixed in acetone for 10 min and incubated with FITC-conjugated goat anti-mouse IgG (H+L chain specific) Ab (Sigma-Aldrich) for 30 min. Pictures were acquired with Nikon SCLIPSS TE2000-S microscope (Nikon) equipped with ACT-1 software (Nikon). Original magnification was ×200.

Statistical analysis

All data are expressed as means ± SD of three independent experiments or from a representative experiment of three independent experiments. The statistical significance of the differences in the experimental data was valued by the Student's t-test. The statistical significance level was set as * $P<0.05$, ** $P<0.01$, *** $P<0.001$.

Author Contributions

Conceived and designed the experiments: WZ JW SX. Performed the experiments: WZ JW. Analyzed the data: WZ JW WX. Contributed reagents/materials/analysis tools: WZ JW BQ WX. Wrote the paper: WZ JW BQ SX.

References

1. Rahman A, Isenberg DA (2008) Systemic lupus erythematosus. N Engl J Med 358: 929–939.
2. Walport MJ (2000) Lupus, DNase and defective disposal of cellular debris. Nat Genet 25: 135–136.
3. Kotzin BL (1996) Systemic lupus erythematosus. Cell 85: 303–306.
4. Savill J, Dransfield I, Gregory C, Haslett C (2002) A blast from the past: clearance of apoptotic cells regulates immune responses. Nat Rev Immunol 2: 965–975.
5. Hoffmann MH, Trembleau S, Muller S, Steiner G (2010) Nucleic acid-associated autoantigens: pathogenic involvement and therapeutic potential. J Autoimmun 34: J178–206.
6. Qiao B, Wu J, Chu YW, Wang Y, Wang DP, et al. (2005) Induction of systemic lupus erythematosus-like syndrome in syngeneic mice by immunization with activated lymphocyte-derived DNA. Rheumatology (Oxford) 44: 1108–1114.
7. Wen ZK, Xu W, Xu L, Cao QH, Wang Y, et al. (2007) DNA hypomethylation is crucial for apoptotic DNA to induce systemic lupus erythematosus-like autoimmune disease in SLE-non-susceptible mice. Rheumatology (Oxford) 46: 1796–1803.
8. Zhang W, Xu W, Xiong S (2010) Blockade of Notch1 signaling alleviates murine lupus via blunting macrophage activation and M2b polarization. J Immunol 184: 6465–6478.
9. Garlanda C, Bottazzi B, Bastone A, Mantovani A (2005) Pentraxins at the crossroads between innate immunity, inflammation, matrix deposition, and female fertility. Annu Rev Immunol 23: 337–366.
10. Bottazzi B, Doni A, Garlanda C, Mantovani A (2010) An integrated view of humoral innate immunity: pentraxins as a paradigm. Annu Rev Immunol 28: 157–183.

11. Lu J, Marnell LL, Marjon KD, Mold C, Du Clos TW, et al. (2008) Structural recognition and functional activation of FcgammaR by innate pentraxins. Nature 456: 989–992.
12. Mold C, Gresham HD, Du Clos TW (2001) Serum amyloid P component and C-reactive protein mediate phagocytosis through murine Fc gamma Rs. J Immunol 166: 1200–1205.
13. Pepys MB, Butler PJ (1987) Serum amyloid P component is the major calcium-dependent specific DNA binding protein of the serum. Biochem Biophys Res Commun 148: 308–313.
14. Breathnach SM, Kofler H, Sepp N, Ashworth J, Woodrow D, et al. (1989) Serum amyloid P component binds to cell nuclei in vitro and to in vivo deposits of extracellular chromatin in systemic lupus erythematosus. J Exp Med 170: 1433–1438.
15. Bickerstaff MC, Botto M, Hutchinson WL, Herbert J, Tennent GA, et al. (1999) Serum amyloid P component controls chromatin degradation and prevents antinuclear autoimmunity. Nat Med 5: 694–697.
16. Bharadwaj D, Mold C, Markham E, Du Clos TW (2001) Serum amyloid P component binds to Fc gamma receptors and opsonizes particles for phagocytosis. J Immunol 166: 6735–6741.
17. Triantafyllopoulou A, Franzke CW, Seshan SV, Perino G, Kalliolias GD, et al. (2010) Proliferative lesions and metalloproteinase activity in murine lupus nephritis mediated by type I interferons and macrophages. Proc Natl Acad Sci USA 107: 3012–3017.
18. Schiffer L, Bethunaickan R, Ramanujam M, Huang W, Schiffer M, et al. (2008) Activated renal macrophages are markers of disease onset and disease remission in lupus nephritis. J Immunol 180: 1938–1947.
19. Hale MB, Krutzik PO, Samra SS, Crane JM, Nolan GP (2009) Stage dependent aberrant regulation of cytokine-STAT signaling in murine systemic lupus erythematosus. PLoS One 4: e6756.
20. Bygrave AE, Rose KL, Cortes-Hernandez J, Warren J, Rigby RJ, et al. (2004) Spontaneous autoimmunity in 129 and C57BL/6 mice-implications for autoimmunity described in gene-targeted mice. PLoS Biol 2: E243.
21. Gillmore JD, Hutchinson WL, Herbert J, Bybee A, Mitchell DA, et al. (2004) Autoimmunity and glomerulonephritis in mice with targeted deletion of the serum amyloid P component gene: SAP deficiency or strain combination? Immunology 112: 255–264.
22. Tamaoki T, Tezuka H, Okada Y, Ito S, Shimura H, et al. (2005) Avoiding the effect of linked genes is crucial to elucidate the role of Apcs in autoimmunity. Nat Med 11: 11–12; author reply 12–13.
23. Napirei M, Karsunky H, Zevnik B, Stephan H, Mannherz HG, et al. (2000) Features of systemic lupus erythematosus in Dnase1-deficient mice. Nat Genet 25: 177–181.
24. Zykova SN, Tveita AA, Rekvig OP (2010) Renal Dnase1 enzyme activity and protein expression is selectively shut down in murine and human membrano-proliferative lupus nephritis. PLoS One 5: e12096.
25. Murray LA, Rosada R, Moreira AP, Joshi A, Kramer MS, et al. (2010) Serum amyloid P therapeutically attenuates murine bleomycin-induced pulmonary fibrosis via its effects on macrophages. PLoS One 5: e9683.
26. Fenton K, Fismen S, Hedberg A, Seredkina N, Fenton C, et al. (2009) Anti-dsDNA antibodies promote initiation, and acquired loss of renal Dnase1 promotes progression of lupus nephritis in autoimmune (NZBxNZW)F1 mice. PLoS One 4: e8474.
27. Emsley J, White HE, O'Hara BP, Oliva G, Srinivasan N, et al. (1994) Structure of pentameric human serum amyloid P component. Nature 367: 338–345.
28. Sorensen IJ, Holm Nielsen E, Schroder L, Voss A, Horvath L, et al. (2000) Complexes of serum amyloid P component and DNA in serum from healthy individuals and systemic lupus erythematosus patients. J Clin Immunol 20: 408–415.
29. Muehrcke RC, Kark RM, Pirani CL, Pollak VE (1957) Lupus nephritis: a clinical and pathologic study based on renal biopsies. Medicine (Baltimore) 36: 1–145.
30. Kuroiwa T, Lee EG (1998) Cellular interactions in the pathogenesis of lupus nephritis: the role of T cells and macrophages in the amplification of the inflammatory process in the kidney. Lupus 7: 597–603.
31. Andrews BS, Eisenberg RA, Theofilopoulos AN, Izui S, Wilson CB, et al. (1978) Spontaneous murine lupus-like syndromes. Clinical and immunopathological manifestations in several strains. J Exp Med 148: 1198–1215.
32. Ito T, Schaller M, Hogaboam CM, Standiford TJ, Sandor M, et al. (2009) TLR9 regulates the mycobacteria-elicited pulmonary granulomatous immune response in mice through DC-derived Notch ligand delta-like 4. J Clin Invest 119: 33–46.
33. Lake FR, Noble PW, Henson PM, Riches DW (1994) Functional switching of macrophage responses to tumor necrosis factor-alpha (TNF alpha) by interferons. Implications for the pleiotropic activities of TNF alpha. J Clin Invest 93: 1661–1669.
34. Sheerin NS, Abe K, Risley P, Sacks SH (2006) Accumulation of immune complexes in glomerular disease is independent of locally synthesized c3. J Am Soc Nephrol 17: 686–696.
35. Chintalacharuvu SR, Wang JX, Giaconia JM, Venkataraman C (2005) An essential role for CCL3 in the development of collagen antibody-induced arthritis. Immunol Lett 100: 202–204.
36. Dupont KM, Sharma K, Stevens HY, Boerckel JD, Garcia AJ, et al. (2010) Human stem cell delivery for treatment of large segmental bone defects. Proc Natl Acad Sci U S A 107: 3305–3310.
37. Xu J, Yun X, Jiang J, Wei Y, Wu Y, et al. (2010) Hepatitis B virus X protein blunts senescence-like growth arrest of human hepatocellular carcinoma by reducing Notch1 cleavage. Hepatology 52: 142–154.
38. Estabrook MM, Jack DL, Klein NJ, Jarvis GA (2004) Mannose-binding lectin binds to two major outer membrane proteins, opacity protein and porin, of Neisseria meningitidis. J Immunol 172: 3784–3792.
39. Chung EY, Liu J, Homma Y, Zhang Y, Brendolan A, et al. (2007) Interleukin-10 expression in macrophages during phagocytosis of apoptotic cells is mediated by homeodomain proteins Pbx1 and Prep-1. Immunity 27: 952–964.
40. Gao B, Duan Z, Xu W, Xiong S (2009) Tripartite motif-containing 22 inhibits the activity of hepatitis B virus core promoter, which is dependent on nuclear-located RING domain. Hepatology 50: 424–433.

16

Genetic Risk Factors in Lupus Nephritis and IgA Nephropathy – No Support of an Overlap

Mai Tuyet Vuong[1,2,3]*, **Iva Gunnarsson**[1], **Sigrid Lundberg**[4], **Elisabet Svenungsson**[1], **Lars Wramner**[5], **Anders Fernström**[6], **Ann-Christine Syvänen**[7], **Lieu Thi Do**[3], **Stefan H. Jacobson**[2], **Leonid Padyukov**[1]

1 Rheumatology Unit, Department of Medicine, Karolinska Institutet, Stockholm, Sweden, **2** Department of Nephrology, Danderyd Hospital, Karolinska Institutet, Stockholm, Sweden, **3** Department of Internal Medicine, Hanoi Medical University, Hanoi, Vietnam, **4** Nephrology Unit, Department of Medicine, Karolinska University Hospital, Stockholm, Sweden, **5** Transplantation Center, Sahlgrenska University Hospital, Göteborg, Sweden, **6** Department of Nephrology, Linköping University Hospital, Linköping, Sweden, **7** Department of Medical Sciences, Uppsala University, Uppsala, Sweden

Abstract

Background: IgA nephropathy (IgAN) and nephritis in Systemic Lupus Erythematosus (SLE) are two common forms of glomerulonephritis in which genetic findings are of importance for disease development. We have recently reported an association of IgAN with variants of *TGFB1*. In several autoimmune diseases, particularly in SLE, *IRF5*, *STAT4* genes and *TRAF1-C5* locus have been shown to be important candidate genes. The aim of this study was to compare genetic variants from the *TGFB1*, *IRF5*, *STAT4* genes and *TRAF1-C5* locus with susceptibility to IgAN and lupus nephritis in two Swedish cohorts.

Patients and Methods: We genotyped 13 single nucleotide polymorphisms (SNPs) in four genetic loci in 1252 DNA samples from patients with biopsy proven IgAN or with SLE (with and without nephritis) and healthy age- and sex-matched controls from the same population in Sweden.

Results: Genotype and allelic frequencies for SNPs from selected genes did not differ significantly between lupus nephritis patients and SLE patients without nephritis. In addition, haplotype analysis for seven selected SNPs did not reveal a difference for the SLE patient groups with and without nephritis. Moreover, none of these SPNs showed a significant difference between IgAN patients and healthy controls. *IRF5* and *STAT4* variants remained significantly different between SLE cases and healthy controls. In addition, the data did not show an association of *TRAF1-C5* polymorphism with susceptibility to SLE in this Swedish population.

Conclusion: Our data do not support an overlap in genetic susceptibility between patients with IgAN or SLE and reveal no specific importance of SLE associated SNPs for the presence of lupus nephritis.

Editor: Syed A. Aziz, Health Canada, Canada

Funding: The support for the project (7500730303 and 75007342) from SIDA Secretariat for Research Cooperation for the bilateral cooperation between Vietnam and Sweden; Swedish Research Council for Medicine, Sweden. The funders had no role in study design, data collection and analysis, decision to publish, or preparation of the manuscript.

Competing Interests: The authors have declared that no competing interests exist.

* E-mail: maituyetvuong@gmail.com

Introduction

Several common gene variations have recently been shown to associate with different autoimmune diseases, particularly Systemic Lupus Erythematosus (SLE). Some nucleotide polymorphisms (SNPs) have been shown to associate with single autoimmune disease, while other SNPs associate with several diseases. Interferon regulatory factor 5 *(IRF5)* polymorphism has been shown to be a risk factor for the development of SLE [1,2,3,4,5], rheumatoid arthritis (RA) [6,7,8,9], multiple sclerosis (MS) [10], Sjögren's syndrome [11] and inflammatory bowel disease [12]. Signal transducers and activator of transcription 4 *(STAT4)* and TNF receptor-associated factor 1-Complement component 5 *(TRAF1-C5)* polymorphisms have been found to associate with both SLE and RA [13,14,15,16]. Recently we reported that transforming growth factor-β1 *(TGFB1)*, an important cytokine gene, is in association with IgA nephropathy (IgAN) [17].

Immunological and biochemical similarities between SLE and IgAN demonstrate a direct link to impaired immune function in both diseases [18]. Patients with lupus nephritis and IgAN both have circulating immune complexes and display anti-C1q antibodies, which might point to certain pathogenic similarities in these glomerular disorders [18,19]. Moreover, lupus nephritis and IgAN are both chronic renal diseases that are classified in the "predominant" inflammatory group, based on morphological similarities [20,21]. We hypothesized that it may be an overlap in genetic susceptibility between lupus nephritis and IgAN and that there could be specific genetic makers associated to the development of nephritis in SLE patients.

To test this hypothesis we compared the genotype, allelic and haplotype frequencies from *IRF5*, *STAT4* and *TRAF1-C5* polymorphisms between IgAN patients and healthy controls, and SLE patients with and without nephritis, from *TGFB1* polymorphisms between SLE patients and healthy controls.

Materials and Methods

Patients and healthy subjects

Two cohorts of patients with SLE or IgAN, altogether 1252 individuals, were included in the present study. The cohort of patients with SLE, consisted of 272 SLE patients, all self-reported Caucasians from 18 to 80 years of age (mean age 45±14 years). 106 SLE patients had biopsy proven nephritis (39%) and 166 SLE patients had no clinical or laboratory signs of nephritis (61%). The control group for SLE patients consisted of 307 healthy age-matched individuals from the same population in Sweden, who were 17 to 70 years old, mean age 44±13 years.

In the IgAN cohort, there were altogether 673 DNA samples, of which 196 samples were obtained from patients with biopsy-proven IgAN, all self-reported Caucasians, and 477 samples were collected from gender- and age matched healthy controls from the same population in Sweden. Patients with Henoch-Schönlein purpura or with other forms of glomerulonephritis and individuals with self-reported non-Caucasian ancestry were excluded in our study. All patients gave written informed consent and the study was approved by the Ethics Committee of the Karolinska University Hospital, Stockholm, Sweden.

DNA extraction, selection of genetic markers, and genotyping

DNA was extracted from EDTA blood samples (5–10 ml) by the "salting out" method, as described elsewhere [22]. The SNPs were selected because they had previously been shown to be associated with SLE [5,14,15], RA [9,13,15], or with IgAN [17]. The SNPs were genotyped by fluorescent single base extension using the multiplex SNPstream system (Beckman Coulter Inc) or by TaqMan allelic discrimination assay (Applied Biosystems, Foster City, U.S.A) (Table 1). All analyzed SNPs were in Hardy-Weinberg equilibrium and the average positive rate of the genotype detection was 97.2%. DNA samples with poor performances in genotyping (<95% successful genotypes) were excluded from the statistical evaluation.

Statistical analysis

To assess genotype, allele and haplotype frequencies, Pearson Chi-square and/or Fisher's Exact Tests were performed when appropriate with PASWStatistics 18.0 Software. Haplotype analysis was carried out by HaploView [23]. Power calculation was performed for two-tail or one-tail tests when appropriate for 5% threshold of significance.

Results

IRF5, STAT4 and TRAF1-C5 polymorphisms did not show an association with susceptibility and/or severity of IgAN

We did not find an association with disease susceptibility for the investigated SNPs in IRF5, STAT4 genes and TRAF1-C5 locus, in both the co-dominant model and the reccessive/dominant model, comparing patients with IgAN and healthy controls. One IRF5 SNP (rs12539741) showed a difference between genotype distribution in IgAN patients and healthy controls in males in the dominant C model (p = 0.04). However, this association was not significant after Bonferroni correction for multiple comparisons. Comparing the allele and haplotype frequencies, we did not observe any significant differences for the SNPs between IgAN patients and controls (Table 2).

TGFB1 polymorphisms did not show an association with susceptibility to SLE or to lupus nephritis

No significant differences in genotype distribution or allele frequencies were observed between SLE patients and healthy controls for four investigated SNPs from the TGFB1 gene. In addition, there was no significant difference between lupus nephritis and healthy controls in both the co-dominant model and the recessive/dominant model of genotype frequencies and allelic frequencies (Table 3). TGFB1 polymorphisms in selected SNPs did not show an association with SLE or with lupus nephritis among SLE patients.

Genetic variations associated with susceptibility to SLE did not correspond to a specific association with lupus nephritis

To determine if SLE-related genetic variants associate specifically with nephritis in SLE patients, we genotyped up to nine variants from the IRF5, STAT4 genes and the TRAF1-C5 locus. We compared genotype frequencies in both the co-dominant

Table 1. Polymorphisms of *TGFB1, IRF5, STAT4* genes, *TRAF1-C5* locus in the study.

Gene	SNP	Position	Chromosome	Chromosome position	Alleles	Methods
STAT4	rs10181656	Intron 3	2q32.2-q32.3	183829287	C/G	TaqMan
IRF5	rs729302	Promoter	7q32	128356196	A/C	SNPstream
IRF5	rs4728142	Promoter	7q32	128361203	A/G	SNPstream
IRF5	rs2004640	The intron-exon border of exon 1B	7q32	128365537	G/T	SNPstream
IRF5	rs3807306	Intron 1	7q32	128367916	G/T	SNPstream
IRF5	rs10954213	3′ UTR	7q32	128376663	A/G	SNPstream
IRF5	rs11770589	Exon 10 3′ UTR	7q32	128376724	A/G	SNPstream
IRF5	rs2280714	3′flanking region	7q32	128381961	C/T	SNPstream
TRAF1-C5	rs3761847	5′ flanking region	9q33-q34	93307696	A/G	TaqMan
TGFB1	rs6957	Downstream 3′genomic region	19q13.1	46522446	C/T	TaqMan
TGFB1	rs2241715	Intron 1	19q13.1	46548726	G/T	TaqMan
TGFB1	rs1982073	Signal sequence of exone 1	19q13.1	46550761	C/T	TaqMan
TGFB1	rs1800469	Promoter	19q13.1	46552136	A/G	TaqMan

Table 2. Allelic frequencies of *IRF5*, *STAT4* and *TRAF1-C5* polymorphisms in IgAN patients and controls.

Gene	SPNs	Association Allele	Control/Patient Ratio Counts	Control/Patient Frequencies	Chi Square	P Value*
STAT4	rs10181656	A	532:388, 206:178	0.578, 0.769	1.927	0.2
IRF5	rs729302	A	629:299, 257:123	0.678, 0.676	0.003	0.9
IRF5	rs4728142	G	505:425, 206:176	0.543, 0.539	0.015	0.9
IRF5	rs2004640	G	444:486, 169:207	0.477, 0.449	0.840	0.4
IRF5	rs3807306	G	455:471, 177:201	0.491, 0.468	0.574	0.4
IRF5	rs10954213	G	342:584, 135:241	0.369, 0.359	0.122	0.7
IRF5	rs11770589	G	475:453, 193:191	0.512, 0.503	0.093	0.8
IRF5	rs2280714	C	294:636, 112:266	0.316, 0.296	0.494	0.5
TRAF1-C5	rs3761847	C	739:197, 297:89	0.790, 0.769	0.651	0.4

*Uncorrected.

model and recessive/dominant model between patients with lupus nephritis and SLE patients without nephritis. We detected no significant differences between these two groups. Moreover, there were no significant differences in allele frequencies of any investigated SNPs (Table 4). We found no differences in haplotype analyses in patients with SLE and healthy controls or between patients with lupus nephritis and SLE patients without nephritis.

Discussion

This is the first investigation to study the importance of *IRF5*, *STAT4* and *TRAF1-C5* gene polymorphisms in patients with IgAN. Our data show no evidence of an association of these genes with the development of IgAN or distinct risk alleles for lupus nephritis in this Swedish population.

According to recent findings, the *IRF5* gene is an important candidate gene in different chronic diseases, especially systemic diseases related to inflammation and autoimmunity. A meta-analysis which included 15 studies regarding *IRF5* gene polymor-

phism and SLE, confirmed the importance of rs2004640 for SLE susceptibility [4]. *TRAF1-C5* and *STAT4* polymorphisms have been shown to associate with RA and SLE, and also with some other autoimmune diseases [5,14,15].

Thus, one might speculate that susceptibility to IgA nephropathy may be due to common variations in *IRF5*, *TRAF1-C5* and *STAT4* genes. Our data do however not confirm this hypothesis. Since no single marker (for *IRF5*, *TRAF1-C5* and *STAT4*), no haplotype associations (for *IRF5*) were detected in patients with IgAN, it is reasonable to rule out a strong influence of these gene polymorphisms in IgAN development or disease progression. We noticed that we have almost 80% power to detect a 10% difference in minor allele frequency (MAF) in our cases and controls. However, due to limited sample size, we cannot exclude minor influences from the investigated gene polymorphism on IgAN, which may also differ in different populations. On the other hand, *TGFB1* polymorphisms were found previously in association with the susceptibility to IgAN [17] but did not show any association with SLE or lupus nephritis in the present study.

Table 3. Allelic frequencies of *STAT4*, *IFR5*, *TRAF1-C5* and *TGFB1* polymorphisms in SLE patients and controls.

Gene	SPNs	Association Allele	Control/Patient Ratio Counts	Control/Patient Frequencies	Chi Square	P Value*
STAT4	rs10181656	C	481:127, 343:201	0.791, 0.631	36.363	1.64E-09
IRF5	rs729302	C	124:248, 105:285	0.333, 0.269	3.722	0.0537
IRF5	rs4728142	G	206:166, 160:230	0.554, 0.410	15.708	7.39E-05
IRF5	rs2004640	G	181:191, 134:256	0.487, 0.344	16.048	6.17E-05
IRF5	rs3807306	G	177:195, 139:251	0.476, 0.356	11.182	8.00E-04
IRF5	rs10954213	G	131:241, 102:288	0.352, 0.262	7.364	0.0067
IRF5	rs11770589	A	195:177, 203:187	0.524, 0.521	0.01	0.9
IRF5	rs2280714	C	115:257, 87:303	0.309, 0.223	7.239	0.007
TRAF1-C5	rs3761847	A	334:258, 277:253	0.564, 0.523	1.946	0.2
TGFB1	rs6957	T	511:89, 453:91	0.852, 0.833	0.772	0.4
TGFB1	rs2241715	G	187:419, 164:378	0.309, 0.303	0.048	0.8
TGFB1	rs1982073	T	224:384, 198:344	0.368, 0.365	0.012	0.9
TGFB1	rs1800469	A	191:417, 162:378	0.314, 0.300	0.269	0.6

*Uncorrected.

Table 4. Allelic frequencies of *STAT4*, *IFR5*, *TRAF1-C5* and *TGFB1* polymorphisms in lupus nephritis against SLE patients without nephritis.

Gene	SPNs	Association Allele	Lupus without nephritis/ Lupus nephritis Ratio Counts	Lupus nephritis/none-nephritis Frequencies	Chi Square	P Value*
STAT4	rs10181656	C	210:122, 133:79	0.633, 0.627	0.015	0.9
IRF5	rs729302	C	65:165, 40:120	0.283, 0.250	0.510	0.5
IRF5	rs4728142	G	97:133, 63:97	0.422, 0.394	0.306	0.6
IRF5	rs2004640	G	87:143, 47:113	0.378, 0.294	2.988	0.1
IRF5	rs3807306	G	87:143, 52:108	0.378, 0.325	1.167	0.3
IRF5	rs10954213	G	65:165, 37:123	0.283, 0.231	1.289	0.3
IRF5	rs11770589	G	113:117, 74:86	0.491, 0.462	0.314	0.6
IRF5	rs2280714	C	59:171, 28:132	0.257, 0.175	3.618	0.06
TRAF1-C5	rs3761847	A	154:166, 99:111	0.481, 0.471	0.049	0.8

*Uncorrected.

There are immunological and biochemical similarities between lupus nephritis and IgAN, and both conditions are associated with immune complex formation and mesangial immune deposits. There are also a number of reports on patients with SLE who develop IgAN [24,25]. However, there was no overlap in genetic risk factors in the here studied genes between SLE and IgAN patients or any specific genetic variants detected comparing lupus patients with or without nephritis.

An association of *TRAF1-C5* locus with SLE was recently detected in a relatively small cohort [14]. However, our data did not show an association between *TRAF1-C5* polymorphism neither in SLE nor in IgAN.

In conclusion, the findings in the present study do not support an overlap in genetic susceptibility between Swedish patients with IgAN or SLE and reveal no specific importance of SLE associated SNPs for presence of lupus nephritis.

Acknowledgments

We would like to thank Eva Jemseby, Per-Anton Westerberg, Susanne Schepull, Micael Gylling, and Per Eriksson for their helpful assistance. We thank the SNP technology platform in Uppsala for genotyping the SNPs in *IRF5*.

Author Contributions

Conceived and designed the experiments: MTV IG SHJ LP. Performed the experiments: MTV ACS LP. Analyzed the data: MTV LP. Contributed reagents/materials/analysis tools: IG SL ES LW AF ACS SHJ LP. Wrote the paper: MTV IG SL ES AF ACS LTD SHJ LP.

References

1. Graham RR, Kozyrev SV, Baechler EC, Reddy MV, Plenge RM, et al. (2006) A common haplotype of interferon regulatory factor 5 (IRF5) regulates splicing and expression and is associated with increased risk of systemic lupus erythematosus. Nat Genet 38: 550–555.
2. Graham RR, Kyogoku C, Sigurdsson S, Vlasova IA, Davies LR, et al. (2007) Three functional variants of IFN regulatory factor 5 (IRF5) define risk and protective haplotypes for human lupus. Proc Natl Acad Sci U S A 104: 6758–6763.
3. Kozyrev SV, Alarcon-Riquelme ME (2007) The genetics and biology of Irf5-mediated signaling in lupus. Autoimmunity 40: 591–601.
4. Lee YH, Song GG (2008) Association between the rs2004640 functional polymorphism of interferon regulatory factor 5 and systemic lupus erythematosus: a meta-analysis. Rheumatol Int.
5. Sigurdsson S, Nordmark G, Goring HH, Lindroos K, Wiman AC, et al. (2005) Polymorphisms in the tyrosine kinase 2 and interferon regulatory factor 5 genes are associated with systemic lupus erythematosus. Am J Hum Genet 76: 528–537.
6. Han SW, Lee WK, Kwon KT, Lee BK, Nam EJ, et al. (2009) Association of Polymorphisms in Interferon Regulatory Factor 5 Gene with Rheumatoid Arthritis: A Metaanalysis. J Rheumatol.
7. Maalej A, Hamad MB, Rebai A, Teixeira VH, Bahloul Z, et al. (2008) Association of IRF5 gene polymorphisms with rheumatoid arthritis in a Tunisian population. Scand J Rheumatol 37: 414–418.
8. Shimane K, Kochi Y, Yamada R, Okada Y, Suzuki A, et al. (2009) A single nucleotide polymorphism in the IRF5 promoter region is associated with susceptibility to rheumatoid arthritis in the Japanese population. Ann Rheum Dis 68: 377–383.
9. Sigurdsson S, Padyukov L, Kurreeman FA, Liljedahl U, Wiman AC, et al. (2007) Association of a haplotype in the promoter region of the interferon regulatory factor 5 gene with rheumatoid arthritis. Arthritis Rheum 56: 2202–2210.
10. Kristjansdottir G, Sandling JK, Bonetti A, Roos IM, Milani L, et al. (2008) Interferon regulatory factor 5 (IRF5) gene variants are associated with multiple sclerosis in three distinct populations. J Med Genet 45: 362–369.
11. Nordmark G, Kristjansdottir G, Theander E, Eriksson P, Brun JG, et al. (2009) Additive effects of the major risk alleles of IRF5 and STAT4 in primary Sjogren's syndrome. Genes Immun 10: 68–76.
12. Dideberg V, Kristjansdottir G, Milani L, Libioulle C, Sigurdsson S, et al. (2007) An insertion-deletion polymorphism in the interferon regulatory Factor 5 (IRF5) gene confers risk of inflammatory bowel diseases. Hum Mol Genet 16: 3008–3016.
13. Plenge RM, Seielstad M, Padyukov L, Lee AT, Remmers EF, et al. (2007) TRAF1-C5 as a risk locus for rheumatoid arthritis-a genomewide study. N Engl J Med 357: 1199–1209.
14. Kurreeman FA, Goulielmos GN, Alizadeh BZ, Rueda B, Houwing-Duistermaat J, et al. (2009) The TRAF1-C5 region on chromosome 9q33 is associated with multiple autoimmune diseases. Ann Rheum Dis.
15. Remmers EF, Plenge RM, Lee AT, Graham RR, Hom G, et al. (2007) STAT4 and the risk of rheumatoid arthritis and systemic lupus erythematosus. N Engl J Med 357: 977–986.
16. Svenungsson E, Gustafsson J, Leonard D, Sandling J, Gunnarsson I, et al. (2009) A STAT4 risk allele is associated with ischemic cerebrovascular events and antiphospholipid antibodies in Systemic Lupus Erythematosus. Ann Rheum Dis.
17. Vuong MT, Lundberg S, Gunnarsson I, Wramner L, Seddighzadeh M, et al. (2009) Genetic variation in the transforming growth factor-{beta}1 gene is associated with susceptibility to IgA nephropathy. Nephrol Dial Transplant.
18. Gunnarsson I, Ronnelid J, Lundberg I, Jacobson SH (1997) Occurrence of anti-C1q antibodies in IgA nephropathy. Nephrol Dial Transplant 12: 2263–2268.
19. Potlukova E, Kralikova P (2008) Complement component c1q antibodies in theory and in clinical practice. Scand J Immunol 67: 423–430.
20. Bhavnani SK, Eichinger F, Martini S, Saxman P, Jagadish HV, et al. (2009) Network analysis of genes regulated in renal diseases: implications for a molecular-based classification. BMC Bioinformatics 10 Suppl 9: S3.
21. Loscalzo J, Kohane I, Barabasi AL (2007) Human disease classification in the postgenomic era: a complex systems approach to human pathobiology. Mol Syst Biol 3: 124.

22. Padyukov L, Hahn-Zoric M, Blomqvist SR, Ulanova M, Welch SG, et al. (2001) Distribution of human kappa locus IGKV2-29 and IGKV2D-29 alleles in Swedish Caucasians and Hong Kong Chinese. Immunogenetics 53: 22–30.

23. Barrett JC, Fry B, Maller J, Daly MJ (2005) Haploview: analysis and visualization of LD and haplotype maps. Bioinformatics 21: 263–265.

24. Basile C, Semeraro A, Montanaro A, Giordano R, De Padova F, et al. (1998) IgA nephropathy in a patient with systemic lupus erythematosus. Nephrol Dial Transplant 13: 1891–1892.

25. Horino T, Takao T, Terada Y IgA nephropathy in a patient with systemic lupus erythematosus. Lupus.

17

Early Vascular Alterations in SLE and RA Patients—A Step towards Understanding the Associated Cardiovascular Risk

Maria José Santos[1,2]*, Diana Carmona-Fernandes[1], Helena Canhão[1,3], José Canas da Silva[2], João Eurico Fonseca[1,3], Victor Gil[4]

1 Rheumatology Research Unit, Instituto de Medicina Molecular da Faculdade de Medicina de Lisboa, Lisbon, Portugal, 2 Rheumatology Department, Hospital Garcia de Orta, Almada, Portugal, 3 Rheumatology and Metabolic Bone Diseases Department, Hospital de Santa Maria, Lisbon, Portugal, 4 Cardiology Department, Hospital Fernando Fonseca, Amadora, Portugal

Abstract

Accelerated atherosclerosis represents a major problem in both systemic lupus erythematosus (SLE) and rheumatoid arthritis (RA) patients, and endothelial damage is a key feature of atherogenesis. We aimed to assess early endothelial changes in SLE and RA female patients (127 SLE and 107 RA) without previous CV events. Biomarkers of endothelial cell activation (intercellular adhesion molecule-1 (sICAM-1), vascular cell adhesion molecule-1 (sVCAM-1), thrombomodulin (TM), and tissue factor (TF)) were measured and endothelial function was assessed using peripheral artery tonometry. Reactive hyperemia index (RHI), an indicator of microvascular reactivity, and augmentation index (AIx), a measure of arterial stiffness, were obtained. In addition, traditional CV risk factors, disease activity and medication were determined. Women with SLE displayed higher sICAM-1 and TM and lower TF levels than women with RA ($p = 0.001$, $p < 0.001$ and $p < 0.001$, respectively). These differences remained significant after controlling for CV risk factors and medication. Serum levels of vascular biomarkers were increased in active disease and a moderate correlation was observed between sVCAM-1 levels and lupus disease activity (rho = 0.246) and between TF levels and RA disease activity (rho = 0.301). Although RHI was similar across the groups, AIx was higher in lupus as compared to RA ($p = 0.04$). Also in active SLE, a trend towards poorer vasodilation was observed ($p = 0.06$). In conclusion, women with SLE and RA present with distinct patterns of endothelial cell activation biomarkers not explained by differences in traditional CV risk factors. Early vascular alterations are more pronounced in SLE which is in line with the higher CV risk of these patients.

Editor: Songtao Shi, University of Southern California, United States of America

Funding: This study was supported by a grant from Fundação para a Ciência e a Tecnologia, Portugal (PIC/IC/82920/2007). The funders had no role in study design, data collection and analysis, decision to publish, or preparation of the manuscript.

Competing Interests: The authors have declared that no competing interests exist.

* E-mail: mjps@netvisao.pt

Introduction

Chronic systemic inflammation predisposes to accelerated atherosclerosis, a risk that is well known in systemic lupus erythematosus (SLE) and in rheumatoid arthritis (RA) patients [1]. Subclinical vascular lesions develop long before atherosclerosis becomes clinically evident, and they progress more rapidly in SLE [2] and RA [3] than in the general population. Traditional cardiovascular (CV) risk factors do not fully explain this enhanced risk, and the disease itself is considered an independent CV risk factor [1]. In addition, the potential contribution of genetic variants to the development of atherosclerosis in RA patients has been recently highlighted [4,5]. However, the reported magnitude of the CV risk is several times higher in SLE than in RA [6–9], and the reason for this divergence is still incompletely understood.

Endothelial damage is considered the first step in the pathogenesis of atherosclerosis. It correlates with disease progression and predicts CV events in the general population [10]. The importance of endothelial cells (ECs) for vascular health is highlighted by its crucial role in maintaining blood fluidity and in regulating vascular tonus and permeability. Under basal conditions ECs express molecules such as thrombomodulin (TM), which prevent platelet aggregation and the activation of the clotting cascade. Further platelet inhibition is achieved as a result of nitric oxide (NO) synthesis, a major vascular relaxant with anti-inflammatory and anti-proliferative properties. During the inflammatory process, ECs undergo changes characterized by enhanced expression of adhesion molecules, increased transendothelial permeability, and loss of antithrombotic properties [11]. Pro-inflammatory cytokines suppress TM expression and promote its cleavage and release into circulation [12]. In addition, they induce the expression of tissue factor (TF), a procoagulant molecule absent from the surface of the intact ECs [13], shifting the balance towards a prothrombotic state. Furthermore, damaged endothelium loses its ability to produce vasodilators, thus adding to the vascular injury. Endothelial dysfunction is potentially a reversible disorder. Indeed, in patients with active RA, the infusion of infliximab, a chimeric antibody against TNF, has been found to improve biomarkers of endothelial activation [14] and transiently ameliorate endothelial function[15].

In vivo, vascular function can be examined non-invasively by quantifying biomarkers of endothelial activation/damage, by measuring the ability of endothelium to release NO in response to various stimuli or by assessing arterial wall stiffness [16]. Previous data indicate impaired endothelial function both in SLE [17] and in RA patients [18] when compared to non-inflammatory controls. Nevertheless it is unclear whether the magnitude of early vascular changes is similar in these two diseases.

Given the clinical and pathophysiological particularities of SLE and RA, we hypothesize that endothelial function is differently disturbed in these two patient groups, which could explain the different CV risk. Thus, the major aim of our study was to compare endothelial cell function between SLE and RA as assessed by the measurement of soluble vascular biomarkers and by endothelial function testing, taking into account the presence of traditional CV risk factors and systemic inflammation.

Materials and Methods

Subjects

Consecutive SLE and RA women fulfilling the ACR classification criteria and free of clinically manifest CV disease were recruited from the rheumatology clinics of Hospital Garcia de Orta, Almada, and Hospital de Santa Maria, Lisbon, between April 2009 and October 2010. A control group of women without systemic inflammatory diseases was also recruited from the local community and evaluated in the same period. Participants were excluded if they were pregnant, breastfeeding, had impaired renal function (defined as serum creatinine >1.5 mg/dl), or had documented ischemic heart disease (previous infarction, revascularization surgery, angina, or heart failure), cerebrovascular disease (stroke or transient ischemic attack) or symptomatic peripheral artery disease. The study was approved by the Ethics Committee of both hospitals and was conducted in accordance with the principles stated in the Declaration of Helsinki. All participants gave written informed consent.

Clinical assessment

Demographic data, disease characteristics, current medication, and CV risk profile including blood pressure, serum lipids, fasting glycemia, smoking habits, and body mass index (BMI) were obtained. Patients were diagnosed with hypertension if the measured blood pressure was repeatedly ≥140/90 mm/Hg or if they used antihypertensive medication. The diagnosis of diabetes was made if fasting glucose level was ≥126 mg/dl, or if patients were under pharmacological treatment. Participants were classified as obese if BMI was ≥30 Kg/m^2. Disease activity was evaluated using the SLE Disease Activity Index 2000 (SLEDAI 2K), [19] and in RA patients 28 joints were examined for tenderness and swelling, and the 4 variable disease activity score (DAS28) was calculated using erythrocyte sedimentation rate [20]. Disease activity was stratified according to the cutoffs of each instrument [20,21]: remission (SLEDAI 2K=0 for SLE or DAS28<2.6 for RA patients), low disease activity (≥1 SLEDAI 2K<4, in the case of SLE, or ≥2.6 DAS28≤3.2, in the case of RA), and active disease (SLEDAI 2K≥4 or DAS28>3.2 for SLE and RA patients, respectively).

Fasting blood samples were obtained before any other procedures for measurement of glucose, uric acid, lipids (total cholesterol, high density lipoprotein (HDL) cholesterol, low density lipoprotein (LDL) cholesterol, and triglycerides), inflammatory mediators (C-reactive protein (CRP) and fibrinogen) and soluble vascular biomarkers (sICAM-1, sVCAM-1, TM, and TF).

Quantification of soluble vascular biomarkers and cytokines

Measurements were performed using commercial enzyme-linked immunosorbent assay (ELISA) based methods according to the manufacturers' instructions. The Human sICAM-1 FlowCytomix Simplex Kit and the Human sVCAM-1 FlowCytomix Simplex Kit (Bender MedSystems GmbH, Vienna, Austria) were used for quantification of adhesion molecules, both using the FlowCytomix^{TM} Technology. Serum levels of TM were measured using the Human Thrombomodulin ELISA Kit (Cell Sciences ®, Canton, MA, USA) and serum levels of TF were quantified using the AssayMax Human Tissue Factor ELISA kit (Assaypro, St Charles, Mo, USA).

Endothelial function tests

Endothelial function was assessed by peripheral artery tonometry (PAT). PAT is a noninvasive operator-independent method that evaluates changes in pulse wave amplitude before and after reactive hyperemia. The inter-day variability of this technique in our department is 11% (data not published). The exam was performed using the EndoPAT 2000 device (Itamar Medical Ltd, Cesarea, Israel) as described elsewhere [22] and by assessors blinded to the clinical diagnosis. Briefly, patients were placed in a quiet room, in supine position, with a specially designed finger probe on the index finger of each hand, and a pressure cuff placed on one arm. Patients were recommended to refrain from smoking and drinking coffee or tea during the previous 24 hours and not to eat for at least 6 hours preceding the exam. PAT was continuously measured during a 10-minute baseline period, for 5 minutes after the pressure cuff was inflated to suprasystolic pressure and for 10 additional minutes following the release of upper arm occlusion. Pressure changes reflecting pulse amplitude were transmitted to a computer and reactive hyperemia index (RHI) was calculated as the ratio of PAT signal amplitude after cuff deflation divided by the amplitude of baseline signal, adjusted for fluctuations in the magnitude of the signal in the contralateral finger [22]. Augmentation index (AIx) was calculated from the mean PAT waveform of the baseline period dividing the amplitude of the second systolic peak by the difference between the second and the first peak.

Statistical analysis

Continuous variables are expressed as means with standard deviations and categorical variables as the number of affected individuals and proportion of the total. Bivariate comparisons of SLE and RA patients were made using Student T-tests, Mann-Whitney, Kruskal-Wallis or χ^2 tests, as appropriate.

The levels of vascular biomarkers, as well as RHI and AIx, were compared between SLE and RA patients first as crude means using the Mann Whitney test, followed by analysis of covariance (ANCOVA) to adjust for significant and clinically relevant baseline covariates. Likewise, in order to assess the effect of disease activity on vascular biomarkers, RHI and AIx, comparisons between remission and active disease were performed.

Correlation between disease activity and endothelial cell function was studied separately in SLE and RA using Spearman correlation coefficient and partial correlations to control for age, disease duration, cardiovascular risk factors and medication.

Statistical analysis was performed assuming a 5% significance level and using SPSS 17 for Windows.

Results

In total 127 women with SLE and 107 with RA, were included in the study. A control group of 124 women, mean age 46.9±13.7 years, 98% Caucasian, and 52% postmenopausal was also evaluated as reference. Demographic and clinical characteristics of SLE and RA patients are shown in Table 1. SLE women were younger and had shorter disease duration (8.4±6.5 years) compared to women with RA (10.7±7.3 years, p = 0.01). All lupus patients were ANA positive and 89% of RA patients were positive either for IgM RF or for anti-citrullinated protein antibodies. The use of antimalarials and aspirin was more common in lupus, while more RA patients received methotrexate. Serum concentration of fibrinogen was higher in SLE (SLE 326±147 mg/dl vs RA 276±101 mg/dl; p = 0.01), but CRP levels were similar in both groups (SLE 1.16±3.2 mg/dl vs 1.06±2.5 mg/dl; p = 0.75).

Vascular biomarkers and endothelial function as assessed by PAT

A distinct pattern of soluble ECs biomarkers was identified in SLE and in RA. While sICAM-1 and TM levels were significantly higher, TF was lower in lupus than in RA patients (Figure 1). Differences in sICAM-1, TM and TF remained significant after adjustment for covariates (Table 2).

Reactive hyperemia was similar in SLE (RHI = 2.135±0.686), in RA (RHI = 2.194±0.810) and in the control population (2.090±0.579), while AIx was significantly higher in SLE as compared to RA (16% vs 11%; p = 0.04), indicating increased arterial wall stiffness in these patients. This increase remained statistically significant after controlling for differences in baseline characteristics (Table 2).

Disease activity and endothelial function

Patients presented a broad range of disease activity. The mean SLEDAI 2K was 3.46±4.5 (range 0 to 21) and the mean DAS28 was 4.19±1.4 (range 1.70 to 7.54). Disease was in remission in 41% of SLE and in 17% of RA cases. 39% of SLE patients presented moderate/high active disease defined as a SLEDAI 2K≥4, and 72% of RA had moderate/high active disease according to the DAS28 definition. Except for prednisolone dosage, which was significantly higher in active SLE and active RA than in remission, demographic characteristics, CV risk profile and medication was comparable in quiescent and active disease.

Overall, serum levels of vascular biomarkers were elevated when disease was active, being statistically significant the differences in sICAM-1, TM and TF levels between active and quiescent SLE and in sICAM-1 and TF levels between active RA and remission (Table 3).

sVCAM-1 showed a significant Spearman and partial correlation with lupus disease activity measured by the SLEDAI (rho 0.246 and 0.361; p = 0.007 and p<0.001 respectively) and TM levels correlated with DAS28 (rho 0.301 and 0.250; p = 0.002 and p = 0.005). In SLE patients there was also a significant correlation between sVCAM-1, TM, TF and ESR (rho 0.246, 0.323 and 0.263; p = 0.01, p = 0.001 and p = 0.01, respectively) and between serum TM levels and CRP (rho 0.315; p = 0.001). No significant correlation was found in RA patients between ESR or CRP and vascular biomarkers.

A trend toward lower RHI was observed in active SLE (1.806±0.16) as compared with remission (2.249±0.13; p = 0.06), but no significant correlation was observed between RHI, AIx and SLEDAI or DAS28.

Discussion

In this comparative study we found distinct patterns of soluble vascular biomarkers in SLE and in RA female patients free from clinically evident CV disease. Lupus patients presented higher serum sICAM-1 and TM levels, while TF was elevated in RA patients. These findings are relevant for understanding the pathophysiology of the increased CV risk in SLE and RA patients, as cell adhesion molecules may represent a link between inflammation and atherosclerosis. In fact, not only are VCAM-1 and ICAM-1 highly expressed on the endothelium overlaying atherosclerotic lesions [23,24], but an increased serum concentration of these molecules is also related to CV risk factors [25] and incident myocardial infarction [26]. In particular, high serum levels of ICAM-1 represent an independent risk factor for atherosclerosis and a predictor of future CV events [26,27]. In addition, we observed significantly increased levels of vascular biomarkers in active disease. These observations are in line with previous studies demonstrating that inflammatory mediators, including TNF, IL-6, interferon-gamma (INFγ) [28], IL-18 [29], but also MCP-1 and MIF [30], upregulate endothelial cell adhesion molecule expression. The fact that SLE patients exhibit higher sICAM-1 and also higher fibrinogen concentrations may be relevant in the initiation and progression of atherosclerosis. Indeed, ICAM-1 serves as a binding site for fibrinogen and promotes adhesion and transendothelial migration of leukocytes [31], an important early step in inflammatory vascular disease. We did not find any difference in VCAM-1 serum levels among the

Table 1. Demographic and clinical characteristics of SLE and RA women.

	SLE (n = 127)	RA (n = 107)	p value
Demographic data			
Age, years	43.9 (13.9)	50.2 (14.1)	0.01
Education, years	8.9 (4.8)	8.3 (5.2)	ns
Caucasians, n (%)	110 (87)	95 (89)	ns
Menopause, n (%)	60 (47)	62 (58)	ns
Traditional CV risk factors			
Current smoker, n (%)	18 (14)	17 (16)	ns
Hypertension, n (%)	51 (40)	37 (35)	ns
Total cholesterol, mg/dl	189.3 (42.8)	204.0 (33.5)	0.005
HDL cholesterol, mg/dl	56.6 (16.1)	63.9 (18.5)	0.002
LDL cholesterol, mg/dl	113.9 (36.6)	123.4 (28.5)	0.04
Triglycerides, mg/dl	125.7 (88.2)	103.1 (42.8)	0.01
Diabetes, n (%)	9 (7)	5 (5)	ns
Obesity, n (%)	33 (26)	33 (31)	ns
Medication			
Antihypertensive, n (%)	51 (40)	32 (30)	ns
Lipid lowering, n (%)	31 (24)	17 (16)	ns
Aspirin, n (%)	28 (22)	6 (6)	<0.001
Hydroxychloroquine, n (%)	97 (74)	20 (19)	<0.001
Methotrexate, n (%)	12 (10)	85 (82)	<0.001
Prednisolone, mg/day	7.8 (10.9)	3.2 (3.5)	0.006

Results are presented as means (SD) or number of affected individuals and (%). SLE – systemic lupus erythematosus; RA – rheumatoid arthritis; CV-cardiovascular; HDL – high density lipoprotein; LDL – low density lipoprotein, ns – non significant.

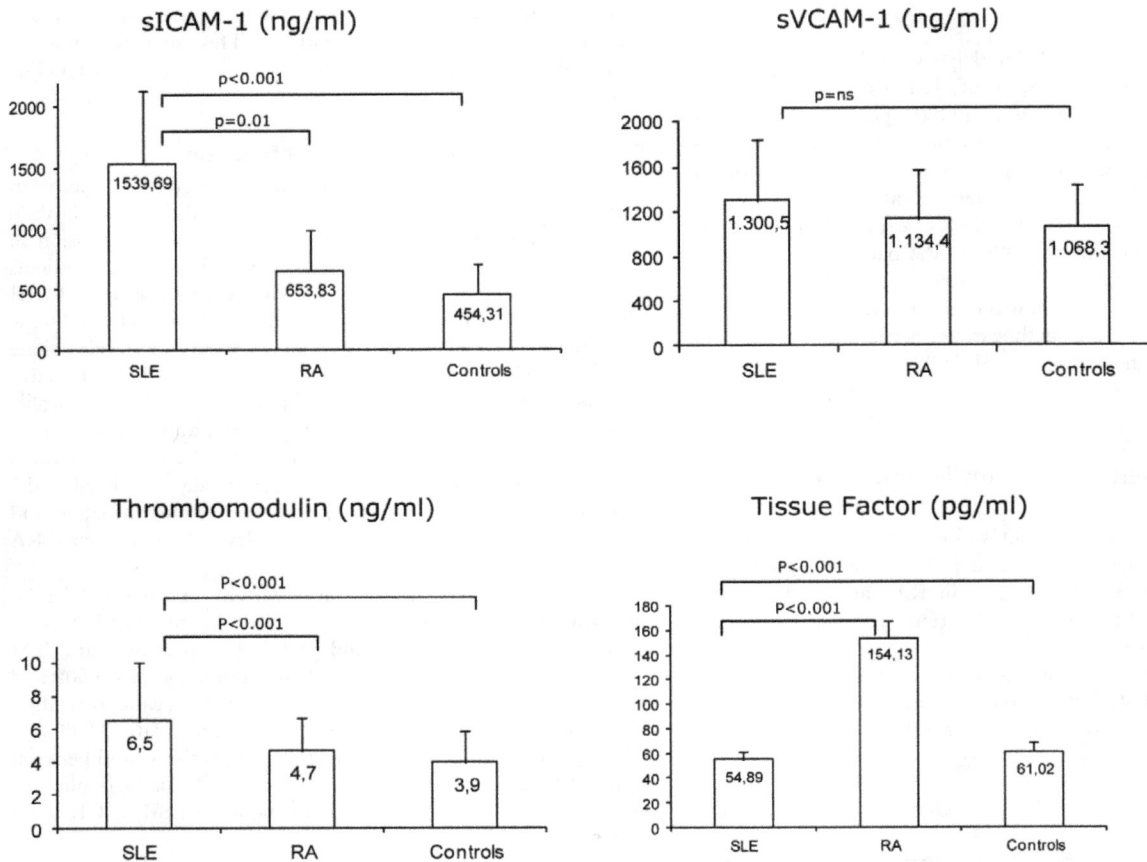

Figure 1. Serum concentrations of vascular biomarkers in SLE and RA patients and non-inflammatory controls. sICAM-1– soluble intercellular adhesion molecule; sVCAM-1 – soluble vascular cell adhesion molecule; RHI–reactive hyperemia index; Aix – augmentation index; SLE – systemic lupus erythematosus; RA – rheumatoid arthritis.

studied groups. In animal models, VCAM-1 expression is considered a major early event in the atherosclerotic process [32], and increased sVCAM-1 levels have been reported in lupus nephritis [33]. However, in RA and SLE patients without renal or vascular disease, serum concentrations of VCAM-1 are similar to the control population and the relationship to atherosclerosis is uncertain [34,35]. Nevertheless, very recently sVCAM-1 was identified as an independent predictor of overall and cardiovascular mortality in SLE[36].

Table 2. Vascular biomarkers and results of PAT assessment in SLE and RA, after controlling for baseline covariates.

	Age adjusted			Adjusted for CV risk factors, disease duration and medication*		
	SLE (n = 127)	RA (n = 107)	p value	SLE(n = 127)	RA(n = 107)	p value
sICAM ng/ml	1436 (600)	778 (651)	0.01	1994(879)	398(898)	0.05
sVCAM, ng/ml	1313 (114)	1129 (125)	0.29	1330 (159)	1160(162)	0.53
TM, ng/ml	6.59 (0.27)	4.54 (0.29)	<0.001	6.47 (0.36)	4.58(0.37)	0.003
TF, pg/ml	56.3 (10.1)	152.6 (10.9)	<0.001	50.1 14.4)	157(14.7)	<0.001
RHI[§]	2.128 (0.08)	2.203 (0.09)	0.53	2.008(0.11)	2.309(0.12)	0.12
Aix[§], %	17.9 (1.9)	9.5 (2)	0.003	20.3 (2.5)	8.3 (2.7)	0.007

Results are presented as estimated marginal means (SE).
*Adjusted for the following covariates: age, disease duration, total cholesterol, HDL, LDL, triglycerides, aspirin, hydroxychloroquine, methotrexate use, and prednisolone dose.
[§]RHI and Aix results refer to 87 women with SLE and 75 with RA.
sICAM-1 – soluble intercellular adhesion molecule; sVCAM-1 – soluble vascular cell adhesion molecule; TM – thrombomodulin; TF – tissue factor; RHI – reactive hyperemia index; Aix – augmentation index.

Table 3. Vascular biomarkers and endothelial function in active disease and in remission.

	SLE (N = 127)			RA (N = 107)		
	Remission	Active	p	Remission	Active	P
sICAM-1	713.9 (147)	1952 (100)	0.04	527 (10.2)	668 (4.7)	0.01
sVCAM-1	1022 (69)	1419 (47)	0.02	1013 (94)	1171 (44)	0.15
TM	6.1 (0.5)	7.2 (0.4)	0.04	4.59 (0.2)	5.01 (0.4)	0.42
TF	54.1 (7.3)	58.6 (1.9)	0.08	126.6 (33)	160.4 (15)	0.03
RHI*	2.249 (0.13)	1.806 (0.16)	0.06	2.444 (0.21)	2.133 (0.10)	0.20
AIx*	14.4 (3.6)	18.5 (2.5)	0.03	12.2 (6.4)	10.8 (2.4)	0.79

Results are expressed as estimated marginal means (SE) adjusted for prednisolone dose.
*RHI and AIx results refer to 87 women with SLE and 75 with RA.
SLE – systemic lupus erythematosus; RA – rheumatoid arthritis; sICAM-1 – soluble inter-cellular adhesion molecule; sVCAM-1 – soluble vascular cell adhesion molecule; TM – thrombomodulin; TF – tissue factor; RHI – reactive hyperemia index; AIx – augmentation index.

There is growing evidence supporting the relationship between inflammation and thrombotic complications of atherosclerosis (atherothrombosis). Interestingly, TM expression, a molecule with anti-coagulant properties, is reduced during the inflammatory process [12], and increased soluble TM levels probably indicate EC injury. Together with increased TF, which is an initiator of the extrinsic coagulation cascade, this environment may raise the thrombogenic activity of plasma and contribute to cardiovascular events. Higher levels of TF in RA patients as compared to SLE patients might be explained by the contribution of TNF to its expression [37]. Nevertheless, serum levels of adhesion molecules, TM, and TF may not accurately translate endothelial functional expression of these molecules, which is a limitation of our work.

A further effect of proinflammatory cytokines on EC is the inhibition of NO synthesis leading to endothelial dysfunction. In the general population, impaired endothelial function is a critical early step in the development of atherosclerosis [38] and predicts the progression of structural arterial disease independently of conventional CV risk factors [39,40]. However, studies of endothelial function in inflammatory rheumatic diseases depicted contradictory results [41–43], and the relevance of endothelial dysfunction for the progression of atherosclerosis in rheumatic

diseases remains uncertain [44–46]. Similarly, the improvement following anti-rheumatic medication is not universally supported by the available literature [18]. Using PAT, we did not find any significant differences in RHI neither between patients and controls, nor between SLE and RA. RHI quantifies changes in pulse wave amplitude in response to reactive hyperemia, a measure of microvascular function. In the general population RHI is an independent predictor of adverse cardiac events [47], but its predictive value in rheumatic diseases has not been established. The fact that we have included only females without previous CV events and normal renal function (relatively low risk population) may in part account for the comparable RHI found in patients and controls. In fact, only in more active SLE cases did RHI show a reduction. The follow up of these patients will allow us to ascertain the predictive value of RHI measured by PAT for the development of CV event in SLE and RA patients.

Lupus patients presented higher AIx than RA patients and this difference remained significant after controlling for covariates. In apparently healthy subjects arterial stiffness is an independent predictor of coronary heart disease and stroke [48], but the predictive value of AIx in rheumatic diseases is unknown. Cardiovascular risk factors and disease related features contribute to arterial stiffening in SLE [49] and RA [50]. Shang et al found a correlation between carotid AIx and SLEDAI [51]. Increased arterial stiffness was also associated with RA disease activity in some, but not all, studies [18]. Increased AIx in SLE women probably indicates a worse vascular condition.

Taken together, our observations add to the evidence that the pathogenesis of atherosclerosis associated with inflammation may differ in SLE and RA. Additionally, we found more pronounced early vascular changes in lupus patients, and when the disease is active, which is in line with the higher risk for CV events documented in these patients.

Acknowledgments

We would like to thank Mrs Célia Monteiro for her help with PAT measurements.

Author Contributions

Conceived and designed the experiments: MJS HC JEF VG. Performed the experiments: MJS DC-F. Analyzed the data: MJS HC JEF JCS VG. Contributed reagents/materials/analysis tools: MJS DC-F VG. Wrote the paper: MJS.

References

1. Symmons DP, Gabriel SE (2011) Epidemiology of CVD in rheumatic disease, with a focus on RA and SLE. Nat Rev Rheumatol 7: 399–408.
2. Thompson T, Sutton-Tyrrell K, Wildman RP, Kao A, Fitzgerald SG, et al. (2008) Progression of carotid intima-media thickness and plaque in women with systemic lupus erythematosus. Arthritis Rheum 58: 835–842.
3. Sodergren A, Karp K, Boman K, Eriksson C, Lundstrom E, et al. (2010) Atherosclerosis in early rheumatoid arthritis: very early endothelial activation and rapid progression of intima media thickness. Arthritis Res Ther 12: R158.
4. Lopez-Mejias R, Gonzalez-Juanatey C, Garcia-Bermudez M, Castaneda S, Miranda-Filloy J, et al. (2012) The lp13.3 genomic region -rs599839- is associated with endothelial dysfunction in patients with rheumatoid arthritis. Arthritis Res Ther 14: R42.
5. Rodriguez-Rodriguez L, Gonzalez-Juanatey C, Garcia-Bermudez M, Vazquez-Rodriguez TR, Miranda-Filloy JA, et al. (2011) CCR5Delta32 variant and cardiovascular disease in patients with rheumatoid arthritis: a cohort study. Arthritis Res Ther 13: R133.
6. Fischer LM, Schlienger RG, Matter C, Jick H, Meier CR (2004) Effect of rheumatoid arthritis or systemic lupus erythematosus on the risk of first-time acute myocardial infarction. Am J Cardiol 93: 198–200.
7. Manzi S, Meilahn EN, Rairie JE, Conte CG, Medsger TA Jr., et al. (1997) Age-specific incidence rates of myocardial infarction and angina in women with

systemic lupus erythematosus: comparison with the Framingham Study. Am J Epidemiol 145: 408–415.
8. Meune C, Touze E, Trinquart L, Allanore Y (2010) High risk of clinical cardiovascular events in rheumatoid arthritis: Levels of associations of myocardial infarction and stroke through a systematic review and meta-analysis. Arch Cardiovasc Dis 103: 253–261.
9. Zoller B, Li X, Sundquist J, Sundquist K (2012) Risk of subsequent coronary heart disease in patients hospitalized for immune-mediated diseases: a nationwide follow-up study from Sweden. PLoS One 7: e33442.
10. Vita JA (2011) Endothelial function. Circulation 124: e906–912.
11. Pober JS, Sessa WC (2007) Evolving functions of endothelial cells in inflammation. Nat Rev Immunol 7: 803–815.
12. Boehme MW, Deng Y, Raeth U, Bierhaus A, Ziegler R, et al. (1996) Release of thrombomodulin from endothelial cells by concerted action of TNF-alpha and neutrophils: in vivo and in vitro studies. Immunology 87: 134–140.
13. Drake TA, Cheng J, Chang A, Taylor FB Jr. (1993) Expression of tissue factor, thrombomodulin, and E-selectin in baboons with lethal Escherichia coli sepsis. Am J Pathol 142: 1458–1470.
14. Gonzalez-Gay MA, Garcia-Unzueta MT, De Matias JM, Gonzalez-Juanatey C, Garcia-Porrua C, et al. (2006) Influence of anti-TNF-alpha infliximab therapy on adhesion molecules associated with atherogenesis in patients with rheumatoid arthritis. Clin Exp Rheumatol 24: 373–379.

15. Gonzalez-Juanatey C, Testa A, Garcia-Castelo A, Garcia-Porrua C, Llorca J, et al. (2004) Active but transient improvement of endothelial function in rheumatoid arthritis patients undergoing long-term treatment with anti-tumor necrosis factor alpha antibody. Arthritis Rheum 51: 447–450.

16. Lane HA, Smith JC, Davies JS (2006) Noninvasive assessment of preclinical atherosclerosis. Vasc Health Risk Manag 2: 19–30.

17. Mak A, Liu Y, Chun-Man Ho R (2011) Endothelium-dependent But Not Endothelium-independent Flow-mediated Dilation Is Significantly Reduced in Patients with Systemic Lupus Erythematosus without Vascular Events: A Metaanalysis and Metaregression. J Rheumatol 38: 1296–1303.

18. Sandoo A, Veldhuijzen van Zanten JJ, Metsios GS, Carroll D, Kitas GD (2011) Vascular function and morphology in rheumatoid arthritis: a systematic review. Rheumatology (Oxford) 50: 2125–2139.

19. Gladman DD, Ibanez D, Urowitz MB (2002) Systemic lupus erythematosus disease activity index 2000. J Rheumatol 29: 288–291.

20. Prevoo ML, van 't Hof MA, Kuper HH, van Leeuwen MA, van de Putte LB, et al. (1995) Modified disease activity scores that include twenty-eight-joint counts. Development and validation in a prospective longitudinal study of patients with rheumatoid arthritis. Arthritis Rheum 38: 44–48.

21. Yee CS, Farewell VT, Isenberg DA, Griffiths B, Teh LS, et al. (2011) The use of Systemic Lupus Erythematosus Disease Activity Index-2000 to define active disease and minimal clinically meaningful change based on data from a large cohort of systemic lupus erythematosus patients. Rheumatology (Oxford) 50: 982–988.

22. Bonetti PO, Barsness GW, Keelan PC, Schnell TI, Pumper GM, et al. (2003) Enhanced external counterpulsation improves endothelial function in patients with symptomatic coronary artery disease. J Am Coll Cardiol 41: 1761–1768.

23. Davies MJ, Gordon JL, Gearing AJ, Pigott R, Woolf N, et al. (1993) The expression of the adhesion molecules ICAM-1, VCAM-1, PECAM, and E-selectin in human atherosclerosis. J Pathol 171: 223–229.

24. Wood KM, Cadogan MD, Ramshaw AL, Parums DV (1993) The distribution of adhesion molecules in human atherosclerosis. Histopathology 22: 437–444.

25. Demerath E, Towne B, Blangero J, Siervogel RM (2001) The relationship of soluble ICAM-1, VCAM-1, P-selectin and E-selectin to cardiovascular disease risk factors in healthy men and women. Ann Hum Biol 28: 664–678.

26. Hwang SJ, Ballantyne CM, Sharrett AR, Smith LC, Davis CE, et al. (1997) Circulating adhesion molecules VCAM-1, ICAM-1, and E-selectin in carotid atherosclerosis and incident coronary heart disease cases: the Atherosclerosis Risk In Communities (ARIC) study. Circulation 96: 4219–4225.

27. Luc G, Arveiler D, Evans A, Amouyel P, Ferrieres J, et al. (2003) Circulating soluble adhesion molecules ICAM-1 and VCAM-1 and incident coronary heart disease: the PRIME Study. Atherosclerosis 170: 169–176.

28. Zhang J, Alcaide P, Liu L, Sun J, He A, et al. (2011) Regulation of endothelial cell adhesion molecule expression by mast cells, macrophages, and neutrophils. PLoS One 6: e14525.

29. Morel JC, Park CC, Woods JM, Koch AE (2001) A novel role for interleukin-18 in adhesion molecule induction through NF kappa B and phosphatidylinositol (PI) 3-kinase-dependent signal transduction pathways. J Biol Chem 276: 37069–37075.

30. Amin MA, Haas CS, Zhu K, Mansfield PJ, Kim MJ, et al. (2006) Migration inhibitory factor up-regulates vascular cell adhesion molecule-1 and intercellular adhesion molecule-1 via Src, PI3 kinase, and NFkappaB. Blood 107: 2252–2261.

31. Languino LR, Duperray A, Joganic KJ, Fornaro M, Thornton GB, et al. (1995) Regulation of leukocyte-endothelium interaction and leukocyte transendothelial migration by intercellular adhesion molecule 1-fibrinogen recognition. Proc Natl Acad Sci U S A 92: 1505–1509.

32. Nakashima Y, Raines EW, Plump AS, Breslow JL, Ross R (1998) Upregulation of VCAM-1 and ICAM-1 at atherosclerosis-prone sites on the endothelium in the ApoE-deficient mouse. Arterioscler Thromb Vasc Biol 18: 842–851.

33. Yao GH, Liu ZH, Zhang X, Zheng CX, Chen HP, et al. (2008) Circulating thrombomodulin and vascular cell adhesion molecule-1 and renal vascular lesion in patients with lupus nephritis. Lupus 17: 720–726.

34. Rho YH, Chung CP, Oeser A, Solus J, Asanuma Y, et al. (2009) Inflammatory mediators and premature coronary atherosclerosis in rheumatoid arthritis. Arthritis Rheum 61: 1580–1585.

35. Rho YH, Chung CP, Oeser A, Solus J, Raggi P, et al. (2008) Novel cardiovascular risk factors in premature coronary atherosclerosis associated with systemic lupus erythematosus. J Rheumatol 35: 1789–1794.

36. Gustafsson J, Simard JF, Gunnarsson I, Elvin K, Lundberg IE, et al. (2012) Risk factors for cardiovascular mortality in patients with systemic lupus erythematosus, a prospective cohort study. Arthritis Res Ther 14: R46.

37. Kirchhofer D, Tschopp TB, Hadvary P, Baumgartner HR (1994) Endothelial cells stimulated with tumor necrosis factor-alpha express varying amounts of tissue factor resulting in inhomogenous fibrin deposition in a native blood flow system. Effects of thrombin inhibitors. J Clin Invest 93: 2073–2083.

38. Kozera L, Andrews J, Morgan AW (2011) Cardiovascular risk and rheumatoid arthritis-the next step: differentiating true soluble biomarkers of cardiovascular risk from surrogate measures of inflammation. Rheumatology (Oxford) 50: 1944–1954.

39. Bonetti PO, Lerman LO, Lerman A (2003) Endothelial dysfunction: a marker of atherosclerotic risk. Arterioscler Thromb Vasc Biol 23: 168–175.

40. Halcox JP, Donald AE, Ellins E, Witte DR, Shipley MJ, et al. (2009) Endothelial function predicts progression of carotid intima-media thickness. Circulation 119: 1005–1012.

41. Hansel S, Lassig G, Pistrosch F, Passauer J (2003) Endothelial dysfunction in young patients with long-term rheumatoid arthritis and low disease activity. Atherosclerosis 170: 177–180.

42. Foster W, Carruthers D, Lip GY, Blann AD (2010) Inflammation and microvascular and macrovascular endothelial dysfunction in rheumatoid arthritis: effect of treatment. J Rheumatol 37: 711–716.

43. Aizer J, Karlson EW, Chibnik LB, Costenbader KH, Post D, et al. (2009) A controlled comparison of brachial artery flow mediated dilation (FMD) and digital pulse amplitude tonometry (PAT) in the assessment of endothelial function in systemic lupus erythematosus. Lupus 18: 235–242.

44. Gonzalez-Juanatey C, Llorca J, Gonzalez-Gay MA (2011) Correlation between endothelial function and carotid atherosclerosis in rheumatoid arthritis patients with long-standing disease. Arthritis Res Ther 13: R101.

45. Gustafsson J, Gunnarsson I, Borjesson O, Pettersson S, Moller S, et al. (2009) Predictors of the first cardiovascular event in patients with systemic lupus erythematosus – a prospective cohort study. Arthritis Res Ther 11: R186.

46. Gonzalez-Gay MA, Gonzalez-Juanatey C, Miranda-Filloy JA, Garcia-Unzueta MT, Llorca J (2012) Lack of association between carotid intimamedia wall thickness and carotid plaques and markers of endothelial cell activation in rheumatoid arthritis patients undergoing anti.TNF therapy. Acta Reumatol Port 37: 155–159.

47. Rubinshtein R, Kuvin JT, Soffler M, Lennon RJ, Lavi S, et al. (2010) Assessment of endothelial function by non-invasive peripheral arterial tonometry predicts late cardiovascular adverse events. Eur Heart J 31: 1142–1148.

48. Mattace-Raso FUS, van der Cammen TJM, Hofman A, van Popele NM, Bos ML, et al. (2006) Arterial Stiffness and Risk of Coronary Heart Disease and Stroke. Circulation 113: 657–663.

49. Selzer F, Sutton-Tyrrell K, Fitzgerald S, Tracy R, Kuller L, et al. (2001) Vascular stiffness in women with systemic lupus erythematosus. Hypertension 37: 1075–1082.

50. Provan SA, Angel K, Semb AG, Mowinckel P, Agewall S, et al. (2011) Early prediction of increased arterial stiffness in patients with chronic inflammation: a 15-year followup study of 108 patients with rheumatoid arthritis. J Rheumatol 38: 606–612.

51. Shang Q, Tam LS, Li EK, Yip GW, Yu CM (2008) Increased arterial stiffness correlated with disease activity in systemic lupus erythematosus. Lupus 17: 1096–1102.

18

Lymphotoxin-LIGHT Pathway Regulates the Interferon Signature in Rheumatoid Arthritis

Jadwiga Bienkowska[1], Norm Allaire[1], Alice Thai[1], Jaya Goyal[1], Tatiana Plavina[1], Ajay Nirula[2], Megan Weaver[3], Charlotte Newman[3], Michelle Petri[4], Evan Beckman[2], Jeffrey L. Browning[2*¤]

1 Translational Medicine, Biogen Idec, Cambridge, Massachusetts, United States of America, 2 Immunobiology, Biogen Idec, Cambridge, Massachusetts, United States of America, 3 Global Clinical Operations, Biogen Idec, Cambridge, Massachusetts, United States of America, 4 Johns Hopkins University School of Medicine, Baltimore, Maryland, United States of America

Abstract

A subset of patients with autoimmune diseases including rheumatoid arthritis (RA) and lupus appear to be exposed continually to interferon (IFN) as evidenced by elevated expression of IFN induced genes in blood cells. In lupus, detection of endogenous chromatin complexes by the innate sensing machinery is the suspected driver for the IFN, but the actual mechanisms remain unknown in all of these diseases. We investigated in two randomized clinical trials the effects on RA patients of baminercept, a lymphotoxin-beta receptor-immunoglobulin fusion protein that blocks the lymphotoxin-αβ/ LIGHT axis. Administration of baminercept led to a reduced RNA IFN signature in the blood of patients with elevated baseline signatures. Both RA and SLE patients with a high IFN signature were lymphopenic and lymphocyte counts increased following baminercept treatment of RA patients. These data demonstrate a coupling between the lymphotoxin-LIGHT system and IFN production in rheumatoid arthritis. IFN induced retention of lymphocytes within lymphoid tissues is a likely component of the lymphopenia observed in many autoimmune diseases.

ClinicalTrials.gov NCT00664716.

Editor: Sylvie Bisser, INSERM U1094, University of Limoges School of Medicine, France

Funding: Biogen Idec conducted, funded and provided infrastructure for these studies and had a role in study design, data collection and analysis, decision to publish, or preparation of the manuscript. The specific roles of the authors are listed in the authors contributions section.

Competing Interests: All authors except MP were salaried employees of Biogen Idec during the conduct of these trials. JB, NA, AT, JG, TP, JO, MW and CN report being current employees of Biogen Idec with an equity interest in the company. AN, EB and JLB are former Biogen Idec employees without equity stakes. MP has received consulting fees from Biogen Idec. There are no patents or marketed products to declare and the drug remains in use in a NIH sponsored clinical study in Sjogren's disease.

* Email: browninj@bu.edu

¤ Current address: Department of Microbiology and Section of Rheumatology, Boston University School of Medicine, Boston, Massachusetts, United States of America

Introduction

Systemic lupus erythematosus (SLE), rheumatoid arthritis (RA), Sjogren's syndrome, systemic sclerosis, myositis and multiple sclerosis patients have circulating blood cells with elevated levels of RNA from IFN-induced genes, i.e. an 'IFN signature' [1–3]. A number of observations point towards a role for IFN in some autoimmune diseases. Notably, risk alleles for SLE include several genes involved in IFN responses. Multiple immunological activities are enhanced by IFN and rodent models of lupus can be accelerated by exogenous IFN. Several rare diseases with lupus-like aspects have mutations in components of the IFN response and are termed 'interferonopathies' [4]. Thus, there is very active interest in whether inhibition of IFN signaling has therapeutic benefit [5]. However, the questions of whether the IFN signature is tightly coupled to the pathology in human disease, which immunological detection systems are engaged and what are the actual cellular sources of the IFN, remain unanswered. Moreover, type I (IFN-α, β, ε, τ and ω), type II (IFN-γ) and type III (IFN-λ) IFNs can induce similar patterns of gene expression despite being produced by different spectra of cell types and being under fundamentally different regulation. The varying distribution of receptors for each IFN type also dictates responsive populations and these aspects further confound the problem.

We have investigated the effects of inhibition of the lymphotoxin-LIGHT system in RA using a soluble lymphotoxin-beta receptor (LTBR, TNFRSF3) immunoglobulin fusion protein called baminercept. LTBR is a central component of a signaling system whereby lymphocytes instruct stromal cells to differentiate into specialized vasculature and certain reticular networks [6–9]. These components form the gateways for lymphocyte entry into organized lymphoid tissues and the reticular scaffolds that guide and position cells for optimal encounters with antigen. As such, adaptive immune responses within the lymphoid organs are impaired to varying degrees in the absence of LTBR signaling. Additionally, the differentiation of critical sentinel macrophages in the subcapsular sinus of the lymph node (LN) and the splenic marginal zone depend on LTBR signaling [10]. More recently, it has become clear that LTBR signaling is interwoven with aspects of myeloid cell homeostasis as well as more innate elements of the immune system such as communication between dendritic cells, innate lymphoid cells and epithelial surfaces especially in mucosal environments [11–15]. Baminercept binds to both LTBR ligands, namely, a membrane bound heterotrimeric lymphotoxin (LT) form LTα1β2 and the ligand called LIGHT (TNFSF14). LIGHT interacts with both LTBR and an additional receptor called HVEM (TNFRSF14) and it has pro-inflammatory roles as well being implicated in aspects of T cell survival [16]. Therefore, baminercept is a dual pathway inhibitor blocking signaling triggered by both membrane LT and LIGHT ligands.

Unexpectedly, we found that baminercept reduced the IFN signature in RA patients. The reduced IFN signature in RA patients following baminercept treatment is the first time outside of high dose steroid therapy that an IFN signature was decreased by a pharmacological treatment not targeting IFN itself. Taken together with the known effects of LTBR inhibition, these studies not only link the LTBR axis to IFN production in man, but also provide potential insight into the nature of the IFN signature.

Results

Baminercept reduces the IFN signature in RA patients

Two randomized phase IIb controlled studies of the effects of baminercept in rheumatoid arthritis were conducted. One study enrolled patients with an inadequate response to disease-modifying antirheumatic drug therapy (DMARD-IR) and the other involved patients with an inadequate response to tumor necrosis factor inhibition (TNF-IR) (flow diagrams Figure 1, patient demographics defined in Supplemental Table 1 in File S1). To examine whether baminercept treatment had an impact on the immune system, the transcriptional profiles of whole blood RNA from all RA patients at 0 and 14 weeks were assessed using Affymetrix microarrays. An unsupervised analysis revealed multiple drug-induced changes that fell into three major clusters. First baminercept treatment led to an increased B cell signature. Second, patients with elevated expression at baseline of a collection of IFN response genes had the signature decreased by baminercept treatment and, third, expression of some genes associated with NK cells were decreased following treatment.

At baseline, roughly 25% of the RA patients in both the DMARD-IR and TNF-IR groups had a high IFN signature (Figure 2) and a 15-gene IFN score was calculated from the genes shown in Figure 2 (Supplemental Table 2 in File S1). Many IFN response gene sets and scores have been utilized in the literature including other sets reported by our group [17]. In general, we found similar results regardless of the selected genes. The IFN signature has been best characterized in SLE and for comparison a control cohort of 292 SLE patients from the Johns Hopkins clinic was analyzed using an identical platform. As expected about 50% of the SLE patients had an elevated IFN signature and the IFN signature in RA patients was slightly weaker than in SLE consistent with a previous study (Supplemental Figure 1 in File S1) [1,3]. Therefore, in terms of the IFN signature, the RA patients in these studies compare favorably to previous analyses.

We divided the patients from the TNF-IR study into four groups- placebo and baminercept treated with baseline low or high IFN signature scores. Figure 3 shows a heat map of the expression changes after 14 weeks for all the genes identified in the unsupervised analysis. There was a general increase in a wide range of B cell associated genes, yet interestingly, IgA1 and IgG3 expression decreased. Baminercept can disrupt follicular dendritic cell networks and germinal center reactions and perhaps this decrease reflects impaired class switching and reduced numbers of

circulating B cells or plasma cells expressing these immunoglobulins. The second cluster of genes is comprised of genes induced by IFN. Patients with a baseline high IFN score displayed substantial decreases in the IFN score following treatment. The third cluster contains multiple NK related genes and these often decreased following baminercept treatment.

To further document the IFN signature, the expression of three IFN stimulated genes, Ly6E, ISG15 and OAS1 was determined by quantitative PCR (qPCR) and an IFN score calculated (Supplemental Table 2 in File S1). The qPCR and microarray scores correlated well (Figure 4a). Figure 4b shows the change in the TNF-IR study following 14 weeks of placebo or baminercept treatment in the 3-gene PCR based IFN score as a function of the pre-treatment IFN score. This analysis revealed a significant interaction between the pre-treatment IFN and treatment, interaction p value = 2×10^{-7}. A substantial reduction in the IFN signature was also observed at 6 weeks. To extend this observation, the 3-gene qPCR IFN signature was determined for patients in DMARD-IR study. Patients were binned into baseline IFN^{high} and IFN^{low} groups based on the 3-gene qPCR IFN score of greater or less than one. The DMARD-IR study had 6 treatment cohorts and only the 70 and 200 mg q2w cohorts were analyzed by qPCR. Baminercept treatment led to a trend towards a reduced IFN signature in both cohorts and combining the two cohorts showed significant reduction (Figure 4c). The biomarker data indicated approximate saturation of the pharmacodynamic response in both these cohorts justifying combining the data (see below and serum LIGHT measurements Supplemental Figure 2 in File S1). We questioned whether the incidence of infectious events could impact the observation and there was little indication that infection rates were substantially increased or decreased following baminercept treatment (Supplemental Table 3 in File S1). Since baminercept potentially dampens the immune system, an increased rate of infection was possible and therefore treatment could have increased the IFN signature. As an increased IFN signature was not observed, infection is not a likely confounder for this result.

To validate further the ability of baminercept treatment to affect an IFN signature, we examined by qPCR the expression of SIGLEC1, another IFN induced gene. In contrast to the genes in the 3-gene panel, it is expressed exclusively in monocytes and, moreover, it is a potential marker of SLE disease severity [18]. Analysis of the SIGLEC1 RNA expression using the qPCR data showed that SIGLEC1 expression was elevated in the IFN high group and baminercept treatment reduced its expression confirming the 3-gene signature analysis (Figure 5a,b). Expression (qPCR) of genes specific for monocytes (SLAMF7, SPARC), DC (CD1E) and plasmacytoid DC (pDC) (CLEC4C and LILRA4) was independent of IFN status.

There is considerable overlap in the expression profiles resulting from type 1 (IFNs α, β and ω) and type II IFN (IFNγ) and, furthermore, each IFN is capable in many contexts of inducing the expression of the other IFN class [19]. An 8 gene IFNγ signature was defined based on genes preferentially induced in blood cells by IFNγ [20]. In our data, there was no significant correlation between the basic IFN and IFNγ signatures suggesting that type I IFNs are dominating in RA (Supplemental Figure 3 in File S1). Two genes, GBP1 and GBP2, were induced selectively by IFNγ in salivary gland epithelial cells, yet in our blood data the GBP1/2 score correlated very well with the basic IFN signature (Supplemental Figure 3 in File S1). In other studies, the GBP1/2 genes are induced by type I IFN in blood cells both in vitro and in vivo in IFN treated hepatitis C and melanoma patients. Our data are consistent with exposure to type I IFN in RA.

RA203 "TNF-IR" Flow Diagram

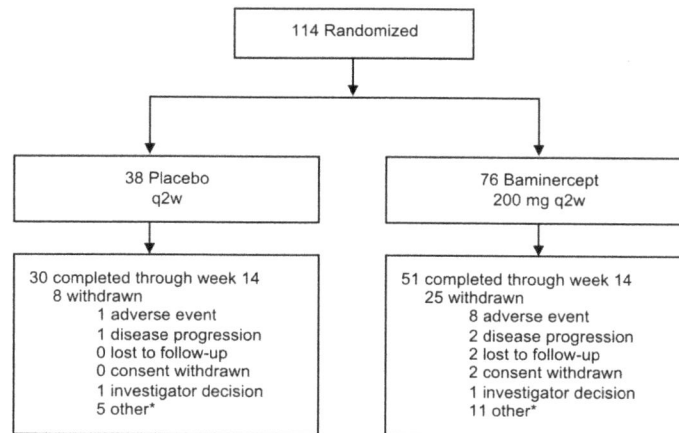

```
                          114 Randomized

        38 Placebo                          76 Baminercept
          q2w                                200 mg q2w

  30 completed through week 14      51 completed through week 14
  8 withdrawn                       25 withdrawn
     1 adverse event                   8 adverse event
     1 disease progression             2 disease progression
     0 lost to follow-up               2 lost to follow-up
     0 consent withdrawn               2 consent withdrawn
     1 investigator decision           1 investigator decision
     5 other*                          11 other*
```

Trial was stopped early due to failed primary endpoint in the parallel RA202 study, hence high discontinuation rate relative to the RA202.

RA202 "DMARD-IR" Flow Diagram

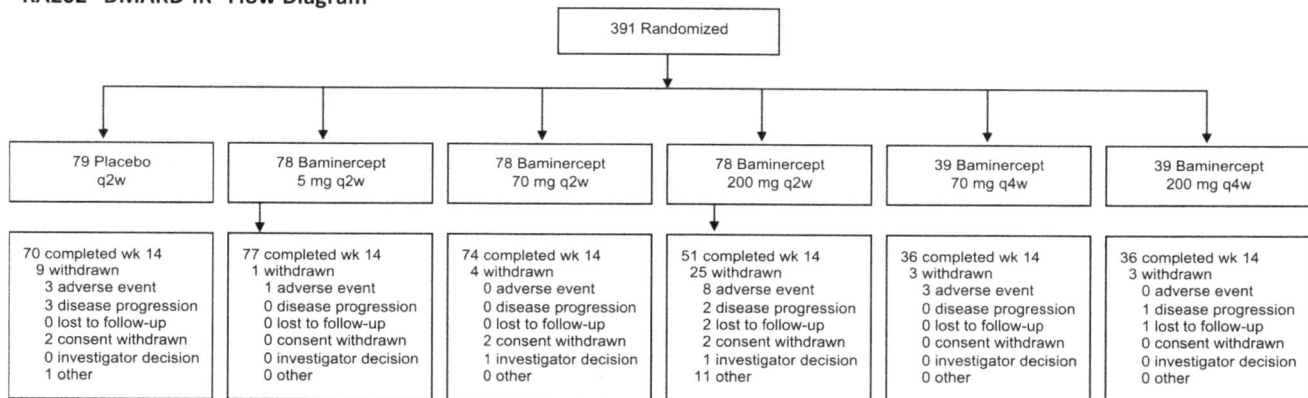

```
                                  391 Randomized

 79 Placebo   78 Baminercept  78 Baminercept  78 Baminercept  39 Baminercept  39 Baminercept
   q2w          5 mg q2w        70 mg q2w       200 mg q2w      70 mg q4w       200 mg q4w

70 completed    77 completed    74 completed    51 completed    36 completed    36 completed
wk 14           wk 14           wk 14           wk 14           wk 14           wk 14
9 withdrawn     1 withdrawn     4 withdrawn     25 withdrawn    3 withdrawn     3 withdrawn
 3 adverse       1 adverse       0 adverse       8 adverse       3 adverse       0 adverse
   event           event           event           event           event           event
 3 disease       0 disease       0 disease       2 disease       0 disease       1 disease
   progression     progression     progression     progression     progression     progression
 0 lost to       0 lost to       0 lost to       2 lost to       0 lost to       1 lost to
   follow-up       follow-up       follow-up       follow-up       follow-up       follow-up
 2 consent       0 consent       2 consent       2 consent       0 consent       0 consent
   withdrawn       withdrawn       withdrawn       withdrawn       withdrawn       withdrawn
 0 investigator  0 investigator  1 investigator  1 investigator  0 investigator  0 investigator
   decision        decision        decision        decision        decision        decision
 1 other         0 other         0 other         11 other        0 other         0 other
```

Figure 1. Flow diagrams for the two clinical trials assessing the effects of baminercept treatment on rheumatoid arthritis patients.

Elevated levels of type I IFN or an IFN-like inducing activity can be found in the sera of a subset of the SLE patients with a transcriptional IFN signature; however, in RA the results range from not detectable to low levels relative to SLE sera [21,22]. We examined serum IFN levels using highly sensitive A549 (more type I IFN selective) or WISH (similar sensitivity to type I and II IFN) cell based reporter assays with an ELISA-based Mx1 protein readout. Analysis of 64 baseline sera from the TNF-IR study including all of the patients with elevated baseline IFN signatures did not reveal IFN activity, whereas substantial activity was readily found in the sera from some SLE patients. Therefore, the blood RNA IFN signature in RA is likely derived from local exposure in organs to IFN.

IFN signature is associated with lymphopenia in both RA and SLE

SLE patients with a high IFN signature tend to be lymphopenic [23]. Using the 15 gene microarray-based IFN signature to group patients at baseline into a high or low IFN status, we observed that both IFN high RA and SLE patients were lymphopenic (Figure 6a). The degree of lymphopenia in IFN high RA patients was not as pronounced as in the comparable SLE group possibly paralleling the relative intensities of the IFN signatures in these two diseases.

In rodents, blockade of the LTBR system leads to lymphocytosis within several weeks most likely due to loss of high endothelial venule addressin expression and reduced entry into the lymph nodes and mucosal environments [24]. Treatment with baminercept led to increased lymphocyte and monocyte counts in the blood of patients with full effect observed within 2–5 weeks (Figure 6b and Supplemental Figures 4 and 5 in File S1). The 5 mg q2w dose was partially active and similar results were seen with both the 70 and 200 mg q2w doses indicating approximate saturation. It is believed that one driver for lymphopenia in SLE may be chronic IFN exposure and prolonged lymphocyte retention within the lymph nodes [25]. To assess whether reduced IFN exposure could contribute to the baminercept induced lymphocytosis, we compared the change in lymphocyte counts in the IFN low and high subsets. Lymphocyte counts increased in both groups following baminercept treatment; however, the magnitude of the change was greater in much of the IFN high subset in the TNF-IR study and trended higher in DMARD-IR

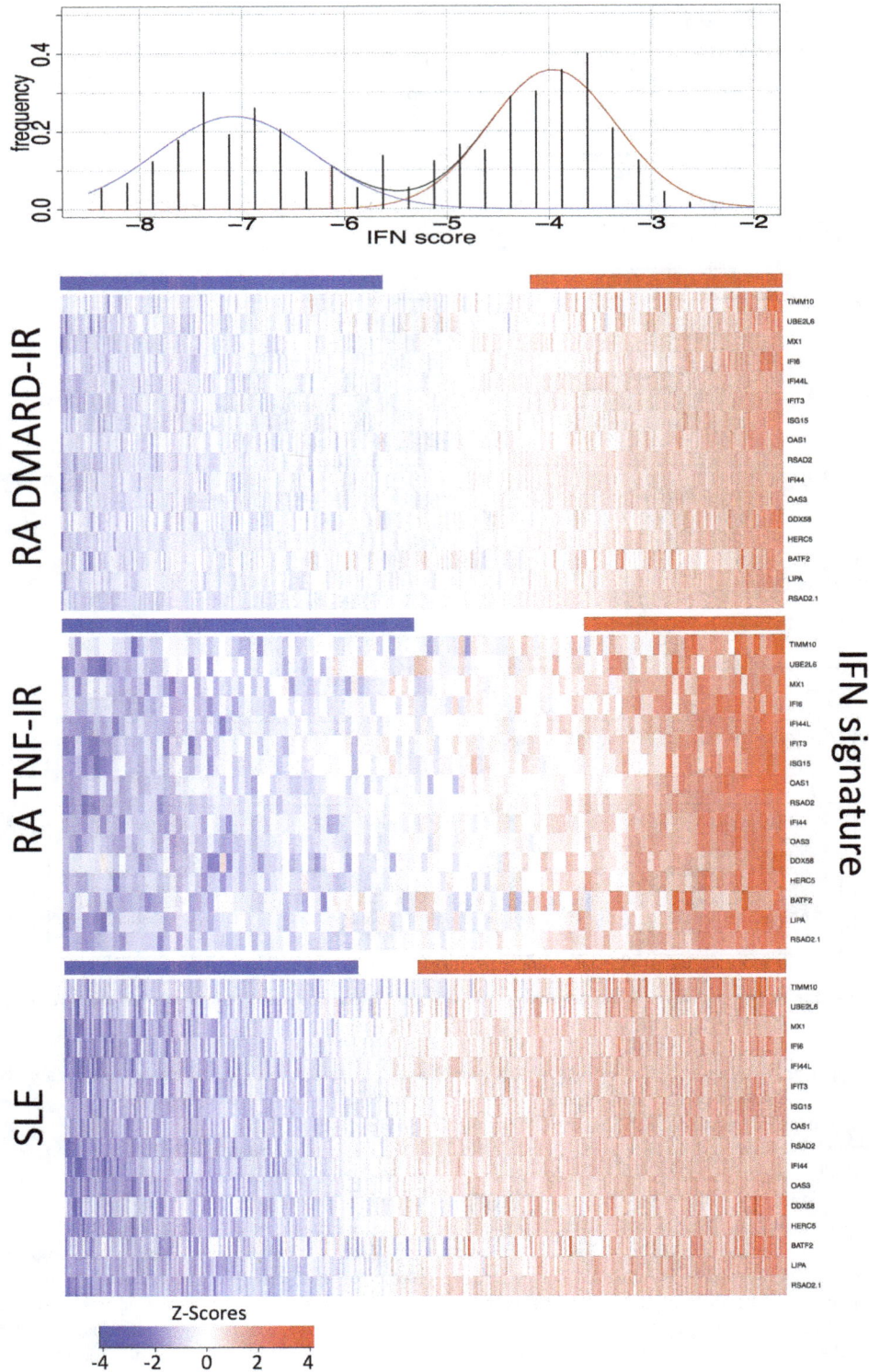

Figure 2. Comparison of the IFN signature in DMARD-IR and TNF-IR RA patients. Baseline heat maps of the RA DMARD-IR, TNF-IR and the SLE cohorts studied in this work. Red indicates increased expression of a panel of 15 IFN inducible genes showing similar percentages of IFN signature positive patients in each RA subgroup (the gene RSAD2 is represented twice). Bars above each map show the clustering as IFN positive (red) or negative (blue) based on assignment to two normal distributions as shown in the top panel with p<0.05. Color bar ranges are as stated for SLE and DMARD-IR, but −3 to 3 for TNF-IR (as per figure 3).

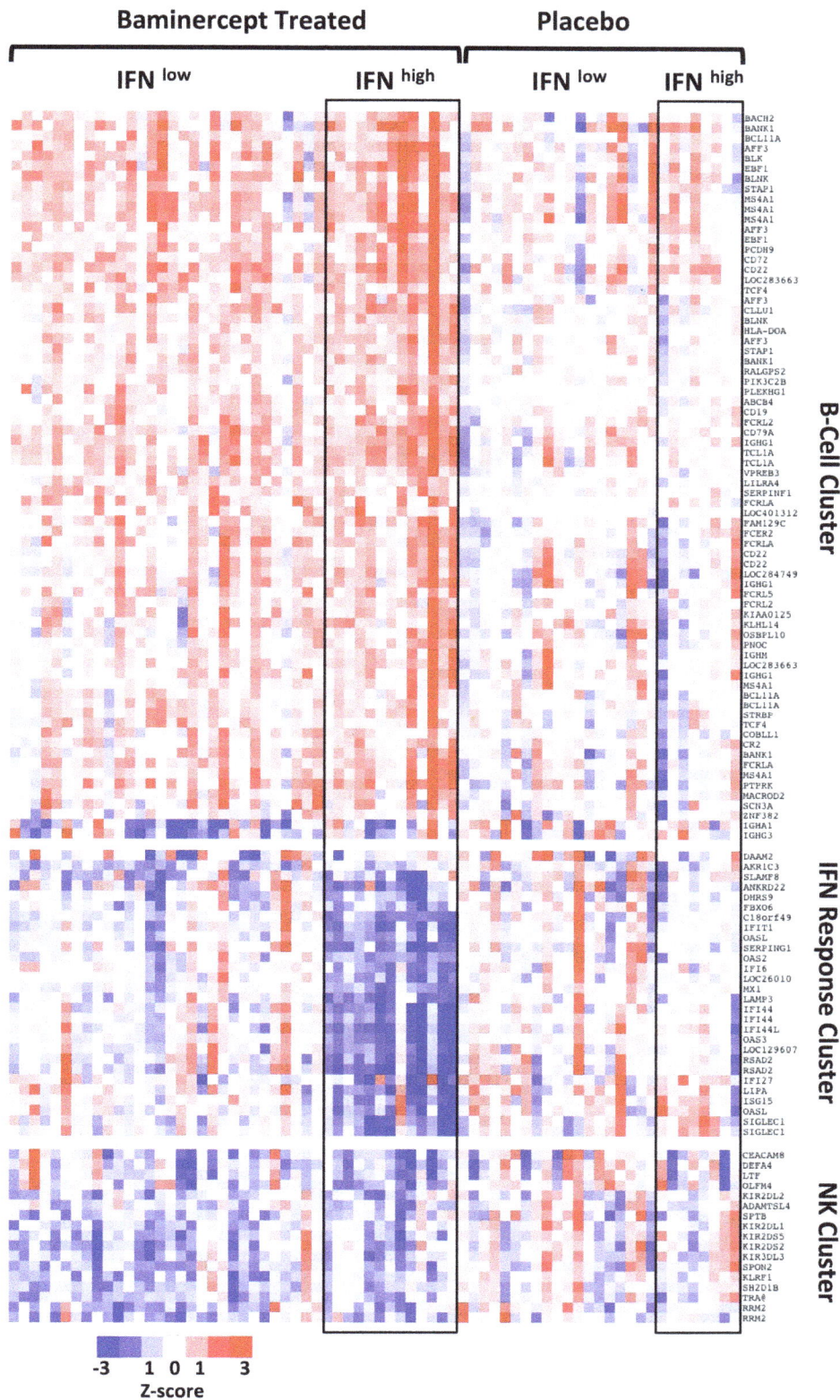

Figure 3. Baminercept induced changes in total blood RNA expression. Heat map showing the change in gene expression after 14 week of either placebo or baminercept treatment. Patients were forced into 4 groups based on treatment and baseline IFN signature. Each of the three gene clusters defined from initial unsupervised clustering are presented separately. The three clusters are characterized by genes associated with B cells, IFN response or NK cells, although some other genes are also present within each category. List only includes genes whose changes were significant (p<0.05), passed FDR and had greater than a 1.5 fold difference in a separate paired sample analysis.

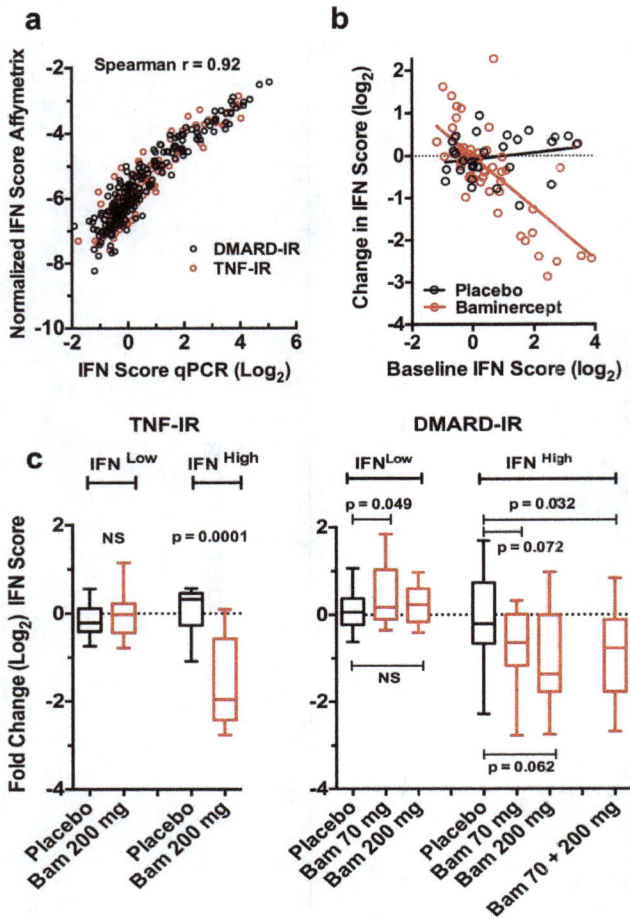

Figure 4. Blockade of the lymphotoxin-LIGHT pathway with baminercept reduces the blood RNA IFN signature in RA patients. a). Analysis of the individual baseline IFN scores as determined using the 15 gene microarray data and a three-gene qPCR score showing excellent correlation. b). Analysis of the change in the 3-gene qPCR IFN score as a function of baseline IFN score following 14 weeks of treatment with 200 mg baminercept q2w in TNF-IR patients, significance is calculated using a linear model of change in IFN score as an interaction of baseline IFN score and treatment (placebo or baminercept). The significance for baseline IFN is $p = 2 \times 10^{-7}$ and for the interaction term $p = 2.3 \times 10^{-7}$. Treatment alone is marginally significant $p = 0.0506$. c). Change in the qPCR-based IFN score at 14 weeks in patients with low vs. high baseline IFN scores (low <1, high >1). Red boxes represent baminercept (Bam) treated patients receiving either 70 or 200 mg q2w (DMARD-IR) or 200 mg q2w (TNF-IR) while black boxes indicate placebo treated patients; n = 20, 50, 11 and 12 (TNF-IR) and 49, 44, 50, 20, 28, 18 and 38 (DMARD-IR) patients in each category in the order listed. P values are from a Mann-Whitney test of placebo vs. baminercept treated patients.

(Figure 6c). These results are consistent with contributions to baminercept induced lymphocytosis from both altered addressin expression and reduced IFN exposure.

In mice, lymphocytosis following LTBR blockade results from elevated T and B cells counts [24]. In these clinical studies, FACS analysis of a small subset of the patients (TNF-IR) showed that B cell numbers were increased roughly 70% over baseline compared to a 24% increase in T cells (Supplemental Figure 6 in File S1). The elevated B cell signature based on the data in figure 3 correlated roughly with the extent of lymphocytosis (r = 0.338, p<

0.0001,) and therefore it is likely that the B cell signature reflects differential lymphocytosis in the baminercept treated cohorts. Furthermore, PCR quantitation of the levels of genes uniquely expressed in lymphocyte subsets revealed some interesting details (Figure 7). RNA levels of CD20 (B cells) increased consistent with the general lymphocytosis, but TCRδ and some natural killer cell specific genes, KLRF1 as well as KLRD1, KIR2DS1 and KIR3DL1 decreased substantially (only a subset of genes identified from the transcriptional profiling were included in the qPCR array). Thus the qPCR data confirmed the decreased NK signature shown in figure 3. Comparison of the change in absolute lymphocyte counts with the change in RNA levels showed a positive correlation with the expression of CD20, TCRα and CD8B RNA (Spearman r values of 0.56, 0.47 and 0.49 respectively), but little correlation with TCRδ (γδ T cells), KLRF1 (NK) and Defensin 3A (immature neutrophils) (r = 0.14, 0.02 and 0.01 respectively). The change in KLRF1 was not coupled to baseline IFN status. In a FACS analysis, B cells and CD4 cell numbers increased, while NK cell numbers trended towards a decrease (Supplemental Figure 6 in File S1). Therefore baminercept appeared to reduce the numbers of immature neutrophils, TCRγδ and NK cells in the blood by a mechanism distinct from the lymphocytosis effects and prior studies in rodents have implicated LTBR in the biology of both TCRγδ and NK cells [26–31]. The decrease in immature neutrophils is intriguing given their propensity to generate chromatin nets and the recent suggestion that nets are a source of citrullinated antigens in RA [32,33].

Given the emphasis on plasmacytoid DC as the source of the IFN signature in SLE, we examined RNA levels in the blood of two known pDC markers, CLEC4C (BDCA2) and LILRA4 (ILT7). LILRA4 levels increased following baminercept treatment, yet CLEC4C levels were unchanged (Supplemental Figure 7 in File S1). CLEC4C appears to be a relatively specific pDC marker, whereas LILRA4 is highly expressed by both pDCs and memory B cells (Immunological Genome). Therefore these data suggest that baminercept does not affect pDC trafficking and increased LILRA4 expression is consistent with the increased numbers of B cells in the blood.

Relationship between IFN status and clinical parameters

After 3 months of treatment, changes in disease status were assessed using the American College of Rheumatology (ACR) scoring system. Overall, baminercept was well tolerated (Supplemental Table 3 in File S1); yet, in neither trial did baminercept treatment substantially increase the ACR scores (Supplemental Table 4 in File S1). Baminercept treatment resulted in a trend towards reduced swollen joint counts (SJC28) in both studies (Supplemental Figure 8 in File S1). Inhibition of TNF or IL-6 significantly decreases ESR and serum CRP levels; however, baminercept did not appreciably lower either serum parameter (Supplemental Figure 9 in File S1).

When patients were grouped based on baseline qPCR IFN status, there was no obvious trend towards a greater reduction in SJC28 in either IFN subgroup in the DMARD-IR study (Supplemental Figure 8 in file S1). The TNF-IR study was too small for such subgrouping. As these studies examined almost 800 patients, an analysis of gender effects was possible and baseline IFN scores were slightly lower in RA males (p = 0.04) and trended slightly lower in males in SLE. No correlation was observed between the IFN high and low groups with baseline swollen joint counts (SJC28), the Disease Activity Score 28 ESR (DAS28 ESR), C-reactive protein, erythrocyte sedimentation rates (ESR), rheumatoid factor titer or anti-CCP positivity (Supplemental Figure 10

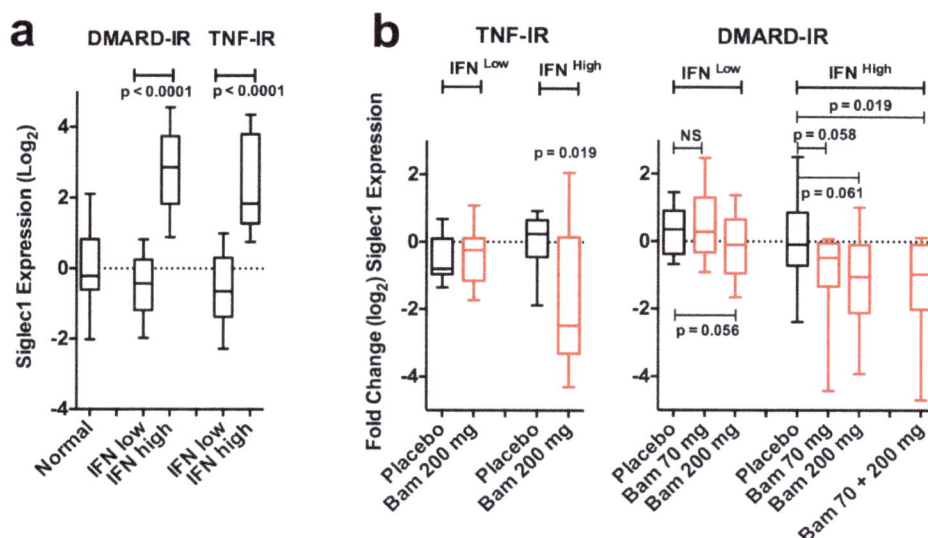

Figure 5. Baminercept treatment lowered RNA expression of the monocyte-associated gene SIGLEC1 in the blood. a). Expression of the monocyte associated gene SIGLEC1 (qPCR determination) is elevated in patients with an elevated IFN signature (qPCR IFN score cut point of 1). b.) SIGLEC1 expression ($\log_2$) was reduced by treatment with baminercept (n's and boxes as per figure 4). P values are from a Mann-Whitney test of placebo vs. baminercept treated patients.

in File S1). Baminercept treatment did not affect total serum IgG, IgM and IgA levels nor were preexisting tetanus toxoid titers altered.

Discussion

We show here that inhibition of the LT/LIGHT pathway reduced not only the global IFN signature, but also RNA levels of SIGLEC1, an IFN-regulated gene expressed only in monocytes. RA and SLE patients with an IFN signature were more lymphopenic and baminercept treatment reversed the lymphopenia. These results demonstrate at the clinical level a fundamental linkage between the LT/LIGHT axis and IFN responses as well as between IFN and lymphopenia. To date, only high dose steroids and anti-interferon-α antibodies have been shown to reduce the signature and the inhibition by anti-IFNα antibodies appears to be partial [34–39]. Neither therapy informs on the nature of the underlying IFN biology. Importantly, a reduction in the IFN signature did not result in diminished arthritis suggesting that the pathology driving the IFN signature is not tightly coupled to the local joint disease. This conclusion needs to be qualified because the trials were insufficiently powered for the IFN positive subset, the treatment duration was relatively short and the levels of inflammatory disease were modest as indicated by the low baseline CRP levels.

The question of what biology is being reflected by the blood IFN signature in RA as well as in other autoimmune diseases remains unanswered. In SLE, the IFN signature is correlated in general with a distinct serological profile, renal disease, and progression to atherosclerosis and disease severity, yet its presence is not obviously linked to any particular immunology [23,40]. Our RA studies and those of others did not reveal obvious differences based on IFN status between the DMARD-IR and TNF-IR cohorts or their clinical or serological features [41,42]. A positive IFN signature in RA has been linked to a poor response to rituximab [43] and a weak or variable correlation with response to TNF inhibition [22,44,45]. In both systemic onset juvenile idiopathic arthritis patients and in Sjogren's syndrome, TNF

inhibition led to an increased IFN signature supporting the hypothesis that TNF- and IFN-driven pathologies may lie at opposite poles of the autoimmune disease spectrum [46,47]. The ability of baminercept to dampen an IFN signature may have been a liability in a TNF dominated setting such as RA.

SLE patients are often lymphopenic and lymphopenia correlated with an elevated IFN signature in both SLE and systemic sclerosis patients [23,48]. Here, we confirmed this association in our SLE cohort and extended it to include RA patients. Lymphopenia could reflect perturbed bone marrow hematopoiesis accompanying systemic inflammation and/or increased retention of lymphocytes in the lymph nodes [49,50]. In the latter mechanism, IFN triggers complex formation between CD69 and sphingosine-1-phosphate receptors thereby inhibiting cell egress into the cortical sinuses [25]. Indeed, administration of IFNβ to multiple sclerosis patients or mice results in lymphopenia [51,52]. Increased retention of lymphocytes in the IFN-rich lymphoid microenvironments would allow more dwell time for productive encounters. Baminercept-induced lymphocytosis most likely has a contribution from restricted entry into the LN and mucosal compartments due to loss of addressin positive high endothelial venules. Baminercept could also reduce lymphopenia by shortening retention times in the LN following reduced IFN exposure. Our data are consistent with contributions from both trafficking and retention components and support the hypothesis that IFN-driven lymphocyte retention in the lymphoid tissues is a substantial component of lymphopenia in autoimmune disease.

The effect of baminercept on the blood IFN signature was largely unanticipated; however, observations from several experimental systems demonstrate that the LT/LIGHT network is entwined with IFN responses to infection [53]. First, murine CMV infection of the spleen induces an early IFN response derived from reticular stromal cells in the marginal zone [31,54,55]. Various aspects of lymphoid reticular stroma are critically dependent upon LTBR signaling and loss of LTBR signaling ablated the initial IFN response to murine CMV infection. Second, SIGLEC1-positive sentinel macrophages in both the LN and splenic environments

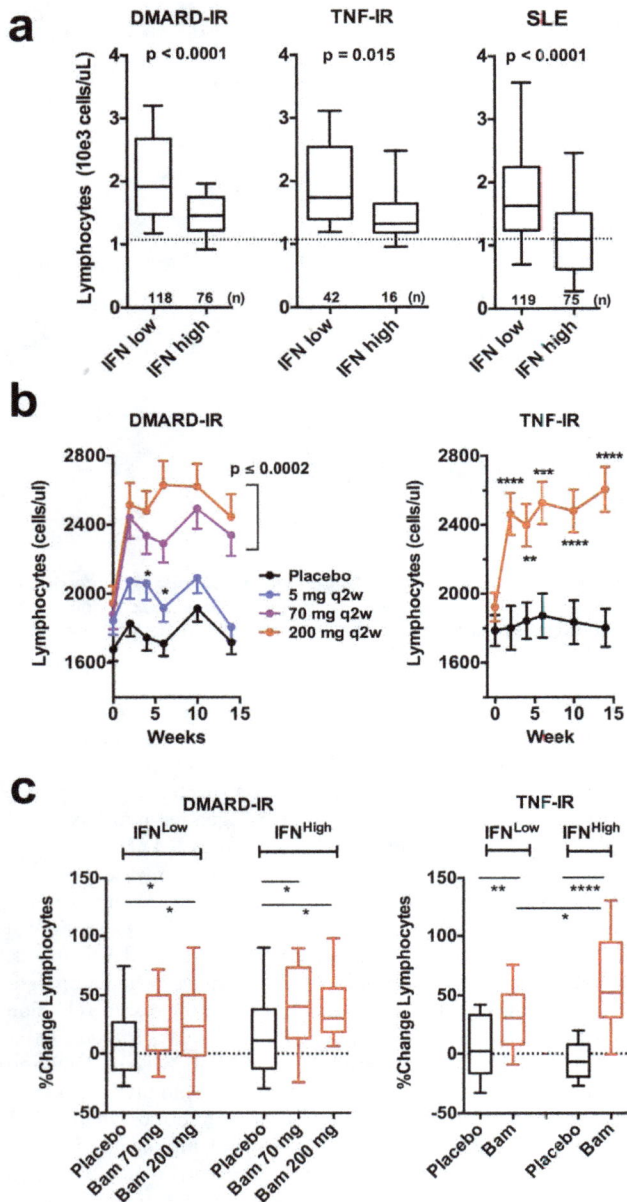

Figure 6. IFN signature positive RA patients are lymphopenic and baminercept treatment resulted in lymphocytosis. a). Patients were segregated based on low and high microarray IFN scores (<−6.5 and>−4.5) and baseline blood lymphocyte counts are plotted. b). Time course of the effects on absolute lymphocyte counts during 14 weeks of baminercept or placebo treatment (means, +/− SEM). All time points in two highest dosed cohorts in DMARD-IR were significant (p< 0.0002), otherwise, significance is indicated by p-values * <0.05, ** < 0.01, *** <0.001 and **** <0.0001. c). Patients were grouped into baseline qPCR IFN signature low or high as in Fig. 1c. Percent change in lymphocyte counts following 14 weeks of treatment with placebo or baminercept is plotted (significance Mann-Whitney in all cases).

survey lymph or blood for immune complexes, lipids, particulates, viruses and sialylated antigens [56–58]. In the case of immune complexes or complement tagged antigens, they capture these elements and route them into the follicle for presentation to B cells.

The differentiation state of these sentinel macrophages is LTBR-dependent [59,60]. Following VSV infection, virus replicates within the LN subcapsular macrophages and the splenic marginal zone metallophilic macrophages triggering IFN production and an effective host response [60–62]. Within the spleen, marginal zone metallophilic macrophages are the major local producers of type I IFN in response to an intravenous HSV challenge [63] and they also generate IFN in response to *Campylobacter jejuni* infection [64]. In a related observation, listeria infection of LTBR-deficient mice failed to generate an IFN response in the spleen [65]. Other LT-dependent sources could include both dendritic cells [11,66–68] as well as follicular dendritic cells where TLRs could be activated following internalization and recycling of antigen [69].

Why is this linkage between the LT and IFN systems manifesting itself in RA? In SLE, a subset of IFN signature high patients has measureable IFN circulating in the blood [21,70]. However, IFN was not detected in the blood of our RA patients and therefore the exposure to IFN must occur while leucocytes traffic through the organs. In RA, robust evidence for a substantial IFN signal in the joints is lacking [3,71,72]. One hypothesis is that lymphocytes become "imprinted" by IFN while trafficking through organized lymphoid microenvironments. Many if not all autoimmune diseases have undercurrents of systemic disease as evidenced by the involvement of additional organ systems, e.g. the lungs in RA, the CNS in SLE, Sjogren's and sarcoidosis, etc. We speculate that LNs draining organs with articular or extra-articular disease, as in lung or glandular involvement in RA, produce IFN as a consequence of sensing signals such as dead cell debris, chromatin complexes, neutrophil nets or antigens as complement tagged or immunoglobulin complexes [69,73]. In this scenario, the amount of IFN exposure would reflect the magnitude of the systemic involvement and may coincide with LN reactivity or even gross lymphadenopathy. Indeed, some association was noted in SLE between lymphoadenopathy and an increased IFN signature [23]. We speculate that baminercept's effects on the IFN signature are due to alteration of the sentinel functions of the lymphoid microenvironments albeit via myeloid or stromal elements.

In conclusion, inhibition of the LTR signaling in RA patients reduced IFN imprinting. The IFN signature is linked to the lymphopenia in RA and SLE supporting a role for IFN in lymphocyte retention in lymphoid organs. Experimentally, the use of viral challenges has revealed much of the linkage between LTBR and IFN responses and, while autoimmune diseases do not have obvious ongoing viral infections, parallels have been drawn between immune responses to virus and chromatin in SLE [74]. Thus, these observations may be highlighting a potential coupling mechanism between tissue damage, debris recognition and an overactive self-reactive immune response. Disruption of LTBR signaling could be a new tool for the investigation and potentially the treatment of certain subgroups in autoimmune diseases.

Experimental Procedures

Patients and Trials

Baminercept is a fusion protein of the extracellular domain of human LTBR coupled to the hinge and Fc domain of human IgG1 [75]. DMARD-IR (104RA202, NCT00664716, EUdraCT 2006-005466-39) was a multicenter, phase IIb, randomized, double-blinded placebo-controlled study of RA patients who had had an inadequate response (IR) to a disease modifying anti-rheumatic drug. In this study 391 RA patients were treated for 14 weeks with subcutaneous injections of placebo q2w (79 patients), 5 mg baminercept (BG9948) q2w (78), 70 mg q2w (78), 70 mg q4w (39), 200 mg q2w (78) or 200 mg q4w (39). 365 patients

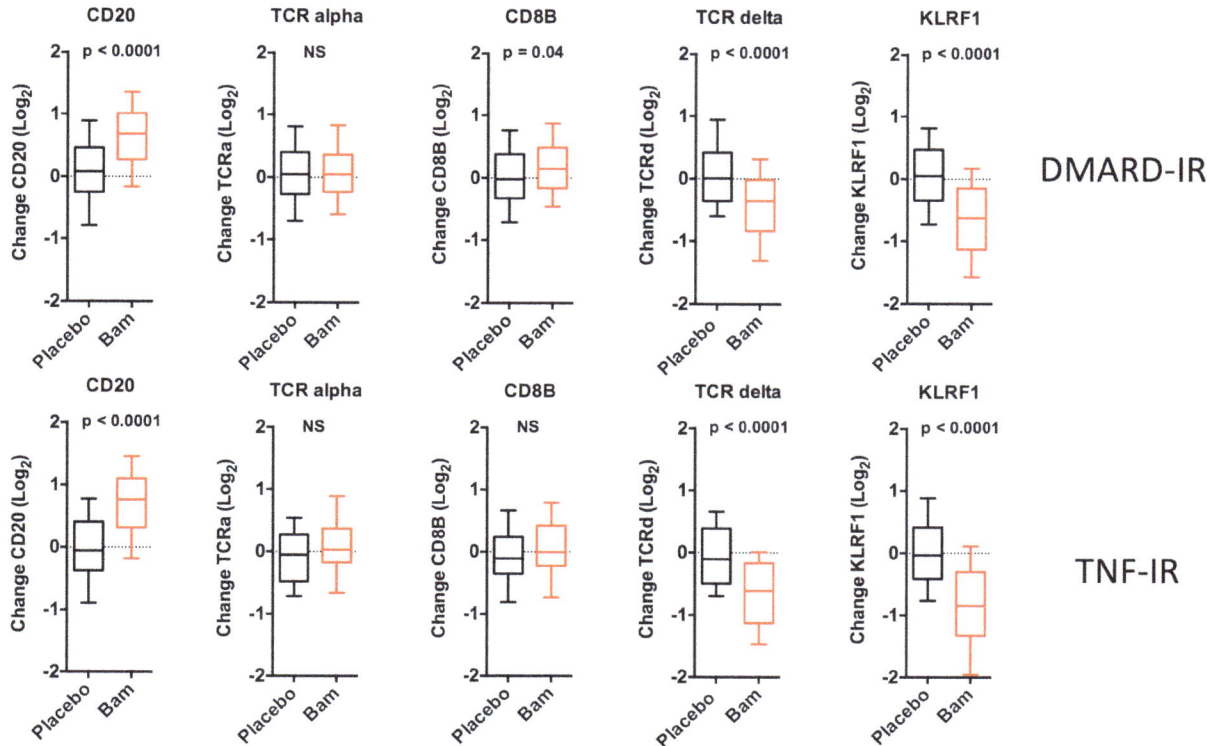

Figure 7. Baminercept alters the levels of RNAs representative of lymphocyte subsets in the blood. Baminercept treatment increased the blood RNA expression (qPCR determination) of genes representing B cells (CD20), T cells (TCRA, CD8B), whereas expression of markers for γδ-T cells (TCRD) and NK cells (KLRF1) decreased. In the DMARD-IR study, data from both 70 and 200 mg 2qw cohorts are pooled.

completed the study. Study was conducted between July 2007 and October 2008 at 58 sites in Argentina, Brazil, Hungary, Mexico, Poland, Romania, Russia and United Kingdom and investigators are listed in the supplemental materials.

TNF-IR (104RA203, NCT00458861, EUdraCT 2006-005467-26) was a multicenter, phase IIb, double-blinded, placebo-controlled study of RA patients who lacked an adequate response to TNF-blocking therapy and had discontinued TNF blocking treatment for at least 90 days. The study dosed 114 patients with subcutaneous injections q2w of either placebo (38) or baminercept 200 mg (76). This study was terminated early due to poor efficacy in the DMARD-IR study; however, 81 patients completed the 3 months of dosing and another 15 patients received at least 2 months of treatment. Study was conducted between March 2007 and October 2008 at 40 sites in the United States, Canada, Belgium and United Kingdom.

Investigators for both baminercept studies are listed in the supplemental materials in File S1. RA patients in both studies were eligible if they met the American College of Rheumatology (ACR) criteria for rheumatoid arthritis and had active RA for at least 6 months. Patients had to have been receiving 10–25 mg methotrexate per week for at least 3 months with a stable dose for the last 4 weeks before entry. Methotrexate therapy was maintained for the duration of the studies. Patients had to have more than 8 swollen and tender joints (66/68 joint count) and either a CRP≥ 1.5 ULN or ESR ≥28 mm/hr at screening. The protocols for these trials re available as supporting information; see Protocol S1 and S2. There is no intent to publish further clinical data from

these studies and the ACR scores (primary trial endpoint) are presented within the supplemental data.

SLE data were from registry (called SPARE) representing a collection of 292 SLE patients from the Hopkins Lupus Center in the US. Patients were eligible if they were aged 18–75 years and met the American College of Rheumatology Revised Criteria for Classification of Systemic Lupus Erythematous. Baseline data were used in this study and patients were under standard clinical practice. Normal controls for RNA analyses were composed of healthy volunteer donors from Biogen Idec. Control group had equal numbers of males and females and was not exactly gender balanced with the predominantly female composition of both the RA and SLE cohorts.

Ethics Statement

The RA studies were approved by the appropriate institutional review boards or ethics committees and all patients provided written informed consent (see supplementary materials in File S1 for a complete listing). All patients from the Hopkins Lupus Center (Johns Hopkins University School of Medicine) provided written informed consent to participate in the SPARE registry and the Johns Hopkins institutional review board approved the study.

Analyses of whole blood RNA

Patient whole blood was collected into PaxGene tubes and analyzed using conventional Affymetrix microarrays and qPCR was performed on the RNA samples using the Fluidigm analyzer. Details for RNA analyses as well as the IFN reporter assays are provided in the Supplemental Materials in File S1. Baseline transcriptional profiling datasets are deposited at GEO, GSE45291.

Supporting Information

File S1 Supporting files. Supplemental Methods and Investigator Listing. Supplemental Table 1, Demographics of the Patients in the RA studies and the SLE registry. Supplemental Table 2, Measurement of IFN signatures. Supplemental Table 3, Incidence of adverse events by preferred term for the combined placebo-controlled studies. Supplemental Table 4, Lack of an appreciable effect of baminercept treatment on ACR scores as assessed at 14 weeks. Supplemental Figure 1, Comparison of IFN signatures in RA and SLE. Supplemental Figure 2, Elevation of serum LIGHT levels in RA patients following baminercept treatment. Supplemental Figure 3, Characteristics of the IFN signatures observed in this study. Elevation of serum LIGHT levels in RA patients following baminercept treatment. Supplemental Figure 4, Characteristics of baminercept induced lymphocytosis in RA patients. Supplemental Figure 5, Relationship between IFN signature and baminercept treatment on blood neutrophil and monocyte counts. Supplemental Figure 6, FACS analysis of the effects of baminercept treatment on peripheral blood lymphocyte subsets. Supplemental Figure 7, Quantitative PCR analysis on whole blood RNA of the effects of baminercept treatment on gene markers of myeloid subsets. Supplemental Figure 8, Effects of baminercept treatment on the Swollen Joint Count 28 (SJC28) scores in the DMARD-IR and TNF-IR studies. Supplemental Figure 9, Little effect of baminercept treatment on CRP levels and Erythrocyte Sedimentation Rates (ESR) in the DMARD-IR and TNF-IR studies. Supplemental Figure 10, The IFN signature status in RA patients does not correlate with clinical or serological parameters.

Checklist S1 CONSORT Checklist.

Protocol S1 Trial Protocol.

Protocol S2 Trial Protocol.

Acknowledgments

We thank the patients who participated in the studies; the investigators and personnel at the study sites, and the members of the baminercept project team, including Paul Chen, Niki Cox, Patrick Cullen, Fred D'Amato, Susan Gawlak, Janet Griffiths, Evangelia Hatzis, Bina Keshaven, Megan Lo, Helena Madden, Nick Messinese, Werner Meier, John O'Gorman, Suezanne Parker, Jitesh Rana, Ann Ranger, Joyce Sobolewski, Cynthia Theodos, Miranda Tighe, Melissa Wojcik and Jim Woodworth. We also thank Larrisa Miller for help with the IFN reporter assay, Susan Kalled and Ronenn Rubinoff for major contributions to the SPARE SLE registry and Ian Rifkin, Carl Ware, Jen Gommerman, Peter Lipsky and Peggy Crow for critique of the manuscript.

Author Contributions

Conceived and designed the experiments: JB JG TP AN MW CN MP EB JLB. Performed the experiments: JB NA AT JG TP AN MW CN MP EB JLB. Analyzed the data: JB JG TP JLB. Contributed to the writing of the manuscript: JB JG TP EB JLB.

References

1. Ronnblom L, Eloranta ML (2013) The interferon signature in autoimmune diseases. Current opinion in rheumatology 25: 248–253.
2. Elkon KB, Wiedeman A (2012) Type I IFN system in the development and manifestations of SLE. Current opinion in rheumatology 24: 499–505.
3. Higgs BW, Liu Z, White B, Zhu W, White WI, et al. (2011) Patients with systemic lupus erythematosus, myositis, rheumatoid arthritis and scleroderma share activation of a common type I interferon pathway. Annals of the rheumatic diseases 70: 2029–2036.
4. Crow YJ (2011) Type I interferonopathies: a novel set of inborn errors of immunity. Annals of the New York Academy of Sciences 1238: 91–98.
5. Kirou KA, Gkrouzman E (2013) Anti-interferon alpha treatment in SLE. Clinical immunology 148: 303–312.
6. Browning JL (2008) Inhibition of the lymphotoxin pathway as a therapy for autoimmune disease. Immunological reviews 223: 202–220.
7. Ware CF (2008) Targeting lymphocyte activation through the lymphotoxin and LIGHT pathways. Immunological reviews 223: 186–201.
8. Remouchamps C, Boutaffala L, Ganeff C, Dejardin E (2011) Biology and signal transduction pathways of the Lymphotoxin-alphabeta/LTbetaR system. Cytokine & growth factor reviews 22: 301–310.
9. Lu TT, Browning JL (2014) Role of the Lymphotoxin/LIGHT System in the Development and Maintenance of Reticular Networks and Vasculature in Lymphoid Tissues. Frontiers in immunology 5: 47.
10. Gray EE, Cyster JG (2012) Lymph node macrophages. Journal of innate immunity 4: 424–436.
11. Summers deLuca L, Gommerman JL (2012) Fine-tuning of dendritic cell biology by the TNF superfamily. Nature reviews Immunology 12: 339–351.
12. De Trez C (2012) Lymphotoxin-beta receptor expression and its related signaling pathways govern dendritic cell homeostasis and function. Immunobiology 217: 1250–1258.
13. Upadhyay V, Fu YX (2013) Lymphotoxin signalling in immune homeostasis and the control of microorganisms. Nature reviews Immunology 13: 270–279.
14. Satpathy AT, Briseno CG, Lee JS, Ng D, Manieri NA, et al. (2013) Notch2-dependent classical dendritic cells orchestrate intestinal immunity to attaching-and-effacing bacterial pathogens. Nature immunology 14: 937–948.
15. Wege AK, Huber B, Wimmer N, Mannel DN, Hehlgans T (2013) LTbetaR expression on hematopoietic cells regulates acute inflammation and influences maturation of myeloid subpopulations. Innate immunity ePub.
16. Steinberg MW, Cheung TC, Ware CF (2011) The signaling networks of the herpesvirus entry mediator (TNFRSF14) in immune regulation. Immunological reviews 244: 169–187.
17. Allaire NE, Bushnell SE, Bienkowska J, Brock G, Carulli J (2013) Optimization of a high-throughput whole blood expression profiling methodology and its application to assess the pharmacodynamics of interferon (IFN) beta-1a or polyethylene glycol-conjugated IFN beta-1a in healthy clinical trial subjects. BMC research notes 6: 8.
18. Rose T, Grutzkau A, Hirseland H, Huscher D, Dahnrich C, et al. (2013) IFNalpha and its response proteins, IP-10 and SIGLEC-1, are biomarkers of disease activity in systemic lupus erythematosus. Annals of the rheumatic diseases 72: 1639–1645.
19. Hall JC, Casciola-Rosen L, Berger AE, Kapsogeorgou EK, Cheadle C, et al. (2012) Precise probes of type II interferon activity define the origin of interferon signatures in target tissues in rheumatic diseases. Proceedings of the National Academy of Sciences of the United States of America 109: 17609–17614.
20. Waddell SJ, Popper SJ, Rubins KH, Griffiths MJ, Brown PO, et al. (2010) Dissecting interferon-induced transcriptional programs in human peripheral blood cells. PloS one 5: e9753.
21. Hua J, Kirou K, Lee C, Crow MK (2006) Functional assay of type I interferon in systemic lupus erythematosus plasma and association with anti-RNA binding protein autoantibodies. Arthritis and rheumatism 54: 1906–1916.
22. Mavragani CP, La DT, Stohl W, Crow MK (2010) Association of the response to tumor necrosis factor antagonists with plasma type I interferon activity and interferon-beta/alpha ratios in rheumatoid arthritis patients: a post hoc analysis of a predominantly Hispanic cohort. Arthritis and rheumatism 62: 392–401.
23. Kirou KA, Lee C, George S, Louca K, Peterson MG, et al. (2005) Activation of the interferon-alpha pathway identifies a subgroup of systemic lupus erythematosus patients with distinct serologic features and active disease. Arthritis and rheumatism 52: 1491–1503.
24. Browning JL, Allaire N, Ngam-Ek A, Notidis E, Hunt J, et al. (2005) Lymphotoxin-beta receptor signaling is required for the homeostatic control of HEV differentiation and function. Immunity 23: 539–550.
25. Cyster JG, Schwab SR (2012) Sphingosine-1-phosphate and lymphocyte egress from lymphoid organs. Annual review of immunology 30: 69–94.
26. Silva-Santos B, Pennington DJ, Hayday AC (2005) Lymphotoxin-mediated regulation of gammadelta cell differentiation by alphabeta T cell progenitors. Science 307: 925–928.
27. Elewaut D, Ware CF (2007) The unconventional role of LT alpha beta in T cell differentiation. Trends in immunology 28: 169–175.
28. Vallabhapurapu S, Powolny-Budnicka I, Riemann M, Schmid RM, Paxian S, et al. (2008) Rel/NF-kappaB family member RelA regulates NK1.1- to NK1.1+

transition as well as IL-15-induced expansion of NKT cells. European journal of immunology 38: 3508–3519.

29. Powolny-Budnicka I, Riemann M, Tanzer S, Schmid RM, Hehlgans T, et al. (2011) RelA and RelB transcription factors in distinct thymocyte populations control lymphotoxin-dependent interleukin-17 production in gammadelta T cells. Immunity 34: 364–374.

30. Van Den Broeck T, Van Ammel E, Delforche M, Taveirne S, Kerre T, et al. (2013) Differential Ly49e expression pathways in resting versus TCR-activated intraepithelial gammadelta T cells. Journal of immunology 190: 1982–1990.

31. Verma S, Wang Q, Chodaczek G, Benedict CA (2013) Lymphoid-tissue stromal cells coordinate innate defense to cytomegalovirus. Journal of virology 87: 6201–6210.

32. Knight JS, Kaplan MJ (2012) Lupus neutrophils: 'NET' gain in understanding lupus pathogenesis. Current opinion in rheumatology 24: 441–450.

33. Khandpur R, Carmona-Rivera C, Vivekanandan-Giri A, Gizinski A, Yalavarthi S, et al. (2013) NETs are a source of citrullinated autoantigens and stimulate inflammatory responses in rheumatoid arthritis. Science translational medicine 5: 178ra140.

34. Lepelletier Y, Zollinger R, Ghirelli C, Raynaud F, Hadj-Slimane R, et al. (2010) Toll-like receptor control of glucocorticoid-induced apoptosis in human plasmacytoid predendritic cells (pDCs). Blood 116: 3389–3397.

35. Guiducci C, Gong M, Xu Z, Gill M, Chaussabel D, et al. (2010) TLR recognition of self nucleic acids hampers glucocorticoid activity in lupus. Nature 465: 937–941.

36. Yao Y, Richman L, Higgs BW, Morehouse CA, de los Reyes M, et al. (2009) Neutralization of interferon-alpha/beta-inducible genes and downstream effect in a phase I trial of an anti-interferon-alpha monoclonal antibody in systemic lupus erythematosus. Arthritis and rheumatism 60: 1785–1796.

37. McBride JM, Jiang J, Abbas AR, Morimoto A, Li J, et al. (2012) Safety and pharmacodynamics of rontalizumab in patients with systemic lupus erythematosus: results of a phase I, placebo-controlled, double-blind, dose-escalation study. Arthritis and rheumatism 64: 3666–3676.

38. Petri M, Wallace DJ, Spindler A, Chindalore V, Kalunian K, et al. (2013) Sifalimumab, a Human Anti-Interferon-alpha Monoclonal Antibody, in Systemic Lupus Erythematosus: A Phase I Randomized, Controlled, Dose-Escalation Study. Arthritis and rheumatism 65: 1011–1021.

39. Higgs BW, Zhu W, Morehouse C, White WI, Brohawn P, et al. (2013) A phase 1b clinical trial evaluating sifalimumab, an anti-IFN-alpha monoclonal antibody, shows target neutralisation of a type I IFN signature in blood of dermatomyositis and polymyositis patients. Annals of the rheumatic diseases 78: 256–262.

40. Huang YL, Chung HT, Chang CJ, Yeh KW, Chen LC, et al. (2009) Lymphopenia is a risk factor in the progression of carotid intima-media thickness in juvenile-onset systemic lupus erythematosus. Arthritis and rheumatism 60: 3766–3775.

41. Cantaert T, van Baarsen LG, Wijbrandts CA, Thurlings RM, van de Sande MG, et al. (2010) Type I interferons have no major influence on humoral autoimmunity in rheumatoid arthritis. Rheumatology 49: 156–166.

42. Thurlings RM, Boumans M, Tekstra J, van Roon JA, Vos K, et al. (2010) Relationship between the type I interferon signature and the response to rituximab in rheumatoid arthritis patients. Arthritis and rheumatism 62: 3607–3614.

43. Raterman HG, Vosslamber S, de Ridder S, Nurmohamed MT, Lems WF, et al. (2012) The interferon type I signature towards prediction of non-response to rituximab in rheumatoid arthritis patients. Arthritis research & therapy 14: R95.

44. Reynier F, Petit F, Paye M, Turrel-Davin F, Imbert PE, et al. (2011) Importance of correlation between gene expression levels: application to the type I interferon signature in rheumatoid arthritis. PloS one 6: e24828.

45. van Baarsen LG, Wijbrandts CA, Rustenburg F, Cantaert T, van der Pouw Kraan TC, et al. (2010) Regulation of IFN response gene activity during infliximab treatment in rheumatoid arthritis is associated with clinical response to treatment. Arthritis research & therapy 12: R11.

46. Palucka AK, Blanck JP, Bennett L, Pascual V, Banchereau J (2005) Cross-regulation of TNF and IFN-alpha in autoimmune diseases. Proceedings of the National Academy of Sciences of the United States of America 102: 3372–3377.

47. Mavragani CP, Niewold TB, Moutsopoulos NM, Pillemer SR, Wahl SM, et al. (2007) Augmented interferon-alpha pathway activation in patients with Sjogren's syndrome treated with etanercept. Arthritis and rheumatism 56: 3995–4004.

48. Assassi S, Mayes MD, Arnett FC, Gourh P, Agarwal SK, et al. (2010) Systemic sclerosis and lupus: points in an interferon-mediated continuum. Arthritis and rheumatism 62: 589–598.

49. de Bruin AM, Libregts SF, Valkhof M, Boon L, Touw IP, et al. (2012) IFNgamma induces monopoiesis and inhibits neutrophil development during inflammation. Blood 119: 1543–1554.

50. Cain DW, Snowden PB, Sempowski GD, Kelsoe G (2011) Inflammation triggers emergency granulopoiesis through a density-dependent feedback mechanism. PloS one 6: e19957.

51. Hartrich L, Weinstock-Guttman B, Hall D, Badgett D, Baier M, et al. (2003) Dynamics of immune cell trafficking in interferon-beta treated multiple sclerosis patients. Journal of neuroimmunology 139: 84–92.

52. Gao J, Majchrzak-Kita B, Fish EN, Gommerman JL (2009) Dynamic accumulation of plasmacytoid dendritic cells in lymph nodes is regulated by interferon-beta. Blood 114: 2623–2631.

53. Gommerman JL, J.L B, C.F W (2014) The Lymphotoxin Network: Orchestrating a Type I Interferon response to optimize adaptive immunity. Cytokine & growth factor reviews in press.

54. Schneider K, Loewendorf A, De Trez C, Fulton J, Rhode A, et al. (2008) Lymphotoxin-mediated crosstalk between B cells and splenic stroma promotes the initial type I interferon response to cytomegalovirus. Cell host & microbe 3: 67–76.

55. Hsu KM, Pratt JR, Akers WJ, Achilefu SI, Yokoyama WM (2009) Murine cytomegalovirus displays selective infection of cells within hours after systemic administration. The Journal of general virology 90: 33–43.

56. Barral P, Polzella P, Bruckbauer A, van Rooijen N, Besra GS, et al. (2010) CD169(+) macrophages present lipid antigens to mediate early activation of iNKT cells in lymph nodes. Nature immunology 11: 303–312.

57. Cyster JG (2010) B cell follicles and antigen encounters of the third kind. Nature immunology 11: 989–996.

58. Klaas M, Crocker PR (2012) Sialoadhesin in recognition of self and non-self. Seminars in immunopathology 34: 353–364.

59. Phan TG, Grigorova I, Okada T, Cyster JG (2007) Subcapsular encounter and complement-dependent transport of immune complexes by lymph node B cells. Nature immunology 8: 992–1000.

60. Moseman EA, Iannacone M, Bosurgi L, Tonti E, Chevrier N, et al. (2012) B cell maintenance of subcapsular sinus macrophages protects against a fatal viral infection independent of adaptive immunity. Immunity 36: 415–426.

61. Honke N, Shaabani N, Cadeddu G, Sorg UR, Zhang DE, et al. (2012) Enforced viral replication activates adaptive immunity and is essential for the control of a cytopathic virus. Nature immunology 13: 51–57.

62. Iannacone M, Moseman EA, Tonti E, Bosurgi L, Junt T, et al. (2010) Subcapsular sinus macrophages prevent CNS invasion on peripheral infection with a neurotropic virus. Nature 465: 1079–1083.

63. Eloranta ML, Alm GV (1999) Splenic marginal metallophilic macrophages and marginal zone macrophages are the major interferon-alpha/beta producers in mice upon intravenous challenge with herpes simplex virus. Scandinavian journal of immunology 49: 391–394.

64. Klaas M, Oetke C, Lewis LE, Erwig LP, Heikema AP, et al. (2012) Sialoadhesin promotes rapid proinflammatory and type I IFN responses to a sialylated pathogen, Campylobacter jejuni. Journal of immunology 189: 2414–2422.

65. Kutsch S, Degrandi D, Pfeffer K (2008) Immediate lymphotoxin beta receptor-mediated transcriptional response in host defense against L. monocytogenes. Immunobiology 213: 353–366.

66. Summers deLuca L, Ng D, Gao Y, Wortzman ME, Watts TH, et al. (2011) LTbetaR signaling in dendritic cells induces a type I IFN response that is required for optimal clonal expansion of CD8+ T cells. Proceedings of the National Academy of Sciences of the United States of America 108: 2046–2051.

67. Lorenzi S, Mattei F, Sistigu A, Bracci L, Spadaro F, et al. (2011) Type I IFNs control antigen retention and survival of CD8alpha(+) dendritic cells after uptake of tumor apoptotic cells leading to cross-priming. Journal of immunology 186: 5142–5150.

68. Spadaro F, Lapenta C, Donati S, Abalsamo L, Barnaba V, et al. (2012) IFN-alpha enhances cross-presentation in human dendritic cells by modulating antigen survival, endocytic routing, and processing. Blood 119: 1407–1417.

69. Heesters BA, Das A, Chatterjee P, Carroll MC (2014) Do follicular dendritic cells regulate lupus-specific B cells? Mol Immunol epub.

70. Yao Y, Liu Z, Jallal B, Shen N, Ronnblom L (2013) Type I interferons in Sjogren's syndrome. Autoimmunity reviews 12: 558–566.

71. Nzeusseu Toukap A, Galant C, Theate I, Maudoux AL, Lories RJ, et al. (2007) Identification of distinct gene expression profiles in the synovium of patients with systemic lupus erythematosus. Arthritis and rheumatism 56: 1579–1588.

72. Yoshida S, Arakawa F, Higuchi F, Ishibashi Y, Goto M, et al. (2012) Gene expression analysis of rheumatoid arthritis synovial lining regions by cDNA microarray combined with laser microdissection: up-regulation of inflammation-associated STAT1, IRF1, CXCL9, CXCL10, and CCL5. Scandinavian journal of rheumatology 41: 170–179.

73. Elkon KB, Santer DM (2012) Complement, interferon and lupus. Curr Opin Immunol 24: 665–670.

74. Migliorini A, Anders HJ (2012) A novel pathogenetic concept-antiviral immunity in lupus nephritis. Nature reviews Nephrology 8: 183–189.

75. Browning JL, Dougas I, Ngam-ek A, Bourdon PR, Ehrenfels BN, et al. (1995) Characterization of surface lymphotoxin forms. Use of specific monoclonal antibodies and soluble receptors. Journal of immunology 154: 33–46.

19

Association between a *C8orf13–BLK* Polymorphism and Polymyositis/Dermatomyositis in the Japanese Population: An Additive Effect with *STAT4* on Disease Susceptibility

Tomoko Sugiura[1], Yasushi Kawaguchi[1]*, Kanako Goto[2], Yukiko Hayashi[2], Takahisa Gono[1], Takefumi Furuya[1], Ichizo Nishino[2], Hisashi Yamanaka[1]

1 Institute of Rheumatology, Tokyo Women's Medical University, Tokyo, Japan, 2 Department of Neuromuscular Research, National Institute of Neuroscience, and Department of Clinical Development, Translational Medical Center, National Center of Neurology and Psychiatry, Tokyo, Japan

Abstract

Background: Accumulating evidence has shown that several non-HLA genes are involved in the susceptibility to polymyositis/dermatomyositis. This study aimed to investigate the involvement of *C8orf13–BLK*, one of the strongest candidate genes for autoimmune diseases, in susceptibility to polymyositis/dermatomyositis in the Japanese population. A possible gene–gene interaction between *C8orf13–BLK* and *STAT4*, which we recently showed to be associated with Japanese polymyositis/dermatomyositis, was also analyzed.

Methods: A single-nucleotide polymorphism in *C8orf13–BLK* (dbSNP ID: rs13277113) was investigated in the Japanese population using a TaqMan assay in 283 polymyositis patients, 194 dermatomyositis patients, and 656 control subjects.

Results: The *C8orf13–BLK* rs13277113A allele was associated with overall polymyositis/dermatomyositis (*P*<0.001, odds ratio [OR] 1.44, 95% confidence interval [CI] 1.19–1.73), as well as polymyositis (*P*=0.011, OR 1.32, 95% CI 1.06–1.64) and dermatomyositis (*P*<0.001, OR 1.64, 95% CI 1.26–2.12). No association was observed between the *C8orf13–BLK* rs13277113A allele and either interstitial lung disease or anti-Jo-1 antibody positivity. The *C8orf13–BLK* rs13277113 A and *STAT4* rs7574865 T alleles had an additive effect on polymyositis/dermatomyositis susceptibility. The strongest association was observed in dermatomyositis, with an OR of 3.07 (95% CI; 1.57–6.02) for the carriers of four risk alleles at the two SNP sites, namely, rs1327713 and rs7574865.

Conclusions: This study established *C8orf13–BLK* as a new genetic susceptibility factor for polymyositis/dermatomyositis. Both *C8orf13–BLK* and *STAT4* exert additive effects on disease susceptibility. These observations suggested that *C8orf13–BLK*, in combination with *STAT4*, plays a pivotal role in creating genetic susceptibility to polymyositis/dermatomyositis in Japanese individuals.

Editor: Ralf Andreas Linker, Friedrich-Alexander University Erlangen, Germany

Funding: This study was supported by autoimmune disease research grants from the Ministry of Health, Labor, and Welfare, Japan and was partly supported by an Intramural Research Grant (23-4, 23-5) for Neurological and Psychiatric Disorders from the National Center of Neurology and Psychiatry. The funders had no role in study design, data collection and analysis, decision to publish, or preparation of the manuscript.

Competing Interests: The authors have declared that no competing interests exist.

* E-mail: y-kawa@ior.twmu.ac.jp

Introduction

Polymyositis and dermatomyositis are rare connective tissue diseases, with unknown etiologies, which belong to the idiopathic inflammatory myopathies (IIMs). The typical clinical features are symmetrical and include proximal weakness of skeletal muscles and infiltrating mononuclear cells seen in muscle biopsies, and may be accompanied by skin rash. The diagnosis of IIMs in 29% of patients is accompanied by other connective tissue diseases (CTDs), such as systemic sclerosis (SSc), systemic lupus erythematosus (SLE), and rheumatoid arthritis (RA) [1], suggesting that IIMs are associated with general autoimmunity.

Although most immunogenetic IIM investigators have focused on the polymorphic genes of the major histocompatibility complex (human leucocyte antigen [HLA]) [2], new genetic markers have been identified outside the HLA region. For example, the R620W polymorphism of the protein tyrosine phosphatase N22 gene (*PTPN22*), one of the most well-documented risk genes for several autoimmune diseases specific for Caucasians [3], was found to be associated with IIMs in British Caucasian patients [4]. Moreover, we have recently shown that a polymorphism (rs7574865) in the signal transducer and activator of transcription 4 gene (*STAT4*) is associated with adult-onset polymyositis and dermatomyositis in a Japanese population [5]. After being identified as a risk gene for

SLE and RA [6], *STAT4* was also associated with susceptibility to a number of other autoimmune diseases, irrespective of ethnicity [7]. These observations strongly suggested that IIMs share an 'autoimmune-prone' genetic background with other autoimmune diseases.

BLK encodes a B lymphoid-specific tyrosine kinase of the Src family, which is involved in B cell receptor-mediated signaling and B cell development [8]. The risk allele (A) of rs13277113 (rs13277113A) within the *C8orf13–BLK* region of chromosome 8p23–p22 was originally identified in SLE patients by a genome-wide association study (GWAS) [9]. This polymorphism is associated with low levels of *BLK* mRNA and high levels of *C8orf13* mRNA, which encodes a ubiquitously expressed gene of unknown function [9]. An association between *C8orf13–BLK* polymorphisms and SLE was first identified in North Americans of European descent and in Swedish populations [9], and was later replicated in both European [10] and Asian populations [11]. Subsequently, other autoimmune diseases, such as SSc [12,13] and RA [14], were shown to be associated with polymorphisms in *C8orf13–BLK*.

The contribution of *C8orf13–BLK* appears to be prominent in Asian populations, in which the risk allele rs13277113A is the major allele. Indeed, the allele frequency of rs13277113A is approximately 0.65 in the Japanese population [11,12], compared with approximately 0.25 in North American and European populations [9,13,14]. In Japanese SLE patients, a positive association between disease susceptibility and this polymorphism in *C8orf13–BLK* was confirmed with an OR of 2.44 [11], whereas the OR was 1.39 in Caucasian populations [9]. A similar increase in OR was observed in Japanese SSc patients compared with Caucasian patients [12,13].

Therefore, genetic variants of *C8orf13–BLK* could strongly contribute to lowering the disease threshold for autoimmune diseases, and particularly in Asian populations. In this study, we investigated whether *C8orf13–BLK* variants contribute to disease susceptibility in Japanese polymyositis/dermatomyositis patients and assessed any potential additive effects between *C8orf13–BLK* and *STAT4* in the susceptibility to polymyositis/dermatomyositis.

Patients and Methods

Subjects

This study was reviewed and approved by the research ethics committees of both the Tokyo Women's Medical University (TWMU) and National Center of Neurology and Psychiatry (NCNP) and complied with the Helsinki Declaration.

We enrolled patients who had probable or definite myositis based on the criteria of Bohan and Peter [15] and who were 18 years of age or older at disease onset. For our study, dermatomyositis patients included those with clinically defined amyopathic dermatomyositis who fulfilled the traditional criteria of Sontheimer [16]. Patients with myositis overlapping with other CTDs, such as RA, SLE, and SSc, were excluded from the study because these CTDs have previously been associated with *C8orf13–BLK* variants [9–14]. Patients with inherited, metabolic, or infectious myopathies and with inclusion body myositis were also excluded. All patients underwent a muscle biopsy.

The polymyositis/dermatomyositis patients were recruited from two different institutions: 138 (46 polymyositis and 92 dermatomyositis patients) were recruited from the Institute of Rheumatology, TWMU (Tokyo, Japan), and 339 (237 polymyositis and 102 dermatomyositis patients) were recruited from the National Institute of Neuroscience, NCNP (Kodaira City, Tokyo, Japan). In total, 477 patients with adult-onset polymyositis/dermatomy-

ositis (69.8% female) were retrospectively investigated, including 283 polymyositis patients (68.3% female) and 194 dermatomyositis patients (71.1% female). The mean ages of the polymyositis and dermatomyositis patients were 51.4 ± 15.8 and 52.3 ± 16.5 y, respectively. None of the patients were genetically related.

As controls, we enrolled healthy unrelated individuals from the Tokyo area (n = 656; 57.1% female; mean age = 38.6 ± 11.9 years). All patients and control subjects were Japanese individuals, and they were living in the central part of mainland Japan (Honshu).

For a sub-analysis of association between the *C8orf13–BLK* rs13277113 polymorphism and the presence or absence of interstitial lung disease (ILD) or serological status, 138 polymyositis/dermatomyositis patients recruited from TWMU were evaluated. The presence of ILD was confirmed or excluded by computed tomography (CT), high-resolution CT, if available, and spirometry. For serological analysis, the only association between the possession of the anti-Jo-1 antibody and *C8orf13–BLK* rs13277113A was analyzed, because not all patients were screened for other myositis-specific autoantibodies (MSAs).

Genotyping

To date, rs13277113 within *C8orf13–BLK* and the related single nucleotide polymorphism (SNP) have shown the strongest association with several autoimmune diseases [9–14]. Given this background, and our previous findings, the *C8orf13–BLK* rs13277113 and *STAT4* rs7574865 genotypes were determined using a TaqMan fluorogenic 5'-nuclease assay, according to the manufacturer's instructions (Applied Biosystems, Carlsbad, CA, USA). End-point fluorescence was measured with an ABI Prism 7900 HT Sequence Detection System (Applied Biosystems). In the disease subgroups and the control group, none of the SNPs deviated from Hardy–Weinberg equilibrium.

Statistical analysis

Association analyses were performed using chi-square tests for 2×2 contingency tables. Bonferroni's correction was applied for association analyses between the *C8orf13–BLK* polymorphism and the three clinical subsets (polymyositis, dermatomyositis, and polymyositis/dermatomyositis patients versus controls) and was expressed as *Pcorr*. The odds ratios (ORs) and 95% confidence intervals (95% CIs) were also determined. A logistic regression model was applied to assess gene–gene interactions between *C8orf13–BLK* rs13277113 and *STAT4* rs7574865 by using SPSS (Statistical Package for the Social Sciences) software version 19.0 (SPSS, Chicago, IL, USA) and to determine the additive effects of these two SNPs. Regression analysis accounted for the combination of the genotypes from both loci; thus, each individual had 0–4 risk alleles when considering both SNP sites. The ORs were computed using a logistic regression model, with individuals carrying 0 or 1 risk allele as a reference. The difference in the *C8orf13–BLK* and *STAT4* risk allele counts between the patients and control subjects was analyzed using Fisher's exact test. Statistical analyses were conducted using SPSS version 19.0 (SPSS).

Power calculations were performed using the Quanto software (http://hydra.usc.edu/gxe/) for case–control analysis, using a significance level of 0.05. Power was calculated to be 0.78 using the ORs previously reported in Japanese collagen disease [12] and the present study, as well as the sample size and risk allele frequency in the present study. Under the same parameter settings, 503 patients would be needed to demonstrate an OR of 1.44, at an alpha of 0.05, with power of 0.8. Similarly, to gain power of 0.9, 665 patients would be needed.

Results

Association of C8orf13–BLK rs13277113 with polymyositis/dermatomyositis in the Japanese population

The frequency of the *C8orf13–BLK* rs13277113 A allele was in good agreement with those previously reported for the Japanese population [11,12]. In the present study, the A (risk) allele of rs13277113 was found in 72% of the chromosomes in the polymyositis patients, 76% in the dermatomyositis patients, and 74% in the polymyositis/dermatomyositis patients. All frequencies in the disease subsets were significantly higher than those in the control subjects (64%; P_{corr} = 0.033, OR 1.32 for polymyositis; P_{corr} = 4.5×10^{-4}, OR 1.64 for dermatomyositis; and P_{corr} = 3.3×10^{-4}, OR 1.44 for polymyositis/dermatomyositis). Comparisons of the genotypes showed association of the rs13277113 A allele in a dominant model with dermatomyositis (rs13277113 A/A or A/G genotype; P_{corr} = 0.0011, OR 4.73). The allele and genotype frequencies are detailed in Table 1.

In the sub-analysis of 138 patients, comprising 46 with polymyositis and 92 with dermatomyositis, the complication of ILD was observed in 46.5% of the polymyositis patients and 66.3% of the dermatomyositis patients; in the combined cohort, 59.8% had ILD. The rs13277113A frequency was equal between patients with ILD (0.75) and those without (0.75). Of the 138 polymyositis/dermatomyositis patients recruited from TWMU, 20.4% were positive for the anti-Jo-1 antibody. The rs13277113A frequency was not statistically significantly different between anti-Jo-1 antibody-positive and antibody-negative patients (0.73 vs. 0.75, respectively). Therefore, no association was found between the rs13277113 polymorphism and the ILD disease phenotype or anti-Jo-1 antibody positivity.

Additive effects of C8orf13–BLK and STAT4

An additive effect of both risk alleles (the *C8orf13–BLK* rs13277113A allele and the *STAT4* rs7574865 T allele) on susceptibility to polymyositis, dermatomyositis, and polymyositis/dermatomyositis was observed (Table 2).

The OR for polymyositis patients carrying four risk alleles was 2.47 (95% CI 1.40–4.35), using individuals with 0 or 1 allele as a reference. The ORs for dermatomyositis gradually increased: 1.71 (95% CI 1.09–2.57) for carriers of two risk alleles, 2.18 (95% CI 1.36–3.48) for carriers of three risk alleles, and 3.07 (95% CI 1.57–6.02) for carriers of four risk alleles. The ORs for the polymyositis/

dermatomyositis patients also gradually increased: 1.64 (95% CI 1.17–2.29) for carriers of three risk alleles and 2.67 (95% CI 1.61–4.42) for carriers of four risk alleles. Therefore, additive effects of *C8orf13–BLK* and *STAT4* were observed, most notably in dermatomyositis.

Discussion

IIMs are clinically and serologically heterogeneous disorders. To date, the genetic basis of IIMs appears to involve at least two major components, viz., HLA regions and non-HLA risk genes common to other autoimmune diseases. The HLA region is associated with overall IIMs susceptibility particularly in Caucasians, in whom the HLA8.1 ancestral haplotype containing DRB1*0301 allele is prevalent, and is tightly linked to production of myositis-specific autoantibodies (MSAs) [2]. However, the association between the HLA region and IIMs is lost in Mexican-American and Korean populations [17]. In the Japanese population, in which the DRB1*0301 allele is rare (0.1–0.2% of the population), DRB1*0803 is weakly associated with susceptibility to IIMs and carriage of anti-aminoacyl-tRNA synthetases (ARS) autoantibodies [18]. Therefore, it seems to be likely that the HLA region is associated with IIM susceptibility to different degrees in different ethnicities, and that it is tightly associated with MSA production. On the other hand, non-HLA risk genes that encode the immune response or cell signaling regulatory proteins are involved in the susceptibility to IIMs, regardless of the presence or not of MSA [2,4,5,19]. Since such risk genes outside of the HLA region are common to other autoimmune diseases, IIMs are likely to share genetic etiology with other autoimmune diseases.

This study presents an association between polymyositis/dermatomyositis and *C8orf13–BLK* rs13277113A in the Japanese population. While preparing this manuscript, data of a GWAS on dermatomyositis in adults and juveniles of European ancestry (n = 1178) were published [19]. According to that study, *BLK* rs2736340 was identified as one of the risk genes for adult and juvenile dermatomyositis in Europeans after screening of 141 non-MHC SNPs that had previously been associated with autoimmune diseases [19]. Because both *BLK* rs2736340 and rs13277113, which were investigated in the present study, are in complete linkage disequilibrium, the risk haplotype identified by GWAS and by the present study are identical. The present Japanese case–control study, as a result, replicated the study of the European GWAS study. To date, few susceptibility genes for IIMs have been

Table 1. Association between *C8orf13–BLK* rs13277113 and polymyositis/dermatomyositis.

Subjects (n)	PM (283)	DM (194)	PM+DM (477)	controls (656)
A allele (frequency)	407 (0.72)	295 (0.76)	702 (0.74)	865 (0.65)
allelic association				
OR (95%CI)	1.32 (1.06–1.64)	1.64 (1.26–2.12)	1.44 (1.19–1.72)	Referent
P	0.011	1.5×10^{-4}	1.1×10^{-4}	-
Corrected P	0.033	4.5×10^{-4}	3.3×10^{-4}	-
A/A+A/G (frequency)	262 (0.92)	189 (0.97)	451 (0.94)	583 (0.89)
genotype association				
OR (95%CI)	1.56 (0.94–2.59)	4.73 (1.88–11.9)	2.17 (1.37–3.46)	Referent
P	N.S.	3.6×10^{-4}	8.8×10^{-4}	-
Corrected P	N.S.	0.0011	0.0026	-

OR: Odds ratio, CI: confidence interval, PM: polymyositis, DM: dermatomyositis, N.S.: not significant.

Table 2. A cumulative effect of risk allele number (*C8orf13–BLK* rs13277113A and *STAT4* rs7574865T) on susceptibility to polymyositis, dermatomyositis, and polymyositis/dermatomyositis.

No. of risk alleles	PM (283)		DM (194)		PM+DM (477)	
	OR (95%CI)	P	OR (95%CI)	P	OR (95%CI)	P
0+1	Referent	-	Referent	-	Referent	-
2	1.12 (0.78–1.62)	N.S.	1.71 (1.09–2.57)	0.017	1.34 (0.98–1.83)	N.S.
3	1.37 (0.91–2.03)	N.S.	2.18 (1.36–3.48)	1.8×10^{-3}	1.64 (1.17–2.29)	3.8×10^{-3}
4	2.47 (1.40–4.35)	1.7×10^{-3}	3.07 (1.57–6.02)	1.1×10^{-3}	2.67 (1.61–4.42)	1.4×10^{-4}

OR: Odds ratio, CI: confidence interval, PM: polymyositis, DM: dermatomyositis, N.S.: not significant.

replicated, except for the HLA 8.1 haplotype in Caucasians, probably due to the different risk allele frequencies in different ethnicities, relatively low disease prevalence, and disease heterogeneity. The present data highlighted the strong contribution of *BLK* to polymyositis/dermatomyositis susceptibility, irrespective of ethnicity.

Accumulating evidence has shown that *BLK* is strongly involved in the development of a wide variety of autoimmune diseases [9–14]. However, it remains unclear how an autoimmune-risk variant within *C8orf13–BLK* influences Blk protein expression, results in altered B cell signaling. Although a risk variant in *C8orf13–BLK* reduces *BLK* mRNA transcript expression in a B cell lymphoblastoid cell line [9], it is unclear whether the variant affects protein expression. However, a recent report showed that the risk variant reduced Blk protein expression in B cells obtained from umbilical cord blood, although not in adult B cell subsets [20]. Reduced Blk expression in the early stage of B cell development may influence B cell receptor signaling, resulting in selection of autoimmune-prone B cells. *Blk*-knockout mice as well as *Blk*$^{+/-}$ mice exhibited an autoimmune phenotype, with a high titer of anti-nuclear antibody production compared with wild-type mice [21]. B cells are strongly involved in the humoral immune response, particularly as it pertains to autoantibody production.

Therefore, the idea that a risk allele of *C8orf13–BLK* is associated with autoantibody production seems to be reasonable. In the present sub-analysis, however, no increase was observed in the frequency of rs13277113A allele carriers in the anti-Jo-1 antibody-positive group of patients. Interestingly, similar results were previously obtained in SLE patients in whom *BLK* risk loci were not found to be associated with anti-DNA antibody production, although this gene increased disease susceptibility overall [22]. In human CD4$^+$ cells, SNP-associated regulation of *BLK* expression has been found [23]. Therefore, although the mechanism underlying the triggering of autoimmune diseases by a *C8orf13–BLK* risk variant remains unknown, it may influence the overall immune response, including auto-reactive B cell selection or T cell function, resulting in altered individual immune response.

We have previously reported *STAT4* rs7574865 is associated with susceptibility to polymyositis/dermatomyositis in Japanese [5]. STAT-4 is a transcription factor that transduces IL-12, IL-23-, and type-1 interferon-mediated signals into Th1 and Th17

differentiation, monocyte activation, and interferon-gamma production [24]. Among many autoimmune disease-related genes, *STAT4* [25,26], *C8orf13–BLK* [11,12], as well as interferon regulatory factor 5 (*IRF5*) [27] seem to be the most representative susceptibility genes in the Japanese population. In particular, the genetic contribution of *C8orf13–BLK* [11], and to a lesser extent, of *STAT4* [25], are greater in the Japanese population compared with the Caucasian population, due to the high prevalence of the risk gene. Although each risk gene has a relatively low OR for disease susceptibility, the carriage of more risk alleles, in several risk genes, appears to increase the risk for disease susceptibility. Such cumulative associations have been shown in other autoimmune diseases [28], and now also here, by the discovery of the additive effect of alleles in *C8orf13–BLK* and *STAT4* in increasing the risk for polymyositis/dermatomyositis.

The major limitation of the present study was the paucity of association studies in clinical subsets, including serological phenotypes. However, despite the rarity of these diseases, we obtained a large sample size, which provided sufficient statistical power for this case–control study. We identified a susceptibility gene, *C8orf13–BLK*, for polymyositis/dermatomyositis. Both *C8orf13–BLK* and *STAT4* additively increased polymyositis/dermatomyositis susceptibility in the Japanese population.

Key messages

- The *C8orf13–BLK* rs13277113A allele is associated with Japanese polymyositis/dermatomyositis.
- *C8orf13–BLK* rs13277113A and *STAT4* rs7574865T exert additive effects in polymyositis/dermatomyositis susceptibility.

Acknowledgments

We thank Mr. Kazutomo Ogata and Ms. Mika Fujita for technical assistance. We also thank Mr. Manabu Kawamoto for helpful suggestions.

Author Contributions

Conceived and designed the experiments: TS YK IN HY. Performed the experiments: TS KG YH TG TF. Analyzed the data: TS YK. Contributed reagents/materials/analysis tools: KG YH TG TF IN. Wrote the paper: TS YK.

References

1. Ramesha KN, Kuruvilla A, Sarma PS, Radhakrishnan VV (2010) Clinical, electrophysiologic, and histopathologic profile, and outcome in idiopathic inflammatory myositis: An analysis of 68 cases. Ann Indian Acad Neurol 13: 250–256.

2. Chinoy H, Lamb JA, Ollier WE, Cooper RG (2011) Recent advances in the immunogenetics of idiopathic inflammatory myopathy. Arthritis Res Ther 13: 216.

3. Kyogoku C, Langefeld CD, Ortmann WA, Lee A, Selby S, et al. (2004) Genetic association of the R620W polymorphism of protein tyrosine phosphatase PTPN22 with human SLE. Am J Hum Genet 75: 504–507.

4. Chinoy H, Platt H, Lamb JA, Betteridge Z, Gunawardena H, et al. (2008) The protein tyrosine phosphatase N22 gene is associated with juvenile and adult idiopathic inflammatory myopathy independent of the HLA 8.1 haplotype in British Caucasian patients. Arthritis Rheum 58: 3247–3254.

5. Sugiura T, Kawaguchi Y, Goto K, Hayashi Y, Tsuburaya R, et al. (2012) Positive association between STAT4 polymorphisms and polymyositis/dermatomyositis in a Japanese population. Ann Rheum Dis 71: 1646–1650.

6. Remmers EF, Plenge RM, Lee AT, Graham RR, Hom G, et al. (2007) STAT4 and the risk of rheumatoid arthritis and systemic lupus erythematosus. N Engl J Med 357: 977–986.

7. Liang YL, Wu H, Shen X, Li PQ, Yang XQ, et al. (2012) Association of STAT4 rs7574865 polymorphism with autoimmune diseases: a meta-analysis. Mol Biol Rep 39: 8873–8882.

8. Dymecki SM, Zwollo P, Zeller K, Kuhajda FP, Desiderio SV (1992) Structure and developmental regulation of the B-lymphoid tyrosine kinase gene blk. J Biol Chem 267: 4815–4823.

9. Hom G, Graham RR, Modrek B, Taylor KE, Ortmann W, et al. (2008) Association of systemic lupus erythematosus with C8orf13–BLK and ITGAM-ITGAX. N Engl J Med 358: 900–909.

10. Fan Y, Tao JH, Zhang LP, Li LH, Ye DQ (2011) Association of BLK (rs13277113, rs2248932) polymorphism with systemic lupus erythematosus: a meta-analysis. Mol Biol Rep 38: 4445–4453.

11. Ito I, Kawasaki A, Ito S, Hayashi T, Goto D, et al. (2009) Replication of the association between the C8orf13–BLK region and systemic lupus erythematosus in a Japanese population. Arthritis Rheum 60: 553–558.

12. Ito I, Kawaguchi Y, Kawasaki A, Hasegawa M, Ohashi J, et al. (2010) Association of the FAM167A-BLK region with systemic sclerosis. Arthritis Rheum 62: 890–895.

13. Gourh P, Agarwal SK, Martin E, Divecha D, Rueda B, et al. (2010) Association of the C8orf13–BLK region with systemic sclerosis in North-American and European populations. J Autoimmun 34: 155–162.

14. Orozco G, Eyre S, Hinks A, Bowes J, Morgan AW, et al. (2011) Study of the common genetic background for rheumatoid arthritis and systemic lupus erythematosus. Ann Rheum Dis 70: 463–468.

15. Bohan A, Peter JB (1975) Polymyositis and dermatomyositis (first of two parts). N Engl J Med 292: 344–347.

16. Sontheimer RD (2002) Would a new name hasten the acceptance of amyopathic dermatomyositis (dermatomyositis sine myositis) as a distinctive subset within the idiopathic inflammatory dermatomyopathies spectrum of clinical illness? J Am Acad Dermatol 46: 626–636.

17. Rider LG, Shamim E, Okada S, Pandey JP, Targoff IN, et al. (1999) Genetic risk and protective factors for idiopathic inflammatory myopathy in Koreans and American whites: a tale of two loci. Arthritis Rheum 42: 1285–1290.

18. Furuya T, Hakoda M, Tsuchiya N, Kotake S, Ichikawa N, et al. (2004) Immunogenetic features in 120 Japanese patients with idiopathic inflammatory myopathy. J Rheumatol 31: 1768–1774.

19. Miller FW, Cooper RG, Vencovsky J, Rider LG, Danko K, et al. (2013) Genome-wide association study of dermatomyositis reveals genetic overlap with other autoimmune disorders. Arthritis Rheum 65: 3239–3247.

20. Simpfendorfer KR, Olsson LM, Manjarrez Orduno N, Khalili H, Simeone AM, et al. (2012) The autoimmunity-associated BLK haplotype exhibits cis-regulatory effects on mRNA and protein expression that are prominently observed in B cells early in development. Hum Mol Genet 21: 3918–3925.

21. Samuelson EM, Laird RM, Maue AC, Rochford R, Hayes SM (2012) Blk haploinsufficiency impairs the development, but enhances the functional responses, of MZ B cells. Immunol Cell Biol 90: 620–629.

22. Chung SA, Taylor KE, Graham RR, Nititham J, Lee AT, et al. (2011) Differential genetic associations for systemic lupus erythematosus based on anti-dsDNA autoantibody production. PLoS Genet 7: e1001323.

23. Murphy A, Chu JH, Xu M, Carey VJ, Lazarus R, et al. (2010) Mapping of numerous disease-associated expression polymorphisms in primary peripheral blood CD4+ lymphocytes. Hum Mol Genet 19: 4745–4757.

24. Watford WT, Hissong BD, Bream JH, Kanno Y, Muul L, et al. (2010) Signaling by IL-12 and IL-23 and the immunoregulatory roles of STAT4. Immunol Rev 202: 139–156.

25. Kawasaki A, Ito I, Hikami K, Ohashi J, Hayashi T, et al. (2008) Role of STAT4 polymorphisms in systemic lupus erythematosus in a Japanese population: a case-control association study of the STAT1-STAT4 region. Arthritis Res Ther 10: R113.

26. Kobayashi S, Ikari K, Kaneko H, Kochi Y, Yamamoto K, et al. (2008) Association of STAT4 with susceptibility to rheumatoid arthritis and systemic lupus erythematosus in the Japanese population. Arthritis Rheum 58: 1940–1946.

27. Kawasaki A, Kyogoku C, Ohashi J, Miyashita R, Hikami K, et al. (2008) Association of IRF5 polymorphisms with systemic lupus erythematosus in a Japanese population: support for a crucial role of intron 1 polymorphisms. Arthritis Rheum 58: 826–834.

28. Koga M, Kawasaki A, Ito I, Furuya T, Ohashi J, et al. (2011) Cumulative association of eight susceptibility genes with systemic lupus erythematosus in a Japanese female population. J Hum Genet 56: 503–507.

20

Anti-Cyclic Citrullinated Peptide Antibody Is Associated with Interstitial Lung Disease in Patients with Rheumatoid Arthritis

Yufeng Yin[1⦾], Di Liang[1⦾], Lidan Zhao[1], Yang Li[1], Wei Liu[2], Yan Ren[1], Yongzhe Li[1], Xiaofeng Zeng[1], Fengchun Zhang[1], Fulin Tang[1], Guangliang Shan[3], Xuan Zhang[1]*

1 Department of Rheumatology, Peking Union Medical College Hospital, Chinese Academy of Medical Sciences and Peking Union Medical College, Beijing, China, **2** Department of Radiology, Peking Union Medical College Hospital, Chinese Academy of Medical Sciences and Peking Union Medical College, Beijing, China, **3** Department of Epidemiology, Institute of Basic Medical Sciences, Chinese Academy of Medical Sciences and Peking Union Medical College, Beijing, China

Abstract

Objective: Patients with rheumatoid arthritis (RA) are at risk to develop RA-associated interstitial lung disease (RA-ILD). This retrospective study aimed to investigate the potential association of the positivity of serum anti-cyclic citrullinated peptide antibody (anti-CCP2) and rheumatoid factor (RF) with RA-ILD in RA patients.

Methods: A total of 285 RA patients were recruited at the inpatient service of Peking Union Medical College Hospital in China between 2004 and 2013. Individual patients were evaluated for the evidence of ILD. The concentrations of serum anti-CCP2 and RF in individual patients were measured. The potential risk factors for ILD in RA patients were assessed by univariate and multivariate models.

Results: There were 71 RA patients with RA-ILD, accounting for 24.9% in this population. The positive rates of anti-CCP2 and RF in the patients with RA-ILD were significantly higher than that in the patients with RA-only (88.7% vs. 67.3%, p<0.001; 84.5% vs. 70.6%, p = 0.02, respectively). Univariate and multivariate logistic regression analysis revealed that RA patients with positive serum anti-CCP2, but not RF, were associated with an increased risk of ILD (crude odds ratio [cOR] 3.83, 95% confidence interval [CI] 1.74–8.43, p<0.001; adjusted odds ratio [aOR] 3.50, 95% CI 1.52–8.04, p<0.001).

Conclusion: Our findings suggest that positive serum anti-CCP2, but not RF, may be associated with RA-ILD in RA patients.

Editor: Song Guo Zheng, Penn State University, United States of America

Funding: This study is supported by the grants of the National Natural Science Foundation of China (30972731, 81172859, 81273312, 81302594), the National High Technology Research and Development Project of China (2011AA020111, 2012AA02A513), the National Major Scientific and Technological Special Project (2012ZX09303006-002), the Research Special Fund for Public Welfare Industry of Health (201202004), the Capital Health Research and Development of Special (2011-4001-02), and the National laboratory Special Fund (2060204). The funders had no role in study design, data collection and analysis, decision to publish, or preparation of the manuscript.

Competing Interests: The authors have declared that no competing interests exist.

* E-mail: zxpumch2003@sina.com

⦾ These authors contributed equally to this work.

Introduction

Patients with rheumatoid arthritis (RA) display high levels of autoantibodies as well as extra-articular manifestations, such as interstitial lung disease (ILD) [1–3]. The RA-related interstitial lung disease (RA-ILD) occurs in nearly 7–10% of the RA patients, and often is associated with a poor prognosis [4,5]. Therefore, the discovery of risk factors contributing to the development of ILD will be of great significance in the prevention and intervention of patients with RA-ILD.

Autoantibodies are valuable biomarkers for the diagnosis of RA and extra-articular manifestations. Antibodies against cyclic citrullinated peptides (anti-CCP2) and rheumatoid factor (RF) have been identified in patients with RA [6]. Previous studies have shown that the specificity and sensitivity of anti-CCP2 detection for the diagnosis of RA are 96–99% and 47–88% respectively,

dependent on the characteristics of the RA population [6,7]. Anti-CCP2 antibodies may be implicated in the pathogenesis of RA and are valuable for evaluating the erosive or non-erosive progression of articular injury in RA patients [8,9]. In addition, anti-CCP2 antibodies have been shown to be highly specific or independently associated with the development of extra-articular manifestations, including ischemic heart disease [10], type 1 diabetes mellitus [11], serositis [12], and subclinical atherosclerosis in patients with RA [13]. RF is another autoantibody most commonly detected in RA [1,14]. Detection of both anti-CCP2 and RF has additional values for the early diagnosis of RA, particularly for those with RA at early stage of the disease process [15].

However, the potential association of anti-CCP2 and RF with the development of ILD in RA patients remains controversial [16–18]. There is little information about whether anti-CCP2 antibodies or RF are associated with ILD in RA patients. In this study, we tested the levels of serum anti-CCP2 and RF in 285 patients with RA and analyzed the potential factors that were correlated with ILD in this population.

Methods

Ethics statement

The experimental protocol was approved by the Institute Review Board of Peking Union Medical College Hospital. All patients provide their written informed consent to participate in this study.

Study population

This study was approved by the Institute Review Board of Peking Union Medical College Hospital. A total of 285 patients with RA were recruited at the inpatient service of the Department of Rheumatology of Peking Union Medical College Hospital from January 2004 to October 2013. All patients fulfilled the criteria for the diagnosis of RA revised by the American College of Rheumatology (ACR) in 1987 [1]. Patients with RA-ILD were diagnosed by the presence of typical features in the lung by high-resolution computerized tomography (HRCT). The chest HRCT scans were evaluated by an expert radiologist in a blinded manner. According to the consensus for idiopathic interstitial pneumonias of the American Thoracic Society/European Respiratory Society (ATS/ERS) [19], the features of HRCT included irregular linear or reticular opacities, ground-glass opacities, consolidation, honeycombing, septal thickening, and traction bronchiectasis or bronchiolectasis. The disease activity of individual patients was evaluated by disease activity score in 28 joints (DAS28) [20,21]. Individuals were excluded if she/he had a history of ILD before the diagnosis of RA, other chronic lung diseases or incomplete medical record.

Clinical assessment

The demographic and clinical data of individual patients were retrospectively reviewed. These data included age, gender, disease duration, and cigarette smoking, co-existent autoimmune diseases, such as systemic lupus erythematosus (SLE), polymyositis/dermatomyositis (PM/DM), systemic sclerosis (SSc) and Sjögren's syndrome. The disease duration was defined from the onset of joint swelling and/or tenderness. Individuals with previous history of treatment with biological or general disease-modifying antirheumatic drugs (DMARDs) and corticosteroids for more than three months were recorded.

Blood samples were obtained from individual patients when they first visited to our institution. The positivity for serum anti-CCP2 (≥25 U/ml) and RF (≥15 IU/ml) in these patients was determined by enzyme linked immunosorbent assay (ELISA) using the specific kit (Euroimmun, Lübeck, Germany) and nephelometry method (Behring, Germany), respectively. The concentrations of serum C-reactive protein (CRP) as well as the value of erythrocyte sedimentation rate (ESR) in individual patients were routinely examined.

Statistical analyses

All values are expressed as the mean ± SD or median with interquartile range (IQR) for normally and non-normally distributed data, respectively. The difference in individual variables between the RA-ILD and RA-only groups was analyzed by univariate model. Comparison of continuous data was performed using independent Student's t and Mann-Whitney non-parametric U test for normal and non-normal data respectively, and of

categorical data using the Pearson Chi-square test or Fisher's exact test. The stratification analyses for age and disease duration were conducted by Cochran-Mantel-Haenszel Chi-square test. The relationship of individual variables with RA-ILD was analyzed using a multivariate logistic regression model with stepwise selected variables. The collinearity of variables was assessed and explained by variance inflation factor (VIF) greater than 4.0 and tolerance less than 0.25 [22]. All statistical analyses were performed using the SPSS software (version 17.0, SPSS Inc., Chicago, IL, USA) and a two-tailed P-value of less than 0.05 was considered statistically significant.

Results

Patients and clinical characteristics

To determine the potential risk factors associated with ILD, a total of 285 patients with RA were recruited. Their demographic and clinical characteristics are summarized in **Table 1**. There were 71 patients with ILD, accounting for 24.9% in this population. The RA-ILD patients were significantly older and had significantly longer duration than that of the RA-only group of patients. However, there was no significant difference in the distribution of gender and in the percentages of smokers between the RA-only and RA-ILD groups of patients.

There was no significant difference in the percentages of complications and treatment history between these two groups of patients. Both groups of patients had similar levels of disease severity, the concentrations of serum CRP and ESR. There were 61 (21.4%) patients who had at least one other connective tissue disease (CTD), including 7 patients with SSc, 41 Sjögren's Syndrome, 4 PM/DM, and 16 SLE. There were 234 (82.1%), 180 (63.2%), 38 (13.3%) and 227 (79.6%) of patients receiving medication of prednisone, methotrexate, biological DMARD, or chemical DMARD, respectively (**Table 1**).

HRCT features and anti-CCP2 and RF status

In 71 patients with RA-ILD, HRCT scans of the lung revealed 48 cases with irregular line or reticular opacities, 22 cases with ground-glass attenuation, 26 cases with basal consolidation, 10 patients with honey-combing, 27 patients with septal thickening and 12 patients with traction bronchiectasis or bronchiolectasis. However, these HRCT characteristics were not significantly associated with the positivity of anti-CCP2 and RF in these patients (**Table 2**).

The relationship between RA-ILD and anti-CCP2 or RF

Characterization of the levels of serum anti-CCP2 and RF revealed that 207 (72.6%) serum samples were positive for anti-CCP2 and 211 (74.0%) were positive for RF in this population. Both the positivity rates of anti-CCP2 and RF were significantly higher (p<0.001 and p=0.02 respectively) in the group of RA-ILD than RA-only (**Table 1**). Cochran-Mantel-Haenszel stratification analyses indicated that the percentages of anti-CCP2 positivity were significantly associated with older age and longer disease duration (OR$_{M-H}$ 3.3, 95% CI 1.5–7.1, p=0.003 and OR$_{M-H}$ 3.9, 95% CI 1.7–8.7, p=0.001, respectively) (**Table 3**).

Univariate and multivariate logistic regression analysis

Univariate logistic regression analysis revealed that age and disease duration were risk factors for RA-ILD (crude odds ratio [cOR] 1.06, 95% CI 1.03–1.09, p<0.001; and cOR 1.04, 95% CI 1.01–1.07, p<0.001 respectively). Treatment with methotrexate (MTX) or other chemical DMARDs was not significantly associated with RA-ILD (cOR 0.58, 95% CI 0.34–1.01,

Table 1. The demographic and clinical characteristics of patients.

Characteristics	All patients	RA-ILD	RA-only	p-value
Patients, n (%)	285 (100)	71 (24.9)	214 (75.1)	—
Age, mean (SD), years	51.7 (13.4)	58.3 (11.2)	49.5 (13.4)	<0.001
Female, n (%)	211 (74.0)	50 (70.4)	161 (75.2)	0.44
Disease duration, median (IQR), years	5.0 (1.0–12.0)	9.0 (2.0–18.0)	4.0 (1.0–10.1)	0.003
Cigarette smoking, n (%)	59 (20.7)	18 (25.4)	41 (19.2)	0.31
Complication With other CTD*, n (%)	61 (21.4)	15 (21.1)	46 (21.5)	1.0
Laboratory test				
Anti-CCP2, n (%)	207 (72.6)	63 (88.7)	144 (67.3)	<0.001
RF, n (%)	211 (74.0)	60 (84.5)	151 (70.6)	0.02
CRP, mean (SD), mg/dL	40.2 (56.3)	42.6 (75.4)	39.4 (48.5)	0.68
ESR, mean (SD), mm/h	56.2 (34.5)	56.6 (33.2)	56.1 (35.0)	0.93
DAS28, mean (SD)	5.4 (1.7)	5.2 (1.8)	5.5 (1.7)	0.13
Treatment history, n (%)				
Prednisone	234 (82.1)	58 (81.7)	176 (82.2)	1.0
Methotrexate	180 (63.2)	38 (53.5)	142 (66.4)	0.07
Biological DMARD	38 (13.3)	6 (8.5)	32 (15.0)	0.23
Chemical DMARD	227 (79.6)	52 (73.2)	175 (81.8)	0.13

RA-ILD: rheumatoid arthritis-associated interstitial lung disease; RA-only: rheumatoid arthritis without interstitial lung disease; IQR: interquartile range; CTD: autoimmune disease; CRP: C-reactive protein; ESR: erythrocyte sedimentation rate; DAS28: disease activity score with 28 joints;
*Other CTD included systemic lupus erythematosus, polymyositis/dermatomyositis, systemic scleroderma and Sjögren's syndrome.

p = 0.05, and cOR 0.61, 95% CI 0.32–1.14, p = 0.12; respectively). The positivity of anti-CCP2 and RF was significantly associated with ILD in RA patients (cOR 3.83; 95% CI 1.74–8.43, p<0.001; and cOR 2.28; 95% CI 1.12–4.61, p = 0.02 respectively). Further stratification of low, moderate and high levels of RF indicated that only high levels of serum RF ($\geq$364.0 IU/ml) were associated with ILD in RA patients (p = 0.02). After adjustment of age and disease duration together with the absence of collinearity (VIF and tolerance were 1.03 and 0.97 respectively) and other related co-variables (**Table 4**), the positivity of anti-CCP2 remained a risk factor for ILD in RA patients (adjusted odds ratio [aOR] 3.50; 95% CI 1.52–8.04, p<0.001), regardless of the level of anti-CCP. However, after adjusting confounding factors including gender, age, disease duration, smoking, medications and other CTD complication, there was no significant association between any level of low, moderate and high positivity of RF and RA-ILD in this population (**Table 4**).

Discussion

The pulmonary manifestations in RA patients was firstly reported half a century ago [23] and affect 10 to 20% of RA patients, which is associated with increased mortality [24]. The ILD has been recognized as the most common complication in the lung of RA patients. In this retrospective study, we evaluated the potential factors that contributed to ILD in RA patients. We found that 24.9% RA patients suffered with ILD, which was higher than that reported [3,4]. The high rate of patients with ILD may be due to long disease duration in a large proportion of our RA patients. Indeed, we found that RA patients with ILD were significantly older and had longer duration than those patients without ILD in this population. Alternatively, the high rate of patients with ILD may stem from unique genetic background.

Some other risk factors for RA-ILD should also be considered in multivariate analysis of the associations of anti-CCP2 positivity with the RA-ILD. Firstly, a previous study has showed that ILD is a severe clinical entity presented in many

Table 2. The relationship between HRCT features and antibody status of anti-CCP2 and RF in patients with RA-ILD.

HRCT feature	Anti-CCP2 (+)	Anti-CCP2 (−)	p	RF (+)	RF (−)	p
Irregular line/reticular opacities, n (%)	43 (68.3)	5 (62.5)	0.71	39 (65.0)	9 (81.8)	0.49
Ground-glass attenuation, n (%)	21 (33.3)	1 (12.5)	0.42	20 (33.3)	2 (18.2)	0.48
Basal consolidation, n (%)	23 (36.5)	3 (37.5)	1.0	20 (33.3)	6 (54.5)	0.19
Honey-combing, n (%)	8 (12.7)	2 (25.0)	0.31	9 (15.0)	1 (9.1)	1.0
Septal thickening, n (%)	24 (38.1)	3 (37.5)	1.0	24 (40.0)	3 (27.3)	0.52
Traction bronchiectasis/bronchiolectasis, n (%)	9 (14.3)	3 (37.5)	0.13	10 (16.7)	2 (18.2)	1.0

Table 3. Stratification analyses of the association of anti-CCP2 with ILD in RA patients.

	RA-ILD	RA-only	OR$_{M-H}$ (CI 95%)	p
Age				
<46 years, n (%)	14 (15.1)	79 (84.9)		
47–58 years, n (%)	19 (19.4)	79 (80.6)	3.3 (1.5–7.1)	0.003
>59 years, n (%)	38 (40.4)	56 (59.6)		
Disease duration				
<1.9 years, n (%)	17 (20.5)	66 (79.5)		
2.0–9.9 years, n (%)	19 (18.6)	83 (81.4)	3.9 (1.7–8.7)	0.001
>10.0 years, n (%)	35 (35.0)	65 (65.0)		

OR$_{M-H}$: Mantel-Haenszel odds ratio. 95% CI: 95% confidence interval. Age and disease duration of all patients were divided into three equal groups.

connective tissue diseases [25]. However, anti-CCP2 has been demonstrated to be extremely specific (96–98%) in patients with RA [26], but only 13.8% with SLE, 2.6% with SSc [27] and 7.5–9% with pSS [28,29]. In our study, 21.4% of patients had at least one other autoimmune disease besides RA and these patients distributed similarly in the RA-only and RA-ILD groups. Further univariate and multivariate analyses revealed that these comorbidities did not affect the significant association of the anti-CCP2 positivity with RA-ILD in this population. Secondly, we stratified patients, according to the radiologic features by HRCT and we found that there was no significant difference in the anti-CCP2 positivity among these subgroups of patients,which was in consistent with a previous report [16]. Thirdly, MTX has been considered as the standard therapy of DMARDs for RA patients. Although MTX has been considered as a low toxic drug, MTX

treatment of patients with pre-existing RA-ILD can cause fatal complication [30]. In our study, we did not observe that treatment with MTX resulted in a fatal outcome. There was no significant difference in the anti-CCP2 positivity between the patients receiving MTX treatment and those without MTX treatment. Thus, MTX treatment may not affect the levels of serum anti-CCP2 in RA patients. Finally, we did not observe that regular smoking was associated with RA-ILD in this population of RA patients, which was in consistent with previous reports [31].

The positivity of anti-CCP2 and RF is valuable for the diagnosis of RA. We found that the percentages of patients with positive anti-CCP2 and/or RF in the RA-ILD group were significantly higher than that in the RA-only group. Further analysis revealed that the percentages of the older patients with anti-CCP2 positivity in the RA-ILD group were significantly higher than that in the RA-only group. The univariate model of logistic regression analyses indicated that the different levels of serum anti-CCP2, but only high levels of RF were associated with ILD in this population of RA patients. Further adjusting other covariates revealed that the positivity of anti-CCP2 was significantly correlated with ILD in RA patients. Our data were in consistent with recent reports in France [18] and Greece [12] and similar to that in Japan [32]. However, there was no significant difference in the positivity of anti-CCP2 between the RA patients with and without ILD in another Japanese population [16] and a Korean population [17]. The difference among these studies may come from difference in patient population, disease definition or methodology for detecting clinical parameters. The variable sensitivity and specificity of the methods for anti-CCP2 detection may also affect its value in evaluating the association with ILD. The significantly higher positivity in the RA-ILD patients indicated that the positivity of anti-CCP2 may be a good biomarker for the diagnosis of ILD in RA patients.

Table 4. Univariate and multivariate analyses of the associations of anti-CCP2 positivity with the RA-ILD.

	Univariate associations			Multivariate associations		
	β	cOR (95% CI)	p	β	aOR (95% CI)	p
Age	0.06	1.06 (1.03–1.09)	<0.001	0.05	1.06 (1.03–1.08)	<0.001
Disease duration	0.04	1.04 (1.01–1.07)	<0.001	0.04	1.04 (1.01–1.07)	0.02
Anti-CCP2						
Seropositive	1.34	3.83 (1.74–8.43)	<0.001	1.25	3.50 (1.52–8.04)	<0.001
Low positive	1.27	3.57 (1.46–8.76)	0.01	1.24	3.46 (1.35–8.89)	0.01
Moderate positive	1.54	4.67 (1.93–11.29)	0.00	1.44	4.22 (1.63–10.90)	0.003
High positive	1.20	3.32 (1.35–8.20)	0.01	1.08	2.96 (1.14–7.67)	0.03
RF						
Seropositive	0.82	2.28 (1.12–4.61)	0.02	−0.04	0.96 (0.38–2.44)	0.93
Low positive	0.74	2.10 (0.91–4.86)	0.08	0.38	1.46 (0.54–3.94)	0.45
Moderate positive	0.75	2.12 (0.93–4.82)	0.07	0.25	1.28 (0.45–3.66)	0.65
High positive	0.97	2.63 (1.16–5.93)	0.02	0.66	1.93 (0.68–5.47)	0.21

Univariate and multivariate associations of anti-CCP2 with the occurrence of RA-ILD was conducted by logistic regression with a backward stepwise model. Covariates in multivariate model included gender, age, disease duration, smoking, medication, and other CTD complication. β: partial regression coefficient; DMARDs: disease-modifying antirheumatic drugs; Anti-CCP2: anti-citrullinated peptide antibody; COR: crude odds ratio; AOR: adjusted odds ratio; 95% CI: 95% confidence interval. Three equal groups of low, moderate and high positive anti-CCP2 were defined as 25.0≤anti-CCP2<271.3 U/ml, 271.3≤anti-CCP2<941.2 U/ml and anti-CCP2≥941.2 U/ml, respectively. Three equal groups of low, moderate and high positive RF were defined as 15.0≤RF<114.0 IU/ml, 114.0≤RF<364.0 IU/ml and RF≥364.0 IU/ml, respectively.

We recognized that our study had limitations. We could not exclude the potential selection bias in our patients although individual patients were diagnosed as having ILD, according to the available diagnostic criteria [33]. Previous studies have estimated the prevalence of ILD in RA patients being about 3.7–33.0% in those without significant abnormal chest X-ray or respiratory symptoms [34–36]. It is possible that we may underestimate the prevalence of ILD in RA patients. In addition, we did exclude individual patients without complete medical records and those developed ILD prior to their RA diagnosis. Moreover, we had no complete medical records of all participants so that we were unable to evaluate whether a delay in treatment of patients with MTX and DMADRs can be a risk factor of ILD in RA patients. Finally, the small sample size in our study may interfere with some results, such as the lack of significant difference in the positivity of anti-CCP2 in different subtypes of ILD in this population. Furthermore,

small sample size can lead to a false positive result and overestimate the magnitude of an association, particularly in a situation with multiple confounding variants. Therefore, further study in a bigger population is warranted to validate the value of anti-CCP2 positivity in evaluating the prognosis of ILD in RA patients.

In summary, we found significantly higher positivity of anti-CCP2 in RA patients with ILD than that in the RA alone patients. Our findings indicated that the positivity of anti-CCP2 is associated with ILD in RA patients.

Author Contributions

Conceived and designed the experiments: YY Yongzhe Li XZ FZ FT XZ. Performed the experiments: YY DL LZ Yang Li WL YR. Analyzed the data: YY DL GS. Contributed reagents/materials/analysis tools: Yongzhe Li XZ FZ FT XZ. Wrote the paper: YY DL.

References

1. Arnett FC, Edworthy SM, Bloch DA, McShane DJ, Fries JF, et al. (1988) The American Rheumatism Association 1987 revised criteria for the classification of rheumatoid arthritis. Arthritis Rheum 31: 315–324. PubMed: 3358796
2. Turesson C, O'Fallon WM, Crowson CS, Gabriel SE, Matteson EL (2003) Extra-articular disease manifestations in rheumatoid arthritis: incidence trends and risk factors over 46 years. Ann Rheum Dis 62: 722–727. PubMed: 12860726
3. Koduri G, Norton S, Young A, Cox N, Davies P, et al. (2010) Interstitial lung disease has a poor prognosis in rheumatoid arthritis: results from an inception cohort. Rheumatology (Oxford) 49: 1483–1489. PubMed: 20223814
4. Olson AL, Swigris JJ, Sprunger DB, Fischer A, Fernandez-Perez ER, et al. (2011) Rheumatoid arthritis-interstitial lung disease-associated mortality. Am J Respir Crit Care Med 183: 372–378. PubMed: 20851924
5. Turesson C, Matteson EL (2004) Management of extra-articular disease manifestations in rheumatoid arthritis. Curr Opin Rheumatol 16: 206–211. PubMed: 15103246
6. Zeng X, Ai M, Tian X, Gan X, Shi Y, et al. (2003) Diagnostic value of anti-cyclic citrullinated Peptide antibody in patients with rheumatoid arthritis. J Rheumatol 30: 1451–1455. PubMed: 12858440
7. Rodriguez-Mahou M, Lopez-Longo FJ, Sanchez-Ramon S, Estecha A, Garcia-Segovia A, et al. (2006) Association of anti-cyclic citrullinated peptide and anti-Sa/citrullinated vimentin autoantibodies in rheumatoid arthritis. Arthritis Rheum 55: 657–661. PubMed: 16874789
8. Rantapää-Dahlqvist S, de Jong BAW, Berglin E, Hallmans G, Wadell G, et al. (2003) Antibodies against cyclic citrullinated peptide and IgA rheumatoid factor predict the development of rheumatoid arthritis. Arthritis & Rheumatism 48: 2741–2749. PubMed: 14558078
9. Reparon-Schuijt CC, van Esch WJ, van Kooten C, Schellekens GA, de Jong BA, et al. (2001) Secretion of anti-citrulline-containing peptide antibody by B lymphocytes in rheumatoid arthritis. Arthritis Rheum 44: 41–47. PubMed: 11212174
10. Lopez-Longo FJ, Oliver-Minarro D, de la Torre I, Gonzalez-Diaz de Rabago E, Sanchez-Ramon S, et al. (2009) Association between anti-cyclic citrullinated peptide antibodies and ischemic heart disease in patients with rheumatoid arthritis. Arthritis Rheum 61: 419–424. PubMed: 19333979
11. Liao KP, Gunnarsson M, Kallberg H, Ding B, Plenge RM, et al. (2009) Specific association of type 1 diabetes mellitus with anti-cyclic citrullinated peptide-positive rheumatoid arthritis. Arthritis Rheum 60: 653–660. PubMed: 19248096
12. Alexiou I, Germenis A, Koutroumpas A, Kontogianni A, Theodoridou K, et al. (2008) Anti-cyclic citrullinated peptide-2 (CCP2) autoantibodies and extra-articular manifestations in Greek patients with rheumatoid arthritis. Clin Rheumatol 27: 511–513. PubMed: 18172572
13. Gerli R, Bartoloni Bocci E, Sherer Y, Vaudo G, Moscatelli S, et al. (2008) Association of anti-cyclic citrullinated peptide antibodies with subclinical atherosclerosis in patients with rheumatoid arthritis. Ann Rheum Dis 67: 724–725. PubMed: 18408112
14. Scott DL (2000) Prognostic factors in early rheumatoid arthritis. Rheumatology (Oxford) 39 Suppl 1: 24–29. PubMed: 11001376
15. Jansen AL, van der Horst-Bruinsma I, van Schaardenburg D, van de Stadt RJ, de Koning MH, et al. (2002) Rheumatoid factor and antibodies to cyclic citrullinated Peptide differentiate rheumatoid arthritis from undifferentiated polyarthritis in patients with early arthritis. J Rheumatol 29: 2074–2076. PubMed: 12375314
16. Inui N, Enomoto N, Suda T, Kageyama Y, Watanabe H, et al. (2008) Anti-cyclic citrullinated peptide antibodies in lung diseases associated with rheumatoid arthritis. Clin Biochem 41: 1074–1077. PubMed: 18638466
17. Jearn LH, Kim TY (2012) Level of anticitrullinated peptide/protein antibody is not associated with lung diseases in rheumatoid arthritis. J Rheumatol 39: 1493–1494. PubMed: 22753807
18. Aubart F, Crestani B, Nicaise-Roland P, Tubach F, Bollet C, et al. (2011) High levels of anti-cyclic citrullinated peptide autoantibodies are associated with co-occurrence of pulmonary diseases with rheumatoid arthritis. J Rheumatol 38: 979–982. PubMed: 21362759
19. American Thoracic Society, European Respiratory Society (2002) American Thoracic Society/European Respiratory Society International Multidisciplinary Consensus Classification of the Idiopathic Interstitial Pneumonias. This joint statement of the American Thoracic Society (ATS), and the European Respiratory Society (ERS) was adopted by the ATS board of directors, June 2001 and by the ERS Executive Committee, June 2001. Am J Respir Crit Care Med 165: 277–304. PubMed: 11790668
20. van der Heijde DM, van 't Hof MA, van Riel PL, Theunisse LA, Lubberts EW, et al. (1990) Judging disease activity in clinical practice in rheumatoid arthritis: first step in the development of a disease activity score. Ann Rheum Dis 49: 916–920. PubMed: 2256738
21. Zhang W, Shi Q, Zhao LD, Li Y, Tang FL, et al. (2010) The safety and effectiveness of a chloroform/methanol extract of Tripterygium wilfordii Hook F (T2) plus methotrexate in treating rheumatoid arthritis. J Clin Rheumatol 16: 375–378. PubMed: 21085018
22. Samouda H, Dutour A, Chaumoitre K, Panuel M, Dutour O, et al. (2013) VAT = TAAT-SAAT: innovative anthropometric model to predict visceral adipose tissue without resort to CT-Scan or DXA. Obesity (Silver Spring) 21: E41–50. PubMed: 23404678
23. Ellman P, Ball RE (1948) Rheumatoid disease with joint and pulmonary manifestations. Br Med J 2: 816–820. PubMed: 18890308
24. Brown KK (2007) Rheumatoid lung disease. Proc Am Thorac Soc 4: 443–448. PubMed: 17684286
25. Castelino FV, Varga J (2010) Interstitial lung disease in connective tissue diseases: evolving concepts of pathogenesis and management. Arthritis Res Ther 12: 213. PubMed: 20735863
26. van Noord C, Hooijkaas H, Dufour-van den Goorbergh BC, van Hagen PM, van Daele PL, et al. (2005) Diagnostic value of anti-cyclic citrullinated peptide antibodies to detect rheumatoid arthritis in patients with Sjogren's syndrome. Ann Rheum Dis 64: 160–162. PubMed: 15608321
27. Morita Y, Muro Y, Sugiura K, Tomita Y (2008) Anti-cyclic citrullinated peptide antibody in systemic sclerosis. Clin Exp Rheumatol 26: 542–547. PubMed: 18799082
28. Tobon GJ, Correa PA, Anaya JM (2005) Anti-cyclic citrullinated peptide antibodies in patients with primary Sjogren's syndrome. Ann Rheum Dis 64: 791–792. PubMed: 15834066
29. Gottenberg JE, Mignot S, Nicaise-Rolland P, Cohen-Solal J, Aucouturier F, et al. (2005) Prevalence of anti-cyclic citrullinated peptide and anti-keratin antibodies in patients with primary Sjogren's syndrome. Ann Rheum Dis 64: 114–117. PubMed: 15231509
30. Saravanan V, Kelly CA (2004) Reducing the risk of methotrexate pneumonitis in rheumatoid arthritis. Rheumatology (Oxford) 43: 143–147. PubMed: 12923285
31. Ayhan-Ardic FF, Oken O, Yorgancioglu ZR, Ustun N, Gokharman FD (2006) Pulmonary involvement in lifelong non-smoking patients with rheumatoid arthritis and ankylosing spondylitis without respiratory symptoms. Clin Rheumatol 25: 213–218. PubMed: 16091838
32. Mori S, Koga Y, Sugimoto M (2012) Different risk factors between interstitial lung disease and airway disease in rheumatoid arthritis. Respir Med 106: 1591–1599. PubMed: 22867979

33. Bongartz T, Nannini C, Medina-Velasquez YF, Achenbach SJ, Crowson CS, et al. (2010) Incidence and mortality of interstitial lung disease in rheumatoid arthritis: a population-based study. Arthritis Rheum 62: 1583–1591. PubMed: 20155830

34. Zrour SH, Touzi M, Bejia I, Golli M, Rouatbi N, et al. (2005) Correlations between high-resolution computed tomography of the chest and clinical function in patients with rheumatoid arthritis. Prospective study in 75 patients. Joint Bone Spine 72: 41–47. PubMed: 15681247

35. Gochuico BR, Avila NA, Chow CK, Novero LJ, Wu HP, et al. (2008) Progressive preclinical interstitial lung disease in rheumatoid arthritis. Arch Intern Med 168: 159–166. PubMed: 18227362

36. Brusselle G (2010) Rheumatoid arthritis and interstitial lung disease. Rheumatology (Oxford) 49: 1425–1426. PubMed: 20223815

21

Association between Sjogren's Syndrome and Respiratory Failure: Put Airway, Interstitia, and Vessels Close Together

Jun-Jun Yeh[1,2,3], Hsuan-Ju Chen[4,5], Tsai-Chung Li[6,7], Yi-Sin Wong[1], Hsien-Chin Tang[1], Ting-Chun Yeh[1], Chia-Hung Kao[8,9]*

1 Department of Family Medicine and Pulmonary Medicine, Ditmanson Medical Foundation Chia-Yi Christian Hospital, Chiayi, Taiwan, 2 Chia Nan University of Pharmacy and Science, Tainan, Taiwan, 3 Meiho University, Pingtung, Taiwan, 4 Management Office for Health Data, China Medical University Hospital, Taichung, Taiwan, 5 College of Medicine, China Medical University, Taichung, Taiwan, 6 Graduate Institute of Biostatistics, College of Management, China Medical University, Taichung, Taiwan, 7 Department of Healthcare Administration, College of Health Science, Asia University, Taichung, Taiwan, 8 Graduate Institute of Clinical Medical Science and School of Medicine, College of Medicine, China Medical University, Taichung, Taiwan, 9 Department of Nuclear Medicine and PET Center, China Medical University Hospital, Taichung, Taiwan

Abstract

Objectives: Few studies have evaluated the association between Sjogren's syndrome (SS) and respiratory failure (RF). Thus, we conducted a retrospective national cohort study to investigate whether Sjogren's syndrome (SS) increases the risk of respiratory failure (RF).

Methods: The cohort consisted of 4954 newly diagnosed patients with SS but without a previous diagnosis of RF, and 19816 patients as the comparison cohort from the catastrophic illnesses registry, obtained from the 2000–2005 period. All of the study participants were followed from the index date to December 31, 2011. We analyzed the association between the risk of RF and SS by using a Cox proportional hazards regression model, controlling for sex, age, and comorbidities.

Results: The overall incidence rate of RF showed a 3.21-fold increase in the SS cohort compared with the comparison cohort. The adjusted HR of RF was 3.04 for the SS cohort compared with the comparison cohort, after we adjusted for sex, age, and comorbidities. The HRs of RF for patients with primary SS and secondary SS compared with the comparison cohort were 2.99 and 3.93, respectively (*P* for trend <.001). The HRs of RF increased as the severity of SS increased, from 2.34 for those with no inpatient care experience to 5.15 for those with inpatient care experience (*P* for trend <.001).

Conclusion: This study indicates that clinical physicians should not only consider secondary SS but also primary SS as a critical factor that increases the risk of RF.

Editor: Antonio Carlos Seguro, University of São Paulo School of Medicine, Brazil

Funding: This study was supported by study projects DMR-102-014 and DMR-102-023 in China Medical University Hospital, the Taiwan Ministry of Health and Welfare Clinical Trial and Research Center of Excellence (MOHW103-TDU-B-212-113002), the Taiwan Ministry Health and Welfare Cancer Research Center for Excellence (MOHW103-TD-B-111-03), and the International Research-Intensive Centers of Excellence in Taiwan (I-RiCE) (NSC101-2911-I-002-303). The funders had no role in the study design, data collection and analysis, decision to publish, or preparation of the manuscript. No additional external funding was received for this study.

Competing Interests: The authors have declared that no competing interests exist.

* Email: d10040@mail.cmuh.org.tw

Introduction

Respiratory failure (RF) remains a common reason for admission to intensive care units (ICUs) [1]. RF is a syndrome characterized by the failure of one or both gas exchange functions of the respiratory system, namely oxygenation and carbon dioxide elimination. In practice, RF is diagnosed when the arterial oxygen tension (PaO_2) is <60 mmHg while breathing air (hypoxemia) or when the arterial carbon dioxide tension ($PaCO_2$) is>50 mm (hypercapnia) [2]. The hypoxemia may be accompanied by

hypercapnia. Furthermore, RF may be an acute RF (ARF) or a chronic RF.[2] RF can arise from an abnormality in any of the components of the respiratory system, including the airways, alveoli, interstitia, and vessels [2,3]. The mortality rate of ARF in critically ill patients is between 40% and 65% [4].

In the general population, Sjogren's syndrome (SS) affects approximately 3%–4% of adults and may be associated with a clinically significant impairment of a person's health and well-being [5]. SS has a broad clinical spectrum, extending from autoimmune exocrinopathy to extraglandular (systemic) diseases affecting the lungs, blood vessels, and lymph nodes [6]. In the absence of other autoimmune diseases, the syndrome is classified as primary SS [7]; when associated with other autoimmune diseases such as rheumatoid arthritis (RA), scleroderma, and systemic lupus erythematosus (SLE), it is classified as secondary SS. Moreover, SS is associated with various diseases of the thyroid gland, diabetes mellitus (DM), and hypertension [8,9]. Despite being a benign autoimmune disease, SS can terminate in a lymphoid malignancy [10]. Previous studies have reported the development of respiratory diseases associated with the interstitial [10–13], alveoli [10,13,14], airways [10,12,13,15], and vessels [10,13,15–18] of the lungs in patients with SS [13,19–21]. Moreover, some studies have associated SS with pulmonary functional impairments, including an obstructive, restrictive, or mixed ventilation [6,12,19].

In recent years, several pathophysiological conditions have been associated with small airway diseases other than chronic obstructive pulmonary disease (COPD) and asthma, including airway infections such as pneumonia and connective tissue diseases such as SS [22]. Exacerbation of COPD, asthma, or pulmonary embolism (PE) [3] may contribute to RF. Moreover, SS may develop from subclinical [12,23–25] to severe deteriorated [26] conditions, because of respiratory lesion such as chronic pulmonary fibrosis [12,13,19] and pulmonary arterial hypertension [3,11,13,18,27]. This is probably the first English literature research to address SS associated with RF in the general population.

Materials and Methods

Data source

Taiwan's National Health Insurance (NHI) is a universal insurance system established in 1996 by the Bureau of National Health Insurance of the Department of Health, and covers nearly 99% of the population in Taiwan. In this study, patient data from 2000 to 2011 were obtained from Taiwan's National Health Insurance Research Database (NHIRD), which contains each patient's information including sex, birthdate, and the registry of medical services. All personal information was encrypted before release to the public to protect patient privacy.

For this study, disease diagnosis was from disease records according to the International Classification of Diseases, 9th Revision, Clinical Modification (ICD-9-CM) in inpatient and catastrophic illnesses registry files.

Data Availability Statement

All data and related metadata are deposited in an appropriate public repository: The study population's data were from Taiwan NHIRD (http://w3.nhri.org.tw/nhird//date_01.html) are maintained by Taiwan National Health Research Institutes (http://nhird.nhri.org.tw/). The National Health Research Institutes (NHRI) is a non-profit foundation established by the government.

Ethics Statement

The NHIRD encrypts patient personal information to protect privacy and provides researchers with anonymous identification numbers associated with relevant claim information, including patients' sex, dates of birth, medical services utilized, and prescriptions. Patient consent is not required for accessing the NHIRD. This study was approved by the Institutional Review Board of China Medical University (CMU-REC-101-012). Our IRB specifically waived the consent requirement.

Study population

We used a retrospective population-based cohort design. The cohort consisted of 4954 newly diagnosed patients with Sjögren syndrome (SS, ICD-9-CM code 710.2) but without a previous diagnosis of RF during 2000–2005 in the catastrophic illnesses registry, and the date of diagnosed SS was defined as the index date. Four participants in the comparison cohort for each patient with SS were randomly selected from insured people without a history of SS and RF, frequency-matched according to age (per 5 y), sex, and index-year. We thus included 4954 patients as the SS cohort and 19 816 patients as the comparison cohort. The primary SS diagnosis was based on the European Study Group on Classification Criteria for Sjogren's Syndrome, a revised version of the European criteria proposed by an American–European study [7]; therein, a secondary SS was defined as a diagnosis of SS in patients with a previous diagnosis of rheumatoid arthritis (RA; ICD-9-CM code 714), systemic lupus erythematosus (SLE; ICD-9-CM code 710.0), scleroderma (ICD-9-CM code 710.1), or primary biliary cirrhosis (PBC; ICD-9-CM code 571.6).

We identified the following as comorbidities before the index date: pneumonia (ICD-9-CM code 480-487), asthma (ICD-9-CM code 493 and 494), hypertension (ICD-9-CM code 401-405), diabetes mellitus (DM, ICD-9-CM code 250), chronic obstructive pulmonary disease (COPD, ICD-9-CM code 491, 492 and 496), pulmonary embolism (PE, ICD-9-CM code 415.1, 639.6 and 673.8), thyroid disease (ICD-9-CM code 240-242 and 244-246), and lymphoma (ICD-9-CM code 200-208).

We identified the first diagnosis of RF (ICD-9-CM 518.81, 518.83, and 518.84) by using hospitalization records as the study endpoint. All of the study participants were followed from the index date to the study endpoint, December 31, 2011, or when the patient withdrew from the insurance system or died.

Statistical analysis

Demographic data, including age (<45, 45–59, and ≥60), sex, and comorbidity, were compared between patients with and without SS by using the chi-square test for categorical variables and the Student's t-test for continuous variables. To estimate the cumulative incidence of RF risks according to SS status, we performed survival analysis by using the Kaplan–Meier method, and significance was determined using the log-rank test. Multivariate Cox proportional hazard regression was used to examine the effect of SS on the risk of RF, which was determined based on the adjusted hazard ratio (HR) with a 95% confidence interval (CI). The multivariable model was used to adjust for age, sex, and comorbidities of pneumonia, asthma, hypertension, DM, COPD, PE, thyroid disease, and lymphoma.

All statistical analyses were performed using the SAS 9.3 statistical package (SAS Institute Inc., NC, USA), and R software (R Foundation for Statistical Computing, Vienna, Austria) was used to plot Kaplan–Meier survival curves; $P<.05$ for 2-tailed tests was considered significant.

Results

In this study, we evaluated 4954 SS patients and 19 816 individuals without SS with a similar average (53 y) and sex ratio (female: 87.08%; Table 1). The SS cohort had a higher proportion of comorbidities, such as pneumonia, asthma, hypertension, DM, COPD, PE, thyroid disease and lymphoma, than did the comparison cohort.

The Kaplan–Meier analysis showed that the cumulative incidence curves of RF were significantly higher in the SS cohort than in the comparison cohort (log-rank test $P<.001$) (Figure 1).

Table 1. Baseline demographic factors and comorbidity of study participants according to sjogren's syndrome status.

Characteristics	Control N = 19,816		SS N = 4,954		p-value
	N	%	n	%	
Gender					0.99
Female	17,256	87.08	4,314	87.08	
Male	2,560	12.92	640	12.92	
Age, years					0.99
<45	5,548	28.00	1,387	28.00	
45–59	7,772	39.22	1,943	39.22	
≥60	6,496	32.78	1,624	32.78	
Mean (SD)	53.32	(14.45)	53.43	(14.36)	0.66
Comorbidity					
Pneumonia	460	2.32	205	4.14	<0.001
Asthma	267	1.35	122	2.46	<0.001
Hypertension	1,516	7.65	473	9.55	<0.001
Diabetes mellitus	909	4.59	190	3.84	0.02
COPD	306	1.54	120	2.42	<0.001
Pulmonary embolism	6	0.03	13	0.26	<0.001
Thyroid disease	203	1.02	169	3.41	<0.001
Lymphoma	15	0.08	15	0.30	<0.001

Abbreviation: COPD, chronic obstructive pulmonary disease; SS, sjogren's syndrome; SD, standard deviation

The overall incidence rate of RF showed a 3.21-fold increase in SS cohort compared with the comparison cohort (6.44 vs 2.01 per 1000 person-y). The adjusted HR of RF was 3.04 (95% CI = 2.57–3.59) for the SS cohort compared with the comparison cohort, after we adjusted for sex, age, and comorbidities (Table 2). In addition, we observed that the death number of discharged in hospitalized patients of respiratory failure were 118 (45.46%) and 0 (0.00%) in the SS and non-SS cohorts (data not show).

Sex-specific analysis revealed that the incidence rates of RF in females and males with SS were 5.10 and 16.40 per 1000 person-years, respectively, which are higher than those in the comparison cohort (1.99 and 2.12 per 1000 person-y, respectively). In addition, compared with the comparison cohort, females exhibited a 2.45-fold (adjusted HR = 2.45, 95% CI = 2.02–2.96) higher risk of developing RF, and males showed a 7.10-fold (adjusted HR = 7.10, 95% CI = 4.83–10.45) higher risk (P for interaction <.001). Compared with comparison cohort, the greatest magnitude of HR was observed in patients with SS aged 60 years and older (8.29, 95% CI = 6.42–10.70). Regardless of the participants' comorbidities, SS patients had a higher HR of RF than the comparison cohort (Table 2).

Table 3 lists the combined effects of SS and comorbidities including pneumonia, hypertension, DM, and COPD on the risk of RF compared with the referent group of no SS and no corresponding comorbidity. We observed a greater magnitude of HRs of RF for patients with SS and pneumonia, hypertension, DM, and COPD compared with patients with no SS and no counterpart comorbidity (HR = 12.54, 95% CI = 8.91–17.65; 11.72, 8.89–15.44; 14.30, 10.12–20.20; and 15.19, 10.26–22.49, respectively).

The HRs of RF for patients with primary and secondary SS compared with the comparison cohort were 2.99 (95% CI = 2.52–3.54) and 3.93 (95% CI = 2.40–6.41), respectively (P for trend < .001) (Table 4). Overall, the HRs of RF increased as the severity of SS increased, from 2.34 (95% CI = 1.92–2.85) for those with no inpatient care experience to 5.15 (4.13–6.42) for those with inpatient care experience compared with the comparison cohort (P for trend <.001).

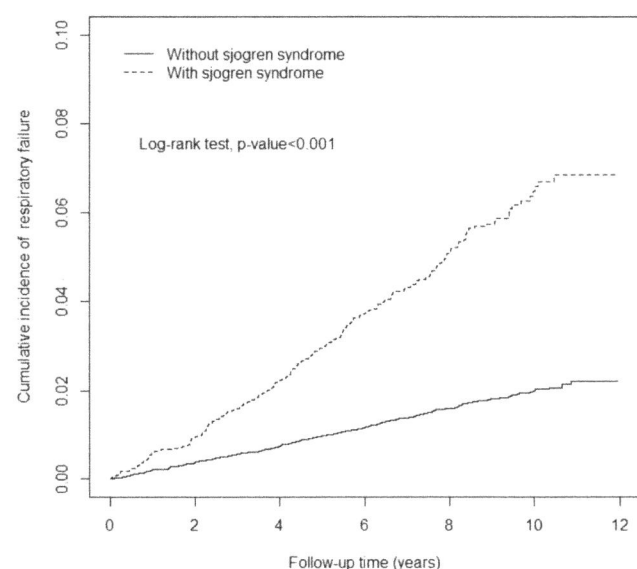

Figure 1. Cumulative incidence curves of respiratory failure for Sjogren syndrome and control Groups.

Table 2. Incidence rates and hazard ratio for respiratory failure according to sjogren's syndrome status stratified by demographic factors and comorbidity.

| | Sjogren's syndrome | | | | | | Compared to non-sjogren's syndrome | |
| | No | | | Yes | | | | |
Characteristics	Case	Person-years	IR	Case	Person-years	IR	Crude HR (95% CI)	Adjusted HR (95% CI)
Overall	317	157919.10	2.01	254	39421.58	6.44	3.21 (2.72-3.78)***	3.04 (2.57-3.59)***
Gender								
Female	277	139081.19	1.99	177	34726.87	5.10	2.56 (2.12-3.09)***	2.45 (2.02-2.96)***
Male	40	18837.91	2.12	77	4694.71	16.40	7.75 (5.29-11.36)***	7.10 (4.83-10.45)***
Age, years								
<45	91	46049.32	1.98	22	11793.58	1.87	0.94 (0.59-1.50)	1.03 (0.63-1.68)
45-59	139	63770.04	2.18	44	15867.92	2.77	1.27 (0.91-1.79)	1.24 (0.88-1.76)
≥60	87	4809.74	1.81	188	11760.08	15.99	8.84 (6.86-11.40)***	8.29 (6.42-10.70)***
Comorbidity status‡								
No	187	141523.81	1.32	133	32877.82	4.05	3.06 (2.45-3.83)***	3.11 (2.49-3.88)***
Yes	130	16395.29	7.93	121	6543.76	18.49	2.34 (1.83-3.00)***	2.25 (1.75-2.89)***

Discussion

The initial findings of this study suggest that the incidence of RF in the primary or secondary SS cohort was higher than that in the non-SS cohort, regardless of sex, age, or comorbidities. In Papathanasiou et al [12], compared with the control participants, the incidence of pulmonary abnormalities in SS was nonsignificant and clinically negligible. By contrast, Strimlan et al [20] observed chest lesions, such as diffuse interstitial fibrosis, recurrent pneumonitis, pleural effusions, and suspected lymphoma or pseudolymphoma, in patients with SS.

The pathophysiology of RF includes the impairment of the airways, alveoli, interstitia, and vessels of the lungs. Further deterioration of the respiratory lesions of SS may lead to progressive changes such as airway obstruction [6,28,29], alveolitis [24,30], pulmonary lymphoma [20], interstitial fibrosis [20], vasculitis [13], or pulmonary arterial hypertension [17,18]. This indicates a positive association of SS with the airways, alveoli, interstitia, and vessels of the lung, which in turn may contribute to the incidence of RF, even without comorbidities [28,31,32].

In our study, the SS cohorts with pneumonia [12,22], hypertension [9,33], DM [8], or COPD [29] exhibited increased risks of RF. In addition, the SS cohort with COPD exhibited the highest IR and HR, and the SS cohort with patients aged ≥60 years exhibited a higher RF incidence than did the non-SS cohort; moreover, concordant findings were observed in other studies investigating elderly patients with comorbidities such as hypertension, DM, or COPD [9,29]. The therapeutic management of the SS cohort with elderly patients could have been complicated by comorbidities and an increased rate of adverse events related to the applied therapeutic agents and polypharmacy. Therefore, effective management of comorbidities, such as COPD, and careful follow-up are necessary for SS patients [34].

The primary SS cohort exhibited a higher incidence of RF than that in the non-SS cohort. Based on Papiris et al, the airway epithelia of the lungs may be the main target of inflammatory lesions in patients with primary Sjogren's syndrome, which may be a common subclinical condition that leads to obstructive small airway physiological abnormalities [35]. Moreover, primary Sjogren's syndrome associated with interstitial lung disease [36] and pulmonary arterial hypertension [18] were the 2 factors that contributed to the development of RF. Furthermore, based on Constantopoulos et al, the cumulative effects of diffuse interstitial lung disease contribute the most to RF in primary SS (25%), followed by small airway disease (22%), desiccation of the upper respiratory tract (17%), and large airway obstruction (8%) [21,28].

Based on the non-SS cohort as a reference, the incidence of RF in the secondary SS cohort exhibited the highest IR and HR. Moreover, a previous study reported a higher incidence of respiratory lesions in the secondary SS cohort than that in the primary SS cohort, which agrees with our findings [37]. Furthermore, another study [12] reported a higher incidence of obstructive airway disease in the secondary SS cohort than in the primary SS cohort, and that obstructive airway disease can contribute to the development of RF [38].

No studies have indicated an association between the frequency of admission and the incidence of RF. In our study, the frequency of admission was higher in the SS cohort than in the non-SS cohort. The patients in the SS cohort at admission may present with RF accompanied by an acute exacerbation of pulmonary fibrosis [39] or pulmonary emboli [40], which may contribute to pulmonary arterial hypertension [26,38,39]. The risk of RF increases with the number of SS exacerbations and admissions [41]. These findings imply a positive association between the

Table 3. Joint effect of SS and comorbidity in association with respiratory failure in study population.

Variable		Case	IR	HR (95% CI)
SS	Pneumonia			
No	No	287	1.85	1.00
No	Yes	30	10.81	4.52 (3.09–6.61)***
Yes	No	216	5.68	3.09 (2.59–3.68)***
Yes	Yes	38	27.93	12.54 (8.91–17.65)***
SS	Hypertension			
No	No	226	1.53	1.00
No	Yes	91	9.34	4.85 (3.75–6.27)***
Yes	No	180	4.97	3.29 (2.71–4.01)***
Yes	Yes	74	22.85	11.72 (8.89–15.44)***
SS	Diabetes			
No	No	260	1.71	1.00
No	Yes	57	10.03	4.58 (3.41–6.14)***
Yes	No	216	5.65	3.32 (2.77–3.97)***
Yes	Yes	38	31.73	14.30 (10.12–20.20)***
SS	COPD			
No	No	285	1.82	1.00
No	Yes	32	18.26	6.62 (4.52–9.67)***
Yes	No	225	5.82	3.21 (2.69–3.82)***
Yes	Yes	29	39.26	15.19 (10.26–22.49)***

Abbreviation: SS, sjogren syndrome; IR, incidence rate, per 10,000 person-years; HR, hazard ratio; CI, confidence interval; COPD, chronic obstructive pulmonary disease. Multivariate-adjusted model including gender, age, and comorbidities.
*** p<0.001.

incidence of RF and recurrent airway inflammation [29,42], interstitial fibrosis [11,41], alveolitis [43], and chronic pulmonary arterial hypertension [18,40], all of which may cause impairment or damage the airways [28,42], interstitia/aleveoli [11,41,43], and pulmonary vessels [40]. These findings indicate poor control as a critical factor for the incidence of RF in patients with SS [19,28,44,45].

The clinical presentation of SS may vary. The onset is insidious [12,43] and usually begins in women aged 40–60 years; however,

it can also affect men and children [46]. The initial manifestations of SS may include asthma, COPD [29], or pneumonia [20,21], which may contribute to the diagnosis of SS [20,21,47]. Concurrently, the subclinical manifestations of SS may delay the diagnosis [23,43,48]. Thus, the initial symptoms of primary SS can be overlooked or misinterpreted easily, and diagnosis can be delayed for several years. Therefore, this study emphasizes the importance of early diagnosis of SS and put the airway, interstitia

Table 4. Incidence and adjusted hazard ratio of respiratory failure in different subgroups and severity sjogren syndrome.

	N	Cases	IR	Crude HR (95% CI)	Adjusted HR (95% CI)
Without sjogren's syndrome	19816	317	2.01	1.00 (Reference)	1.00 (Reference)
Subgroups of sjogren's syndrome					
Primary sjogren syndrome	4672	237	6.37	3.17 (2.68–3.76)***	2.99 (2.52–3.54)***
Secondary sjogren syndrome‡	282	17	7.60	3.78 (2.32–6.16)***	3.93 (2.40–6.41)***
Sjogren syndrome					
Hospital admissions					
No	3,743	147	4.92	2.45 (2.01–2.98)***	2.34 (1.92–2.85)***
Yes	1,211	107	11.23	5.60 (4.50–6.97)***	5.15 (4.13–6.42)***

Abbreviation: IR, incidence rate, per 1,000 person-years; HR, hazard ratio; CI, confidence interval.
Adjusted HR: adjusted for age, gender, and comorbidity in Cox proportional hazards regression
‡A secondary SS was defined a diagnosis of SS in patients with a previous diagnosis of rheumatoid arthritis (ICD-9-CM code 714), systemic lupus erythematosus (SLE; ICD-9-CM code 710.0), scleroderma (ICD-9-CM code 710.1), or primary biliary cirrhosis (ICD-9-CM code 571.6).
*** p<0.001.

and vessels close together in the development of RF among the patients with primary SS or secondary SS.

Limitations

Several limitations must be considered when interpreting the findings of this study. The NHIRD provides no detailed lifestyle information, such as smoking, body mass index, and physical activity, all of which were potential confounding factors for this study. However, the treatment and lifestyle modifications of patients with SS may implicate these factors in the accelerated development of respiratory lesions in SS. In addition, our study data provided no information on the SS severity scale, including disease activity, functional impairment, and physical damage [49]. Another limitation was the lack of individual information of drugs' use in the database, including pilocarpine, hydroxychloroquine, and glucocorticosteroids, which were the possible risk factors for respiratory failure could have been used to adjust for the outcomes of interest. However, Taiwan launched a national health insurance (NHI) in 1995, operated by a single-buyer, the government. Medical reimbursement specialists and peer review should scrutinize all insurance claims. Therefore, under the reimbursement coverage of NHI, every patient with SS in this study should already receive the standard treatments for SS including systemic steroid or other immunosuppressive drugs. Despite our meticulous study design to control for the confounding factors, a key limitation of this study is the potential for bias caused by possible unmeasured or unknown confounders.

Strengths

The strength of this study is that it provides a nationwide, population-based, longitudinal cohort study on the risk of RF in Asian patients with SS. The outcomes of the cohort study in the general population may be similar to those in the "real world". [50] Thus, the findings of this study can be generalized to the general population.

Conclusion

In conclusion, this nationwide study investigating approximately 4954 patients with SS with 19 816 follow-up person-years reveals that patients with SS exhibit a 3.04-fold increased risk of developing RF compared with the general population. These findings highlight the importance of a multidisciplinary team adopting an integrated approach to the intervention of the potential risk factors for patients with SS. Early diagnosis of SS and initiation of treatment for these patients may prevent the development of RF in patients with pulmonary SS, thereby preventing the need for ICU admission.

Author Contributions

Conceived and designed the experiments: JJY CHK. Performed the experiments: JJY HJC CHK. Analyzed the data: JJY HJC CHK. Contributed reagents/materials/analysis tools: CHK. Wrote the paper: JJY HJC TCL YSW HCT TCY CHK.

References

1. Afessa B, Keegan MT, Mohammad Z, Finkielman JD, Peters SG (2004) Identifying potentially ineffective care in the sickest critically ill patients on the third ICU day. Chest 126: 1905–1909.
2. Roussos C, Koutsoukou A (2003) Respiratory failure. Eur Respir J Suppl 47: 3s–14s.
3. Gunning KEJ (2003) Pathophysiology of Respiratory Failure and Indications for Respiratory Support. Surgery (Medicine Publishing) 21: 72–76.
4. Lewandowski K, Metz J, Deutschmann C, Preiss H, Kuhlen R, et al. (1995) Incidence, severity, and mortality of acute respiratory failure in Berlin, Germany. Am J Respir Crit Care Med 151: 1121–1125.
5. Thomas E, Hay EM, Hajeer A, Silman AJ (1998) Sjogren's syndrome: a community-based study of prevalence and impact. Br J Rheumatol 37: 1069–1076.
6. Segal I, Fink G, Machtey I, Gura V, Spitzer SA (1981) Pulmonary function abnormalities in Sjogren's syndrome and the sicca complex. Thorax 36: 286–289.
7. Vitali C, Bombardieri S, Jonsson R, Moutsopoulos HM, Alexander EL, et al. (2002) Classification criteria for Sjogren's syndrome: a revised version of the European criteria proposed by the American-European Consensus Group. Ann Rheum Dis 61: 554–558.
8. Humbert P, Dupond JL (1988) [Multiple autoimmune syndromes]. Ann Med Interne (Paris) 139: 159–168.
9. Pérez-De-Lis M, Akasbi M, Sisó A, Diez-Cascon P, Brito-Zerón P, et al. (2010) Cardiovascular risk factors in primary Sjogren's syndrome: a case-control study in 624 patients. Lupus 19: 941–948.
10. Sarkar PK, Patel N, Furie RA, Talwar A (2009) Pulmonary manifestations of primary Sjogren's syndrome. Indian J Chest Dis Allied Sci 51: 93–101.
11. Deheinzelin D, Capelozzi VL, Kairalla RA, Barbas Filho JV, Saldiva PH, et al. (1996) Interstitial lung disease in primary Sjogren's syndrome. Clinical-pathological evaluation and response to treatment. Am J Respir Crit Care Med 154: 794–799.
12. Papathanasiou MP, Constantopoulos SH, Tsampoulas C, Drosos AA, Moutsopoulos HM (1986) Reappraisal of respiratory abnormalities in primary and secondary Sjogren's syndrome. A controlled study. Chest 90: 370–374.
13. Fischer A, du Bois R (2012) Interstitial lung disease in connective tissue disorders. Lancet 380: 689–698.
14. Papiris SA, Kalomenidis I, Malagari K, Kapotsis GE, Harhalakis N, et al. (2007) Extranodal marginal zone B-cell lymphoma of the lung in Sjogren's syndrome patients: reappraisal of clinical, radiological, and pathology findings. Respir Med 101: 84–92.
15. Kokosi M, Riemer EC, Highland KB (2010) Pulmonary involvement in Sjogren syndrome. Clin Chest Med 31: 489–500.
16. Kikuchi A, Okai T, Taketani Y (1996) Pulmonary embolism associated with Sjogren's syndrome in pregnancy. J Obstet Gynaecol Res 22: 421–423.
17. Asherson RA, Cervera R (2007) Pulmonary hypertension, antiphospholipid antibodies, and syndromes. Clin Rev Allergy Immunol 32: 153–158.
18. Launay D, Hachulla E, Hatron PY, Jais X, Simonneau G, et al. (2007) Pulmonary arterial hypertension: a rare complication of primary Sjogren syndrome: report of 9 new cases and review of the literature. Medicine (Baltimore) 86: 299–315.
19. Ito I, Nagai S, Kitaichi M, Nicholson AG, Johkoh T, et al. (2005) Pulmonary manifestations of primary Sjogren's syndrome: a clinical, radiologic, and pathologic study. Am J Respir Crit Care Med 171: 632–638.
20. Strimlan CV, Rosenow EC 3rd, Divertie MB, Harrison EG Jr (1976) Pulmonary manifestations of Sjogren's syndrome. Chest 70: 354–361.
21. Constantopoulos SH, Papadimitriou CS, Moutsopoulos HM (1985) Respiratory manifestations in primary Sjogren's syndrome. A clinical, functional, and histologic study. Chest 88: 226–229.
22. Burgel PR, Bergeron A, de Blic J, Bonniaud P, Bourdin A, et al. (2013) Small airways diseases, excluding asthma and COPD: an overview. Eur Respir Rev 22: 131–147.
23. Wallaert B, Hatron PY, Grosbois JM, Tonnel AB, Devulder B, et al. (1986) Subclinical pulmonary involvement in collagen-vascular diseases assessed by bronchoalveolar lavage. Relationship between alveolitis and subsequent changes in lung function. Am Rev Respir Dis 133: 574–580.
24. Salaffi F, Manganelli P, Carotti M, Baldelli S, Blasetti P, et al. (1998) A longitudinal study of pulmonary involvement in primary Sjogren's syndrome: relationship between alveolitis and subsequent lung changes on high-resolution computed tomography. Br J Rheumatol 37: 263–269.
25. Wright SA, Convery RP, Liggett N (2003) Pulmonary involvement in Sjogren's syndrome. Rheumatology (Oxford) 42: 697–698.
26. Naffaa M, Mazor Y, Azzam ZS, Yigla M, Guralnik L, et al. (2013) Fulminant pneumonitis: a clue to autoimmune disease. Isr Med Assoc J 15: 195–197.
27. Fernández-Pérez ER, Yilmaz M, Jenad H, Daniels CE, Ryu JH, et al. (2008) Ventilator settings and outcome of respiratory failure in chronic interstitial lung disease. Chest 133: 1113–1119.
28. Ismael S, Wermert D, Dang-Tran KD, Venot M, Fagon JY, et al. (2014) Severe excessive dynamic airway collapse in a patient with primary Sjogren's syndrome. Respir Care Respir Care. 2014;59:e156–9.
29. Newball HH, Brahim SA (1977) Chronic obstructive airway disease in patients with Sjogren's syndrome. Am Rev Respir Dis 115: 295–304.
30. Dalavanga YA, Constantopoulos SH, Galanopoulou V, Zerva L, Moutsopoulos HM (1991) Alveolitis correlates with clinical pulmonary involvement in primary Sjogren's syndrome. Chest 99: 1394–1397.
31. Chung WS, Lin CL, Ho FM, Li RY, Sung FC, et al. (2014) Asthma increases pulmonary thromboembolism risk: a nationwide population cohort study. Eur Respir J 43: 801–807.
32. Konstantinides SV (2014) Asthma and pulmonary embolism: bringing airways and vessels closer together. Eur Respir J 43: 694–696.

33. Juarez M, Toms TE, de Pablo P, Mitchell S, Bowman S, et al. (2014) Cardiovascular risk factors in women with primary Sjögren's syndrome: United Kingdom primary Sjögren's syndrome registry results. Arthritis Care Res (Hoboken). 66: 757–64.

34. Moerman RV, Bootsma H, Kroese FG, Vissink A (2013) Sjogren's syndrome in older patients: aetiology, diagnosis and management. Drugs Aging 30: 137–153.

35. Papiris SA, Maniati M, Constantopoulos SH, Roussos C, Moutsopoulos HM, et al. (1999) Lung involvement in primary Sjogren's syndrome is mainly related to the small airway disease. Ann Rheum Dis 58: 61–64.

36. Nannini C, Jebakumar AJ, Crowson CS, Ryu JH, Matteson EL (2013) Primary Sjögren's syndrome 1976–2005 and associated interstitial lung disease: a population-based study of incidence and mortality. BMJ Open 3: e003569.

37. Vitali C, Tavoni A, Viegi G, Begliomini E, Agnesi A, et al. (1985) Lung involvement in Sjogren's syndrome: a comparison between patients with primary and with secondary syndrome. Ann Rheum Dis 44: 455–461.

38. Fukumura A, Ogawa N, Simoyama K, Karasawa H, Okada J, et al. (2001) [A case of Sjogren's syndrome with dermatomyositis who died of rapidly progressive interstitial pneumonia]. Ryumachi 41: 37–43.

39. Tuder RM, Lee SD, Cool CC (1998) Histopathology of pulmonary hypertension. Chest 114: 1S–6S.

40. Chung WS, Lin CL, Sung FC, Hsu WH, Chen YF, et al. (2014) Increased Risks of Deep Vein Thrombosis and Pulmonary Embolism in Sjogren Syndrome: A Nationwide Cohort Study. J Rheumatol 41: 909–15.

41. Enomoto Y, Takemura T, Hagiwara E, Iwasawa T, Fukuda Y, et al. (2013) Prognostic factors in interstitial lung disease associated with primary Sjogren's syndrome: a retrospective analysis of 33 pathologically-proven cases. PLoS ONE 8: e73774.

42. Chiorini JA, Cihakova D, Ouellette CE, Caturegli P (2009) Sjogren syndrome: advances in the pathogenesis from animal models. J Autoimmun 33: 190–196.

43. Pirildar T, Gumuser G, Ruksen E, Sakar A, Dinc G, et al. (2010) Assessment of alveolar epithelial permeability with Tc-99m DTPA aerosol scintigraphy in patients with Sjogren syndrome. Rheumatol Int 30: 599–604.

44. Yazisiz V, Arslan G, Ozbudak IH, Turker S, Erbasan F, et al. (2010) Lung involvement in patients with primary Sjogren's syndrome: what are the predictors? Rheumatol Int 30: 1317–1324.

45. Vij R, Strek ME (2013) Diagnosis and treatment of connective tissue disease-associated interstitial lung disease. Chest 143: 814–824.

46. Franklin DJ, Smith RJ, Person DA (1986) Sjogren's syndrome in children. Otolaryngol Head Neck Surg 94: 230–235.

47. Usuba FS, Lopes JB, Fuller R, Yamamoto JH, Alves MR, et al. (2014) Sjogren's syndrome: An underdiagnosed condition in mixed connective tissue disease. Clinics (Sao Paulo) 69: 158–162.

48. Gomes Pde S, Juodzbalys G, Fernandes MH, Guobis Z (2012) Diagnostic Approaches to Sjogren's syndrome: a Literature Review and Own Clinical Experience. J Oral Maxillofac Res 3: e3.

49. Meiners PM, Vissink A, Kroese FG, Spijkervet FK, Smitt-Kamminga NS, et al. (2014) Abatacept treatment reduces disease activity in early primary Sjogren's syndrome (open-label proof of concept ASAP study). Ann Rheum Dis 73: 1393–6.

50. Booth CM, Rapoport B (2011) Uptake of novel medical therapies in the general population. Curr Oncol 18: 105–108.

22

Organic Solvents as Risk Factor for Autoimmune Diseases

Carolina Barragán-Martínez, Cesar A. Speck-Hernández, Gladis Montoya-Ortiz, Rubén D. Mantilla, Juan-Manuel Anaya, Adriana Rojas-Villarraga*

Center for Autoimmune Diseases Research (CREA), School of Medicine and Health Sciences, Universidad del Rosario, Bogota, Colombia

Abstract

Background: Genetic and epigenetic factors interacting with the environment over time are the main causes of complex diseases such as autoimmune diseases (ADs). Among the environmental factors are organic solvents (OSs), which are chemical compounds used routinely in commercial industries. Since controversy exists over whether ADs are caused by OSs, a systematic review and meta-analysis were performed to assess the association between OSs and ADs.

Methods and Findings: The systematic search was done in the PubMed, SCOPUS, SciELO and LILACS databases up to February 2012. Any type of study that used accepted classification criteria for ADs and had information about exposure to OSs was selected. Out of a total of 103 articles retrieved, 33 were finally included in the meta-analysis. The final odds ratios (ORs) and 95% confidence intervals (CIs) were obtained by the random effect model. A sensitivity analysis confirmed results were not sensitive to restrictions on the data included. Publication bias was trivial. Exposure to OSs was associated to systemic sclerosis, primary systemic vasculitis and multiple sclerosis individually and also to all the ADs evaluated and taken together as a single trait (OR: 1.54; 95% CI: 1.25–1.92; p-value<0.001).

Conclusion: Exposure to OSs is a risk factor for developing ADs. As a corollary, individuals with non-modifiable risk factors (i.e., familial autoimmunity or carrying genetic factors) should avoid any exposure to OSs in order to avoid increasing their risk of ADs.

Editor: Sudha Chaturvedi, Wadsworth Center, United States of America

Funding: This project did not have any specific funding, but the work was supported by the School of Medicine and Health Sciences, Universidad del Rosario. The funders had no role in study design, data collection and analysis, decision to publish, or preparation of the manuscript.

Competing Interests: The authors have declared that no competing interests exist.

* E-mail: adrirojas@gmail.com

Introduction

Autoimmune diseases (ADs) are initiated by the loss of immune tolerance and mediated through T or B cell activation leading to tissue damage. ADs share clinical signs and symptoms, physio-pathological mechanisms, and genetic factors [1]. They are complex diseases caused by the interaction between genetic, epigenetic, and environmental factors over time [2,3].

Despite the difficulties in defining environmental risk factors that lead to immunopathology, the number of candidates proposed for specific ADs is continuously growing as new evidence is reported for infectious agents, chemicals, physical factors, adjuvants, and hormones [4–15]. A significant body of research has pointed out that, for autoimmunity to occur, the genetic background warrants to be combined with environmental injuries and novel associations has been described as the case of the air pollution [5,16]. However these environmental factors often explain only a small number of cases, and, on their own, they are not sufficient to cause the disease [5].

Solvents are liquids that dissolve a solid, liquid or gas. They can be broadly classified into two categories: organic and inorganic. Organic solvents (OSs) are compounds whose molecules contain carbon. They may be broken down further into aliphatic-chain compounds, such as n-hexane, and aromatic compounds with a 6-carbon ring, such as benzene or xylene. OSs arose in the latter half of the 19th century from the coal-tar industry. Common uses for OSs are: dry cleaning (e.g., tetrachloroethylene), paint thinner (e.g., toluene, turpentine), nail polish removers and glue solvents (acetone, methyl acetate, ethyl acetate), spot removers (e.g., hexane, petrol ether), detergents (citrus turpenes), perfumes (ethanol), nail polish and chemical synthesis [17]. In contrast, the use of inorganic solvents (other than water) is typically limited to research in chemistry and some technological processes.

The applications of OSs became more diversified in both developed and developing countries. Research in this area began in 1957 when the first patients developing a scleroderma-like syndrome after exposure to vinyl chloride, epoxy resins, trichloroethylene (TCE), perchloroethylene and other mixed solvents were reported [18,19]. Nevertheless, few published studies have analyzed the wide spectrum of ADs in subjects exposed to OSs. Therefore, we aimed to analyze the evidence of an association between the exposure to OSs and the development of AD through a systematic literature review and a meta-analysis. In addition, a comprehensive review concerning the mechanisms by which OSs exposure induces immunological alterations is presented.

Methods

Literature Search

The search was done using the following databases: PubMed, SCOPUS, SciELO and LILACS and took into account articles published up to February 2012. We followed the PRISMA guidelines for meta-analysis of observational studies [20] in our data extraction, analysis, and reporting (Text S1).

The most relevant terms regarding OSs exposure were suggested by an expert chemical engineer specialist in industrial hygiene. The following Medical Subject Heading (MeSH) terms were used: "systemic vasculitis," "vasculitis," "rheumatoid arthritis," "lupus," "multiple sclerosis," "scleroderma," "systemic sclerosis," "antiphospholipid syndrome," "Sjögren's syndrome," "dermatomyositis," "polymyositis," "myasthenia gravis," "Churg-Strauss syndrome," "giant cell arteritis," "microscopic polyangiitis," "cryoglobulinemia," "polyarteritis nodosa," "Wegener granulomatosis," "inflammatory bowel diseases," "anemia, pernicious," "thyroiditis, autoimmune," "celiac disease," "juvenile rheumatoid arthritis," "vitiligo," "primary biliary cirrhosis," "biliary cirrhosis," "primary sclerosing cholangitis," "autoimmune hepatitis," "transverse myelitis," "relapsing polychondritis," "Addison disease," "glomerulonephritis," "idiopathic thrombocytopenic purpura," "psoriatic arthritis," "spondylitis, ankylosing," "sarcoidosis," "Raynaud's disease," "connective tissue disease," and "autoimmune disease." Each one of them was cross-referenced with the following MeSH terms: "solvent," "tetrachloroethylene," "trichloroethylene," "trichloroethane," "perchlorethylene," "toluene," "vinyl chloride," "acetone," "ethylacetate," "turpentine," "benzene," "5-hydroxytryptophan," "diethylpropion," "fenfluramine," and "hair dye." Furthermore, we used 'text words' if there was no MeSH term such as in the cases of "hexane," "white spirit," "urea formaldehyde," and "nail polish."

In addition, each MeSH term was translated into DeCS (Health Sciences Descriptors), the tool that permits navigation between records and sources of information through controlled concepts and organized in Portuguese, Spanish and English, in order to search the SciElo and LILACS databases. No limits regarding language, period of publication, or publication type were taken into account. Those references from the articles that seemed to be relevant for our review were hand-searched. Authors of publications to which full text access was unavailable were contacted via e-mail.

In addition, a systematic search was done in the PubMed database up to February 2012 looking for the molecular mechanisms by which OSs may alter immune responses and induce the developing of ADs. The search was restricted to: (1) studies in humans and mice, (2) restricted by title and (3) English language, (4) articles published in the last 20 years, (5) studies in ADs (6) studies including the term autoimmunity, (7) studies including the term "immune system". All of the search strategies included MeSH terms: "Tetrachloroethylene", "Trichloroethylene", "Trichloroethanes", "Perchlorethylene", "Toluene", "Vinyl Chloride", "Acetone", "Ethylacetate", "Turpentine", "Benzene", "5-Hydroxytryptophan", "Diethylpropion", "Fenfluramine", "Hair Dyes", "Hexane", "Immune System", and "autoimmunity". Furthermore, we used key words if there was no MeSH term such as in the cases of "white spirit", "urea formaldehyde", "nail polish and "autoimmune diseases". The exclusion criteria were the following: 1) Articles related to immune alterations due to allergic responses in solvent exposure, 2) articles related to cytotoxic and genotoxic effects of solvent in cancer progression, 3) articles in a language other than English, 4)

reviews, 5) comments and case reports that did not report any biological implication related to solvent exposure.

Study Selection, Data Extraction, and Quality Assessment

Inclusion criteria for the systematic review were the following: any types of study that used accepted classification criteria for ADs and had information about exposure to OSs explicitly listed as a category.

Articles were excluded from the analysis if they included the same data that were published in another study.

Abstracts and full text articles were reviewed in the search for eligible studies. Two reviewers did the search independently while applying the same selection criteria. The two resulting databases were compared and disagreements resolved by consensus. For articles in languages other than English or Spanish, translations of abstracts or full text articles were reviewed to determine eligibility.

Each eligible study was classified as: review, case report, case series, cohort, or case-control. Inclusion criteria for the meta-analysis were applied to publications that provided epidemiologic data on risk factors [relative risks (RR) and odds ratios (OR) with confidence intervals (CI)] or that provided information that let us calculate these data. For cohort studies, the requirements were the number of subjects exposed, the number unexposed, and the number of subjects who developed the disease in each of the two cases. For case-control studies, the requirements were the number of subjects with AD that were exposed and not exposed, and the number of controls that were exposed and not exposed. In those instances where the study had not reported the number of subjects in each group, either the RR or the OR with the CI, at least, must have been reported in order for them to be included in the meta-analysis calculations.

Studies were excluded from the meta-analysis if the groups were not clearly defined, e.g. case- controls studies with likely AD diagnosis in control subjects or exposed cohorts with low specificity for OS.

For each eligible study, the type of exposure and exposure assessment was analyzed regarding the source of information (census, database, interview, mailed questionnaires, etc.) and classified as follows: "qualitative" if it was stated by the subject or interviewer on questionnaires measured by the quality of exposure rather than its quantity, "quantitative" if it was related to a number or quantity, and "semi-quantitative" if it was expressed as a quantity susceptible of measurement but was not related to a number. Quantitative assessment was sub-classified in "indirect quantitative" if it was defined by an estimate from a register of specific jobs at risk or calculated using a job-exposure matrix formula, and "direct quantitative" if the OS was directly measured in the environment or as a biomarker in the subject. Furthermore it was extracted the information that described the condition of exposure (e.g occupation, living characteristics.)

The quality and strength of scientific evidence was evaluated supporting an etiologic relationship between ADs and the proposed risk factor. In this investigation, a quantitative scoring system based on the Bradford Hill criteria was used [21]. The quantitative Bradford Hill score (qBHs) is divided into categorical ratings of the overall strength of causal association as follows: 0 to 6 points was considered poor or no causal association; 7 to 14 points was considered moderate or inconclusive causal association, and 15 to 21 points was considered a strong causal association. No study was excluded from the review based on this assessment.

Meta-analysis

Data were analyzed using the Comprehensive Meta-Analysis version 2 program (Biostat, Englewood, NJ, 2004). Calculations were carried out for the whole group of articles depending on the binary data available for any AD: number of subjects and risk data (OR and RR with the corresponding 95% CI). Effect size was calculated based on studies that only showed the OR and respective 95% CI and the raw data from case-control and cohort studies. A second effect size was calculated independently with studies that only showed the RR and the respective 95% CI and the raw data from cohort studies. Different study designs were used to compute the same effect size since the effect size had the same meaning in all studies and were comparable in relevant aspects. Thus, this study was able to transform all values to log values (log odds ratio and standard error), which were used in the pooled analysis. This approach prevented the omission of studies that used an alternative measure.

A sensitivity analysis was done in which the meta-analysis results of the studies as a whole was compared to the same meta-analysis with one study excluded in each round to determine how robust the findings were. It was also done to evaluate the impact of decisions that lead to different data being used in the analysis and whether the conclusions reached might differ substantially if a single study or a number of studies were omitted.

Additional meta-analyses were done for studies with complex data structure and non-cumulative results if the information for the different effects was not totally independent. Thus, articles showing multiple independent subgroups within a study were considered in these analyses (i.e. different definitions of the disease, gender differences, toxic exposure or more than one comparison group within a study). To compare effects across subgroups we typically use subgroup as the unit of analysis in an independent meta-analysis.

Supplementary analyses were done for the association between each specific AD and OSs exposure. Additional analyses were also done grouping the data according to the exposure assessment category.

ORs were grouped by weighing individual ORs by the inverse of their variance. For each analysis, the final effect OR and 95% CI were obtained by means of both random and fixed effect models. The selection of the computational model was done based on the expectation that the studies shared a common effect size. The random effect model was preferred because it accepts that there is a distribution of true effect sizes rather than one true effect and assigns a more balanced weight to each study. It was also used because all the studies were considered to be unequal in terms of specific ADs.

Heterogeneity was calculated by means of Cochran's (Q) and Higgins's ($I2$) tests. The $I2$ test showed the proportion of observed dispersion that was real rather than spurious and was expressed as a ratio ranging from 0% to 100%. $I2$ values of 25%, 50%, and 75% were qualitatively classified as low, moderate, and high respectively. A significant Q-statistic (p<0.10) indicated heterogeneity across studies. Publication bias was determined using Funnel plots and Egger's regression asymmetry tests, and additional tests were applied if it was found.

Results

The search with the defined MeSH Terms in PubMed, SCOPUS, SciELO, and LILACS [DeCS Terms] retrieved 531 articles. Using text words, 794 articles were found in PubMed, SCOPUS, SciELO and LILACS. Nine additional records were identified through references (Figure 1).

After duplicates were removed, there were 575 potentially relevant articles. Based on title or abstract, 143 were chosen for full text review. Six full text publications were not found and the authors of these publications or authors of publications that referenced them (e.g. [22]) were contacted. Of these, 4 articles were sent via e-mail [23–26] and one by post mail [27]. It was not possible to get full text access to one article [28]. One hundred and three articles described exposure to OSs as a category and used accepted classification criteria for ADs. Of these, 3 were meta-analysis [29–31], 29 were reviews, 5 case series [32–36], 15 case reports [37–51], and 51 epidemiological studies. Thirty-three of the epidemiological studies were finally included in the meta-analysis (Table 1) [7,23,26,27,52–80]. Because of lack of information, 18 epidemiological studies [25,81–97] were not included in the meta-analysis (Table S1). Eight studies were not included because lack of information about the number of subjects with confirmed AD; two case-control studies were not included because lack of information about exposure in control subjects; one case-control study was excluded because control subjects had likely an AD diagnosis; three cohort studies were not included because lack of information about the number of unexposed and how many developed AD. Four studies were excluded because exposure data had low specificity for OS.

Types of exposure and exposure assessments are described in table 1 for each study. The average qBHs for the total publications included in the meta-analysis was 14.25 points (SD, 1.586; range, 11–17 points; 99% CI, 13.528–14.972) reflecting a categorical rating of moderate relationship.

We found a significant association between OSs exposure and the increased risk of developing an autoimmune trait by evaluating all ADs as a single group. Figure 2 shows the forest plot corresponding to the meta-analysis including the most relevant outcome per author where the final common effect size based on a random model was statistically significant (OR: 1.54; 95% CI: 1.25–1.92; p-value<0.001). The results of different measures for heterogeneity calculated for the analysis showed in Figure 2 were as follows: Q-value: 132.1; degree of freedom (Q):30; p-value<0.0001; I-squared: 77.3%; Tau-Squared 0.19. The relative weight of each study is included in the forest plot (Figure 2)

There were 5 studies showing complex data structure with different and non-cumulative results where the information for the different effects was not totally independent [52,57,70,76,78]. Then, 22 additional meta-analyses including 30 articles and the different outcomes of four of the above mentioned studies were calculated independently [57,70,76,78]. These analyses included five from Diot et al. 2002 [76] (different toxic exposure measured: chlorinate, ketones, aromatic, toluene, TCE), one from Nelson et al. 1994 [57] (control not disabled population) and Purdie et al. 2011 [70] (a different cutoff point to disease criteria) and fifteen from Thompson et al. 2002 [78] (different toxic exposure measured: toluene, benzene, white spirit, perchlorethylene, TCE, trichlorethane, vinyl chloride, urea formaldehyde, meta-phenylenediamene, bicromade, aromatic hydrocarbons, aliphatic hydrocarbons, fenfluramine, diethylpropion, L5 OH-tryptophan). In these meta-analyses, the studies that provided uniquely RR data were not included [52,54] for statistical reasons. All these additional meta-analyses showed a significant association between the exposure to OSs and ADs as a trait (Figures S1, S2, S3, S4, S5, S6, S7, S8, S9, S10, S11, S12, S13, S14, S15, S16, S17, S18, S19, S20, S21, S22). After doing a sensitivity analysis excluding one study at a time, the results were similar to the cumulative analysis (Figures S23 and S24).

A second effect size was calculated based on data from two studies showing RR data [52,54] with raw data from cohort

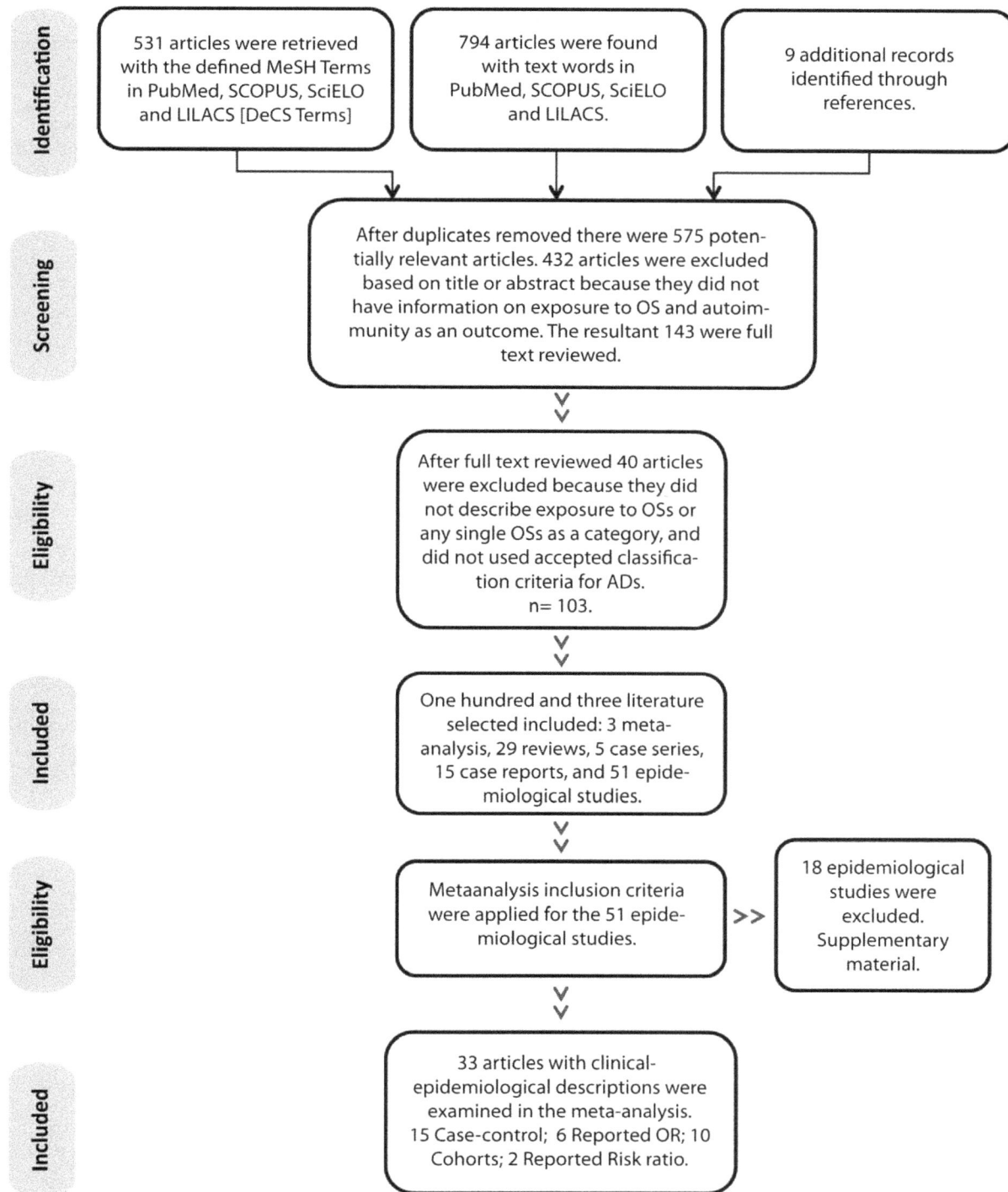

Figure 1. Systematic Review Results. Footnote: OSs: organic solvents; AD: autoimmune disease; OR: odds ratio.

studies [26,55,56,63–66,70]; this effect size was not significant (OR: 1.62; 95% CI: 0.99–2.65; p-value:0.051) (Figure S25). The results of different measures for heterogeneity calculated for the analysis showed in Figure S25 were as follows: Q-value: 42.01; degree of freedom (Q):11; p-value<0.001; I-squared: 73.8%; Tau-Squared 0.40.

Additional analysis limited to the association between each specific AD and OSs exposure presented significant associations in the random model. For MS, the OR was 1.53 with 95& CI 1.03–2.29 and p value: 0.035, with fifteen studies included. For primary systemic vasculitis (PSV), the OR was 3.15 with 95% CI: 1.56–6.36 and p-value: 0.001, with one study included in the cumulative analysis for this disease. Systemic sclerosis (SSc) showed these

Table 1. Characteristics of the studies examined in the meta-analysis.

First author and year of publication	AD	Study population and control group	Assessment of exposure	Outcome	qBHs (max. score 21)
		-Country	- Method used to get the information (questionnaire, database)		
		-Method used to identify cases and controls-Number (N).	- Terms of the exposure estimate (qualitative, semi-quantitative, quantitative indirect)		
		-Study design	-Type of exposure		
Lundberg et al. 1994 [52]	AS RA	Sweden. From the computer-based census was extracted a cohort according to the occupational status ten years before the observation. N = 375,035 men and 140,139 women. Using the hospital discharge register the study population was observed from 1981–1983 and rheumatoid diseases cases extracted. N = 896 males and 629 females for RA; 79 males and 13 females for AS; for myosic 23 males and 14 females; for SSc 47 males and 24 females; 36 males and 57 females for SLE, 31 males and 6 females for vasculitis. Study design: retrospective cohort.	Job-exposure matrix with two categories of intensity for OS (semi-quantitative). Substantial use designated occupations where the average amount of solvent handled per year was estimated to 100 litters or more, e.g. house painters. Limited use designed occupations in which average amount of solvent handled was estimated 1–99 litters, e.g. house carpenters.	Increased relative risk for workers in occupations with substantial use of OS. Painters showed increased isk for AS.	16
Fored et al. 2004 [53]	GN	Sweden. Cases identified from the NPR (1996–1998) men and women whose creatinine level exceeded 300 mmol/L and 250 mmol/L, respectively, physicians at each hospital treating patients determined case eligibility by reviewing medical records N = 217. Control subjects randomly selected from the NPR and frequency-matched according to age and gender. Study design: population based case-control study.	Face to face interview by occupational hygienists (not blinded). Senior occupational hygienist estimated the intensity and cumulative lifetime exposure to OS using an accepted rating and arithmetic method (quantitative indirect). Seventy percent of the case patients and 62% of the control subjects reported exposure during manufacturing work, largest group: metal workers.	Adjusted OR 0.96 (95% CI 0.68–1.34)	12
Sesso et al. 1990 [54]	GN	Brazil. Cases: 17 patients with rapidly progressive GN associated with OS exposure and 34 matched hospital controls. Renal histo ogic findings suggest immune complex mediated injury. Study design: Case-control.	Self-report OS exposure (qualitative) was defined as 1 hour or more weekly for 3 consecutive months or longer. Increased risk was detected in exposed to fuels.	Relative risk = 5 (95% IC 1.14–22)	15
Flodin et al. 2003 [55]	MS	Sweden. Cases were identified among The Nurse Union through an appeal published in the union magazine. The occupational group they focused was Nurse anesthetists. Among the subjects who replied, Nurse anesthetists with MS diagnosis were identified. To confirm MS medical files were requested N = 10. Study design: retrospective cohort.	A questionnaire requested qualitative information about years and kind of work tasks, and type of anesthetics they had used.	Increased MS risk was detected in nurse anesthetists.	17
Stenager et al. 2003 [26]	MS	Denmark. In a nationwide study on the isk of MS in Danish nurses were identified nurse anesthetists with confirmed cases of MS. Expected number of MS was calculated in an age- and sex-matched population. Study design: retrospective cohort.	Qualitative data was assessed using a national register of nurses and the Danish Multiple Sclerosis Register.	Nurse anesthetist had no increased risk	11
Amaducci et al. 1982 [56]	MS	Italy. Cases were identified from a register of MS patients and interviewed to establish their last occupation before the disease onset. Five cases of MS were employed in shoe and leather industry. Relative risk was calculated between shoe and leather workers and the general population of Florence. Study design: retrospective cohort.	Data on general population and people employed in the shoe and leather industry of Florence were obtained from Census.	Increased risk among shoe and leather industry workers (4.81)	13

Table 1. Cont.

First author and year of publication	AD	Study population and control group	Assessment of exposure	Outcome	qBHs (max. score 21)
Nelson et al. 1994 [57]	MS	USA. Cases identified by reviewing medical records of employees taking medical disability at any of eight automobile assembly plants located in Michigan and Ohio N = 20. Controls chosen from employees who took disability retirement for disorders other than those of interest. Study design: Case- control.	Semi-quantitative exposure indices were assigned by two industrial hygienists and expressed in years working in solvent exposed tasks.	OR 2.0 (95% CI 0.6–6.9)	15
Grønning et al. 1993 [58]	MS	Norway. Cases were patients living in Hordaland with clinical MS onset between 1976–86 N = 139. Controls comprised patients admitted to the hospital with other diagnosis matched on age, sex and residence N = 161. Distributions among type of work and type of OS were similar among cases and controls. Study design: case- control.	Face to face questionnaire that elicited detailed information about exposure to OS and number of years of exposure. Exposure index was calculated using Ravnskov formula (quantitative indirect). Main occupational exposure to OS occurred at mechanical, oil, textile, wood-working, paint, printing, plastic and rubber industries.	OR 1.55 (95% CI 0.83–2.90)	15
Zorzon et al. 2003 [59][bc]	MS	Italy. Cases were consecutive patients who were being seen in routine follow-up at the Multiple Sclerosis Center of the University of Trieste N = 140. Control group was formed by sex and age matched blood donors N = 131. Controls were similar to cases in area of residence and ethnicity. Study design: case- control.	Face to face interview (blinded) collected detailed information related to occupational exposures (qualitative). Exposure was considered when lasting >5 years.	OR 0.8 (95% CI 0.5–1.4)	14
Juntunen et al. 1989 [60]	MS	Finland. From the Finish Twin Cohort 21 cases of MS were extracted and records reviewed by a neurologist. Only 2 pairs were concordant. The comparison group was formed by the co-twins. Study design: Nested case control.	Face to face interview by a specialist on occupational medicine. Exposure was estimated and roughly classified (semi-quantitative).	No statistically significant association of exposure.	13
Flodin U et al. 1988 [27]	MS	Sweden. Cases were obtained from the patient files of the neurologic clinics of the General Hospital of Linköping N = 83. Control group was already available as primarily utilized for cancer studies, and randomly drawn from the population registers N = 467. Study design: Case- control.	Mailed questionnaire. A minimum criterion of one year was required for exposure time. Semi-quantitative score was obtained based on Ravnskov method.	Mantel-Haenezel Rate Radio 2 (90% CI 0.9–4)	14
Koch-Henriksen et al. 1989 [61]	MS	Canada. Case group N = 187. Control group N = 187. Case- ascertainment and selection of controls: NA. Study design: population based case-control study.	Questionnaire about industrial OS exposure (qualitative).	No significant association	14
Casetta et al. 1994 [23]	MS	Italy. Cases: definite MS patients living in the province of Ferrara N = 104. Two matched control groups, one from hospitalized patients and the other from general population. Study design: Case- control.	Face to face blind interview about occupational history before the age of onset (qualitative).	OR 4 (95% CI 1.48–11.11)	14
Landtblom et al. 1993 [62]	MS	Sweden. Cases collected from the files of the neurological department of the hospitals Jönköping and Kalmar N = 91. Controls were randomly drawn from population registers of the administrative provinces of Jönköping and Kalmar N = . Study design: population based case-control study.	Mailed questionnaire focused on occupational exposures. A minimum criterion of one year was required for exposure time. Semi-quantitative score was obtained based on Ravnskov method.	Mantel-Haenszel Rate Radio 2.8 (95% CI 0.9–8)	15

Table 1. Cont.

First author and year of publication	AD	Study population and control group	Assessment of exposure	Outcome	qBHs (max. score 21)
Landtblom et al. 2006 [63]	MS	Sweden. From the 1985 census were identified nurse anesthetists (N = 907) and compared to other nurses (N = 39,703) and teachers (N = 20,053). Age restriction to the interval of 35–50. Cases: MS diagnosis or disability pension due to MS (N = 168). Study design: retrospective cohort.	In the census each person had to declare which occupation held. Based on this information nurse anesthetists, potentially exposed to OS, were identified (qualitative).	Cumulative incidence rate ratio was increased in female nurse anesthetists (statistically no significant)	15
Mortensen et al. 1998 [64]	MS	Denmark. From the 1970 census "solvent-exposed men" group was extracted N = 124,766. "Unexposed men" cohort comprised electricians, bricklayers, and butchers N = 87,501. After a 20 years of follow-up 87 MS cases presented among presumed to be exposed. Study design: cohort.	Census contains information of the occupational status and qualitative data of exposure. House painters, carpenters, and typographers are the occupations with the longest exposure.	There was no important difference in the standardize morbidity ratio between occupational groups.	14
Riise et al. 2002 [65]	MS	Norway. Three cohorts of 11,542 painters; 36,899 construction workers and 9,314 food-processing were followed from 1970 to1986. A total of 9 painters, 12 construction workers and 6 food-workers received pension because of MS. Study design: cohort.	Workers potentially exposed to OS (qualitative data) were identified by the 1970 national census.	The relative risk 95% CI for painters compared with workers not exposed to OS was 2	15
Riise et al. 2011 [66]	MS	Norway. From the Registry of Employers and Employees was extracted a cohort of 27,900 offshore petroleum workers, 42,657 onshore petroleum workers and 365,805 referents. The total cohort was linked to the nationwide Norwegian MS registry including all cases of MS with onset after the start of their working engagement. Study design: retrospective cohort.	Offshore workers of the petroleum industry with suspected OS exposure (qualitative data) included technicians, laboratory engineers and control operators involved in the production process and 'drilling and well maintenance offshore'.	There was no increased risk of MS among offshore workers	12
Gershwin et al. 2005 [67]	PBC	USA. Between November 1999 and June 2004 a total of 1,090 patients with PBC were refereed from 23 referral medical centers. Referring physicians re-evaluated anonymized clinical information in 100 randomly selected enrolled patients. Controls were selected by random digit dialing and matched for sex, age, race, and geographical area. Study design: case-control.	Telephone interview included over 180 questions and 300 sub-questions, including exposure data (semi-quantitative). PBC patients reported to use hair dye 38±50 times/year and nail polish 29±65 times/year.	A history of nail polish was associated with PBC AOR 1.002 (95% CI 1.00–1.003).	15
Lane et al. 2003 [68]	PSV	UK. Cases: PSV diagnosed between May 1988 and july 2000 identified from a prospective vasculitis register. Case notes were reviewed for clinical and laboratory details N = 103. Controls N = 220 hospital inpatients and outpatients with non-inflammatory musculoskeletal disease, matched to the age of the case at the time of interview. Controls were excluded if personal history of AD. Study design: case –control.	Face to face structured questionnaire. To defined occupational OS exposure was used the Steenland job exposure matrix (quantitative indirect).	A history of OS was associated with PSV; OR 2.7 (95%IC 1.1–6.6) a nd WG 3.4 (1.3–8.9)	15
De Roos et al. 2005 [69]	RA	USA. The Agricultural Health Study is a cohort of licensed pesticide applicators and their spouses. From this cohort RA diagnosis were validated among women who had self-reported RA, N = 136 physician-confirmed cases were matched by age to 5 controls. Controls were selected from among women in the cohort except those who had reported any AD. Study design: Nested case-control.	Information was available from the Agricultural Health Study questionnaires (qualitative).	Risk of RA was not associated with OS; OR 0.6 (95% CI 0.3–1.5)	14

Table 1. Cont.

First author and year of publication	AD	Study population and control group	Assessment of exposure	Outcome	qBHs (max. score 21)
Purdie et al. 2011 [70]	RD	New Zeeland. Technicians, scientist, and laboratory assistants working in medical laboratories were assessed for RD using the UK Scleroderma Study group questionnaire. RD rates in solvent-exposed histology, cytology, and transfusion medicine (N = 301) were compared with unexposed medical laboratory workers from transfusion medicine. Study design: retrospective cohort.	Laboratory workers self-report history of exposure to OS including frequency and years working (semi-quantitative). Higher rates of RD, particularly, for those who had worked with xylene, toluene or acetone.	OR 8.8 (95% CI 1.9–41.1)	16
Cooper et al. 2004 [71]	SLE	USA. Cases: Carolina Lupus Study included resent diagnosed patients identified through community based rheumatologist practices in the study area N = 265. Population based controls were identified through driver license records and were f requency matched to the cases by age, sex, and state N = 355. Study designed: case-control.	In 60 minutes in person interview, job history and specific questions about potential exposure were asked. Three reviewers (one industrial hygienist and 2 epidemiologist) reviewed the job and task description and qualified the exposure in 5 categories (likely-high, possible-high, possible-moderate, indirect, none).	There was no evidence of association between occupational exposure to OS and SLE	11
Cooper et al. 2010 [72]	SLE	Canada. Cases: recruited from 11 rheumatology centers across Canada N = 258. Control randomly selected from phone number listings and matched by age, sex, and area of residence N = 263. Study design: case-control.	30–45 minutes telephone interview assessed work history and specific potential exposures (qualitative). Strong associations were seen with work as an artist working with paints, dyes or developing film (1), and applying nail polish (2).	(1) OR 3.9 (95% 1.3–12.3) (2) OR 10.2 (95%CI 1.3–81.5)	15
Finckh et al. 2006 [7]	SLE	USA. cases: women with SLE were identified through both community screening and hospital data-bases in 4 predominant African American neighborhoods N = 95. Controls were female residents of the same area who participated in one of the screening events but were negative for SLE N = 191. Study design: population based case-control.	Data were collected using in-person interviews (qualitative). A detailed lifetime work history followed by a structured checklist involving specific jobs likely to involve exposure to solvents (e.g. wood finishes, paints, dry-cleaning, pottery).	OR 1.04 (95% 0.34–3.2)	13
Nietert et al. 1998 [73]	SSc	USA. Cases: From March 1995 to February 1997 were included patients being seen in the rheumatology clinics N = 178. Controls diagnosed with osteoarthritis, gout and fibromyalgia were selected during the same time period N = 200. Study design: case-control.	Data were collected using in-person nterviews. Semi-quantitative score were assigned by computerized method, based on the occupational and industrial classification.	OR 2.9 (95% CI 1.1–7.1)	15
Bovenzi et al. 1995 [74]	SSc	Italy. Cases: from the computerized admission files of all of the local hospitals from 1976 to 1991 N = 21. Clinical records were obtained and verify. With the same database system, for each case, 2 age and gender matched referents. Study design: case-control.	Blinded interview with a structured questionnaire, which included exposure to OS. The subjects were allocated into the various exposure categories (semi-quantitative) by 2 occupational physicians who were blinded. Minimum criterion of six months was required for exposure duration.	OR 9.28 (95% CI 0.48–74.1) for men; 2.11 (0.20–22.0) for women	16
Bovenzi et al. 2004 [75]	SSc	Italy. Cases: N = 55 (46 female, 9 male) recruited at Institute of Internal Medicine of University of Hospital Verona, patients affected with localized scleroderma were not included. Controls N = 171 among patients admitted in the same study period to the Institute of Orthopedics with other diagnosis different to any AD. Study design: case-control.	In-person interview and structured questionnaire focused on occupational history. Explicit questions referenced to potential exposure to OS. The occupational history was reviewed and qualified (semi-quantitative) by an expert in industrial hygiene and occupational health, blind to case-control condition.	Female teachers OR 3.4 (95% CI 1.2–10.1) Textile workers OR 2.1 (95% CI 1.0–4.6)	14

Table 1. Cont.

First author and year of publication	AD	Study population and control group	Assessment of exposure	Outcome	qBHs (max. score 21)
Diot et al. 2002 [76]	SSc	France. Cases admitted consecutively to the department of Internal Medicine from 1998 to 2000 N = 80. For each case, two age, gender, and smoking habits (frequency and quantity) matched controls. Study design: case-control.	A semi-quantitative score were calculated, by a committee of six experts, based on probability, intensity, daily frequency, and duration of exposure for each period of employment. Final cumulative score was obtained.	Significant associations were observed for TCE, toluene, aromatic solvents, ketones, white spirit, epoxy resins and welding fumes.	15
Maître et al. 2004 [77]	SSc	France. Cases: 10 men and 33 women diagnosed between 1995 and 1999 and 206 age and sex matched controls, randomly selected from general population. Study design: case-control.	Mailed questionnaire and phone interview. The questions included occupational details and suspect forms of exposure. Every job was classified by a group of experts according to the potential level of exposure on a 3-level scale (semi-quantitative). The criteria used for this classification were likelihood, duration, intensity and percentage of working time exposed.	Solvents were linked to SSc OR 3.2 (95% CI 1.5–6.6) in both men and women	15
Thompson et al. 2002 [78]	SSc	Canada. Cases: N = 91 patients identified in a rheumatology outpatient practice. Controls N = 154 derived from the same practice, same rheumatologist, and matched by age and sex, did not have SSc. Study design: case-control.	Mail questionnaire with specific questions of employment information and chemical exposure (semi-quantitative) at workplace or home. Exposure rates in both groups were low.	There were no differences in type of employment between the 2 groups.	11
Silman et al. 1992 [79]	SSc	UK. Cases recruited from registers of patients with SSc from different centers, N = 56 men. Controls: (1) patients were asked to provide three male friends within 5 years of age and (2) general practitioner was approached to provide the names of three male patients, age matched. Study design: case-control.	Postal questionnaire for self-report exposure. Occupational exposure was assessed in two ways. First, detailed history of occupations was assessed, blinded to the case or control status, by an experienced occupational hygienist and scored (semi-quantitative) for nil, possible, or probable exposure. Secondly the subjects were asked to recall exposure to a detailed list of solvents.	No significant increase in exposure to OS was noted.	13
Czirják et al. 1989 [80]	SSc	Hungary. Cases from hospital data N = 61, with controls matched for age and sex. Study design: case-control.	Self-reported exposure (qualitative) to: benzene, isopropyl alcohol, ethyl acetate. Risk related to length of exposure but not data on risk by intensity.	OR 23.18 (95% CI 2.97–180.79)	17

AD: autoimmune disease, qBHs: Quantitative score of the Bradford Hills Criteria for causation. AS: ankylosing spondylitis. RA: rheumatoid arthritis. SSc: systemic sclerosis. SLE: systemic lupus erythematous, OS: Organic solvent. GN: glomerulonephritis,NPR: National population Register; N: number of subjects in each group. OR 95% CI: Odds ratio with 95% confident interval. MS: multiple sclerosis. NA: not available data. PBC: primary biliary cirrhosis. AOR: Adjusted odds ratio. PSV: primary systemic vasculitis, WG: Wegener's granoulomatosis. RD: Raynaud's disease. TCE: trichloroethylene.

results OR: 2.54; 95% CI: 1.23–5.14; p-value: 0.011, with eight studies included (Figure 3). Primary biliary cirrhosis (PBC) was positively associated but not statistically significant (OR: 1.002; 95% CI: 1–1.004; p-value: 0.092).

The analyses according to the exposure assessment category are shown in figure S26. There were three groups included. Two of them were not significant: qualitative (OR: 1.29; 95% CI: 0.84–1.98; p-value 0.231) and quantitative indirect (OR: 1.69; 95% CI: 0.90–3.16; p-value 0.101) and one was significant: semi-quantitative [(OR: 1.48; 95% CI: 1.17–1.87; p-value 0.001). Heterogeneity: Q-value: 56.7; degree of freedom (Q):13; p-value<0.0001; I-squared: 77%; Tau-Squared 0.19]. The total heterogeneity between the three groups for the random effects analysis was not significant [Q-value: 0.60; degree of freedom (Q):2; p-value: 0.741]

Evidence of significant publication bias was identified using the Egger test (p-value 2-tailed: 0.002; intercept: 1.09) for the meta-analysis which included studies that report OR with its respective

95% CI and raw data from case control and cohort designed studies. The Funnel plot showing the standard error on the Y axis is shown in Figure S27. Therefore, a second analysis was run in a search for publication bias. The classic fail-safe analysis indicated that 279 missing studies would give a p-value of >0.05. Begg and Mazumdar rank correlation was not significant (p-value 2-tailed: 0.16) and the trim and fill adjustment did not suggest a lower risk than the original analysis [adjusted values (11 studies trimmed) point estimate 1.03 (0.83–1.28), Q value: 227]. Based on all the analyses for publication bias, we consider the impact of bias in the present meta-analyses trivial.

Since 1977, 20 publications including case-reports and case series (Table S2) have reported 37 cases of AD possibly being triggered by OSs. We also found 3 previous meta-analyses. The first was published in 1996 by Landtblom AM et al [29] and concerned OSs exposure as a cause of Multiple Sclerosis (MS).

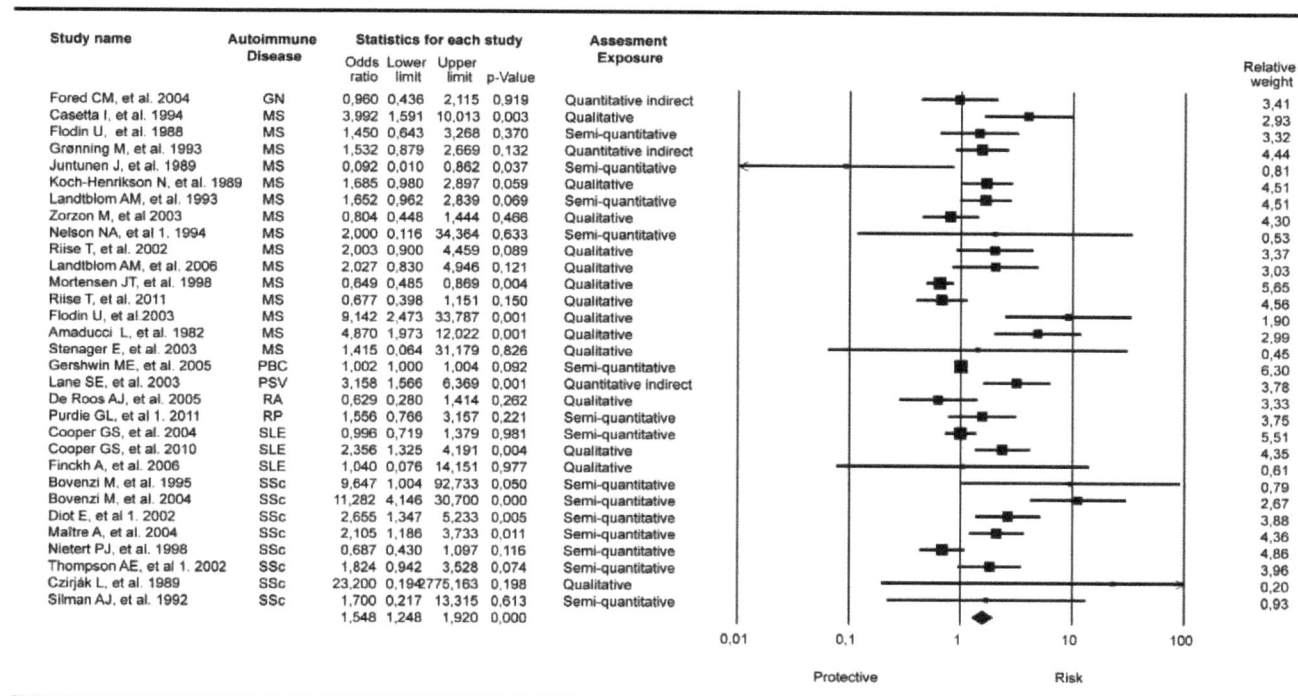

Figure 2. Forest plot of studies meta-analyzed: association between organic solvents and autoimmune disease as a trait. Footnote: final common effect size based on a random model. Odds Ratio (95%CI) with raw data from case control and cohort designed studies were included. The most relevant outcome per author was included. The relative weight of each study is included. GN: glomerulonephritis; MS: multiple sclerosis; PBC: primary biliary cirrhosis; PSV: primary systemic vasculitis; RA: rheumatoid arthritis; RP: Raynaud disease; SLE: systemic lupus erythematosus; SSc: systemic sclerosis. Diot, et al 1: organic solvent as a whole; Thompson AE, et al 1: turpentine exposure (the most significant result); Nelson NA, et al 1. 1994: disabled population; Purdie GL, et al 1. 2011 confirmed RP population.

They found 13 studies and reported an overall RR of 1.7 (with a 95% CI of 1.1–2.4). Later in 2001, Aryal BK et al [30] published a meta-analysis of SSc and solvent exposure. Eight studies met inclusion criteria, and the RR was reported to be 2.91 (with a 95% CI of 1.60 to 5.30). Kettaneh A et al in 2007 [31] published the most recent meta-analysis about occupational exposure to solvents and gender-related risk of SSc, they found a statistically significant association of SSc with OS exposure (OR 2.4; 95% CI 1.7–3.4: P = 0.002) and concluded that whereas SSc affects women predominantly, among subjects with occupational exposure to OS, men are at a higher risk of developing the disease than women. All the studies included in these publications were examined in our analysis. No meta-analysis evaluating ADs as a trait was found.

Regarding the systematic search for the OSs molecular mechanisms related to responses of immune system and ADs, with defined MeSH Terms and text words, retrieved 893 articles. After duplicates were removed, we obtained 827 articles of which 86 were included according to the inclusion criteria. The results are described in detail in Tables S3 and S4 and inclusion/exclusion criteria are described on Figure S28. Table 2 shows selected articles, representing main molecular processes related with OSs exposure and their potential implication on immune system or autoimmune pathologies. We found that the effects of OSs on the immune system include lymphoproliferation, autoantibody production, Th1 and Th17 responses, oxidative stress, protein modification as well as effects on gene expression.

Discussion

Our results indicate that OS exposure is a risk factor for developing ADs. Even though the individual meta-analyses (i.e. each AD considered separately) disclosed significant association for MS, PSV and SSc (Figure 3), the direction and significance of this association did not change when all ADs, considered as a single trait, were analyzed (Figure 2).Different combinations of factors involved in the generation of autoimmunity produce diverse clinical pictures within the wide spectrum of ADs (mosaic of autoimmunity) [2]. Our study, which takes into account both OSs as a whole and each solvent separately, reinforces this as well as the fact that ADs might share several common mechanisms(i.e., the autoimmune tautology) [98]. However, the term "separately," which is used to refer to the studies that analyze only one solvent, is not the most biologically appropriate because most of the solvents are a mixture [99].

Our meta-analysis with ORs as the measure of association including 31 articles regarding 8 ADs showed a significant relationship of OSs exposure with ADs (OR: 1.54; 95% CI: 1.25–1.92; p-value<0.001) and that with RRs as the measure of association including 10 articles and 5 ADs showed a near significant relationship (OR: 1.62; 95% CI: 0.99–2.65; p-value:0.051). When each AD was considered individually, there were also significant results with MS, PSV, SSc and PBC, although the latter was positively associated but not statistically significant.

A systematic and comprehensive review of the effects of OSs on the immune system is shown in Table 2. OSs are capable of altering cellular proliferation, apoptosis and tissue-specific function [100–126]. Both the amount and duration of OSs exposure are

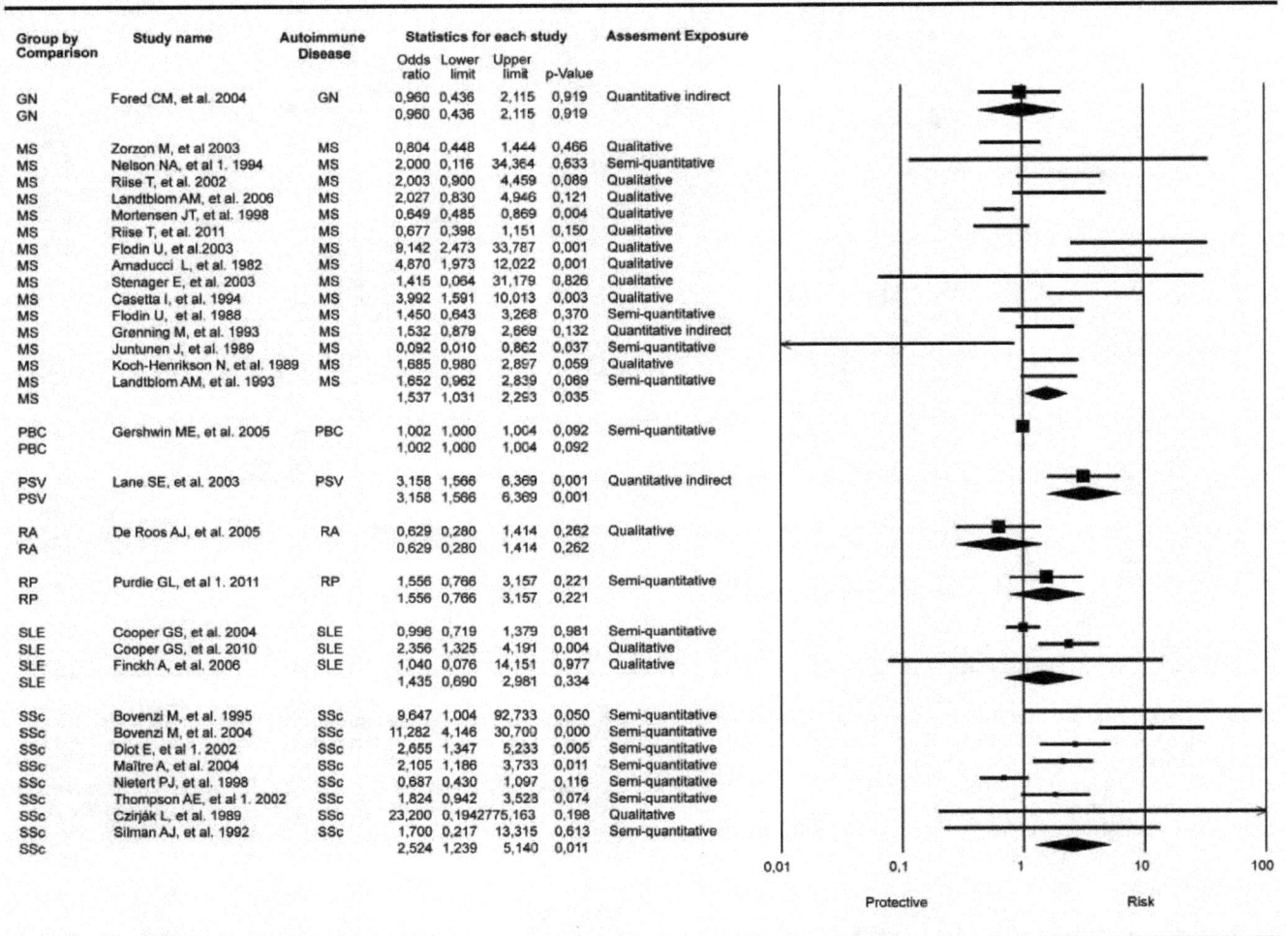

Figure 3. Forest plot of studies meta-analyzed grouping by comparison of specific autoimmune diseases. Footnote: random effect model showing significant association between SSC and OSs exposure. PBC and PSV included only one study (100% of the weight). Q value for SSc analysis: 33,7, I^2:79,2, Degree of freedom (Q):7, p-value<0,0001. GN: glomerulonephritis; MS: multiple sclerosis; PBC: primary biliary cirrhosis; PSV: primary systemic vasculitis; RA: rheumatoid arthritis; RP: raynaud disease; SLE: systemic lupus erythematosus; SSc: systemic sclerosis. Diot, et al 1: organic solvent as a whole; Thompson AE, et al 1: turpentine exposure (the most significant result); Purdie GL, et al 1: confirmed RP population; Nelson NA, et al 1. 1994: disabled population.

essential in pathology causation. Chronic exposure to OSs might lead to deposits in an organ and consequently to immune infiltration, similar to what is observed in ADs. The self-proteins that are modified by OSs may become immunogenic, recognized as foreign, and then initiate an inflammatory response and tissue injury. In this regard and according with our results, there are similar pathways operating on the incidence of ADs, but there are also specific mechanism that could lead to the particular manifestations of each AD; for instance, lymphocyte infiltration and immunoglobulin's deposits in SLE, and enzymatic alteration and scleroderma-specific antibody subsets in SSc [86,106,109].

Ketones are the most common OS used by the general population. Acetone, the simplest example of the ketones, is a commonly used solvent and is the active ingredient in nail polish remover and some paint thinners. It has been suggested that nail polish use may be associated with PBC [67]. These data are intriguing in view of the xenobiotic hypothesis proposed for the development of PBC with specific halogenated compounds. These compounds could increase the immunogenicity of mitochondrial

proteins and induce anti-mitochondrial antibodies in animal models [127]. In fact, only one clinical study was included in the meta-analysis regarding PBC and nail polish exposure disclosing a positive associated but not statistically significant [67]. More studies involving PBC patients searching for this association could be useful.

Long term exposure to OSs seems to foster massive hepatic mononuclear infiltration leading to autoimmune hepatitis although it is important to highlight that this infiltration is the first step in the immunopathogenesis of not only autoimmune hepatitis but also the rest of the ADs [108]. As shown by Cai et al [109], lymphocyte infiltration was found in the pancreas, lungs, and kidneys in addition to the liver.

In autoimmune thyroid disease, it is probable that solvents may interfere with iodine transportation and induce oxidative stress that leads to an inflammatory response to the thyroid gland [128].

The relevance of our results rely in the fact that relation between SSc and environmental exposure, especially involving OSs is significant. Mice MRL+/+, an autoimmunity susceptible

Table 2. Effects of the exposition to organic solvents on experimental models.

OS	EFFECTS ON PHENOTYPE	REFERENCES
TCE - DCAD	Lymphoproliferative reaction, ANAs and anti-cardiolipin autoantibodies production (Mouse).	[100]
TCE, PCE	Protein modification, TCE binds covalently with some proteins or lipids and form adducts (Rat, Mouse).	[101][102][103][104][105]
TCE	Splenocytes of mice treated with TCE secreted higher levels of IL-17 and IL-21. Protein adducts stimulate the activation of Th17 cells.	[125]
TCE	Production of ROS and NO, activation T cells; cellular infiltration (Mouse, Human Keratinocytes).	[109][111][126]
TCE	The low exposure to TCE generates a Th1-like cytokine responses and ANAs production; High-Exposure, increase CD44high T cells subsets with ability of IFN-γ secretion and cellular infiltration (Mouse).	[107]
TCE	Increase of CD4+ and CD8+ T cells population (Mouse).	[110]
TCE	Inhibition of cellular apoptosis of naive CD4+ and CD8+ T cells subset; anti-histone autoantibodies production (Mouse).	[111]
TCE-TCAH	Inhibition of lymphocyte apoptosis in the thymus through decrease FasL or peripheral lymphocyte (Mouse).	[112]
TCE + HgCl2	Anti-Hsp90 autoantibodies and antibodies against liver proteins production (Mouse).	[114]
TCE−DCVC	High-doses cause cellular necrosis. Low-doses produces changes in the transcription of several genes involved in apoptosis and cellular proliferation (Human).	[115]
TCE	Low-doses cause DNA-hypermetylation on cardiac myoblasts (Rat).	[116]
Benzene	Decrease of T cells population (cellular immunity) (American kestrels Birds).	[117]
Benzene	Decrease in number of CD4+ and CD8+ T cells, B cells, granulocyte and platelets (Human).	[118]
Benzene	Increase of ROS production and induction of DNA-fragmentation (Human).	[119]
Benzene	Changes in gene transcription involved in apoptosis, oxidative stress, cellular cycle and cytokine production (Mouse).	[121]
Toluene	High-doses affect the IFN-γ, IL.-4 and IL-13 production by T cells and increases TNF-α expression (Human PBMCs).	[122]
Toluene-hexane- Methyl ethyl Ketone	Produce oxidative stress (Human Jurkat Cells).	[123]
TCE −Benzene- HgCl2	Changes in gene expression with effects on cellular proliferation, apoptosis and tissue-specific function (Rat).	[124]

In parenthesis is shown the model where the effect was studied. OS: Organic solvent; TCE: Trichloroethylene; DCAC: dichloroacetyl chloride; TCAH: Trichloroacetaldehyde hydrate; HgCl2: Mercuric Chloride; DCVC: dichlorovinyl-l-cysteine; PCE: Perchloroethylene; ROS: Reactive Oxygen Species; NO: Nitric Oxide; ANA: Anti-Nuclear Antibodies; TNF-α: Tumor Necrosis Factor alpha; IFN-γ: Interferon Gama; IL-4: Interleukin 4.

strain, when exposed to TCE increase the total IgG serum concentration, antinuclear antibodies (ANAs) and anticardiolipin autoantibodies [100]. On the other hand, in an in vitro model of human epidermal keratinocytes, was possible to determinate that TCE not only stimulates reactive oxygen species release, but also it stimulates nitric oxide synthesis by nitric oxide synthase. These cellular changes may contribute to the physiopathological process that lead to skin injury such as shown in SSc [106]. The biological mechanisms by which OSs may induce the development of ADs support the results observed trough the meta-analysis.

Concerning MS, when an independent analysis was done for each disease, MS show a significant association with OSs exposure. These results are like those reported by Landtblom et al [29], in their 1996 meta-analysis. Landtblom et al implemented a Mantel-Haenszel RR calculation. The main differences between their analysis and ours rely on the statistical approach because the Mantel-Haenszel method for combining OR is an alternative to the fixed-effect inverse variance method and we developed a random effect model. Our meta-analysis included 15 MS studies, 7

new to the previous meta-analysis [26,55,59,63–66] published between 1994 and 2012.

The precise mechanisms responsible for the development of environmentally-induced autoimmune disorders are unknown. Although many hypotheses for the occurrence of autoimmune phenomena after various environmental exposures have been proposed, none of the hypotheses is completely supported by direct causal evidence. Also, mechanisms thought to be involved in the initiation of the disease process might differ from the mechanisms believed to exacerbate an established illness. However, the experimental approaches have been able to identify different environmental factors that use the same toxicity paths and mechanisms and either individually or jointly can have strong effects on molecular signaling pathways, immune responses or regulation mechanisms actively involved in health and disease (Figure 4 and Table 2).

It could be suggested that, as described for autoimmune/ inflammatory syndrome induced by adjuvants, the toxic effect

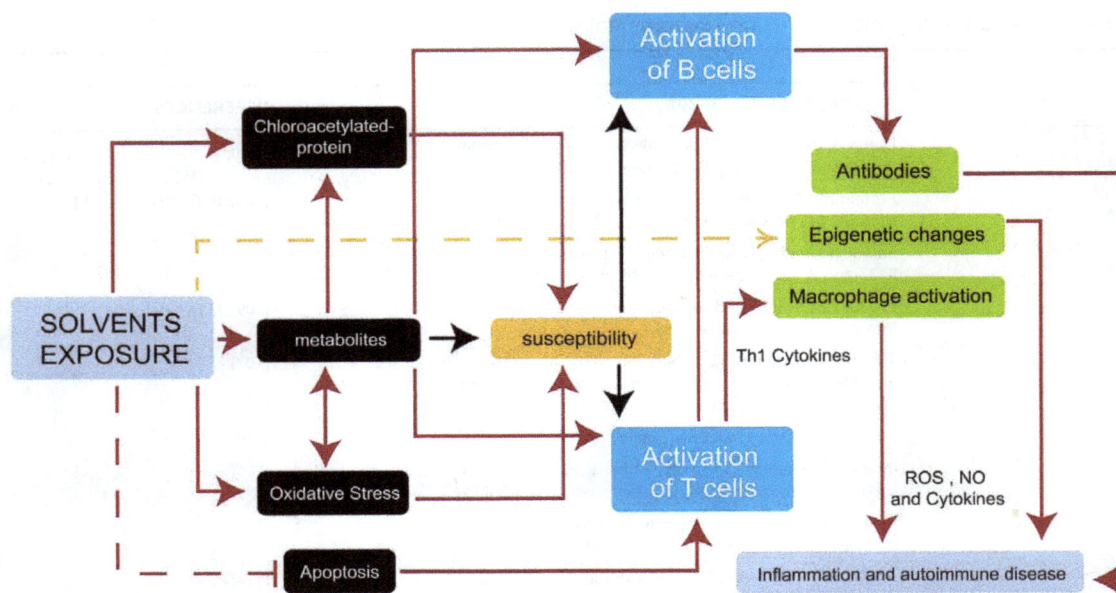

Figure 4. Potential molecular mechanisms implicated in solvent autoimmune disease development. Footnote: Solid red arrows represent known paths. Yellow dashed arrow represents hypothetical mechanisms (warranting future research), and red dashed line represents an inhibited process. In susceptible individuals, activation paths are stronger (black arrows). See text for details. ROS: Reactive oxygen Species; NO: Nitric Oxide.

influences the appearance of these conditions only in subjects who are genetically susceptible [13].

Study Limitations

Significant differences between case-control and cohort models were found. This fact can be explained by the limitations of each of these methodologies [129]. The following are the limitations in case-control studies. (I) the information about exposure is primarily based on interviews and may be subject to recall bias. (II) Validating the information on exposure can be difficult or even impossible. (III) By definition, case-control studies evaluate a single disease. (IV) The selection of an appropriate control group might be difficult. Most of the studies ignored the common origin of ADs and this generates the possibility of including patients with an underlying autoimmune condition as controls.

Most of the cohort studies included in our meta-analysis were retrospective. This implied that: (I) data was collected before the research hypothesis was defined leading to inaccurate data for the research. (II) The crude information was taken from databases or census. Therefore, the report on the exposure is not a direct quantification of the exposure. (III) The outcome information came from databases or medical records, but the subjects were not examined and this can lead to misdiagnosis. The explanation for why the result in the meta-analysis that included studies that reported the RR and raw data from cohort studies was not significant could be based on the abovementioned information as well as the low power due to a small sample size.

Exposure misclassification is a major problem when assessing the roll of environmental factors in complex diseases. Most individuals are not aware of the specific agents to which they have been exposed, and databases do not provide further information. None of the studies included in this meta-analysis employed an objective method of exposure assessment. Only two studies retrieved in this search [83,85] reported a direct-quantitative measure of exposure (i.e. TCE in concentrations from 6 to over

500 parts-per-billion [83]). After performing the analyses according to the exposure assessment category (figure S26) the final common effect size remained significantly associated as risk factor.

A significant effort is necessary to determine the proper way to test the causal factors for autoimmunity. Nevertheless, we believe that identifying the causal pathways of toxics already known to be associated with generating autoimmunity is a breakthrough. Standardizing the pathways as validated biomarkers would lead to more accurate studies. Future research on environmental exposure will enhance our knowledge of the common mechanisms associated with ADs.

In conclusion, an association between OSs exposure and ADs was observed. This approach could be applied to any study of the association between exposure to other toxics and ADs. Although OSs exposure has not yet been sufficiently investigated, in order to clarify their roles in ADs pathogenesis, there is a need to study their relationship with genes associated, whether involved in protection or susceptibility to each AD and their effects on development of the autoimmune process.

Supporting Information

Figure S1 Forest plot of supplementary meta-analyses. Footnote: final common effect size based on a random model. Odds Ratio (95%CI) with raw data from case control and cohort designed studies were included. Studies that provided uniquely RR data were not included for statistical reasons. Each different outcome of the studies with complex data structure was included.GN: glomerulonephritis; MS: multiple sclerosis; PBC: primary biliary cirrhosis; PSV: primary systemic vasculitis; RA: rheumatoid arthritis; RP: Raynaud disease; SLE: systemic lupus erythematosus; SSc: systemic sclerosis. The complex data structure and non-cumulative results of articles showing multiple independent or dependent subgroups included in the analysis was S1 Diot E, et al.2 2002 Exposition to chlorinate.

Figure S2   Forest plot of supplementary meta-analyses.
Final common effect size based on a random model. The studies included and abbreviations are the same as in Figure S1 with the exception of Diot E, et al.3 2002. Exposition to ketones.

Figure S3   Forest plot of supplementary meta-analyses.
Final common effect size based on a random model. The studies included and abbreviations are the same as in Figure S1 with the exception of Diot E, et al.4 2002. Exposition to aromatic.

Figure S4   Forest plot of supplementary meta-analyses.
Final common effect size based on a random model. The studies included and abbreviations are the same as in Figure S1 with the exception of Diot E, et al.5 2002. Exposition to toluene.

Figure S5   Forest plot of supplementary meta-analyses.
Final common effect size based on a random model. The studies included and abbreviations are the same as in Figure S1 with the exception of Diot e, et al.6. Exposition to TCE.

Figure S6   Forest plot of supplementary meta-analyses.
Final common effect size based on a random model. The studies included and abbreviations are the same as in Figure S1 with the exception of Nelson NA, et al 2. 1994 control population.

Figure S7   Forest plot of supplementary meta-analyses.
Final common effect size based on a random model. The studies included and abbreviations are the same as in Figure S1 with the exception of Purdie GL, et al 2. 2011 including confirmed and possible Raynaud.

Figure S8   Forest plot of supplementary meta-analyses.
Final common effect size based on a random model. The studies included and abbreviations are the same as in Figure S1 with the exception of Thompson AE, et al. 2002 10. Exposition to Bicromade.

Figure S9   Forest plot of supplementary meta-analyses.
Final common effect size based on a random model. The studies included and abbreviations are the same as in Figure S1 with the exception of Thompson AE, et al. 2002 11. Exposition to Toluene.

Figure S10   Forest plot of supplementary meta-analyses.
Final common effect size based on a random model. The studies included and abbreviations are the same as in Figure S1 with the exception of Thompson AE, et al. 2002 12. Exposition to Aromatic hydrocarbons.

Figure S11   Forest plot of supplementary meta-analyses.
Final common effect size based on a random model. The studies included and abbreviations are the same as in Figure S1 with the exception of Thompson AE, et al. 2002 13. Exposition to Aliphatic hydrocarbons.

Figure S12   Forest plot of supplementary meta-analyses.
Final common effect size based on a random model. The studies included and abbreviations are the same as in Figure S1 with the exception of Thompson AE, et al. 2002 14. Exposition to Fenfluramine.

Figure S13   Forest plot of supplementary meta-analyses.
Final common effect size based on a random model. The studies included and abbreviations are the same as in Figure S1 with the exception of Thompson AE, et al. 2002 15. Exposition to Diethylpropion.

Figure S14   Forest plot of supplementary meta-analyses.
Final common effect size based on a random model. The studies included and abbreviations are the same as in Figure S1 with the exception of Thompson AE, et al. 2002 16. Exposition to L5 Ohtryptophan.

Figure S15   Forest plot of supplementary meta-analyses.
Final common effect size based on a random model. The studies included and abbreviations are the same as in Figure S1 with the exception of Thompson AE, et al. 2002 2. Exposition to Benzene.

Figure S16   Forest plot of supplementary meta-analyses.
Final common effect size based on a random model. The studies included and abbreviations are the same as in Figure S1 with the exception of Thompson AE, et al. 2002 3. Exposition to White spirit.

Figure S17   Forest plot of supplementary meta-analyses.
Final common effect size based on a random model. The studies included and abbreviations are the same as in Figure S1 with the exception of Thompson AE, et al. 2002 4. Exposition to Perchlorethylene.

Figure S18   Forest plot of supplementary meta-analyses.
Final common effect size based on a random model. The studies included and abbreviations are the same as in Figure S1 with the exception of Thompson AE, et al. 2002 5. Exposition to Trichlorethylene.

Figure S19   Forest plot of supplementary meta-analyses.
Final common effect size based on a random model. The studies included and abbreviations are the same as in Figure S1 with the exception of Thompson AE, et al. 2002 6. Exposition to Trichlorethane.

Figure S20   Forest plot of supplementary meta-analyses.
Final common effect size based on a random model. The studies included and abbreviations are the same as in Figure S1 with the exception of Thompson AE, et al. 2002 7. Exposition to vinyl chloride.

Figure S21   Forest plot of supplementary meta-analyses.
Final common effect size based on a random model. The studies included and abbreviations are the same as in Figure S1 with the exception of Thompson AE, et al. 2002 8. Exposition to Urea formaldehyde.

Figure S22   Forest plot of supplementary meta-analyses.
Final common effect size based on a random model. The studies included and abbreviations are the same as in Figure S1 with the exception of Thompson AE, et al. 2002 9. Exposition to Meta-phenylenediamene.

Figures S23 Sensitivity analysis. Footnote: Odds Ratio (95%CI) excluding one study at a time. CI: confidence interval. Diot, et al 1: organic solvent as a whole; Thompson AE, et al 1: turpentine exposure (the most significant result); Purdie GL, et al 1: confirmed RP population; Nelson NA, et al 1. 1994: disabled population.

Figures S24 Cumulative analysis. Footnote: Odds Ratio (95%CI) The most relevant outcome per author was included. CI: confidence interval. Diot, et al 1: organic solvent as a whole; Thompson AE, et al 1: turpentine exposure (the most significant result); Purdie GL, et al 1: confirmed RP population; Nelson NA, et al 1. 1994: disabled population.

Figure S25 Forest plot of studies showing RR data and raw data from cohort studies. Footnote: final common effect size based on a random model. Risk Ratio (95%CI). CI: confidence interval; AS: Ankylosing spondylitis; GN: glomerulonephritis; MS: multiple sclerosis; RA: rheumatoid arthritis; RP: Raynaud disease; SLE: systemic lupus erythematosus; SSc: systemic sclerosis. Lundberg I, et al. 1 1994 painters AS; Lundberg I, et al. 3 1994 Substantial RA men; Lundberg I, et al. 5 1994 substantial RA women; Purdie GL, et al 1: confirmed RP population.

Figure S26 Forest plot of studies showing OR data according to the exposure assessment category. Footnote: Odds Ratio (95%CI). The most relevant outcome per author was included. GN: glomerulonephritis; MS: multiple sclerosis; PBC: primary biliary cirrhosis; PSV: primary systemic vasculitis; RA: rheumatoid arthritis; RP: Raynaud disease; SLE: systemic lupus erythematosus; SSc: systemic sclerosis. Diot, et al 1: organic solvent as a whole; Thompson AE, et al 1: turpentine exposure (the most significant result); Purdie GL, et al 1: confirmed RP population; Nelson NA, et al 1. 1994: disabled population.

Figure S27 Funnel Plot of standard error by log odds ratio. Footnote: X-axis: Log odds ratio. Y-axis: Standard Error.

Figure S28 Systematic Review Results for OSs molecular mechanisms related to responses of immune system and ADs. Footnote: ADs: Autoimmune Diseases.

Text S1 PRISMA 2009 Checklist. PRISMA: Preferred Reporting Items for Systematic Reviews and Meta-Analyses.

Table S1 Studies not included in the Meta-analysis. Footnote: AD: Autoimmune Disease; C-C: Case Control Study; OS: Organic Solvent; SSc: Systemic Sclerosis or Scleroderma; SLE: Systemic Lupus Erythematous; MS: Multiple Sclerosis; PSV: Primary systemic vasculitis; RA: Rheumatoid Arthritis; PBC: Primary Biliary Cirrhosis; GN: Glomerulonephritis; y/o: years old; VC: vinyl chloride; TCE: trichloroethylene; PCE: Perchlorethylene; RDX: Royal Demolition explosive; EEG: electroencephalographic study; PVC: polyvinyl chloride; ESRD: End Stage Renal Disease.

Table S2 Case reports and case series. Footnote: AD: Autoimmune Disease; OS: Organic Solvent; SSc: Systemic Sclerosis or Scleroderma; SLE: Systemic Lupus Erythematous; MS: Multiple Sclerosis; PSV: Primary systemic vasculitis; RA: Rheumatoid Arthritis; RD: Raynaud Disease; PBC: Primary Biliary Cirrhosis; GN: Glomerulonephritis; Anti- GBM: Anti-glomerular basement membrane antibody; PM/DM: Polimiositis/Dermatomiositis; y/o: years old; VC: vinyl chloride; TCE: trichloroethylene; PCE: Perchlorethylene; Jo-1: anti-histidyl-t-RNA synthetase.

Table S3 Search strategy related to solvent exposure and immune alterations.

Table S4 Effects of the exposition to organic solvents on experimental models.

Acknowledgments

We would like to thank our colleagues Jenny Amaya-Amaya, Zayrho DeSanVicente-Celis, Manuel Amador-Patarroyo, Catalina Herrera-Diaz, Jorge Cardenas Roldan, Juliana M. Giraldo-Villamil, Juan C. Castellanos, Omar-Javier Calixto, and Julian Caro M. for their fruitful contributions. We specially thank professors Yolanda Torres and Carlos E. Trillos for his advice, and Cesar Mantilla, chemical engineer specialist in industrial hygiene for his advice. We also thanks the reviewers for their fruitful criticism. This work was supported by Universidad del Rosario, Bogota, Colombia.

Author Contributions

Conceived and designed the experiments: ARV JMA RDM. Performed the experiments: CBM ARV JMA. Analyzed the data: ARV CBM. Contributed reagents/materials/analysis tools: CBM CSH GMO RDM JMA ARV. Wrote the paper: CBM CSH GMO RDM JMA ARV. Interpreted the possible pathways: GMO CSH.

References

1. Anaya JM (2010) The autoimmune tautology. Arthritis research & therapy 12: 147. doi:10.1186/ar3175.
2. Anaya JM, Corena R, Castiblanco J, Rojas-Villarraga A, Shoenfeld Y (2007) The kaleidoscope of autoimmunity: multiple autoimmune syndromes and familial autoimmunity. Expert review of clinical immunology 3: 623–635. doi:10.1586/1744666X.3.4.623.
3. Selmi C, Leung PSC, Sherr DH, Diaz M, Nyland JF, et al. (2012) Mechanisms of environmental influence on human autoimmunity: A national institute of environmental health sciences expert panel workshop. Journal of autoimmunity. Available: http://www.ncbi.nlm.nih.gov/pubmed/22749494. Accessed 19 October 2012.
4. Rook G (2011) Hygiene Hypothesis and Autoimmune Diseases. Clinical reviews in allergy & immunology: 5–15. doi:10.1007/s12016-011-8285-8.
5. Youinou P, Pers J-O, Gershwin ME, Shoenfeld Y (2010) Geo-epidemiology and autoimmunity. Journal of autoimmunity 34: J163–7.
6. Pigatto PD, Guzzi G (2010) Linking mercury amalgam to autoimmunity. Trends in immunology 31: 45–48. doi:10.1016/j.it.2009.12.004.
7. Finckh A, Cooper GS, Chibnik LB, Costenbader KH, Watts J, et al. (2006) Occupational silica and solvent exposures and risk of systemic lupus erythematosus in urban women. Arthritis and rheumatism 54: 3648–3654.
8. Kiyohara C, Washio M, Horiuchi T, Tada Y, Asami T, et al. (2009) Cigarette smoking, N-acetyltransferase 2 polymorphisms and systemic lupus erythematosus in a Japanese population. Lupus 18: 630–638.
9. Shoenfeld Y, Aharon-Maor A, Sherer Y (1997) Smoking and immunity: an additional player in the mosaic of autoimmunity. Scandinavian Journal of Immunology 45: 1–6.
10. Cooper GS, Gilbert KM, Greidinger EL, James JA, Pfau JC, et al. (2008) Recent advances and opportunities in research on lupus: environmental influences and mechanisms of disease. Environmental health perspectives 116: 695–702.
11. Chang C, Gershwin ME (2010) Drugs and autoimmunity A contemporary review and mechanistic approach. Journal of autoimmunity 34: J266–75.

12. Barbara G, Cremon C, Carini G, Bellacosa L, Zecchi L, et al. (2011) The immune system in irritable bowel syndrome. Journal of neurogastroenterology and motility 17: 349–359.

13. Shoenfeld Y, Agmon-Levin N (2011) "ASIA" - autoimmune/inflammatory syndrome induced by adjuvants. Journal of autoimmunity 36: 4–8. Available: http://www.ncbi.nlm.nih.gov/pubmed/20708902. Accessed 13 March 2012.

14. Shoenfeld Y, Selmi C, Zimlichman E, Gershwin ME (2008) The autoimmunologist: geoepidemiology, a new center of gravity, and prime time for autoimmunity. Journal of autoimmunity 31: 325–330. Available: http://www.ncbi.nlm.nih.gov/pubmed/18838248. Accessed 13 April 2012.

15. Chighizola C, Meroni PL (2012) The role of environmental estrogens and autoimmunity. Autoimmunity reviews 11: A493–501. Available: http://www.ncbi.nlm.nih.gov/pubmed/22172713. Accessed 19 October 2012.

16. Farhat SC, Silva CA, Orione MA, Campos LM, Sallum AM, et al. (2011) Air pollution in autoimmune rheumatic diseases: a review. Autoimmun Rev 11: 14–21. doi:S1568-9972(11)00150-9 [pii] 10.1016/j.autrev.2011.06.008 [doi].

17. Gourley M, Miller FW (2007) Mechanisms of disease: Environmental factors in the pathogenesis of rheumatic disease. Nature clinical practice Rheumatology 3: 172–180.

18. Garabrant DH, Dumas C (2000) Epidemiology of organic solvents and connective tissue disease. Arthritis research 2: 5–15.

19. Miller FW, Alfredsson L, Costenbader KH, Kamen DL, Nelson LM, et al. (2012) Epidemiology of environmental exposures and human autoimmune diseases: Findings from a National Institute of Environmental Health Sciences Expert Panel Workshop. Journal of autoimmunity. doi:10.1016/j.jaut.2012.05.002.

20. Moher D, Liberati A, Tetzlaff J, Altman DG (2009) Preferred reporting items for systematic reviews and meta-analyses: the PRISMA statement. Bmj 339: b2535–b2535. doi:10.1136/bmj.b2535.

21. Lozano-Calderón S, Anthony S, Ring D (2008) The quality and strength of evidence for etiology: example of carpal tunnel syndrome. The Journal of hand surgery 33: 525–538. doi:10.1016/j.jhsa.2008.01.004.

22. Marrie RA (2004) Reviews Environmental risk factors in multiple sclerosis aetiology. Neurology 3: 709–718.

23. Casetta I, Granieri E, Malagu S, Tola MR, Paolino E, et al. (1994) Environmental risk factors and multiple sclerosis: a community-based, case-control study in the province of Ferrara, Italy. Neuroepidemiology 13: 120–128.

24. Garnier R, Bazire A, Chataigner D (2006) Sclérodermie et exposition professionnelle aux solvants organiques. Archives des Maladies Professionnelles et de l'Environnement 67: 488–504. doi:ADMP-06-2006-67-3-1250-3274-101019-200518826.

25. Hopkins RS, Indian RW, Pinnow E, Conomy J (1991) Multiple sclerosis in Galion, Ohio: prevalence and results of a case-control study. Neuroepidemiology 10: 192–199. Available: http://www.ncbi.nlm.nih.gov/pubmed/1745329. Accessed 9 January 2012.

26. Stenager E, Brønnum-Hansen H, Koch-Henriksen N (2003) Risk of multiple sclerosis in nurse anaesthetists. Multiple Sclerosis 9: 427–428.

27. Flodin U (1988) Multiple sclerosis, solvents, and pets. Archives of neurology 47: 128.

28. Zachariae H, Bjerring P, Søndergaard KH, Halkier-Sørensen L (1997) Occupational systemic sclerosis in men. Ugeskrift For Laeger 159: 2687–2689.

29. Landtblom AM, Flodin U, Söderfeldt B, Wolfson C, Axelson O (1996) Organic solvents and multiple sclerosis: a synthesis of the current evidence. Epidemiology (Cambridge, Mass) 7: 429–433.

30. Aryal BK, Khuder S, Schaub E (2001) Meta-analysis of systemic sclerosis and exposure to solvents. American journal of industrial medicine 40: 271–274.

31. Kettaneh A, Al Moufti O, Tiev K, Chayet C, Tolédano C, et al. (2007) Occupational exposure to solvents and gender-related risk of systemic sclerosis: a metaanalysis of case-control studies. The Journal of rheumatology 34: 97–103.

32. Fernández J, Sanz-Gallén PNS (2010) Seguimiento de dos pacientes con glomerulonefritis iga mesangial con antecedentes de exposición a tóxicos (cadmio y disolventes orgánicos) Follow-up of two patients with mesangial IgA glomerulonephritis exposed to cadmium and organic solvents. 33: 309–314.

33. Savige JA, Dowling J, Kincaid-Smith P (1989) Superimposed glomerular immune complexes in anti-glomerular basement membrane disease. American journal of kidney diseases: the official journal of the National Kidney Foundation 14: 145–153. Available: http://www.ncbi.nlm.nih.gov/pubmed/2757019. Accessed 9 January 2012.

34. Brautbar N, Richter ED, Nesher G (2004) Systemic vasculitis and prior recent exposure to organic solvents: report of two cases. Archives of environmental health 59: 515–517. Available: http://www.ncbi.nlm.nih.gov/pubmed/16425661. Accessed 9 January 2012.

35. Calvani N, Silvestris F, Dammacco F (n.d.) Familial systemic sclerosis following exposure to organic solvents and the possible implication of genetic factors. Annali italiani di medicina interna: organo ufficiale della Società italiana di medicina interna 16: 175–178. Available: http://www.ncbi.nlm.nih.gov/pubmed/11692907. Accessed 9 January 2012.

36. Petkova V, Nakova L, Matakeva M (1992) [A clinical observation of vinyl chloride-induced disease]. Problemi na khigienata 17: 195–199. Available: http://www.ncbi.nlm.nih.gov/pubmed/1364541. Accessed 9 January 2012.

37. Reis J, Dietemann JL, Warter JM, Poser CM (2001) A case of multiple sclerosis triggered by organic solvents. Neurological sciences official journal of the Italian Neurological Society and of the Italian Society of Clinical Neurophysiology 22: 155–158.

38. Amaducci L, Arfaioli C, Inzitari D, Martinetti MG (1978) Another possible precipitating factor in multiple sclerosis: the exposure to organic solvents. Bollettino dell'Istituto sieroterapico milanese 56: 613–617.

39. Magnavita N, Bergamaschi A, Garcovich A, Giuliano G (1986) Vasculitic Purpura in Vinyl Chloride Disease: A Case Report. Angiology 37: 382–388.

40. Ohtsuka T (2009) Organic solvent-induced myopathy simulating eosinophilic fasciitis and/or dermatomyositis. The Journal of dermatology 36: 358–359.

41. Serratrice J, Granel B, Pache X, Disdier P, De Roux-Serratrice C, et al. (2001) A case of polymyositis with anti-histidyl-t-RNA synthetase (Jo-1) antibody syndrome following extensive vinyl chloride exposure. Clinical rheumatology 20: 379–382. Available: http://www.ncbi.nlm.nih.gov/pubmed/11642524. Accessed 9 January 2012.

42. Benzarti A, Amor AB, Euch DE, Mbazaa A, Osmen AB, et al. (2010) Sclérodermie systémique et exposition professionnelle aux solvants organiques «perchloréthylène». À propos d'un cas Systemic sclerosis and occupational exposure to organic solvents: " Perchlorethylene ", a case. Occupational and Environmental Medicine 50: 501–508.

43. Hinnen U, Schmid-Grendelmeier P, Müller E, Elsner P (1995) [Exposure to solvents in scleroderma: disseminated circumscribed scleroderma (morphea) in a painter exposed to perchloroethylene]. Schweizerische medizinische Wochenschrift 125: 2433–2437. Available: http://www.ncbi.nlm.nih.gov/pubmed/8553031. Accessed 9 January 2012.

44. Garcia-Zamalloa AM, Ojeda E, Gonzalez-Beneitez C, Goni J, Garrido A (1994) Systemic sclerosis and organic solvents: early diagnosis in industry. Annals of the Rheumatic Diseases 53: 618.

45. Bottomley WW, Sheehan-Dare RA, Hughes P, Cunliffe WJ (1993) A sclerodermatous syndrome with unusual features following prolonged occupational exposure to organic solvents. The British journal of dermatology 128: 203–206. Available: http://www.ncbi.nlm.nih.gov/pubmed/8457454. Accessed 9 January 2012.

46. Tibon-Fisher O, Heller E, Ribak J (1992) [Occupational scleroderma due to organic solvent exposure]. Harefuah 122: 530–532, 551. Available: http://www.ncbi.nlm.nih.gov/pubmed/1398326. Accessed 9 January 2012.

47. Brasington RD, Thorpe-Swenson AJ (1991) Systemic sclerosis associated with cutaneous exposure to solvent: case report and review of the literature. Arthritis & Rheumatism 34: 631–633.

48. Karamfilov T, Buslau M, Dürr C, Weyers W (2003) [Pansclerotic porphyria cutanea tarda after chronic exposure to organic solvents]. Der Hautarzt; Zeitschrift für Dermatologie, Venerologie, und verwandte Gebiete 54: 448–452.

49. Pralong P, Cavailhes A, Balme B, Cottin V, Skowron F (2009) [Diffuse systemic sclerosis after occupational exposure to trichloroethylene and perchloroethylene]. Annales de dermatologie et de vénéréologie 136: 713–717.

50. Sparrow GP (1977) A connective tissue disorder similar to vinyl chloride disease in a patient exposed to perchloroethylene. Clinical and experimental dermatology 2: 17–22.

51. Czirják L, Pócs E, Szegedi G (1994) Localized scleroderma after exposure to organic solvents. Dermatology (Basel, Switzerland) 189: 399–401. Available: http://www.ncbi.nlm.nih.gov/pubmed/7873829. Accessed 9 January 2012.

52. Lundberg I, Alfredsson L, Plato N, Sverdrup B, Klareskog L, et al. (1994) Occupation, occupational exposure to chemicals and rheumatological disease. A register based cohort study. Scandinavian journal of rheumatology 23: 305–310.

53. Fored CM, Nise G, Ejerblad E (2004) Absence of association between organic solvent exposure and risk of chronic renal failure: a nationwide population-based case-control study. Journal of the: 180–186. doi:10.1097/01.ASN.0000103872.60993.06.

54. Sesso R, Stolley PD, Salgado N, Pereira AB, Ramos OL (1990) Exposure to hydrocarbons and rapidly progressive glomerulonephritis. Brazilian journal of medical and biological research Revista brasileira de pesquisas medicas e biologicas Sociedade Brasileira de Biofisica et al 23: 225–233.

55. Flodin U, Landtblom A-M, Axelson O (2003) Multiple sclerosis in nurse anaesthetists. Occupational and environmental medicine 60: 66–68.

56. Amaducci L, Arfaioli C, Inzitari D, Marchi M (1982) Multiple sclerosis among shoe and leather workers: an epidemiological survey in Florence. Acta neurologica Scandinavica 65: 94–103.

57. Nelson NA, Robins TG, White RF, Garrison RP (1994) A case-control study of chronic neuropsychiatric disease and organic solvent exposure in automobile assembly plant workers. Occupational and environmental medicine 51: 302–307.

58. Grønning M, Albrektsen G, Kvåle G, Moen B, Aarli JA, et al. (1993) Organic solvents and multiple sclerosis: a case-control study. Acta Neurologica Scandinavica 88: 247–250.

59. Zorzon M, Zivadinov R, Nasuelli D, Dolfini P, Bosco A, et al. (2003) Risk factors of multiple sclerosis: a case-control study. Neurological sciences: official journal of the Italian Neurological Society and of the Italian Society of Clinical Neurophysiology 24: 242–247.

60. Juntunen J, Kinnunen E, Antti-Poika M, Koskenvuo M (1989) Multiple sclerosis and occupational exposure to chemicals: a co-twin control study of a nationwide series of twins. British journal of industrial medicine 46: 417–419.

61. Koch-Henriksen N (1989) An epidemiological study of multiple sclerosis. Familial aggregation social determinants, and exogenic factors. Acta neurologica Scandinavica Supplementum 124: 1–123.

62. Landtblom AM, Flodin U, Karlsson M, Palhagen S, Axelson O, et al. (1993) Multiple sclerosis and exposure to solvents, ionizing radiation and animals. Scandinavian Journal of Work, Environment & Health 19: 399–404.

63. Landtblom A-M, Tondel M, Hjalmarsson P, Flodin U, Axelson O (2006) The risk for multiple sclerosis in female nurse anaesthetists: a register based study. Occupational and Environmental Medicine 63: 387–389.

64. Mortensen JT, Brønnum-Hansen H, Rasmussen K (1998) Multiple sclerosis and organic solvents. Epidemiology (Cambridge, Mass) 9: 168–171. Available: http://www.ncbi.nlm.nih.gov/pubmed/9504285. Accessed 9 January 2012.

65. Riise T, Moen BE, Kyvik KR (2002) Organic solvents and the risk of multiple sclerosis. Epidemiology (Cambridge, Mass) 13: 718–720. Available: http://www.ncbi.nlm.nih.gov/pubmed/12410015. Accessed 9 January 2012.

66. Riise T, Kirkeleit J, Aarseth JH, Farbu E, Midgard R, et al. (2011) Risk of MS is not associated with exposure to crude oil, but increases with low level of education. Multiple sclerosis (Houndmills, Basingstoke, England) 17: 780–787. doi:10.1177/1352458510397686.

67. Gershwin ME, Selmi C, Worman HJ, Gold EB, Watnik M, et al. (2005) Risk factors and comorbidities in primary biliary cirrhosis: a controlled interview-based study of 1032 patients. Hepatology 42: 1194–1202.

68. Lane SE, Watts RA, Bentham G, Innes NJ, Scott DGI (2003) Are environmental factors important in primary systemic vasculitis? A case-control study. Arthritis and rheumatism 48: 814–823.

69. De Roos AJ, Cooper GS, Alavanja MC, Sandler DP (2005) Rheumatoid arthritis among women in the Agricultural Health Study: risk associated with farming activities and exposures. Annals of epidemiology 15: 762–770. doi:10.1016/j.annepidem.2005.08.001.

70. Purdie GL, Purdie DJ, Harrison A (2011) Raynaud's Phenomenon in medical laboratory workers who work with solvents. The Journal of rheumatology 38: 1940–1946.

71. Cooper GS, Parks CG, Treadwell EL, Clair EW (2004) Occupational Risk Factors for the Development of Systemic Lupus Erythematosus. Journal of Rheumatology Oct;31(10): 1928–1933.

72. Cooper GS, Wither J, Bernatsky S, Claudio JO, Clarke A, et al. (2010) Occupational and environmental exposures and risk of systemic lupus erythematosus: silica, sunlight, solvents. Rheumatology (Oxford, England) 49: 2172–2180.

73. Nietert PJ, Sutherland SE, Silver RM, Pandey JP, Knapp RG, et al. (1998) Is occupational organic solvent exposure a risk factor for scleroderma? Arthritis & Rheumatism 41: 1111–1118.

74. Bovenzi M, Barbone F, Betta A, Tommasini M, Versini W (1995) Scleroderma and occupational exposure Short Communications Scleroderma and occupational exposure. Health (San Francisco) 21: 289–292.

75. Bovenzi M, Barbone F, Pisa FE, Betta A, Romeo L, et al. (2004) A case-control study of occupational exposures and systemic sclerosis. International Archives of Occupational and Environmental Health 77: 10–16.

76. Diot E, Lesire V, Guilmot JL, Metzger MD, Pilore R, et al. (2002) Systemic sclerosis and occupational risk factors: a case-control study. Occupational and environmental medicine 59: 545–549.

77. Maître A, Hours M, Bonneterre V, Arnaud J, Arslan MT, et al. (2004) Systemic sclerosis and occupational risk factors: role of solvents and cleaning products. The Journal of 31.

78. Thompson AE, Pope JE (2002) Increased prevalence of scleroderma in southwestern Ontario: a cluster analysis. Increased Prevalence of Scleroderma in Southwestern Ontario: A Cluster Analysis. Journal of Rheumatology 29.

79. Silman AJ, Jones S (1992) What is the contribution of occupational environmental factors to the occurrence of scleroderma in men? Annals of the rheumatic diseases 51: 1322–1324.

80. Czirják L, Bokk A, Csontos G, Lörincz G, Szegedi G (1989) Clinical findings in 61 patients with progressive systemic sclerosis. Acta dermatovenereologica 69: 533–536.

81. Black CM, Welsh KI, Walker AE, Bernstein RM, Catoggio LJ, et al. (1983) Genetic susceptibility to scleroderma-like syndrome induced by vinyl chloride. Lancet 1: 53–55.

82. Landtblom A, Wastenson M, Ahmadi A, Söderkvist P (2003) Multiple sclerosis and exposure to organic solvents, investigated by genetic polymorphisms of the GSTM1 and CYP2D6 enzyme systems. Neurological sciences : official journal of the Italian Neurological Society and of the Italian Society of Clinical Neurophysiology 24: 248–251. doi:10.1007/s10072-003-0148-5.

83. Kilburn KH, Warshaw RH (1992) Prevalence of symptoms of systemic lupus erythematosus (SLE) and of fluorescent antinuclear antibodies associated with chronic exposure to trichloroethylene and other chemicals in well water. Environmental Research 57: 1–9.

84. Souberbielle BE, Martin-Mondiere C, O'Brien ME, Carydakis C, Cesaro P, et al. (1990) A case-control epidemiological study of MS in the Paris area with particular reference to past disease history and profession. Acta neurologica Scandinavica 82: 303–310.

85. Hathaway JA, Buck CR (1977) Absence of health hazards associated with RDX manufacture and use. Journal of occupational medicine: official publication of the Industrial Medical Association 19: 269–272. Available: http://www.ncbi.nlm.nih.gov/pubmed/323432. Accessed 9 January 2012.

86. Povey A, Guppy MJ, Wood M, Knight C, Black CM, et al. (2001) Cytochrome P2 polymorphisms and susceptibility to scleroderma following exposure to organic solvents. Arthritis and rheumatism 44: 662–665. Available: http://www.ncbi.nlm.nih.gov/pubmed/11263781. Accessed 9 January 2012.

87. Albert DA, Albert AN, Vernace M, Sebastian JK, Hsia EC (2005) Analysis of a Cluster of Cases of Wegener Granulomatosis. JCR: Journal of Clinical Rheumatology 11: 188–193.

88. Brogren CH, Christensen JM, Rasmussen K (1986) Occupational exposure to chlorinated organic solvents and its effect on the renal excretion of N-acetyl-beta-D-glucosaminidase. Archives of toxicology Supplement = Archiv für Toxikologie Supplement 9: 460–464. Available: http://www.ncbi.nlm.nih.gov/pubmed/3468929. Accessed 9 January 2012.

89. Goldman JA (1996) Connective tissue disease in people exposed to organic chemical solvents: systemic sclerosis (scleroderma) in dry cleaning plant and aircraft industry workers. Journal of clinical rheumatology: practical reports on rheumatic & musculoskeletal diseases 2: 185–190.

90. Koischwitz D, Marsteller HJ, Lackner K, Brecht G, Brecht T (1980) [Changes in the arteries in the hand and fingers due to vinyl chloride exposure (author's transl)]. RöFo: Fortschritte auf dem Gebiete der Röntgenstrahlen und der Nuklearmedizin 132: 62–68. Available: http://www.ncbi.nlm.nih.gov/pubmed/6446500. Accessed 9 January 2012.

91. Sińczuk-Walczak H, Głuszcz M (1982) [Various aspects of the clinical and electroencephalographic studies in workers chronically exposed to vinyl chloride]. Medycyna pracy 33: 349–354. Available: http://www.ncbi.nlm.nih.gov/pubmed/7182717. Accessed 9 January 2012.

92. Hotz P, Thielemans N, Bernard A (1993) Serum laminin, hydrocarbon exposure, and glomerular damage. British journal of: 1104–1110.

93. Hsieh H-I, Chen P-C, Wong R-H, Wang J-D, Yang P-M, et al. (2007) Effect of the CYP2E1 genotype on vinyl chloride monomer-induced liver fibrosis among polyvinyl chloride workers. Toxicology 239: 34–44.

94. Jacob S, Héry M, Protois J-C, Rossert J, Stengel B (2007) Effect of organic solvent exposure on chronic kidney disease progression: the GN-PROGRESS cohort study. Journal of the American Society of Nephrology: JASN 18: 274–281. doi:10.1681/ASN.2006060652.

95. Jacob S, Hery M, Protois J-C, Rossert J, Stengel B (2007) New insight into solvent-related End Stage Renal Disease: occupations, products and types of solvents at risk. Occupational and environmental medicine. Available: http://www.pubmedcentral.nih.gov/articlerender.fcgi?artid=2095352&tool=pmcentrez&rendertype=abstract. Accessed 30 December 2011.

96. Prince MI, Ducker SJ, James OF (2010) Case-control studies of risk factors for primary biliary cirrhosis in two United Kingdom populations. Gut 59: 508–512. doi:10.1136/gut.2009.184218.

97. Magnant J, de Monte M, Guilmot JL, Lasfargues G, Diot P, et al. (2005) Relationship between occupational risk factors and severity markers of systemic sclerosis. The Journal of rheumatology 32: 1713–1718.

98. Anaya J-M, Rojas-Villarraga A, García-Carrasco M (2012) The autoimmune tautology: from polyautoimmunity and familial autoimmunity to the autoimmune genes. Autoimmune diseases 2012: 297193. Available: http://www.pubmedcentral.nih.gov/articlerender.fcgi?artid=3362807&tool=pmcentrez&rendertype=abstract. Accessed 29 October 2012.

99. United States Department of Labor: Safety and Health Topics | Solvents (n.d.).

100. Khan MF, Kaphalia BS, Prabhakar BS (1995) Trichloroethene-induced autoimmune response in female MRL+/+ mice. Toxicology and applied 134: 155–160. doi:10.1006/taap.1995.1179.

101. Halmes NC, Perkins EJ, McMillan DC, Pumford NR (1997) Detection of trichloroethylene-protein adducts in rat liver and plasma. Toxicology letters 92: 187–194.

102. Cai P, Konig MF, Khan MF, Kaphalia BS, Ansari GA (2007) Differential immune responses to albumin adducts of reactive intermediates of trichloroethene in MRL+/+ mice. Toxicology and applied 220: 278–283. doi:10.1016/j.taap.2007.01.020.

103. Wang G, König R, Ansari GAS, Khan MF (2008) Lipid peroxidation-derived aldehyde-protein adducts contribute to trichloroethene-mediated autoimmunity via activation of CD4+ T cells. Free radical biology & medicine 44: 1475–1482. Available: http://www.pubmedcentral.nih.gov/articlerender.fcgi?artid=2440665&tool=pmcentrez&rendertype=abstract. Accessed 9 January 2012.

104. Wang G, Ansari GAS, Khan MF (2007) Involvement of lipid peroxidation-derived aldehyde-protein adducts in autoimmunity mediated by trichloroethene. Journal of toxicology and environmental health Part A 70: 1977–1985. Available: http://www.ncbi.nlm.nih.gov/pubmed/17966069. Accessed 9 January 2012.

105. Grune T, Michel P, Sitte N, Eggert W, Albrecht-Nebe H, et al. (1997) Increased levels of 4-hydroxynonenal modified proteins in plasma of children with autoimmune diseases. Free radical biology & medicine 23: 357–360.

106. Wang G, Cai P, Ansari GAS, Khan MF (2007) Oxidative and nitrosative stress in trichloroethene-mediated autoimmune response. Toxicology 229: 186–193. Available: http://www.pubmedcentral.nih.gov/articlerender.fcgi?artid=1945101&tool=pmcentrez&rendertype=abstract. Accessed 5 January 2012.

107. Griffin JM, Blossom SJ, Jackson SK, Gilbert KM, Pumford NR (2000) Trichloroethylene accelerates an autoimmune response by Th1 T cell activation in MRL +/+ mice. Immunopharmacology 46: 123–137.

108. Griffin JM, Gilbert KM, Lamps LW, Pumford NR (2000) CD4(+) T-cell activation and induction of autoimmune hepatitis following trichloroethylene

treatment in MRL+/+ mice. Toxicological sciences: an official journal of the Society of Toxicology 57: 345–352.

109. Cai P, König R, Boor PJ, Kondraganti S, Kaphalia BS, et al. (2008) Chronic exposure to trichloroethene causes early onset of SLE-like disease in female MRL +/+ mice. Toxicology and applied pharmacology 228: 68–75. Available: http://www.pubmedcentral.nih.gov/articlerender.fcgi?artid = 2442272&tool = pmcentrez&rendertype = abstract. Accessed 9 January 2012.

110. Peden-Adams MM, Eudaly JG, Heesemann LM, Smythe J, Miller J, et al. (2006) Developmental immunotoxicity of trichloroethylene (TCE): studies in B6C3F1 mice. Journal of environmental science and health Part A, Toxic/ hazardous substances & environmental engineering 41: 249–271. Available: http://www.ncbi.nlm.nih.gov/pubmed/16484062. Accessed 9 January 2012.

111. Blossom SJ, Doss JC (2007) Trichloroethylene alters central and peripheral immune function in autoimmune-prone MRL(+/+) mice following continuous developmental and early life exposure. Journal of immunotoxicology 4: 129–141. Available: http://www.ncbi.nlm.nih.gov/pubmed/18958721. Accessed 9 January 2012.

112. Blossom SJ, Gilbert KM (2006) Exposure to a metabolite of the environmental toxicant, trichloroethylene, attenuates CD4+ T cell activation-induced cell death by metalloproteinase-dependent FasL shedding. Toxicological sciences : an official journal of the Society of Toxicology 92: 103–114. Available: http://www.ncbi.nlm.nih.gov/pubmed/16641322. Accessed 7 December 2011.

113. Gilbert KM, Pumford NR, Blossom SJ (2006) Environmental contaminant trichloroethylene promotes autoimmune disease and inhibits T-cell apoptosis in MRL(+/+) mice. Journal of immunotoxicology 3: 263–267. doi:10.1080/15476910601023578.

114. Gilbert KM, Rowley B, Gomez-Acevedo H, Blossom SJ (2011) Coexposure to mercury increases immunotoxicity of trichloroethylene. Toxicological sciences: an official journal of the Society of Toxicology 119: 281–292. Available: http://www.pubmedcentral.nih.gov/articlerender.fcgi?artid = 3023566&tool = pmcentrez&rendertype = abstract. Accessed 30 September 2011.

115. Lash LH, Putt DA, Hueni SE, Horwitz BP (2005) Molecular markers of trichloroethylene-induced toxicity in human kidney cells. Toxicology and applied pharmacology 206: 157–168. Available: http://www.ncbi.nlm.nih.gov/pubmed/15967204. Accessed 9 January 2012.

116. Palbykin B, Borg J, Caldwell PT, Rowles J, Papoutsis AJ, et al. (2011) Trichloroethylene induces methylation of the Serca2 promoter in H9c2 cells and embryonic heart. Cardiovascular toxicology 11: 204–214. doi:10.1007/s12012-011-9113-3.

117. Olsgard ML, Bortolotti GR, Trask BR, Smits JEG (2008) Effects of inhalation exposure to a binary mixture of benzene and toluene on vitamin a status and humoral and cell-mediated immunity in wild and captive American kestrels. Journal of toxicology and environmental health Part A 71: 1100–1108. Available: http://www.ncbi.nlm.nih.gov/pubmed/18569622. Accessed 9 January 2012.

118. Lan Q, Zhang L, Li G, Vermeulen R, Weinberg RS (2004) Hematotoxicity in workers exposed to low levels of benzene. Science 306: 1774–1776. doi:10.1126/science.1102443.

119. Emara AM, El-Bahrawy H (2008) Green tea attenuates benzene-induced oxidative stress in pump workers. Journal of immunotoxicology 5: 69–80. Available: http://www.ncbi.nlm.nih.gov/pubmed/18382860. Accessed 9 January 2012.

120. Seaton MJ, Schlosser P, Medinsky MA (1995) In vitro conjugation of benzene metabolites by human liver: potential influence of interindividual variability on benzene toxicity. Carcinogenesis 16: 1519–1527.

121. Park H-J, Oh JH, Yoon S, Rana SVS (2008) Time Dependent Gene Expression Changes in the Liver of Mice Treated with Benzene. Biomarker insights 3: 191–201. Available: http://www.pubmedcentral.nih.gov/articlerender.fcgi?artid = 2688356&tool = pmcentrez&rendertype = abstract. Accessed 9 January 2012.

122. Wichmann G, Mühlenberg J, Fischäder G, Kulla C, Rehwagen M, et al. (2005) An experimental model for the determination of immunomodulating effects by volatile compounds. Toxicology in vitro: an international journal published in association with BIBRA 19: 685–693. doi:10.1016/j.tiv.2005.03.012.

123. McDermott C, Allshire A, van Pelt F, Heffron JJA (2008) In vitro exposure of jurkat T-cells to industrially important organic solvents in binary combination: interaction analysis. Toxicological sciences: an official journal of the Society of Toxicology 101: 263–274. Available: http://www.ncbi.nlm.nih.gov/pubmed/17982160. Accessed 9 January 2012.

124. Hendriksen PJM, Freidig AP, Jonker D, Thissen U, Bogaards JJP, et al. (2007) Transcriptomics analysis of interactive effects of benzene, trichloroethylene and methyl mercury within binary and ternary mixtures on the liver and kidney following subchronic exposure in the rat. Toxicology and applied pharmacology 225: 171–188. Available: http://www.ncbi.nlm.nih.gov/pubmed/17905399. Accessed 9 January 2012.

125. Wang G, Wang J, Fan X, Ansari GAS, Khan MF (2012) Protein adducts of malondialdehyde and 4-hydroxynonenal contribute to trichloroethene-mediated autoimmunity via activating Th17 cells: dose- and time-response studies in female MRL+/+ mice. Toxicology 292: 113–122. doi:10.1016/j.tox.2011.12.001.

126. Shen T, Zhu Q-X, Yang S, Ding R, Ma T, et al. (2007) Trichloroethylene induce nitric oxide production and nitric oxide synthase mRNA expression in cultured normal human epidermal keratinocytes. Toxicology 239: 186–194. Available: http://www.ncbi.nlm.nih.gov/pubmed/17719164. Accessed 19 June 2011.

127. Rieger R, Gershwin ME (2007) The X and why of xenobiotics in primary biliary cirrhosis. Journal of autoimmunity 28: 76–84. doi:10.1016/j.jaut.2007.02.003.

128. Duntas LH (2008) Environmental factors and autoimmune thyroiditis. Nature clinical practice Endocrinology & metabolism 4: 454–460. Available: http://www.ncbi.nlm.nih.gov/pubmed/18607401. Accessed 22 November 2011.

129. Noordzij M, Dekker FW, Zoccali C, Jager KJ (2009) Study designs in clinical research. Nephron Clinical Practice 113: c218–c221. Available: http://www.ncbi.nlm.nih.gov/pubmed/19690439. Accessed 22 November 2012.

Permissions

List of Contributors

Laura L. Vines, Melissa A. Bates
Department of Food Science and Human Nutrition, Diagnostic Center for Population and Animal Health, Michigan State University, East Lansing, Michigan, United States of America
Center for Integrative Toxicology, Diagnostic Center for Population and Animal Health, Michigan State University, East Lansing, Michigan, United States of America

James J. Pestka
Department of Food Science and Human Nutrition, Diagnostic Center for Population and Animal Health, Michigan State University, East Lansing, Michigan, United States of America
Center for Integrative Toxicology, Diagnostic Center for Population and Animal Health, Michigan State University, East Lansing, Michigan, United States of America
Department of Microbiology and Molecular Genetics, Diagnostic Center for Population and Animal Health, Michigan State University, East Lansing, Michigan, United States of America

Kaiyu He
Center for Integrative Toxicology, Diagnostic Center for Population and Animal Health, Michigan State University, East Lansing, Michigan, United States of America
Department of Microbiology and Molecular Genetics, Diagnostic Center for Population and Animal Health, Michigan State University, East Lansing, Michigan, United States of America

Ingeborg Langohr
Division of Anatomic Pathology, Diagnostic Center for Population and Animal Health, Michigan State University, East Lansing, Michigan, United States of America

Maggie Eidson, Justin Wahlstrom
Department of Pediatrics, Memorial Sloan-Kettering Cancer Center, New York, New York, United States of America

Aimee M. Beaulieu
Immunology Program, Sloan-Kettering Institute, Memorial Sloan-Kettering Cancer Center, New York, New York, United States of America

Derek B. Sant'Angelo
Immunology Program, Sloan-Kettering Institute, Memorial Sloan-Kettering Cancer Center, New York, New York, United States of America
Weill Graduate School of Medical Sciences of Cornell University, New York, New York, United States of America
Gerstner Graduate School of Biomedical Sciences, Memorial Sloan-Kettering Cancer Center, New York, New York, United States of America

Bushra Zaidi, Jianda Yuan
Ludwig Center for Cancer Immunotherapy, Immunology Program, Memorial Sloan-Kettering Cancer Center, New York, New York, United States of America

Steven E. Carsons
Division of Rheumatology, Allergy and Immunology, Department of Medicine, Winthrop- University Hospital, Mineola, New York, United States of America

Peggy K. Crow
Rheumatology Division, Mary Kirkland Center for Lupus Research, Hospital for Special Surgery, New York, New York, United States of America
Weill Graduate School of Medical Sciences of Cornell University, New York, United States of America

Jedd D. Wolchok
Department of Medicine, Memorial Sloan-Kettering Cancer Center, New York, New York, United States of America

Bernhard Horsthemke, Dagmar Wieczorek
Institut fuer Humangenetik, Universitaetsklinikum Essen, Essen, Germany

Xiang Zhang, Shuk-mei Ho
Department of Environmental Health, University of Cincinnati, Cincinnati, Ohio, United States of America

Ravichandran Panchanathan, Hui Shen, Divaker Choubey
Department of Environmental Health, University of Cincinnati, Cincinnati, Ohio, United States of America
Cincinnati Veterans Affairs Medical Center, Cincinnati, Ohio, United States of America

Pragya Yadav
Department of Chemistry, The City College of New York and the Graduate Center of the City University of New York, New York, New York, United States of America
The Ph.D. program in Biochemistry, The City College of New York and the Graduate Center of the City University of New York, New York, United States of America

Paul Gottlieb, Linda Spatz
The Ph.D. program in Biochemistry, The City College of New York and the Graduate Center of the City University of New York, New York, United States of America
The Graduate School of Biology, The City College of New York, New York, United States of America
Department of Microbiology and Immunology, Sophie Davis School of Biomedical Education, The City College of New York, New York, United States of America

Hoa Tran, Roland Ebegbe, Rita H. Lewis
The Graduate School of Biology, The City College of New York, New York, United States of America

Hui Wei, Alice Mumbey-Wafula, Atira Kaplan, Elina Kholdarova
Department of Microbiology and Immunology, Sophie Davis School of Biomedical Education, The City College of New York, New York, United States of America

Ali S. Khashan, Louise C. Kenny, Uzma Mahmood, Keelin O'Donoghue
Anu Research Centre, Department of Obstetrics and Gynaecology, Cork University Maternity Hospital, University College Cork, Wilton, Cork, Republic of Ireland

Thomas M. Laursen, Preben B. Mortensen
National Centre for Register-Based Research, University of Aarhus, Aarhus, Denmark

Tine B. Henriksen
Perinatal Epidemiology Research Unit, Department of Paediatrics, Aarhus University Hospital, Aarhus, Denmark

Jeannie L. Te, Igor M. Dozmorov, Kim L. Nguyen, Joshua W. Cavett, Jennifer A. Kelly, Gail R. Bruner, Joshua O. Ojwang
Department of Arthritis and Immunology, Oklahoma Medical Research Foundation, Oklahoma City, Oklahoma, United States of America

John B. Harley
Department of Arthritis and Immunology, Oklahoma Medical Research Foundation, Oklahoma City, Oklahoma, United States of America
Department of Medicine, University of Oklahoma Health Sciences Center, Oklahoma City, Oklahoma, United States of America
United States Department of Veterans Affairs Medical Center, Oklahoma City, Oklahoma, United States of America

Joel M. Guthridge
Department of Clinical Immunology, Oklahoma Medical Research Foundation, Oklahoma City, Oklahoma, United States of America

Frédéric Reynier, Fabien Petit, Malick Paye, Fanny Turrel-Davin, Pierre-Emmanuel Imbert, Arnaud Hot, Bruno Mougin
Joint Unit Hospices Civils de Lyon - bioMérieux, Hôpital Edouard Herriot, Lyon, France

Pierre Miossec
Joint Unit Hospices Civils de Lyon - bioMérieux, Hôpital Edouard Herriot, Lyon, France
Department of Clinical Immunology and Rheumatology and immunogenomics and Inflammation Research Unit EA 4130, University of Lyon, Hôpital Edouard Herriot, Lyon, France

Jean-Eric Alard, Sophie Hillion
EA2216 "Immunology and Pathology" and IFR 148 ScInBioS, Universitéde Brest and UniversitéEuropéenne de Bretagne, Brest, France

Alain Saraux, Jacques-Olivier Pers, Pierre Youinou, Christophe Jamin
EA2216 "Immunology and Pathology" and IFR 148 ScInBioS, Universitéde Brest and UniversitéEuropéenne de Bretagne, Brest, France
Centre Hospitalier Universitaire, Brest, France

Loïc Guillevin
Department of Internal Medicine, Hôpital Cochin, Paris, France

Lunan Wang, Rui Zhang, Kuo Zhang, Jinming Li
National Center for Clinical Laboratories, Beijing Hospital, Beijing, People's Republic of China

Wenli Li, Wei Wang, Shipeng Sun, Yu Sun, Yang Pan
National Center for Clinical Laboratories, Beijing Hospital, Beijing, People's Republic of China
Graduate School, Peking Union Medical College, Chinese Academy of Medical Sciences, Beijing, People's Republic of China

Svetlana N. Zykova anders A. Tveita
Department of Biochemistry, Institute of Medical Biology, Medical Faculty, University of Tromsø, Tromsø, Norway

Ole Petter Rekvig
Department of Biochemistry, Institute of Medical Biology, Medical Faculty, University of Tromsø, Tromsø, Norway
Department of Rheumatology, University Hospital of Northern Norway, Tromsø, Norway

Nam Hoon Kwon, Jin Young Lee, Seung Jae Jeong
Center for Medicinal Protein Network and Systems Biology, College of Pharmacy, Seoul National University, Seoul, Republic of Korea

Sunghoon Kim
Center for Medicinal Protein Network and Systems Biology, College of Pharmacy, Seoul National University, Seoul, Republic of Korea
Department of Molecular Medicine and Biopharmaceutical Sciences, Graduate School of Convergence Science and Technology, Seoul National University, Suwon, Republic of Korea

Jung Min Han
Center for Medicinal Protein Network and Systems Biology, College of Pharmacy, Seoul National University, Seoul, Republic of Korea
Research Institute of Pharmaceutical Sciences, College of Pharmacy, Seoul National University, Seoul, Republic of Korea

Hee Jung Jung, Hyeong Rae Kim
Cancer & Infectious Disease Research Center, Bio-Organic Science Division, Korea Research Institute of Chemical Technology, Dae Jeon, Republic of Korea

Zihai Li
Center for Immunotherapy of Cancer and Infectious Diseases, University of Connecticut School of Medicine, Farmington, Connecticut, United States of America

Bengt Zöller, Xinjun Li, Kristina Sundquist
Center for Primary Health Care Research, Lund University/Region Skåne, Clinical Research Centre, Skåne University Hospital, Malmö, Sweden

Jan Sundquist
Center for Primary Health Care Research, Lund University/Region Skåne, Clinical Research Centre, Skåne University Hospital, Malmö, Sweden
Stanford Prevention Research Center, Stanford University School of Medicine, Stanford, California, United States of America

Klara Martinsson, Per Hultman
Division of Molecular and Immunological Pathology (AIR), Department of Clinical and Experimental Medicine, Linköping University, Linköping, Sweden

Thomas Skogh
Rheumatology Unit (AIR), Department of Clinical and Experimental Medicine, Linköping University, Linköping, Sweden

Jan-Ingvar Jönsson
Experimental Hematology Unit, Department of Clinical and Experimental Medicine, Linköping University, Linköping, Sweden

Seyed Ali Mousavi
Medical Genetics Laboratory, Department of Medical Genetics, Rikshospitalet University Hospital, Oslo, Norway

Trond Berg
Department of Molecular Biosciences, University of Oslo, Oslo, Norway

Simone Mader andreas Lutterotti, Franziska Di Pauli, Bettina Kuenz, Kathrin Schanda, Thomas Berger, Markus Reindl
Clinical Department of Neurology, Innsbruck Medical University, Innsbruck, Austria

Aboul-Enein, Wolfgang Kristoferitsch
Department of Neurology, SMZ-Ost Donauspital, Vienna, Austria

Fahmy, Michael Khalil, Maria K. Storch
Department of Neurology, Medical University of Graz, Graz, Austria

Sven Jarius
Division of Molecular Neuroimmunology, Department of Neurology, University of Heidelberg, Heidelberg, Germany

Weijuan Zhang, Jin Wu, Bin Qiao, Wei Xu
Institute for Immunobiology and Department of Immunology, Shanghai Medical College, Fudan University, Shanghai, People's Republic of China

Sidong Xiong
Institute for Immunobiology and Department of Immunology, Shanghai Medical College, Fudan University, Shanghai, People's Republic of China
Institutes of Biology and Medical Sciences, Soochow University, Suzhou, People's Republic of China

Iva Gunnarsson, Elisabet Svenungsson, Leonid Padyukov
Rheumatology Unit, Department of Medicine, Karolinska Institutet, Stockholm, Sweden

Mai Tuyet Vuong
Rheumatology Unit, Department of Medicine, Karolinska Institutet, Stockholm, Sweden
Department of Nephrology, Danderyd Hospital, Karolinska Institutet, Stockholm, Sweden
Department of Internal Medicine, Hanoi Medical University, Hanoi, Vietnam

Stefan H. Jacobson
Department of Nephrology, Danderyd Hospital, Karolinska Institutet, Stockholm, Sweden

Lieu Thi Do
Department of Internal Medicine, Hanoi Medical University, Hanoi, Vietnam

Sigrid Lundberg
Nephrology Unit, Department of Medicine, Karolinska University Hospital, Stockholm, Sweden

Lars Wramner
Transplantation Center, Sahlgrenska University Hospital, Göteborg, Sweden

Anders Fernström
Department of Nephrology, Linköping University Hospital, Linköping, Sweden

Ann-Christine Syvänen
Department of Medical Sciences, Uppsala University, Uppsala, Sweden

Diana Carmona-Fernandes
Rheumatology Research Unit, Instituto de Medicina Molecular da Faculdade de Medicina de Lisboa, Lisbon, Portugal

Maria JoséSantos
Rheumatology Research Unit, Instituto de Medicina Molecular da Faculdade de Medicina de Lisboa, Lisbon, Portugal
Rheumatology Department, Hospital Garcia de Orta, Almada, Portugal

Helena Canhão, João Eurico Fonseca
Rheumatology Research Unit, Instituto de Medicina Molecular da Faculdade de Medicina de Lisboa, Lisbon, Portugal
Rheumatology and Metabolic Bone Diseases Department, Hospital de Santa Maria, Lisbon, Portugal

José Canas da Silva
Rheumatology Department, Hospital Garcia de Orta, Almada, Portugal

Victor Gil
Cardiology Department, Hospital Fernando Fonseca, Amadora, Portugal

Jadwiga Bienkowska, Norm Allaire, Alice Thai, Jaya Goyal, Tatiana Plavina
Translational Medicine, Biogen Idec, Cambridge, Massachusetts, United States of America

Ajay Nirula, Evan Beckman, Jeffrey L. Browning
Immunobiology, Biogen Idec, Cambridge, Massachusetts, United States of America

Megan Weaver, Charlotte Newman
Global Clinical Operations, Biogen Idec, Cambridge, Massachusetts, United States of America

Michelle Petri
Johns Hopkins University School of Medicine, Baltimore, Maryland, United States of America

Tomoko Sugiura, Yasushi Kawaguchi, Takahisa Gono, Takefumi Furuya, Hisashi Yamanaka
Institute of Rheumatology, Tokyo Women's Medical University, Tokyo, Japan

Kanako Goto, Yukiko Hayashi, Ichizo Nishino
Department of Neuromuscular Research, National Institute of Neuroscience and Department of Clinical Development, Translational Medical Center, National Center of Neurology and Psychiatry, Tokyo, Japan

Yufeng Yin, Di Liang, Lidan Zhao, Yan Ren, Yongzhe Li, Xiaofeng Zeng, Fengchun Zhang, Fulin Tang, Xuan Zhang Yang Li
Department of Rheumatology, Peking Union Medical College Hospital, Chinese Academy of Medical Sciences and Peking Union Medical College, Beijing, China

Wei Liu
Department of Radiology, Peking Union Medical College Hospital, Chinese Academy of Medical Sciences and Peking Union Medical College, Beijing, China

Guangliang Shan
Department of Epidemiology, Institute of Basic Medical Sciences, Chinese Academy of Medical Sciences and Peking Union Medical College, Beijing, China

Yi-Sin Wong, Hsien-Chin Tang, Ting-Chun Yeh
Department of Family Medicine and Pulmonary Medicine, Ditmanson Medical Foundation Chia-Yi Christian Hospital, Chiayi, Taiwan

Jun-Jun Yeh
Department of Family Medicine and Pulmonary Medicine, Ditmanson Medical Foundation Chia-Yi Christian Hospital, Chiayi, Taiwan
Chia Nan University of Pharmacy and Science, Tainan, Taiwan
Meiho University, Pingtung, Taiwan

Hsuan-Ju Chen
Management Office for Health Data, China Medical University Hospital, Taichung, Taiwan
College of Medicine, China Medical University, Taichung, Taiwan

Tsai-Chung Li
Graduate Institute of Biostatistics, College of Management, China Medical University, Taichung, Taiwan
Department of Healthcare Administration, College of Health Science, Asia University, Taichung, Taiwan

Chia-Hung Kao
Graduate Institute of Clinical Medical Science and School of Medicine, College of Medicine, China Medical University, Taichung, Taiwan
Department of Nuclear Medicine and PET Center, China Medical University Hospital, Taichung, Taiwan

Carolina Barragán-Martínez, Cesar A. Speck-Hernández, Gladis Montoya-Ortiz, Rubén D. Mantilla, Juan-Manuel Anaya, Adriana Rojas-Villarraga
Center for Autoimmune Diseases Research (CREA), School of Medicine and Health Sciences, Universidad del Rosario, Bogota, Colombia

Index

www.ingramcontent.com/pod-product-compliance
Lightning Source LLC
Chambersburg PA
CBHW070154240326

41458CB00126B/4596